Introductory Textbook of Psychiatry

Second Edition

Introductory Textbook of Psychiatry

Second Edition

Nancy C. Andreasen, M.D., Ph.D.
Andrew H. Woods Professor of Psychiatry
Director, Mental Health Clinical Research Center

Donald W. Black, M.D.
Associate Professor
Department of Psychiatry
The University of Iowa College of Medicine
Iowa City, Iowa

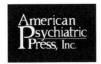

Washington, DC
London, England

Copyright © 1995 American Psychiatric Press, Inc.
ALL RIGHTS RESERVED
Manufactured in the United States of America on acid-free paper
98 97 96 95   4 3 2 1
Second Edition

American Psychiatric Press, Inc.
1400 K Street, N.W., Washington, DC   20005

Diagnostic criteria and other DSM-IV material included in this book are reprinted with permission from the *Diagnostic and Statistical Manual of Mental Disorders*, Fourth Edition. Copyright 1994 American Psychiatric Association.

Library of Congress Cataloging-in-Publication Data

Andreasen, Nancy C.
    Introductory textbook of psychiatry / Nancy C. Andreasen, Donald
W. Black. — 2nd ed.
        p.   cm.
    Includes bibliographical references and index.
    ISBN 0-88048-704-6 (hard : alk. paper). — ISBN 0-88048-705-4
    (soft : alk. paper)
    1. Psychiatry.   I. Black, Donald W., 1956-   .   II. Title.
    [DNLM: 1. Mental Disorders.   WM 100 A557i 1995]
    RC454.A427   1995
    616.89—dc20
    DNLM/DLC
    for Library of Congress   94-44481
                                                                    CIP

British Library Cataloguing in Publication Data
A CIP record is available from the British Library.

Contents

Section III
Special Topics

Section IV
Treatments

Preface to the Second Edition

Only four years have elapsed since the publication of the first edition of this textbook in 1991. Yet the worlds of medicine and psychiatry have changed with astonishing rapidity during that short interval, and the changes appear likely to accelerate.

Health care reform, viewed by many as health care destruction, is transforming the way that physicians treat their patients and organize their practices. Primary care is recovering recognition as the heart of medicine, and specialization is becoming less valued. If this reduces fragmentation of care, for patients a frustration at best and a bane at worst, medical care will be improved. On the other hand, managed care also appears to be making unwanted and sometimes undesirable intrusions into decision making. As physicians, we believe that the health and well-being of our patients should be our guiding compass, and economic incentives (including our own) should be secondary. We refuse to consider this position old-fashioned or naive.

Where does psychiatry stand in this rapidly changing environment? Although it is not a primary care discipline to the same extent as pediatrics or internal medicine, it will play a major role in a health care system that emphasizes the importance of primary care. Mental illnesses, after all, are very common. Only physicians in laboratory specialties such as pathology or radiology can avoid encountering the patients who have them. Family practitioners, internists, surgeons, pediatricians, and obstetrician/gynecologists are all certain to have to work with patients with depression or substance abuse almost daily. Other mental illnesses, such as schizophrenia, Alzheimer's disease, and anorexia nervosa, are also extremely common. The primary care physician must be able to diagnose mental illnesses on a regular basis and either treat them or refer patients to a psychiatrist as appropriate. In either situation a good grasp of psychiatry is mandatory. The treating psychiatrist, on the other hand, will also no doubt increasingly deliver more primary care to the patients in his or her practice. Just as the obstetrician/gynecologist is the only physician that many women see regularly, thereby de facto becoming a primary care provider, a psychiatrist is also often the only physician that many patients see regularly. The distinction between psychiatry and primary care is likely to become increasingly blurred as psychiatrists assume more responsibility for the general health of the patients whom they see regularly.

The field of psychiatry has experienced many exciting new developments that permit it to be responsive to these challenges. Forty years ago, mental illnesses were untreatable and hopeless. The modern psychiatrist has a large arsenal of effective medications and other treatments, which now give most mental illnesses a better prognosis than cancer or cardiac disease. Further, the past few years have produced many new medications that are further enhancing our ability to care for patients. Just during the short interval since the first edition of this book, we have acquired risperidone for schizophrenia, paroxetine for obsessive-compulsive disorder, and venlafaxine for depression. Psychotherapeutic techniques also continue to be refined and better matched to the disorders for which they are most effective, as in the case of interpersonal psychotherapy for depression. In the area of diagnosis, the fourth edition of the *Diagnostic and Statistical Manual of Mental Disorders* (DSM-IV) was published in 1994, continuing the tradition of providing precise, objective, and optimally validated methods for defining and diagnosing mental illnesses.

The scientific basis of psychiatry also continues to grow and develop. Neuroimaging techniques now give us a direct window on the brain, permitting us to see with our own eyes the underlying physiology of mental activities such as remembering, feeling sadness, or making a decision. The psychiatrist using these techniques to map the brain is engaged in a voyage of discovery not unlike that of the early explorers who sought a trade route to India and instead discovered America. Textbooks of neuroscience are already being rewritten as truisms based on the older lessons of lesion studies or Brodmann cytoarchitectonics are found to be wrong. The chemical systems of the brain are also being remapped, and the mechanisms of drug action in the in vivo intact brain are being discovered. We can now visualize how the medications that we prescribe block various classes of receptors in the brain and exert their therapeutic effects. The 1990s have been declared the decade of the brain, and rightly so. Neuroscience and psychiatry are exploring the last uncharted territory in the human body. It is an incredibly exciting time to work in these fields.

Inevitably, all this growth in knowledge has required the appearance of a second edition of our textbook. Each chapter has been extensively updated to provide the most current information available about the various disorders and their treatments. Several new chapters have been added and additional topics are covered, including legal issues in psychiatry, sleep disorders, impulse control disorders, and violence. We have been gratified by the response to the first edition by our readers, who provided many helpful comments and criticisms that we have collected and responded to as best we can. Our medical students deserve special thanks, for they have proved to be a fertile testing ground—a focus group, if you will—to explore new ideas for further improving the book. Among the changes we have incorporated: more tables, additional case examples (and follow-up news on some of our first edition patients!), more complete coverage of mental disorders described in the DSM, and use of the latest criteria.

We have also been gratified that our book has enjoyed widespread acceptance and is used all over the United States, as well as in many foreign countries. Although some critics have suggested that the book is "biological," we refuse to be pigeonholed. If a descriptive term must be used, we prefer the terms *objective*, *empirical*, or *scientific*. Granted, we do not advocate slavish or unthinking adherence to outdated theory. Nor do we advocate uncritical acceptance of poorly grounded "facts." An objective, practical, and dynamic approach has shaped our approach to patient care: if well-grounded data exist to guide us, we shall use them. Where data do not exist, we shall use common sense, seeking new knowledge continuously and using it as it becomes available.

Psychiatry is sometimes considered fuzzy, imprecise, or not accountable. One of our objectives in this book has been to convey to students of all types that psychiatry is not only exciting, fun, and interesting, but also that it can be (and usually is) clearheaded, careful, and credible. After all, the reliability of diagnosing schizophrenia is higher than that of diagnosing rheumatoid arthritis, not to mention systemic lupus or multiple sclerosis. The cost-effectiveness of treating depression and mania is well established, and the treatment is far more gratifying to administer than treatments for stroke, back pain, or many forms of cancer. Of course, some trendy or silly ideas are sometimes put forth by psychiatrists, thereby calling into question the credibility of the field as a whole. But the majority provide the type of competent and well-founded diagnosis and treatment that we believe this book advocates. Psychiatry as a field and the illnesses that it treats are far from silly. These illnesses are common, important, potentially devastating, and often gratifyingly responsive to good care and management.

Our hope is that students reading this book will learn to share our excitement about the practice of psychiatry and our curiosity about its scientific foundations. We psychiatrists have a unique opportunity to spend time with our patients, to get to know them personally, and to work with an interdisciplinary team. Modern psychiatrists wear many hats. They must understand diagnosis, pathophysiology, and the latest drug therapies; at the same time, psychiatrists must possess empathy, be able to counsel and comfort distraught patients, and learn to help patients function in their day-to-day lives. A typical day's work may involve prescribing medication to a depressed patient, helping a teenager come to grips with the effect of having an alcoholic parent, and guiding a severely handicapped schizophrenic patient toward receiving needed social services. All this is not easy, but it can be enormously rewarding, particularly when students are able to follow their patients long enough to observe that for most the treatment actually works! Nothing is more satisfying than restoring a disabled person to independent functioning or a suffering person to freedom from mental pain.

We encourage students to read the introductory chapters first, to gain a working background of concepts and vocabulary and to learn interviewing techniques. Students should then feel free to skip around and read chapters or sections of chapters that apply to their particular patients—or sections that are simply interesting and fun to read. Enjoy!

Preface to the First Edition

Students sometimes begin working in psychiatry with a set of preconceptions about what it is, preconceptions shaped by the fact that information about psychiatry is omnipresent in popular culture. Taxi drivers, CEOs, teachers, and ministers often feel qualified to offer information and advice about how to handle "psychiatric problems," even though they may be unaware of distinctions as fundamental as the difference between psychiatry and psychology. These two disciplines are blurred together in the popular mind, and the term *psychiatry* evokes a potpourri of associations—Freud's couch, Jack Nicholson receiving electroconvulsive therapy in *One Flew Over the Cuckoo's Nest*, or Dr. Ruth discussing sexual adjustment on television. These images and associations tend to cloak psychiatry with an aura of vagueness, imprecision, muddleheadedness, and mindless coercion. It is unfortunate that such preconceptions are so pervasive, but fortunate that most of them are in fact in error, as students who use this book in conjunction with studying psychiatry in a clinical setting will soon discover.

What is psychiatry? It is the branch of medicine that focuses on the diagnosis and treatment of mental illnesses. Some of these illnesses are very serious, such as schizophrenia, Alzheimer's disease, or the various mood disorders. Others may be less serious, but still very significant, such as adjustment disorders or personality disorders. Psychiatry differs from psychology by virtue of its medical orientation. Its primary focus is illness or abnormality, as opposed to normal psychological functioning; the latter is the primary focus of psychology. Of course, abnormal psychology is a small branch within psychology, just as understanding normality is necessary for the psychiatrist to recognize and treat abnormal functioning. As a discipline within medicine, the primary purposes of psychiatry are to define and recognize illnesses, to identify methods for treating them, and ultimately to develop methods for discovering their causes and implementing preventive measures.

Psychiatry during the last decade of the 20th century may be the most exciting discipline within medicine. Contemporary psychiatry is exciting for a variety of reasons. First, psychiatrists are specialists who work with the most interesting organ within the body, the brain. The brain is intrinsically fascinating because it controls nearly all aspects of functioning within the rest of the body, as well as the way people interact with and relate to one another. Psychiatry has received enormous support during recent years through the burgeoning of neuroscience, which has provided psychiatrists with the tools by which they can understand brain anatomy, chemistry, and physiology, thereby gradually developing a scientific base that will permit them to understand human emotion and behavior and to develop methods for treating abnormalities in these domains.

Yet, as psychiatry evolves into a relatively high-powered science, it remains a very clinical and human branch within medicine, and therefore a very rewarding field for students who have chosen medicine because they wish to have contact with patients. The clinician working in psychiatry must spend time with his or her patients and learn about them as human beings as well as as individuals who have illnesses or problems. Learning the life stories of individual people is fun and interesting; as one colleague once said, "It amazed me when I realized that I would get paid for asking people things that everybody always wants to know about anyway!"

Finally, psychiatry has enormous breadth. As a scientific discipline, it ranges from the highly detailed facts of molecular biology to the abstract concepts of the mind. As a clinical discipline, it ranges from the absorbingly complex disturbances that characterize illnesses such as schizophrenia to the understandable fearfulness shown by young children when they must separate from their parents and attend school or be left with a baby-sitter. It can be very scientific and technical, as in the frontier-expanding research currently occurring in molecular genetics or neuroimaging; but it can also be very human and personal, as when a clinician listens to a patient's story and experiences the pleasure of being able to offer help by providing needed insights or even simple encouragement and support.

This book is intended as a tool to help you learn from your patients and from your teachers. We have tried to keep it simple, clear, and factual. References are provided for students who want to explore in more depth the topics covered in the various chapters. We have written this book primarily for medical students and residents during the first several years of their training, although we anticipate that it may also be useful to individuals seeking psychiatric training from the perspectives of other disciplines such as nursing or social work. We hope that, using this book as a tool, students of all ages and types will learn to enjoy working with psychiatric patients and with the art and science of contemporary psychiatry as much as we do.

Section I

Background

Chapter 1

History of Psychiatry

What curiosity, that delicate little plant, needs more than
anything, besides stimulation, is freedom.

Albert Einstein

To understand some of the conceptual tensions in modern psychiatry, as well as the somewhat confused attitudes of contemporary society toward mentally ill persons, it is helpful to examine current situations and thinking in the light of their historical background. Over many centuries a complicated and conflicting array of attitudes has been built up, and many of these still affect our current perceptions and ideas.

Mental Illness in Biblical and Classical Times

Mental illnesses are among the first diseases to have been recognized as discrete illnesses. The concept of cancer or even congestive heart failure is relatively new compared with the concept of mental illness. Perhaps the oldest medical document in existence, the Eber Papyrus (probably composed in 1900 B.C.), contains references to specific syndromes such as depression. Biblical writings also contain descriptions of individuals with major mental illnesses; for example, in I Samuel, Saul is portrayed as falling into a serious depression, for which he is treated with soothing music.

By classical times, a full classification of mental illnesses had been devel-

3

oped. These included melancholia (depression), mania (a variety of psychotic states), delirium (mental confusion accompanied by fever), and hysteria (sudden unexplained episodes of somatic illness involving pain, sensory loss, paralysis, etc.). Although Greek and Roman physicians generally recognized these as major classes of mental illness, they could not agree on their specific causes. Hippocrates, for example, argued that mental illnesses, as well as all other cognitive and emotional functions, derived principally from the brain. Galen and his followers believed that mental illnesses were due to imbalances in quantities of body fluids. Melancholia, for example, was due to an excess of black bile, whereas other abnormalities arose from imbalances in the other three main fluids or humors of the body (blood, phlegm, and yellow bile). Still others argued for an "organ theory" of disease and believed that specific dysfunctions could be attributed to abnormalities in specific organs; delirium or mania, for example, were brain abnormalities, whereas hysteria was due to a wandering uterus.

Although physicians in classical times had their major or minor differences about both the nosology and pathophysiology of major mental illnesses, they rather consistently shared the belief that these illnesses were physical in nature. Although the Greeks developed highly sophisticated theories about the nature of the spirit, soul, or mind, they nevertheless believed that illnesses such as mania or melancholia were due to aberrations in the body rather than the soul or spirit. This led in turn to humane practices for the treatment of serious mental illnesses, involving rest and peaceful surroundings.

Medieval and Renaissance Attitudes

As Roman civilization declined and finally fell, enlightened attitudes about mental illness declined as well. The barbarian tribes that conquered Rome had no interest in maintaining learning or education, leading to massive destruction of the libraries that summarized classical knowledge about science and literature. Europe gradually struggled out of these "Dark Ages," largely through the influence of the Christian church, but the new prevailing world view was not conducive to enlightenment about human illness in general or mental illness in particular. The emphasis was on saving souls, not bodies.

In this environment, mentally ill persons were often believed to be possessed by the Devil rather than to have some form of illness. Witches, warlocks, and demons in disguise were very real to the people of the Middle Ages. Various types of misfortune or suffering were often perceived as just punishments meted out through divine intervention as a consequence of sinful behavior. Thus, it was easy to believe that a person who fell into the deep despondency of depression, and who was experiencing a delusion of sin and guilt, was spiritually rather than physically ill. A person with the agitation and mental confusion that often accompany severe psychosis could easily be seen as possessed by diabolical forces. Such individuals were often "treated" through the church rather than through medicine, and many were tortured or burned at the stake. The church published texts, such as the *Malleus Maleficarum* (or the *Hammer of Witches*) to explain how such possessed individuals could be identified and killed, because they were considered to be dangerous to society. As late as the seventeenth century, the reigning monarch in England, James I, wrote a book on this topic, *Demonologie*. The last witch was hanged in England in 1684, but witch trials continued in the United States in Salem into the eighteenth century.

The Renaissance, the rebirth of interest in classical learning that began in Italy in the fifteenth century and spread throughout the rest of Europe during the next 100 years, brought a refreshing new light to this rather dim atmosphere. Artists rediscovered the study of anatomy, forbidden by the church, in order to better depict the human body. Authoritarian teachings were questioned. The new physics of Copernicus and Galileo displaced humans and the earth from the center of the universe. Doctors began to believe what their eyes and their inferences taught them, in contrast to arbitrary dogma that was obviously in error.

A few brave voices began to suggest that mental illnesses were diseases rather than forms of possession and bewitchment. In 1584, Reginald Scot published *The Discoverie of Witchcraft*, in which he argued that individuals accused of witchcraft were not in fact possessed by demons, but were instead mentally ill, and that their own descriptions of being possessed represented false products of their fevered imaginations and thus should be considered as delusions. Two years later, in 1586, a physician, Timothy Bright, published the first textbook about mental illness to appear in English, *The Treatise of Melancholie*. In this book he described the classic symptoms of depression and their tendency to alternate with the periods of being "high" (in a way that anticipated later descriptions of manic-depressive illness) and argued that the symptoms of mental illness were "naturall perturbations" that "altered either brayne or hart." Although these revolutionary ideas did not instantly gain wide acceptance, the foundations of modern psychiatry were being laid.

The Dawn of Scientific Psychiatry

Serious mental illnesses tended to be relatively chronic and incapacitating, especially in an era when no good treatments were available. If mentally ill persons were not burned at the stake, some other disposition had to be made. Hospitals or asylums were an alternative solution. To refer to the institutions created for mentally ill persons during the seventeenth and eighteenth centuries as hospitals or asylums is, however, by and large a misnomer. Patients were in fact typically incarcerated, and many were not only locked in but were also locked up in chains. Making matters worse, often distinctions were not clearly made between the mentally ill, the criminal, the mentally retarded, and the economically unfortunate. The desire to spare rich people from being forced to observe the suffering of poor, handicapped, or seriously ill people seems to be a persistent human failing, although hardly an appealing one.

The seeds of skepticism and doubt sown during the Renaissance flowered into rebellion and revolution during the era of the Enlightenment in the eighteenth century. All over the world the weak, deprived, and powerless sought to take back their rights and to seize authority from the rich and powerful. The United States led the way with the first revolution of modern times, declaring all men to be created equal. The revolutionary movement in America sparked others in France, Italy, and elsewhere.

Philippe Pinel, a leader of the French Revolution, is usually considered to be the founding father of modern psychiatry. In 1793, he was named director of the Bicêtre, the hospital in Paris for insane men. Soon afterward he instituted a grand, symbolic change by removing the chains that bound the patients to the walls at the Bicêtre and instituted a new type of treatment that he referred to as "moral treatment." (This meant treating patients in ways that were morally and ethically sensitive rather than attempting to teach them "morality.") He was later made director of the corresponding hospital for women, the Salpêtrière. In addition to attempting to treat patients with kindness and decency, Pinel also tried to approach the study of mentally ill persons scientifically. As he describes his efforts in his *Treatise on Insanity* (1806):

> I, therefore, resolved to adopt that method of investigation which has invariably succeeded in all the departments of natural history, viz. To notice successively every fact, without any other object than that of collecting materials for future use; and to endeavor, as far as possible, to divest myself of the influence, both of my own prepossessions and the authority of others. (p. 2)

The *Treatise on Insanity* contains detailed case histories of individual patients so clearly described that they are instantly diagnosable as classic cases of what we now call schizophrenia or manic-depressive illness 200 years later.

In addition to introducing psychotherapy, in the form of moral treatment, and stressing the importance of empirical observation, Pinel also applied the scientific method to the study of psychiatry. He established epidemiological methods for recording numbers of cases, instituted follow-up studies so that the natural history of diseases could be observed, and used whatever scientific technology he had at hand to understand the pathophysiology of mental diseases. His approaches became the standard methods in most enlightened psychiatric facilities throughout Europe and the United States in the nineteenth century.

Thus, a new specialty within medicine was created, consisting of doctors who chose to specialize in the care of mentally ill persons. They became known as *psychiatrists*, which means literally "healers of the mind." Psychiatry was one of the first disciplines within medicine to identify itself as a specialty. This was no doubt a consequence of both the large numbers of patients with mental illness and the special needs and challenges that they presented.

Psychiatry also got off to an early start in the United States. Perhaps because the creation of the United States was based on the ideals of the Enlightenment (most of the Founding Fathers such as Franklin, Washington, and Jefferson were adherents of the ideals of the Age of Reason), American attitudes toward mental illness were very progressive early in U.S. history. Benjamin Rush, a physician who specialized in the care of mentally ill persons, also signed the Declaration of Independence and founded the first psychiatric hospital in America more than 200 years ago (the Pennsylvania Hospital). The American Psychiatric Association was founded more than 150 years ago, in 1844; and its official journal, *The American Journal of Psychiatry*, is the oldest medical specialty journal in the United States and one of the oldest medical journals as well. The American Psychiatric Association was created through the collaboration of 13 people who were in charge of hospitals specifically dedicated to the care of mentally ill persons; they agreed to meet regularly and to share their experiences in caring for people with illnesses that caused them to lose their capacity to reason clearly. In this era nearly every physician was a family practitioner. But even at that time it was recognized that caring for mentally ill persons required special skills. The early writings of these 13 founders of the American Psychiatric Association contain an interesting combination of emphasis on empirical description, the study of neuroanatomy, and the value of compassion.

The First Era of Neuroscience

While psychiatry was establishing itself as a medical specialty, a new subdivision within science was also emerging. During the nineteenth century, clinical observations and technological developments converged to create an era when the brain was studied scientifically for the first time.

Some of the landmark achievements of the first era of neuroscience are summarized in Table 1–1. One major aspect was the mapping of specific cortical

Table 1–1.   Some major discoveries in the first era of neuroscience

Year	Discovery
1861	Broca: The identification of "Broca's area"
1868	Harlow: Description of Phineas Gage and the role of the frontal cortex
1870	Fritsch and Hitzig: Lateralization of motor function
1876	Wernicke: The localization of language comprehension
1897	Dax: The lateralization of language
1909	Brodmann: Maps of cortical cytoarchitecture
1920s	Penfield: Mapping of cognitive and motor functions with microelectrodes
1921	Foix: Localization of Parkinson's in the substantia nigra
1937	Papez: Description of the limbic system

functions in the human brain. The initial observations focused on the specificity of language systems in the brain, beginning in 1837 with the observation of Marc Dax that left-sided injury tended to be associated with aphasia and right with hemiparesis. A steady progression of discoveries ensued. More specific language functions were mapped, as Paul Broca observed that posterior frontal lesions led to impaired speech but intact comprehension, and Carl Wernicke observed that more posterior lesions in the parietal cortex (now recognized as language association regions) led to impaired comprehension with fluent but garbled and incomprehensible speech. Well-defined motor and sensory regions were subsequently recognized as well. The vast area of the frontal cortex, anterior to the central sulcus, was observed to mediate a variety of higher cognitive and emotional functions that distinctly differentiate human personality and behavior, such as social judgment, long-term planning, and the capacity to form close emotional attachments.

These various observations about human cerebral specialization were achieved through a combination of clinical observation and developments in the basic sciences. Most of the observations about language function were made through the study of stroke patients, and the role of the prefrontal cortex in governing human personality was first identified through the famous case of Phineas Gage, who sustained a major lesion to his frontal lobes in an accident. (This case is further discussed in Chapters 5 and 6.) The motor cortex was mapped through the developing science of neurophysiology.

Basic neuroscience was also making major strides, as the brain was being studied systematically for the first time: anatomically, microscopically, and functionally. A variety of staining techniques were developed that permitted scientists to examine the cellular structure of the brain and begin to explore the neural networks that connected various regions. Nissl, Golgi, and Weigert provided methods for visualizing neuronal cell bodies, axons, and dendrites. Subsequently, Brodmann used these staining techniques to systematically map structural differentiation within the brain and to relate it to specific types of cortical function. His detailed maps of differentiations in cell layers and structures permitted the identification of the more primitive paleocortex (such as is found in the limbic system) as distinct from the neocortex and also permitted the identification of different types of cell layers in cortical regions specialized for different functions, such as sensory perception versus motor activity.

These advances did not escape the notice of forward-looking individuals in the new discipline of psychiatry. While still a student and trainee, young Sigmund Freud attempted to develop a new staining technique for nerve cells that was never successful; later he wrote a treatise on aphasia in children and worked in pharmacology by examining the potential therapeutic effects of cocaine.

One of the greatest departments of psychiatry of all time was assembled in Munich at the turn of the century under the leadership of Emil Kraepelin, who joins Phillipe Pinel as a major founding father of modern psychiatry. If Pinel was the founder of the psychosocial tradition in psychiatry, Kraepelin was the founder of the neuroscience tradition.

Emil Kraepelin and some of the members of his Department of Psychiatry in Munich are shown in Figure 1–1. (Brodmann, also a member of this department for a time, is not in this particular picture.) Kraepelin had made a commitment

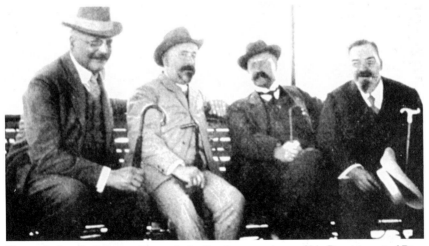

Figure 1–1. Emil Kraepelin, seated with other members of his Department of Psychiatry, near the Starnberger lake. From *left* to *right:* Alzheimer, Kraepelin, Gaupp, and Nissl (circa 1908). Reprinted with permission from Hippius H: Kraepelin's Memoirs. New York, Raven, 1989, p 257.

to study psychiatry from the time he was in his late teens. He began his career in Dorpat, a city in the Baltic region that was part of Russia at the time, and then progressed to become a professor in Heidelberg and later in Munich. His vision of psychiatry was that it should combine careful clinical description with good basic neuroscience. His own interest was cognitive psychology, and he did some of the earliest work examining the effects of drugs on learning and memory. He also had the vision to recognize the importance of neuropathology and brain science, however, and he recruited some of the best scientific minds available to work with him to identify the mechanisms of major mental illnesses. At its peak, his team included Kraepelin himself, Alzheimer, Brodmann, Nissl, and several less well known scientists. The productivity of this group is remarkable. Perhaps even more remarkable is the fact that most of these men were active clinicians who cared for patients during the day and worked in their laboratories at night. All were close friends, and all shared the goal of unraveling the mechanisms of the incapacitating brain diseases that eventually came to be known as schizo-phrenia, Alzheimer's disease, paranoia, and manic-depressive illness.

Kraepelin himself was a superb clinician and teacher who provided us with the classification of major mental illnesses that we still use. Combining informa-tion about age at onset with the natural history and longitudinal course of disor-ders, he differentiated dementia praecox (now referred to as schizophrenia) from dementia in elderly persons (now referred to as Alzheimer's disease), paranoia (now referred to as delusional disorder), and manic-depressive illness (now re-ferred to as bipolar affective disorder). He did this by observing that some indi-viduals develop intellectual deterioration at a young age and fail to recover, whereas others develop this deterioration relatively late in life; he decided the former had a discrete illness that he referred to as dementia praecox, whereas the latter had a very different illness because of their long period of intact function-ing before the onset of dementia. He distinguished between dementia praecox and manic-depressive illness because the former had a relatively chronic course leading to deterioration, whereas the latter was typically episodic with full remis-sion between episodes of psychosis.

As Kraepelin and others within his department laid out this nosological structure, they applied the techniques of neuroscience to the study of postmor-tem brain specimens from patients they had known during life. Alzheimer ob-served that the elderly demented patients had characteristic neuropathological lesions, consisting of plaques and tangles; these became the neuropathological indicator of what we now know as Alzheimer's disease. Similar characteristic lesions were sought in patients with schizophrenia and manic-depressive illness, but none were found, although occasional abnormalities were noted in both fron-tal and temporal regions. Kraepelin and his group were convinced that the major mental illnesses would ultimately be understood in terms of aberrations in neural functions. The goals that they set for themselves at the turn of the nineteenth century remain those that we have set for ourselves at the turn of the twentieth century.

In this era, achievements were also being made for the first time in the domain of somatic therapy. Working in Vienna, another contemporary of Freud and Kraepelin, Julius Wagner von Jauregg, accidentally observed in 1887 that infection with malaria had a beneficial effect on patients with psychosis. This observation eventually led him to conduct a formal set of experiments 20 years later in which he infected with malaria a group of patients who had syphilis, a disorder largely under the care of psychiatrists because of its severe cognitive, behavioral, and emotional symptoms. The treatment was so effective that Von Jauregg was later awarded a Nobel Prize for this discovery in 1927. Malarial treatment for syphilis remained a standard part of the therapeutic armamentarium until the discovery of penicillin. In the early twentieth century other relatively crude and nonspecific treatments were also developed. These included the introduction of insulin shock therapy as a treatment for psychosis by Manfred Sakel in 1927 and the later development of electroshock therapy by Cerletti and Bini in 1938. Although most of the older forms of somatic therapy have now been supplanted by more specific methods of modulating brain chemistry through medications (see Chapter 26), electroconvulsive therapy is still widely used and highly effective in a small subgroup of psychiatric patients who primarily have severe mood disorders.

The Development of Psychoanalysis

Psychoanalysis was developed in the late nineteenth and early twentieth centuries. Because of the widespread popular appeal of psychoanalysis, its history is much better known than that of the neuroscience traditions of psychiatry. It is important to realize, however, that psychoanalysis actually had its beginnings within the tradition of neuroscience. Sigmund Freud, the founder of the psychoanalytic method, spent his early career thinking about cerebral specialization, higher cortical functions, and their relationship to the symptoms of mental illness. He embodied this thinking in a treatise, A *Project for a Scientific Psychology*, in which he suggested that most specific symptoms of mental illness could be understood in terms of brain mechanisms.

However, methods for investigating brain-behavior relationships were still relatively limited in the early twentieth century, consisting largely of neuroanatomy and neuropathology, with only a modest amount of neuropharmacology and neurophysiology. Thus, Freud himself turned to another fruitful avenue, the observation of clinical phenomena combined with speculations and hypotheses about their underlying psychic mechanisms. Unlike Kraepelin and his group, Freud was less interested in symptoms of psychosis and more interested in the symptoms referred to as conversion or hysterical phenomena. These symptoms consisted of peculiar, unexplained pains and paralyses experienced by many individuals in the early twentieth century.

Freud's earliest thoughts on this subject, contained in *Studies on Hysteria* (coauthored with Josef Breuer), contained the fundamental ideas that were the basis for what was later to become the extensive field of psychoanalysis. On the basis of his own experience in treating patients who had the sudden onset of paralyses or seizures with no obvious physical cause, he speculated that these symptoms could be due to some type of trauma occurring early in life that remained embedded in the psyche and caused irritation: "The memory of the trauma acts like a foreign body which long after its entry must continue to be regarded as an agent that is still at work." (p. 6) He observed that releasing these embedded memories, either through hypnosis or through free association, sometimes led to the remission of symptoms. This led to Freud and Breuer's famous pronouncement: "Hysterics suffer mainly from reminiscences." (p. 7)

These early ideas led to the extensive development of theories of psychological structure and function, such as the id, ego, and superego, as well as a variety of methods of psychotherapy for manipulating psychological structures and functions and reducing symptoms. Psychoanalysis also extensively explored human sexuality, a courageous step at a time when most people were bound by rigid Victorian inhibitions about what they were allowed to say, think, and do. Because of its imagination and courage, the work of Freud and his disciples gained widespread respect. The methods that he developed for clinical management of milder psychiatric syndromes gained popularity and are still in use today, mostly in modified form.

The Second Era of Neuroscience

The term *neuroscience* did not in fact exist during the nineteenth or early twentieth century. Kraepelin, Alzheimer, Nissl, and Brodmann would have described themselves as "brain scientists." By the early to mid-twentieth century, however, a new array of techniques had been developed that permitted brain scientists to go far beyond the simple processes of looking at neurons under the microscope or studying the gross structure of the brain. Developments in neuropharmacology, neurochemistry, molecular biology, and a variety of other related fields have been extraordinary. These developments led to the founding of a society of neuroscience in 1970, so that scientists working in the diverse areas related to the nervous system could meet and communicate with one another. By the mid-1990s, the Society for Neuroscience had gained more than 20,000 members, making it one of the largest scientific organizations in the United States. The vast array of techniques now available for studying the nervous system has rekindled the strong connections between psychiatry and neuroscience. Many psychiatrists believe that the dream (shared by Kraepelin and Freud) of understanding mental phenomena in terms of neural mechanisms now lies within our reach.

The growth of knowledge and expertise in neuroscience can be easily summarized by examining the history of Nobel Prize awards since their inception. Table 1–2 lists Nobel Prizes awarded in neuroscience and psychiatry. Early awards were given for microscopic techniques and for clinical achievements. Two awards, the prize to Wagner von Jauregg for malarial treatment of syphilis and to Moniz for the development of prefrontal leukotomy to treat schizophrenia, were purely clinical. Others were given more recently in basic areas that laid important foundations for clinical applications, such as Axelrod's studies of neurotransmission within the catecholamine system. The listing in Table 1–2 indicates that there has been a steady increase in prizes awarded in the area of neuroscience during the past several decades.

For any Nobel Prize given in any single year, there are of course dozens of other equally deserving individuals who have made major contributions to science and clinical practice. For example, Nobel Prizes have not been awarded for positron-emission tomography, a far more powerful imaging technique than computerized tomography, or for either neuroleptic drugs or antidepressants, which have been far more lasting and powerful ameliorators of human suffering than prefrontal leukotomy. Nevertheless, this list of Nobel laureates indicates that our knowledge base in neuroscience and its clinical applications has been steadily advancing.

Within psychiatry as a specialized discipline, the major sources of impact from neuroscience have been neuropharmacology and neurochemistry. Coupled with the overall development in neuroscience, the discovery of relatively potent pharmacological treatments for major mental illnesses has also served to reawaken interest in clinical neurobiology. The discovery of chlorpromazine by Delay and Deniker in 1952 indicated that drugs could be developed that would have a powerful calming effect on psychotic and agitated patients. This discovery led rapidly to the development of a variety of neuroleptic drugs that are used for the treatment of psychosis. By the late 1950s, a second new specific class of medications had been developed, the antidepressants, the prototype of which is imipramine. Antianxiety drugs such as meprobamate were also developed. By the early 1960s it had become clear to psychiatrists that an entire new discipline,

Table 1–2. Nobel Prizes awarded in neuroscience and psychiatry

Year	Investigators	Discovery
1906	Camillo Golgi and Santiago Ramón y Cajal	Work on structure of the nervous system
1927	Julius Wagner von Jauregg	Discovery of the therapeutic importance of malaria inoculation in dementia paralytica
1932	Edgar D. Adrian and Sir Charles Scott Sherrington	Discoveries regarding function of the neurons
1936	Sir Henry H. Dale and Otto Loewi	Discoveries relating to the chemical transmission of nerve impulses
1944	Joseph Erlanger and Herbert S. Gasser	Research on the differentiated function of single nerve fibers
1949	Walter Rudolf Hess	Discovery of the functional organization of the midbrain as coordinator of the activities of the internal organs
1949	Antonio Egas Moniz	Discovery of therapeutic value of leukotomy in certain psychoses
1963	Sir John C. Eccles, Sir Alan Lloyd Hodgkin, and Andrew F. Huxley	Study of the transmission of nerve impulses along a nerve fiber (or relationship between inhibition of nerve cells and repolarization of a cell's membrane)
1970	Julius Axelrod, Sir Bernard Katz, and Ulf von Euler	Discoveries concerning the chemistry of nerve transmission
1971	Earl Wilbur Sutherland, Jr.	Study of hormones, the chemical substances that regulate virtually every body function
1977	Rosalyn S. Yalow	Radioimmunoassay
1977	Roger C. L. Guillemin and Andrew V. Schally	Production of peptide hormones in the brain
1979	Earl Hounsfield and Sir Allan M. Cormack	Development of computed tomography scanning
1981	Roger Sperry, David H. Hubel, and Tosten N. Wiesel	Studies on the function of the corpus callosum (split brain research, functions of left and right hemispheres); discoveries on the organization of the visual system
1986	Rita Levi-Montalcatini and Stanley Cohen	Discovery of nerve growth factor

psychopharmacology, was at their feet and that this discipline provided a powerful alternative to the techniques of psychotherapy that had been their major means of treating patients up to this point. Psychopharmacology (also referred to as neuropharmacology or neuropsychopharmacology) was clearly not only a tool for treatment, but also a tool for studying brain chemistry and for developing new classifications of diseases based on patients' responses to specific drugs that manipulated specific classes of chemicals within the brain.

These developments have placed psychiatry in the 1990s squarely within the traditions of medicine and neuroscience. To an interest in neuropharmacology have been added interests in neuroimaging and molecular biology. Modern students of psychiatry must simultaneously view their patients on multiple planes: as human beings who have particular symptoms (psychological), as individuals living within a social and cultural context (social), as products of the genetic endowments given them by their parents and coded in their chromosomes (genetic-molecular), and as individuals whose ideas and emotions are both the product and the producers of a complex set of chemical events in their brains (neurochemical-neuroanatomical).

The Mind/Body Problem in Psychiatry

As this brief summary of the history of psychiatry indicates, people have not consistently agreed about the origins of mental illness or the appropriate areas of expertise for the clinicians who treat mental illness. Although the historical origins of psychiatry are clearly biological, in that the first individuals to identify and define mental illness in classical times believed that these illnesses were physical in origin, for many centuries people have also believed mental illnesses to be caused by a disease of the spirit or psyche. From the Middle Ages up through the eighteenth or nineteenth century, mentally ill persons were perceived as spiritually or morally diseased. Although the bulk of contemporary psychiatrists no longer hold this belief, there are literally centuries of misunderstanding that must be forgotten or eliminated. Old ideas do not die easily, and consequently mental illnesses tend to be stigmatized or misunderstood. The role of psychiatry is confused as well. Many laypersons still view psychiatrists as literally doctors of the mind or soul.

This misunderstanding has also been enhanced by the long-standing controversy about the relationship between the mind and the body. Many religions teach that there is a soul or spirit that exists independently of the body and that survives it after death. People who think concretely and metaphorically tend to see soul or spirit as a tiny ghost sitting somewhere in the body (usually in the brain in modern thinking) and moving or guiding its actions. The existence of the spirit or soul is fundamentally a philosophical or religious issue, not a scientific or medical one. There is simply no way to prove or disprove the existence of the soul and its continuing existence after death. That is a matter of faith.

On at least one level, it is clear that what is commonly referred to as the mind is simply the summation of a variety of electrical and chemical events occurring in the brain. Thinking, believing, remembering, feeling, tasting, and all the other cognitive, sensory, and behavioral functions that human beings experience are fundamentally determined at the molecular level, within a context of neural networks. These events do not exist independently of external environmental influences, but rather are influenced by and reactive to them. Head injuries damage neurons and cause new networks to be developed. Perceptions and experiences are encoded and remembered, and this learning and memory affect later cognitive events. Thus, mental phenomena, often referred to as "mind," can and must be understood in terms of the brain.

The study of psychiatry—the branch of medicine devoted to the study of mental illnesses—is, therefore, a discipline dedicated to the investigation of abnormalities in brain function. The clinical appearance of these abnormalities may be florid and obvious, as in the case of psychosis. The abnormalities may be subtle and mild, as in the case of personality disorders. Ultimately the drive of modern psychiatry is to develop a comprehensive understanding of normal brain function at levels that range from mind to molecule, and to determine how aberrations in these normal functions (produced either endogenously through genetic coding or exogenously through environmental influences) lead to the development of symptoms of mental illnesses.

Bibliography

Ackerknecht EH: Short History of Psychiatry. New York, Hafner, 1968

Alexander FG, Selesnick ST: The History of Psychiatry: An Evaluation of Psychiatric Thought and Practice From Prehistoric Times to the Present. New York, Harper & Row, 1966

Andreasen NC: The Broken Brain: The Biological Revolution in Psychiatry. New York, Harper & Row, 1984

Andreasen NC (ed): Am J Psychiatry 151 (Sesquicentennial Edition supplement, June), 1994

Breuer J, Freud S: The Standard Edition of the Complete Psychological Works of Sigmund Freud, Vol 2, Studies on Hysteria. Translated and edited by Strachey J. London, Hogarth Press, 1955

Gilman SL: Seeing the Insane. New York, Wiley, 1982

Kraepelin E: Lectures on Clinical Psychiatry. London, Bailliere, Tindall & Cox, 1904

Pichot P: A Century of Psychiatry. Paris, Editions Roger Dacosta, 1983

Pinel P: A Treatise on Insanity. London, Messrs Cadell & Davies, Strand, 1806

Rush B: Two Essays on the Mind. Philadelphia, PA, Charles Cist, 1786

Zilboorg G: A History of Medical Psychology. New York, Norton, 1941

Self-Assessment Questions

1. Describe Greek attitudes toward mental illness. What were the four humors?
2. Describe attitudes toward mentally ill persons during the Middle Ages. How long ago was the last witch known to be tormented or burned at the stake?
3. Describe the ideas and accomplishments of Philippe Pinel.
4. Who was Emil Kraepelin? Name two eminent neuroscientists who were members of his department.
5. Wagner von Jauregg and Moniz received Nobel Prizes for clinical achievements. What were they? Describe two achievements more recent than theirs that received Nobel Prizes and that provide a link between neuroscience and psychiatry.

Chapter 2

Diagnosis and Classification

Knowledge keeps no better than fish.

Alfred North Whitehead

Beginning students of psychiatry are often puzzled about what is expected of them when they are asked to make a diagnosis. This is because two major traditions for observing and understanding patients have historically coexisted within psychiatry: the biomedical model and the psychodynamic model. The biomedical model is closely allied with general medicine and stresses diagnosing discrete illnesses or disorders. The psychodynamic model, on the other hand, stresses the importance of understanding the patient's symptoms and behavior in terms of underlying psychological processes (referred to as psychodynamics). A psychiatrist applying the biological or medical model attempts to determine whether the patient has one of the group of commonly recognized disorders, such as schizophrenia or bipolar illness, and then plans the care of the patient accordingly, often by prescribing medications. A psychiatrist applying the psychodynamic model attempts to understand why patients present with a particular complaint, often in terms of relationships with parents or early life experiences, and then seeks to help patients change their maladaptive behavior or reduce their psychological pain by helping them understand and readjust these dynamics. This is often done with psychotherapy.

Although these two traditions were once relatively polarized, they have become increasingly unified in the modern practice of psychiatry, which usually stresses the importance of an integrated *biopsychosocial model*. This model emphasizes the importance of evaluating all aspects of a patient's symptoms and experiences: examining both biological and psychological processes as they occur within a particular social and personal context. The heart of this examination begins, however, with attempting to recognize the particular pattern of symptoms and experiences that leads to the recognition of a specific psychiatric diagnosis, expressed in a nomenclature and classification system that has been developed with considerable care and rigor during the past two decades. This system, published as the *Diagnostic and Statistical Manual of Mental Disorders*, Fourth Edition (DSM-IV; American Psychiatric Association 1994), provides the basis for diagnosis and classification in psychiatry.

The Fundamental Purpose of Diagnosis and Classification

The fundamental purpose of diagnosis and classification is to isolate a group of discrete disease entities, each of which is characterized by a distinct pathophysiology and/or etiology. Ideally, all diseases in medicine would be defined in terms of etiology. For most illnesses, however, we do not know or understand the specific etiology. By and large, a full understanding of etiology is limited to the infectious diseases, in which the etiology is exposure to some infectious agent to a degree that the body's immune mechanisms are overwhelmed. (And even in this instance, our knowledge of immune mechanisms is incomplete.) We also understand the etiology of a variety of hereditary metabolic diseases, such as phenylketonuria (PKU). We have been able to define these diseases in terms of a specific metabolic defect (e.g., failure to metabolize phenylalanine) and have traced that metabolic defect down to a specific genetic locus that produces an abnormal protein. The case of PKU, however, illustrates how complex the search for causes can actually be. We now know that there are two forms of PKU; both are characterized by failure to metabolize phenylalanine, but they involve two different enzymes within the metabolic pathway. Thus, even for a simple disease with a recognized metabolic defect, increasing knowledge can also increase complexity. Now this simple disease must be understood as two different diseases with two different specific causes at the molecular level.

For most diseases, however, our understanding is at the level of pathophysiology rather than etiology. Diseases are defined in terms of the mechanisms that produce particular symptoms, such as infarction in the myocardium, inflammation in the joints, or abnormal regulation of insulin production.

In the areas of pathophysiology and etiology, psychiatry has more uncharted territory than the rest of medicine. Most of the disorders or diseases diagnosed in psychiatry are *syndromes:* collections of symptoms that tend to occur together and that appear to have a characteristic course and outcome. Much of the current investigative research in psychiatry is directed toward the goal of identifying the pathophysiology and etiology of major mental illnesses, but this goal has been achieved for only a few disorders (Alzheimer's disease, multi-infarct dementia, Huntington's disease, and substance-induced syndromes such as amphetamine psychosis or Wernicke-Korsakoff syndrome).

Purposes of Diagnosis in Psychiatry

Even though they do not contain information about specific mechanisms or causes for an identified group of symptoms, diagnoses in psychiatry serve a variety of important purposes. Thus, making a careful diagnosis is as fundamental in psychiatry as it is in the remainder of medicine.

Diagnosis helps to simplify our thinking and reduce the complexity of clinical phenomena in psychiatry.   Psychiatry is a diverse field, and symptoms of mental illness encompass a broad range of emotional, cognitive, and behavioral abnormalities. The use of diagnoses introduces order and structure to this complexity. Disorders are divided into broad classes based on common features (e.g., psychosis, substance abuse, dementia, anxiety). The overall structure of the current psychiatric classification system used in this text is summarized in Table 2–1.

Within each of the major classes, specific syndromes are then further delineated (e.g., dividing substance-related disorders in terms of the type of substance involved, dividing the dementias into Alzheimer's disease and vascular dementia). The existence of broad groups of diagnostic categories, subdivided into specific disorders, creates a structure within the apparent chaos of clinical phenomena and makes mental illnesses easier to learn about and understand. Although diagnoses are not necessarily defined in terms of etiology or pathophysiology, they are typically defined in terms of syndromal clinical features. Thus, this creation of order out of chaos does not misrepresent reality in the process of facilitating understanding.

Psychiatric diagnoses facilitate communication between clinicians.   When physicians give a patient's symptoms a specific diagnosis, such as bipolar mood disorder, they are making a specific statement about the clinical picture with which that particular patient presents. A diagnosis concisely summarizes information for all other clinicians who subsequently examine the patient's records,

Table 2–1.   DSM-IV classification

Disorders usually evident in infancy, childhood, or adolescence
Mental retardation
  Mild
  Moderate
  Severe
  Profound
  Severity unspecified
Learning disorders
  Reading disorder
  Mathematics disorder
  Disorder of written expression
  Learning disorder not otherwise
    specified
Motor skills disorder
Communication disorders
  Expressive language disorder
  Mixed receptive-expressive language
    disorder
  Phonological disorder
  Stuttering
  Communication disorder not otherwise
    specified
Pervasive developmental disorders
  Autistic disorder
  Rett's disorder
  Childhood disintegrative disorder
  Asperger's disorder
  Pervasive developmental disorder not
    otherwise specified
Attention-deficit and disruptive behavior
  disorders
  Attention-deficit hyperactivity
    disorder
  Conduct disorder
  Oppositional defiant disorder
  Attention-deficit hyperactivity disorder
    not otherwise specified
  Disruptive behavior disorder not
    otherwise specified
Feeding and eating disorders of infancy
  or early childhood
  Pica
  Rumination disorder
  Feeding disorder of infancy or early
    childhood
Tic disorders
  Tourette's disorder
  Chronic motor or vocal tic disorder

  Transient tic disorder
  Tic disorder not otherwise specified
Elimination disorders
  Encopresis
  Enuresis
Other disorders of infancy, childhood, or
  adolescence
  Separation anxiety disorder
  Selective mutism
  Reactive attachment disorder of
    infancy or early childhood
  Stereotypic movement disorder
  Disorders of infancy, childhood, or
    adolescence not otherwise
    specified

Delirium, dementia, and amnestic and other cognitive disorders
Delirium
  Delirium due to a general medical
    condition
  Substance-induced delirium
  Delirium due to multiple etiologies
  Delirium not otherwise specified
Dementia
  Dementia of Alzheimer's type
  Vascular dementia
  Dementia due to human immuno-
    deficiency virus (HIV) disease
  Dementia due to head trauma
  Dementia due to Parkinson's disease
  Dementia due to Huntington's disease
  Dementia due to Pick's disease
  Dementia due to Creutzfeldt-Jakob
    disease
  Dementia due to other general
    medical conditions
  Substance-induced persisting
    dementia
  Dementia due to multiple etiologies
  Dementia not otherwise specified
Amnestic disorders
  Amnestic disorder due to a general
    medical condition
  Substance-induced persisting
    amnestic disorder
  Amnestic disorder not otherwise
    specified
Other cognitive disorders

Table 2–1. DSM-IV classification *(continued)*

Mental disorders due to a general medical condition
Catatonic disorder due to a general medical condition
Personality change due to a general medical condition
Mental disorder not otherwise specified due to a general medical condition

Substance-related disorders
Substance abuse
Substance intoxication
Substance withdrawal
Alcohol-related disorders
Amphetamine (or amphetamine-like)-related disorder
Caffeine-related disorders
Cannabis-related disorders
Cocaine-related disorders
Hallucinogen-related disorders
Inhalant-related disorders
Nicotine-related disorders
Opioid-related disorders
Phencyclidine (or phencyclidine-like)-related disorders
Sedative-, hypnotic-, or anxiolytic-related disorders
Polysubstance-related disorder
Other (or unknown) substance-related disorders

Schizophrenia and other psychotic disorders
Schizophrenia
    Paranoid type
    Disorganized type
    Catatonic type
    Undifferentiated type
    Residual type
Schizophreniform disorder
Schizoaffective disorder
Delusional disorder
Brief psychotic disorder
Shared psychotic disorder (folie à deux)
Psychotic disorder due to a medical condition
Substance-induced psychotic disorder

Psychotic disorder not otherwise specified

Mood disorders
Mood episodes
    Major depressive episode
    Manic episode
    Mixed episode
    Hypomanic episode
Depressive disorders
    Major depressive disorder
    Dysthymic disorder
    Depressive disorder not otherwise specified
Bipolar disorders
    Bipolar I disorder
    Bipolar II disorder
    Cyclothymic disorder
    Bipolar disorder not otherwise specified
Other mood disorders
    Mood disorders due to a general medical condition
    Substance-induced mood disorder
    Mood disorder not otherwise specified

Anxiety disorders
Panic attack
Agoraphobia
Panic disorder without agoraphobia
Panic disorder with agoraphobia
Agoraphobia without history of panic disorder
Specific phobia
Social phobia
Obsessive-compulsive disorder
Posttraumatic stress disorder
Acute stress disorder
Generalized anxiety disorder
Anxiety disorder due to a general medical condition
Substance-induced anxiety disorder
Anxiety disorder not otherwise specified

Somatoform disorders
Somatization disorder
Undifferentiated somatoform disorder
Conversion disorder

Table 2–1. DSM-IV classification *(continued)*

Somatoform disorders
Pain disorder
Hypochondriasis
Body dysmorphic disorder
Somatoform disorder not otherwise
  specified

Factitious disorder

Dissociative disorders
Dissociative amnesia
Dissociative fugue
Dissociative identity disorder
Depersonalization disorder
Dissociative disorder not otherwise
  specified

Sexual and gender identity disorders
Sexual dysfunctions
  Sexual desire disorders
  Sexual arousal disorders
  Orgasmic disorders
  Sexual pain disorders
  Sexual dysfunction due to a general
    medical condition
  Substance-induced sexual
    dysfunction
  Sexual dysfunction not otherwise
    specified
Paraphilias
  Exhibitionism
  Fetishism
  Frotteurism
  Pedophilia
  Sexual masochism
  Sexual sadism
  Transvestic fetishism
  Voyeurism
  Paraphilia not otherwise specified
Gender identity disorders
Sexual disorder not otherwise specified

Eating disorders
Anorexia nervosa

Bulimia nervosa
Eating disorder not otherwise
  specified

Sleep disorders
Primary sleep disorders
  Dyssomnias
  Parasomnias
Sleep disorder related to another mental
  disorder
Sleep disorder due to a general medical
  condition
Substance-induced sleep disorder

**Impulse-control disorders not elsewhere
classified**
Intermittent explosive disorder
Kleptomania
Pyromania
Pathological gambling
Trichotillomania
Impulse-control disorder not otherwise
  specified

Adjustment disorders

Personality disorders
Paranoid personality disorder
Schizoid personality disorder
Schizotypal personality disorder
Antisocial personality disorder
Borderline personality disorder
Histrionic personality disorder
Narcissistic personality disorder
Avoidant personality disorder
Dependent personality disorder
Obsessive-compulsive personality
  disorder
Personality disorder not otherwise
  specified

**Other conditions that may be a focus of
clinical attention**

or to whom the patient is referred. A diagnosis of bipolar mood disorder, for example, indicates that

- The patient has had at least one episode of mania.
- During that episode of mania the patient will have experienced a characteristic group of symptoms such as elated mood, increased energy, racing thoughts, rapid speech, grandiosity, and poor judgment.
- The patient has probably had episodes of depression as well, characterized by sadness, insomnia, decreased appetite, feelings of worthlessness, and other typical depressive symptoms.

The use of diagnostic categories gives clinicians a kind of shorthand through which they can summarize large quantities of information relatively easily.

Diagnoses help to predict the outcome of the disorder.   Many psychiatric diagnoses are associated with a characteristic course and outcome. For example, bipolar illness is usually episodic, with periods of relatively severe abnormalities in mood interspersed with periods of near normality or complete normality. Most patients with bipolar disorder have a relatively good outcome. Other types of disorders, such as schizophrenia or personality disorders, typically run a more chronic course. Diagnoses are a useful way of summarizing the clinician's expectations about the patient's course of illness in the future.

Diagnoses are often used to decide on an appropriate treatment.   As psychiatry has advanced clinically and scientifically, relatively specific treatments for particular disorders or groups of symptoms have been developed. For example, neuroleptic drugs are typically used to treat psychoses. Thus, they are used for disorders such as schizophrenia, in which psychosis is typically prominent, as well as forms of mood disorder in which psychotic symptoms occur. A diagnosis of mania suggests the use of medications such as lithium carbonate or carbamazepine. Some relatively targeted medications are now available, such as clomipramine for obsessive-compulsive disorder or alprazolam for panic disorder.

Diagnoses are used to assist in the search for pathophysiology and etiology. Clinical researchers use diagnoses to reduce heterogeneity in their samples and to separate groups of patients who may share a mechanism or cause that produces their symptoms. Patients who share a relatively specific set of symptoms, such as severe schizophrenia characterized by negative symptoms, are often hypothesized to have a disorder that is mechanistically or etiologically distinct. Knowledge about specific groupings of clinical symptoms can be related to knowledge about brain specialization and function in order to formulate hypotheses about the neurochemical or anatomical substrates of a particular disorder. Ideally, the use of diagnoses defined on the basis of the clinical picture will lead ultimately to diagnoses that serve the fundamental purpose of identifying causes.

Other Purposes of Diagnosis

Beyond these clinical uses, diagnostic systems also have other purposes. Although physicians prefer to conceptualize their relationships with patients in terms of care and treatment, diagnoses are used by health care providers, attorneys, epidemiologists, and insurance companies. Each time a clinician makes a diagnosis and records it, he or she must do so with an awareness of the other nonclinical uses to which it may be put.

Diagnoses are used to monitor treatment and to make decisions about reimbursement.   As care has become increasingly managed, predetermined guidelines (diagnosis-related groups, or DRGs) have been set that define how long a hospitalization or treatment course a specific diagnosis should require. In some regions, physicians or their assistants must spend hours on the phone or writing letters if their patient's course of treatment appears to exceed the preset guidelines. This situation will probably not change the physician's diagnosis, but it has certainly changed the autonomy that physicians once enjoyed.

Diagnoses are used by attorneys in malpractice suits and in other litigation. Although psychiatrists are the least sued among medical specialists, lawsuits are a concern for all specialists in our litigious society. Some diagnoses, such as depression, carry with them a clear set of risks, such as suicide. Clinicians must be aware of those risks and clearly document that they have provided appropriate care. As DSM has made the diagnostic system of psychiatry more open and available, both lawyers and patients have learned much more about psychiatric nosology. A physician called into court must expect to defend a recorded diagnosis with appropriate documentation that the various criteria have been assessed and are met.

Diagnoses are used by health care epidemiologists to determine the incidence and prevalence of various diseases throughout the world.   This is a somewhat more constructive use of diagnosis. Diagnoses recorded in hospital or clinic charts are translated into a standard system established by the World Health Organization: the International Classification of Diseases (ICD). This system is used to track regional differences in disease patterns, as well as changes over time.

Diagnoses are used to make decisions about insurance coverage. A carelessly made diagnosis, be it of hypertension or depression, may make it difficult for a patient to obtain life insurance or future health care insurance. Diagnoses are also sometimes used to make decisions about employment, admission to college, and other important opportunities. Because mental illnesses may be subject to discrimination and misunderstanding, these diagnoses involve a particular risk. The clinician must obviously walk a fine line—perhaps impossibly fine.

Development of the *Diagnostic and Statistical Manual of Mental Disorders*

The process of diagnosis in psychiatry is partially simplified by the fact that the national professional organization to which most psychiatrists belong, the American Psychiatric Association (APA), has formulated a manual that summarizes all the diagnoses used in psychiatry, specifies the symptoms that must be present to make a given diagnosis, and organizes these diagnoses together into a classification system. This manual is entitled the *Diagnostic and Statistical Manual of Mental Disorders* (DSM). Over the years it has gone through four major revisions (DSM-I, DSM-II, DSM-III, and DSM-IV). Currently, diagnoses in psychiatry are based on DSM-IV, which was revised during the 1990s and published in 1994.

Psychiatry is the only specialty in medicine that has so consistently and comprehensively formalized the diagnostic processes for the disorders within its domain. This precision and structure are particularly important in psychiatry because it lacks recognized etiologies for most disorders and lacks specific laboratory diagnostic tests as well. Consequently, diagnosis relies largely on the patient's presenting symptoms and history. Without such structure, the diagnostic process could become confused and fuzzy.

The impetus to organize DSM began during World War II. For the first time, psychiatrists from all over the United States were brought together in clinical settings that required them to communicate clearly with one another. It became apparent that diagnostic practices varied widely throughout the United States, no doubt reflecting a diversity of training. After World War II, the Veterans Administration attempted to design a relatively comprehensive diagnostic system for its own use. Shortly thereafter, the APA convened a task force to develop a diagnostic manual for use in all of American psychiatry. The product was DSM-I, which was published in 1952. The second revision, DSM-II, was published in 1968.

Compared with DSM-III and DSM-IV, the more recent manuals, DSM-I and DSM-II were relatively simple. The definitions of disorders and the overall classification system were designed by a small group of clinicians who convened, discussed their clinical experiences, and decided together on appropriate categories and defining features. Definitions tended to be brief, descriptive, and relatively vague. For example, the definition of manic-depressive illness in DSM-II was as follows:

Manic-Depressive Illnesses (Manic-Depressive Psychoses)

These disorders are marked by severe mood swings and a tendency to remission and recurrence. Patients may be given this diagnosis in the absence of a previous history of affective psychosis if there is no obvious precipitating event. This disorder is divided into three major subtypes: manic type, depressed type, and circular type. (p. 8)

These handbooks were relatively small. DSM-I contained 132 pages, and DSM-II contained 119 pages.

DSM-III, by contrast, represented a major change—and, most clinicians would concur, a major improvement. Because of their vagueness and imprecision, the definitions in DSM-I and DSM-II did not adequately fulfill many of the purposes summarized above. In particular, the descriptions were not specific enough to facilitate communication among clinicians and to delineate one disorder from another. Although the purpose of DSM-I and DSM-II was to ensure that a psychiatrist in Peoria, Illinois, meant the same thing by a diagnosis of schizophrenia as a psychiatrist on Park Avenue in New York City or in Laguna Beach, California, this was clearly not the case.

A number of research investigations had examined diagnostic agreement among clinicians. They had made it clear that, using DSM-I or DSM-II guidelines, different clinicians would give different diagnoses for the same patient. Naturally, this lack of consensus and agreement about how to diagnose patients called the credibility of psychiatry into question. These research studies of poor agreement, completed during the 1960s, coincided with the development of relatively specific new medications such as neuroleptics and antidepressants. When relatively specific treatments for particular disorders became available, it was clearly important to define the disorders well so that appropriate treatment would be prescribed.

When the Task Force on DSM-III was appointed in 1972, its members decided to set a new agenda for the development of the DSMs. Many members of this task force were eminent researchers with expertise in disciplines such as pharmacology and genetics. Thus, they were especially aware of the importance of diagnostic precision. At their first meetings, they decided to formulate a set of rules by which they would abide:

- They would attempt to formulate specific diagnostic criteria that would be as objective as possible to define each of the disorders included in the manual.
- They would make their decisions about defining criteria and overall organizational structure on the basis of existing research data whenever possible.
- They would not resort to anecdotal approaches or simple clinical opinion if at all possible.
- They would include a glossary to define terms used in the text.
- In addition to the criteria, they would provide clinicians with information that would assist them in understanding specific disorders better, such as population frequency, gender ratio, and longitudinal course.
- They would provide a set of references that would support their decisions.

Apart from the last rule, which was not feasible because of the large quantity of references that would have been needed, these rules were followed relatively closely.

When DSM-III finally appeared in 1980, it was widely recognized as a major innovation. Although some clinicians complained that it was boring or dull, most appreciated its objectivity. For the first time, the methods by which a psychiatric diagnosis could be made were relatively clear. The process has been somewhat facetiously referred to as the "Chinese-menu approach" to diagnosis. Most of the time, the criteria require that a specified subset from a listed group of symptoms be present in order to make a diagnosis (e.g., select "two from column one and three from column two," as on some Chinese menus). For example, in contrast to the rather vague definition of manic-depressive illness above, the DSM-III definition of major depressive disorder was as follows:

Diagnostic Criteria for Major Depression

A. One or more major depressive episodes
B. Has never had a manic episode

Diagnostic Criteria for Major Depressive Episode

A. Dysphoric mood or loss of interest or pleasure in all or almost all usual activities and pastimes. The dysphoric mood is characterized by symptoms such as the following: depressed, sad, blue, hopeless, low, down in the dumps, irritable. The mood disturbance must be prominent and relatively persistent, but not necessarily the most dominant symptom, and does not include momentary shifts from one dysphoric mood to another dysphoric mood, e.g., anxiety to depression to anger, such as are seen in states of acute psychotic turmoil. (For children under 6, dysphoric mood may have to be inferred from a persistently sad facial expression.)

B. At least four of the following symptoms have been present nearly every day for a period of at least 2 weeks (in children under 6, at least three of the first four).
   1. poor appetite or significant weight loss (when not dieting) or increased appetite or significant weight gain (in children under 6, consider failure to make expected weight gains)
   2. insomnia or hypersomnia
   3. psychomotor agitation or retardation (but not merely subjective feelings of restlessness or being slowed down) (in children under 6, hypoactivity)
   4. loss of interest or pleasure in usual activities, or decrease in sexual drive not limited to a period when delusional or hallucinating (in children under 6, signs of apathy)
   5. loss of energy; fatigue
   6. feelings of worthlessness, self-reproach, or excessive or inappropriate guilt (either may be delusional)
   7. complaints or evidence of diminished ability to think or concentrate, such as slowed thinking, or indecisiveness not associated with marked loosening of associations or incoherence
   8. recurrent thoughts of death, suicidal ideation, wishes to be dead, or suicide attempt

C. Neither of the following dominates the clinical picture when an affective syndrome is absent (i.e., symptoms in criteria A and B above):
   1. preoccupation with a mood-incongruent delusion or hallucination (see definition below)
   2. bizarre behavior

D. Not superimposed on schizophrenia, schizophreniform disorder, or a paranoid disorder

E. Not due to any organic mental disorder or uncomplicated bereavement (pp. 213–214, 218)

DSM-III was the first effort by a medical specialty to provide a comprehensive and detailed diagnostic manual in which all disorders were defined by highly specific criteria. DSM-III was a hefty tome: 494 pages long. DSM-III changed the practice of psychiatry in many ways. Its main value was to introduce substantial improvements in psychiatric diagnosis, which have been carried forward in the more recent DSM-IV revision. But the treatment of previous muddleheadedness has not been without some untoward side effects as well.

Advantages and Disadvantages of the DSM III/IV Approach

The DSM-III/IV approach has many advantages compared with the earlier DSMs. These advantages can be summarized as follows:

DSM III/IV substantially improved the reliability of diagnosis. Reliability, a biometric concept, refers to the ability of two observers to agree on what they see. It is measured by a variety of statistical methods, such as percent agreement, correlation coefficients, and the kappa statistic, which corrects for chance agreement. The reliability of DSM-III was assessed in field trials and found to be relatively good. The original field-trial data for some diagnostic categories, based on kappa, are summarized in Table 2–2. (A kappa of .8 or greater is considered very good, and a kappa greater than .5 is considered acceptable.) The kappas in Table 2–2 are generally in this range. By contrast, percent agreements (which are not even corrected for chance agreement) for disorders such as depression or schizophrenia had been estimated to be as low as 20%–30% in several studies

Table 2–2. Kappa coefficients of agreement for DSM-III Axes I and II diagnostic classes for adults (18 and older)

	Phase 1 (*n* = 339)		Phase 2 (*n* = 331)	
	Kappa	% of sample	Kappa	% of sample
Axis I				
Disorders usually first evident in infancy, childhood, or adolescence	.65	5.3	.73	3.6
Organic mental disorders	.79	11.8	.76	10.0
Substance use disorders	.86	21.2	.80	21.2
Schizophrenic disorders	.81	17.7	.81	23.3
Paranoid disorders	.66	1.2	.75	1.5
Psychotic disorders not elsewhere classified	.64	11.2	.69	6.7
Affective disorders	.69	43.1	.83	38.7
Anxiety disorders	.63	9.1	.72	8.8
Somatoform disorders	.54	3.8	.42	3.3
Dissociative disorders	.80	0.9	−.003	0.6
Psychosexual disorders	.92	2.1	.75	1.5
Factitious disorders	.66	1.2	−.005	0.9
Disorders of impulse control not elsewhere classified	.28	1.8	.80	1.8
Adjustment disorder	.67	12.1	.68	8.5
Psychological factors affecting physical condition	.62	3.2	.44	2.1
Overall kappa for Axis I	.68		.72	
Axis II			1.2	
Specific developmental disorders			.40	1.2
Personality disorders	.56	59.9	.65	49.8
Overall kappa for Axis II	.56		.64	

completed before DSM-III was available. Similar assessments of reliability were also completed for the DSM-IV revisions and documented ongoing improvement in reliability.

The DSM III/IV approach has clarified the diagnostic process and facilitated history taking.   Because DSM III/IV specifies exactly which symptoms must be present to make a diagnosis, as well as the characteristic course of disorders whenever this is appropriate, it is highly objective. During the 1970s, many psychiatrists received predominantly psychodynamic training, which deemphasized a medical approach to diagnosis. This approach stressed the importance of recognizing underlying psychological processes rather than objective signs and symptoms. Although clinically useful, this approach is more subjective, is difficult to teach to beginners, and requires substantial training. DSM III/IV provided a simpler approach that brought signs and symptoms back to the forefront of evaluation. Its criteria systematically specify which signs must be observed and which symptoms must be inquired about. This structured approach also makes it an excellent teaching tool for medical students and residents.

DSM III/IV also clarified and facilitated the process of differential diagnosis. Because it is so explicit, DSM III/IV helps clinicians decide which symptoms must be present to rule in or to rule out a particular diagnosis. For example, it specifies that a diagnosis of schizophrenia cannot be made if a full mood syndrome is present. Likewise, a diagnosis cannot be made if some type of drug of abuse, such as amphetamine, has led to the presence of psychotic symptoms. Not only are differential diagnostic issues embedded in the criteria, but the text of DSM III/IV also contains a relatively detailed discussion of the differential diagnosis for each disorder.

Every paradise has its serpent and poisoned apple. Every treatment has its unwanted side effects. Thus, DSM III/IV also has certain problems and disadvantages.

The increased precision sometimes gives clinicians and researchers a false sense of certainty about what they are doing.   DSM III/IV criteria are simple provisional agreements, arrived at by a group of experts, on what characteristic features must be present to make a diagnosis. Although the criteria are based on data whenever possible, the available data are often inadequate for building the criteria totally on a scientific database. Thus, the selection of signs and symptoms is often relatively arbitrary. The diagnoses themselves are certainly arbitrary. They will remain arbitrary as long as we are ignorant about pathophysiology and etiology. Medical students and residents often crave certainty (as do many physicians long out of training), and so they want very much to believe that a given DSM III/IV diagnosis refers to some "real thing." Thus, these DSM editions sometimes lead clinicians to lapse into petty and pointless debates about whether a patient "really" is depressed if he or she does or does not meet the criteria in these editions. The criteria should be seen for what they are: a useful tool that introduces structure but is arbitrary in essence. They should be applied with a healthy sense of skepticism.

DSM III/IV may sacrifice validity for reliability.   Whereas reliability refers to the capacity of individuals to agree on what they see, validity refers to the capacity to make useful predictions. In particular, the validity of a medical diagnostic system refers to its ability to predict prognosis and outcome, response to treatment, and ultimately etiology. Put simply, reliability refers to whether something can be measured precisely, whereas validity refers to whether it is worth measuring at all. Psychodynamically oriented clinicians have objected that DSM III/IV have sacrificed some of psychiatry's most clinically important concepts, because psychodynamic explanations and descriptions are by and large excluded from these editions. Biologically oriented psychiatrists have objected to the lack of validity in DSM III/IV as well. In this instance, they point to the arbitrary nature of the definitions, which are not rooted in information about biological causes.

Overview of DSM Nosology

As Table 2–1 indicates, the various diagnoses that can be given to psychiatric patients are divided among a substantial number of main categories or headings. A more detailed description of the various diagnoses under these headings appears in Section II of this book, where specific diagnoses are discussed in detail.

Disorders usually first evident in infancy, childhood, or adolescence include a large variety of conditions that typically begin before adulthood. They include developmental disorders such as mental retardation and a variety of specific learning, motor, and communication disabilities. They also include pervasive developmental disorders such as autism and other related conditions. The attention-deficit and disruptive behavior disorders include some of the most common conditions seen in children, such as attention-deficit/hyperactivity disorder and conduct disorders (the juvenile delinquency of the *I Love Lucy* era). This category also includes disorders involving motor activity that occur in children (e.g., Tourette's disorder and other tic syndromes) and disorders of basic biological processes such as eating and elimination. Some disorders that are often observed in children and adolescents, such as depression or schizophrenia, are not classified here because the preponderance of individuals with these diagnoses are adults, and the clinical syndromes are essentially the same in both children and adults.

Delirium, dementia, and amnestic and other cognitive disorders include the various dementias such as Alzheimer's disease, vascular dementia, Huntington's disease, and Creutzfeldt-Jakob disease. This category also includes delirium, which is subspecified according to its cause (e.g., secondary to a general medical condition or to some type of drug). The common theme in this particular category is that a cause or pathophysiological mechanism is usually clearly recognized. It may be a pathogen such as human immunodeficiency virus (HIV), a drug such as alcohol, or a general medical illness such as myxedema. The disorders in this category are also characterized by abnormalities in higher cortical functions such as memory or abstract thinking.

Substance-related disorders include the various conditions that occur as a consequence of substance use. These syndromes are subdivided into abuse, intoxication, and withdrawal, on the basis of the pattern of use, the acuity of recent dose, and the presence of physiological dependence. The specific type of drug being used or abused is also identified.

Schizophrenia and other psychotic disorders include a group of conditions characterized by the presence of abnormalities in perception (hallucinations) and in inferential thinking (delusions) as well as other symptoms that reflect difficulties in distinguishing between what is real and what is unreal and that are referred to as psychotic. Schizophrenia is a severe psychotic disorder that is among the most common psychiatric disorders. A variety of other psychotic conditions are also classified in this category, such as substance-induced psychosis.

Mood disorders are also among the most common conditions seen in psychiatry. They are divided into two broad groups. The bipolar conditions are characterized by at least one episode of mania (and typically episodes of depression as well), whereas the depressive disorders involve only depression (and therefore are sometimes referred to as unipolar disorders).

Anxiety disorders also include a variety of very common conditions, such as panic disorder, agoraphobia, social phobia, obsessive-compulsive disorder, posttraumatic stress disorder, and generalized anxiety disorder.

Somatoform disorders represent a category in which the patient has a variety of physical complaints for which no specific etiology can be found. They include conversion disorder (e.g., unexplained paralyses, seizures), hypochondriasis, and somatization disorder (a disorder characterized by multiple somatic complaints and sometimes referred to as Briquet's syndrome).

Factitious disorders are feigned disorders in which the patient produces the symptoms intentionally; either physical or psychological symptoms may be feigned.

Dissociative disorders are a grouping of conditions that are relatively uncommon, although they have been diagnosed with increasing frequency during recent years. They include dissociative identity disorder (formerly called multiple personality disorder), dissociative fugue, dissociative amnesia, and depersonalization disorder. The essential feature of these disorders is a disturbance in identity, memory, or consciousness that cannot be explained on a physical basis.

Sexual disorders include conditions often referred to as sexual deviations (paraphilias), such as exhibitionism, pedophilia, sexual masochism, and sexual sadism. They also include specific sexual dysfunctions, such as difficulty in achieving erection or orgasm, premature ejaculation, and dyspareunia.

Eating disorders include anorexia nervosa and bulimia nervosa. Patients with anorexia nervosa have a pathological desire to be excessively thin and develop a syndrome characterized by weight loss and emaciation. Those with bulimia nervosa maintain normal weight but use vomiting or other methods (e.g., laxative use) as a way to control the effects of binge-eating behavior.

Sleep disorders are divided into dyssomnias and parasomnias. The dyssomnias are disorders of initiating or maintaining sleep, such as insomnia and hypersomnia. The parasomnias include conditions more "psychological" in nature, such as nightmares, sleep terrors, and sleepwalking. These conditions are particularly common in children but are grouped with the sleep disorders to maintain consistency.

Impulse-control disorders include a variety of conditions involving poor impulse control, such as kleptomania, pathological gambling, and pyromania.

Adjustment disorders include a group of disorders involving a painful or maladaptive reaction to some specific stress, such as divorce, marital discord, or loss of a job. The adjustment disorders are further subdivided according to the type of symptomatology that the patient experiences, such as anxiety, depression, or physical complaints.

Personality disorders refer to conditions in which personality traits become maladaptive. The personality disorders are divided into three clusters. Cluster A consists of personality disorders that are symptomatically (and perhaps etiologically) related to psychotic disorders, such as paranoid personality disorder, schizoid personality disorder, and schizotypal personality disorder. Cluster B includes personality disorders sometimes referred to as "acting out." People with these personality disorders are often somewhat difficult to deal with because they are erratic, unpredictable, overemotional, and self-centered. They include antisocial, borderline, histrionic, and narcissistic personality disorders. Cluster C consists of personality disorders characterized by fearfulness and anxiety. They include avoidant, dependent, and obsessive-compulsive personality disorders.

The DSM classification system is multiaxial. The term *multiaxial* refers to a system that characterizes patients in multiple ways so that the clinician is encouraged to evaluate all aspects of the patient's health and social background. The five axes used to code patient characteristics are summarized in Table 2–3.

Axis I is used to indicate the major syndromes, such as schizophrenia, bipolar disorder, and panic disorder. If several diagnoses are present, all can be noted.

Axis II is used to code disorders that arise relatively early in life and persist; specifically, mental retardation and personality disorders are coded on this axis. This is seen as a way of calling the clinician's attention to these conditions, which are often ignored (particularly the personality disorders). Patients may of course have both Axis I and Axis II diagnoses (e.g., major depressive disorder and borderline personality disorder).

Axis III is used to code the various medical conditions that the patient has (e.g., hypertension, diabetes, thyroid disease) that may be relevant to his or her care. Axis III is an important component of diagnosis because it calls the clinician's attention to medical conditions that might interact with the various psychiatric disorders the patient has. It also alerts the clinician to the fact that the patient might be on medications to treat these conditions that could interact with any psychoactive drugs prescribed.

Axis IV codes the various psychosocial and environmental problems that may interact with the patient's psychiatric and general medical illnesses. Whenever possible, the clinician notes the specific stressor and codes its level of severity. Axis IV serves to alert the clinician to any personal factors that might be relevant to the patient's diagnosis (e.g., the exacerbation of depression produced by living with an alcoholic spouse) or that raise problems in care and management (e.g., homelessness). The coding for the severity of psychosocial and environmental problems, along with some typical examples that serve as anchor points, is summarized in Table 2–4.

Axis V provides a global assessment of the overall level of functioning and psychological health of the patient. It includes various indices of social, psychological, and occupational functioning. These are coded on the Global Assessment of Functioning (GAF) Scale, which ranges from 1 to 90, with 90

Table 2–3.   Multiaxial system of DSM-IV

Axis I	Clinical disorders
	Other conditions that may be a focus of clinical attention
Axis II	Personality disorders
	Mental retardation
Axis III	General medical conditions
Axis IV	Psychosocial and environmental problems
Axis V	Global assessment of functioning

representing absent or minimal symptoms. The GAF Scale is summarized in Table 2–5. (The use of this scale provides the clinician with some indication of the patient's overall prognosis, because high-functioning individuals typically have a better outcome.)

How to Become Familiar With the DSM System

The DSM system is obviously large and complex. Beginning clinicians should not attempt to master everything at once. Rather, they should focus on the major and common conditions that are frequently seen either in psychiatric practice or in primary care settings. They should become very familiar with the diagnostic criteria for a few common conditions such as schizophrenia, major depression, dementia, anxiety disorders, and personality disorders. A few sets of symptom criteria (e.g., major depression) should be committed to memory, simply because they are used so often in so many different clinical settings. The system is too vast to commit all of it to memory, however, and so the clinician should not feel concerned about the need to refer to the criteria frequently when evaluating patients' symptoms and making diagnoses.

Table 2–4. DSM-IV severity of psychosocial stressors scale

		Examples of stressors	
Code	Term	Acute events	Enduring circumstances
1	None	No acute events that may be relevant to the disorder	No enduring circumstances that may be relevant to the disorder
2	Mild	Broke up with boyfriend or girlfriend; started or graduated from school; child left home	Family arguments; job dissatisfaction; residence in high-crime neighborhood
3	Moderate	Marriage; marital separation; loss of job; retirement; miscarriage	Marital discord; serious financial problems; trouble with boss; being a single parent
4	Severe	Divorce; birth of first child	Unemployment; poverty
5	Extreme	Death of spouse; serious physical illness diagnosed; victim of rape	Serious chronic illness in self or child; ongoing physical or sexual abuse
6	Catastrophic	Death of child; suicide of spouse; devastating natural disaster	Captivity as hostage; concentration camp experience
0	Inadequate information, or no change in condition		

Table 2–5. DSM-IV Global Assessment of Functioning (GAF) Scale

Consider psychological, social, and occupational functioning on a hypothetical continuum of mental health to illness. Do not include impairment in functioning due to physical (or environmental) limitations.

Code Note: Use intermediate codes when appropriate, e.g., 45, 69, 72.

90
|
81

Absent or minimal symptoms (e.g., mild anxiety before an exam), **good functioning in all areas, interested and involved in a wide range of activities, socially effective, generally satisfied with life, no more than everyday problems or concerns** (e.g., an occasional argument with family members).

80
|
71

If symptoms are present, they are transient and expectable reactions to psychosocial stressors (e.g., difficulty concentrating after family argument); **no more than slight impairment in social, occupational, or school functioning** (e.g., temporarily falling behind in schoolwork).

70
|
61

Some mild symptoms (e.g., depressed mood and mild insomnia) **OR some difficulty in social, occupational, or school functioning** (e.g., occasional truancy, or theft within the household), **but generally functioning pretty well, has some meaningful interpersonal relationships.**

60
|
51

Moderate symptoms (e.g., flat affect and circumstantial speech, occasional panic attacks) **OR moderate difficulty in social, occupational, or school functioning** (e.g., few friends, conflicts with co-workers).

50
|
41

Serious symptoms (e.g., suicidal ideation, severe obsessional rituals, frequent shoplifting) **OR any serious impairment in social, occupational, or school functioning** (e.g., no friends, unable to keep a job).

40
|
|
31

Some impairment in reality testing or communication (e.g., speech is at times illogical, obscure, or irrelevant) **OR major impairment in several areas, such as work or school, family relations, judgment, thinking, or mood** (e.g., depressed man avoids friends, neglects family, and is unable to work; child frequently beats up younger children, is defiant at home, and is failing at school).

30
|
|
21

Behavior is considerably influenced by delusions or hallucinations OR serious impairment in communication or judgment (e.g., sometimes incoherent, acts grossly inappropriately, suicidal preoccupation) **OR inability to function in almost all areas** (e.g., stays in bed all day; no job, home, or friends).

20
|
|
11

Some danger of hurting self or others (e.g., suicide attempts without clear expectation of death, frequently violent, manic excitement) **OR occasionally fails to maintain minimal personal hygiene** (e.g., smears feces) **OR gross impairment in communication** (e.g., largely incoherent or mute).

10
|
1

Persistent danger of severely hurting self or others (e.g., recurrent violence) **OR persistent inability to maintain minimal personal hygiene OR serious suicidal act with clear expectation of death.**

0 **Inadequate information.**

Bibliography

American Psychiatric Association: Diagnostic and Statistical Manual of Mental Disorders. Washington, DC, American Psychiatric Association, 1952

American Psychiatric Association: Diagnostic and Statistical Manual of Mental Disorders, 2nd Edition. Washington, DC, American Psychiatric Association, 1968

American Psychiatric Association: Diagnostic and Statistical Manual of Mental Disorders, 3rd Edition. Washington, DC, American Psychiatric Association, 1980

American Psychiatric Association: Diagnostic and Statistical Manual of Mental Disorders, 4th Edition. Washington, DC, American Psychiatric Association, 1994

Feighner JP, Robins E, Guze SB, et al: Diagnostic criteria for use in psychiatric research. Arch Gen Psychiatry 26:57–63, 1972

Feinstein AR: ICD, POR, and DRGs: unsolved scientific problems in the nosology of clinical medicine. Arch Intern Med 148:2269–2274, 1988

Frances AJ, Widiger TA, Pincus HA: The development of DSM-IV. Arch Gen Psychiatry 46:373–375, 1989

Kendler KS: Toward a scientific psychiatric nosology: strengths and limitations. Arch Gen Psychiatry 47:969–973, 1990

King LS: Medical Thinking: A Historical Preface. Princeton, NJ, Princeton University Press, 1982

Pincus HA, Frances A, Davis WW, et al: DSM-IV and new diagnostic categories: holding the line on proliferation. Am J Psychiatry 149:112–117, 1992

Robins E, Guze SB: Establishment of diagnostic validity in psychiatric diagnosis: its application to schizophrenia. Am J Psychiatry 126:983–987, 1970

Spitzer RL, Endicott J, Robins E: Research Diagnostic Criteria: rationale and reliability. Arch Gen Psychiatry 35:773–782, 1978

Spitzer RL, Williams JBW, Skodol AE: DSM-III: the major achievements and an overview. Am J Psychiatry 137:151–164, 1980

Tischler GL (ed): Diagnosis and Classification in Psychiatry: A Critical Appraisal of DSM-III. Cambridge, England, Cambridge University Press, 1987

Wilson M: DSM-III and the transformation of American psychiatry—a history. Am J Psychiatry 150:399–410, 1993

Wing JK, Cooper JE, Sartorius N: The Measurement and Classification of Psychiatric Symptoms. Cambridge, Cambridge University Press, 1974

World Health Organization: International Statistical Classification of Diseases and Related Health Problems, 10th Revision. Geneva, Switzerland, World Health Organization, 1992

Self-Assessment Questions

1. What is the overall purpose of diagnosis and classification in medicine generally? Give several examples of diseases for which this purpose has been achieved. Describe the extent to which it has been achieved in psychiatry.
2. Describe some of the specific purposes of psychiatric diagnosis.
3. Describe some of the changes introduced by DSM-III.
4. Define the concepts of reliability and validity.
5. Describe the advantages of the DSM approach. What are some of its disadvantages?
6. What is meant by the term *multiaxial*? List the five axes that are included in DSM-IV.

Chapter 3

Interviewing and Assessment

Festina lente
Make haste slowly

A Latin proverb

Because so much of psychiatric diagnosis depends at present on clinical history, the ability to interview and to take an accurate history is one of the most fundamental skills in psychiatry. Demands placed on the interviewer will vary, depending on the type of illness the patient has and its severity. Patients with milder syndromes, such as anxiety disorders or personality disorders, are usually more capable of describing their symptoms and past history clearly and articulately. The severely ill depressed, manic, or psychotic patient presents a real challenge. These patients may speak in a disorganized manner, be very distractible, be uninterested or uncooperative, or even be mute. Clinicians may have to depend on informants, such as family members or friends, in addition to the patient.

Interviewing Techniques

Although the demands of the interview may vary depending on the patient and the illness, some techniques are common to most interviewing situations.

Establish rapport as early in the interview as possible. It is often best to begin by asking the patient about himself—what kind of work he does, where he goes to school, what he is studying, how old he is, whether he is married or single, and what kinds of things he does for fun. Questions about these topics should not be asked in a manner that seems to grill the patient, but rather in a way that indicates that the interviewer is genuinely interested in getting to know the patient. The overall tone of the opening of the interview should, therefore, convey warmth and friendliness. After rapport has been established, the interviewer should then inquire about what kind of problem the patient has been having, what brought him to the clinic, or why he came into the hospital.

The interviewer needs to determine the patient's chief complaint. Sometimes this complaint will be helpful and explicit (e.g., "I've been feeling very depressed," or "I've been having a pain in my head that other doctors can't explain"). At other times the chief complaint may be relatively vague and require a number of follow-up questions (e.g., "I don't know why I'm here—my family brought me," "I've been having trouble at work"). When the replies are not particularly explicit, the interviewer will need to follow up his or her initial questions with others that will help determine the nature of the patient's problem (e.g., "What kinds of things have been bothering your family?" "What kind of trouble at work?"). The initial portion of the interview, devoted to eliciting the chief complaint, should take as long as is necessary to determine the patient's primary problem. When the patient is a clear, logical informant, let her tell her story as freely as possible without interruption. When she is a relatively poor informant, the interviewer will need to be active and directive.

Use the chief complaint to develop a provisional differential diagnosis. As in the rest of medicine, once the patient's primary problem has been determined, the interviewer begins to construct in his or her mind a range of explanations as to the specific diagnosis that might lead to that particular problem. For example, if the patient indicates that he has been hearing voices, the differential diagnosis includes a variety of disorders that produce this type of psychotic symptom, such as schizophrenia, schizophreniform disorder, psychotic mania, substance abuse involving hallucinogens, or alcoholic hallucinosis. Being able to develop a differential diagnosis, of course, requires some knowledge of the various types of psychiatric disorders and their characteristic symptoms. As in the rest of medicine, skill in making a differential diagnosis increases with knowledge and experience. Overall, however, it may be comforting to realize that the fundamental process of interviewing and diagnosing is the same in psychiatry as it is in internal medicine or neurology.

Rule the various diagnostic possibilities out or in by using more focused and detailed questions. The existence of DSM-IV is particularly helpful in this regard. If the patient's chief complaint has suggested three or four different possible diagnoses, the interviewer can determine which is most relevant by referring to the diagnostic criteria for those disorders. Thus, the interviewer determines what additional symptoms are present besides those already enumerated when the chief complaint was elicited. The interviewer inquires about the course and onset of the symptoms and the existence of physical or psychological precipitants such as drugs, alcohol, or personal losses.

Follow up vague or obscure replies with enough persistence to accurately determine the answer to the question. Some patients, particularly psychotic patients, have great difficulty answering questions clearly and concisely. They may say "yes" or "no" to every question asked. When a pattern of this sort is observed, the patient should be repeatedly asked to describe his experiences as explicitly as possible. For example, if the patient says that she hears voices, she should be asked to describe them in more detail—whether they are male or female, what they say, and how often they occur. The greater the level of detail the patient is able to provide, the more confident the clinician can feel that the symptom is truly present. Because making a diagnosis of schizophrenia or other major psychiatric disorder has important prognostic implications, the clinician should not hastily accept an answer that suggests vaguely that the patient may have a particular symptom of a disorder.

Let the patient talk freely enough to observe how tightly his thoughts are connected. Most patients should be allowed to talk for at least 3 or 4 minutes in the course of any psychiatric interview without interruption. Of course, the very laconic patient will not be able to do this, but most can. The coherence of the pattern in which the patient's thoughts are presented may provide major clues to the type of problem that he is experiencing. For example, patients with mania, schizophrenia, or depression may have any one of a variety of types of "formal thought disorder." (See "Definitions of Common Signs and Symptoms and Methods for Eliciting Them" later in this chapter.) Coherence of thought may also be helpful in making a differential diagnosis between dementia or depression.

Use a mixture of open and closed questions. An interviewer can learn a great deal about the patient by mixing up types of questions, just as a good pitcher mixes up his pitches. Open-ended questions permit the patient to ramble and become disorganized, whereas closed questions determine whether the patient can come up with the specifics when pressed. These are important indicators as to whether the patient is conceptually disorganized or confused, whether she is being evasive, or whether she is answering randomly or falsely. The content of the questions should be mixed as well. For example, at some point in the interview, the interviewer will probably want to drop his or her objective style of interviewing and focus on some personal topic that is affect-laden, such as sexual or interpersonal relationships. These questions will give the interviewer important clues about the patient's capacity to show emotional responsiveness. Evaluating the patient's mood and affect is a fundamental aspect of the psychiatric evaluation, as is evaluating the coherence of her thinking and communication.

Don't be afraid to ask about topics that you or the patient might find difficult or embarrassing. Beginning interviewers sometimes find it hard to ask about topics such as sexual relationships, sexual experiences, or even use of alcohol or drugs. Yet all this information is part of a complete psychiatric interview and must be included. Nearly all patients expect doctors to ask these questions and are not offended. Likewise, beginning interviewers are sometimes embarrassed to ask about symptoms of psychosis, such as hearing voices. To the interviewer, these symptoms seem so "crazy" that the patient might be insulted by being asked about them. Again, however, information of this type is basic and cannot be avoided. If John Hinckley, Jr.'s psychiatrist had been more aggressive in inquiring about delusions, a diagnosis of schizophrenia might have been made before the assassination attempt on President Reagan occurred, and a great deal of misery could thereby have been avoided. If the patient seems "obviously" not psychotic, questions about psychotic symptoms should still be asked—and in an unapologetic manner. If the patient seems amused or annoyed, then the interviewer can explain that he or she must cover all kinds of questions to provide a comprehensive evaluation of each patient.

Don't forget to ask about suicidal thoughts. This is another topic that may seem to fall into the "embarrassing" category. Nevertheless, suicide is a common outcome of many psychiatric illnesses, and it is incumbent on the interviewer to ask about it. The subject can be broached quite tactfully by a question such as "Have you ever felt life isn't worth living?" The topic of suicide can then be approached gradually, leading to questions such as "Have you ever thought about taking your life?" Further tips on interviewing the suicidal patient are provided in Chapter 20.

Give the patient a chance to ask questions at the end. From the patient's point of view, there is nothing more frustrating than being interviewed for an hour and then being ushered out of the office or examining room with his own questions unanswered. The questions that a patient asks often tell

a great deal about what is on his mind (or not on his mind). Thus, these questions may be quite helpful in the differential diagnostic process. Even if not helpful, they are significant to the patient and therefore intrinsically important.

Conclude the initial interview by conveying a sense of confidence and, if possible, of hope. Thank the patient for providing so much information. Compliment her, in whatever way it can be done sincerely, on having told her story well. Indicate that you now have a much better understanding of her problems, and conclude by indicating that you will do what you can to help her. If you already have a relatively good idea that her problem is one that is amenable to treatment, explain that to her. At the end of the initial interview, if you are uncertain about diagnosis or treatment, indicate that you have learned a great deal, but that you need to think about her problem some more and perhaps gather more information before arriving at a recommendation.

Components of a Psychiatric Interview and Assessment

An initial psychiatric evaluation serves several purposes. One is to formulate an impression as to the patient's diagnosis or differential diagnosis and to begin to generate a treatment plan. The second purpose is to produce a written document for the patient's record that contains information organized in a standard, readable, and easily interpretable way. The initial interview is often therapeutic as well, in that it permits the clinician to establish a relationship with the patient and to reassure him that help will be provided.

The outline of that written record is summarized in Table 3–1. As Table 3–1 indicates, a standard psychiatric evaluation is very similar to those used in the rest of medicine, with some minor modifications. The content of the present illness and past history is focused primarily on psychiatric symptoms, whereas the family history includes more information about psychiatric illnesses in the family. Family history and social history also include more sociodemographic and personal information than is recorded in the standard medical history. The mental status examination is typically only included in psychiatric and neurological evaluations.

Identification of Patient and Informants

Identify the patient by stating her age, handedness, race, gender, marital status, and occupational status. Indicate whether the patient was the sole informant or whether additional history was obtained from family members or previous psychiatric records. Indicate whether the patient was self-referred, was brought in at the request of family members, or was referred by a physician; if the latter, specify

Table 3–1.   Outline of the psychiatric evaluation

Identification of patient and informants	General medical history
Chief complaint	Mental status examination
History of present illness	General physical examination
Past history	Neurological examination
Family history	Diagnostic impression
Social history	Treatment and management plan

which family members or physician. In addition, indicate how reliable the informants appear to be.

Chief Complaint

Begin by stating the patient's chief complaint in his own words. An additional sentence or two of amplifying information may also be provided, particularly if the patient's chief complaint is relatively vague.

History of Present Illness

Provide a concise history of the illness or problem that brought the patient in for treatment. Begin by describing the onset of the symptoms. If this is the patient's first episode, first psychiatric evaluation, or first hospital admission, that should be stated early in the history of the present illness. Indicate how long ago the first symptoms began, the nature of their onset (e.g., acute, insidious), and whether the onset was precipitated by any particular life events or problems. If the latter, these events or problems should be described in some detail. Likewise, medical conditions that may have served as precipitants should be described. If drug or alcohol abuse was a potential precipitant, that should also be noted.

The evolution of the patient's various symptoms should be described. A systematic summary of all symptoms present, in a form useful for making a differential diagnosis of the present illness, should be provided. This listing of symptoms should reflect the criteria included in DSM-IV and should specify both which symptoms are present and which symptoms are absent. The description of symptoms should not be limited to those included in DSM-IV diagnostic criteria, however, because these typically do not provide a full description of the range of symptoms that patients have (i.e., they are minimal, not comprehensively descriptive). The description of the present illness should also indicate the degree of incapacity that the patient is experiencing as a consequence of her symptoms, as well as the influence of the symptoms on her personal and family life. Any treatments the patient has received for the present illness should be noted, including doses, duration of treatments, and effectiveness of the specific medications, because these will often dictate what the next step will be.

History

The history has two main components: history of past psychiatric illness and personal history.

History of past psychiatric illness provides a summary of past illnesses, problems, and their treatment. In patients with complex histories and chronic psychiatric illnesses, this portion of the history will be quite extensive. It should begin by noting the number of past hospitalizations or episodes and the age at which the patient was first seen for psychiatric evaluation. Thereafter, past episodes should be described in chronological order, with some information about duration of episodes, types of symptoms present, severity of symptoms, and treatments received (and response to treatment). If a characteristic pattern is present (e.g., episodes of mania are always followed by episodes of depression, or past depressive episodes consistently responded to a particular medication), this pattern should be noted, because it provides useful prognostic information. If the patient's memory for past symptoms is relatively poor, this should also be noted. If the bulk of the past history is obtained from old records rather than from the patient himself, this should be recorded. Confirmation by family members of types and patterns of symptoms and number of episodes should also be noted.

Personal history provides a narrative description of the patient's life history in a concise manner. It includes information about where the patient was born, where she grew up, and the nature of her early life adjustment. If she had problems during childhood, such as temper tantrums, school phobia, or delinquency, these should be noted. Her relationship with her parents should be described, as well as her relationship with her siblings. Psychosexual development, such as age of first sexual experience, should also be described. Information about familial religious or cultural attitudes that is relevant to the patient's condition should be noted. Educational history should be summarized, including information about how far the patient went in school, how well she performed, and what her academic interests were. Some description should be provided of her interest and participation in extracurricular activities and her interpersonal relationships during adolescence and early adulthood. Work history and military history should also be summarized. Certain areas may need more emphasis and detail, depending on the chief complaint and diagnostic formulation.

Family History

The age and occupation of both parents and all siblings should be noted, as should the age and education or occupation of all children (if applicable). If any of these first-degree relatives has a history of any mental illness, the specific illness should be mentioned, along with information about treatment, hospitalization, and long-term course and outcome. It may be necessary to run through specific disorders, because many patients will not recognize alcoholism or criminality, for example, as emotional problems: "Do any blood relatives have a history of alcoholism, criminality, drug abuse, severe depression, or suicide attempts or suicide? Have any ever had psychiatric hospitalization or institutionalization?

Have any ever taken 'nerve pills' or seen psychiatrists, psychologists, or counselors?" The interviewer should obtain as much information as possible about mental illness in second-degree relatives as well. Any relevant information about the family's social, cultural, or educational background may also be included in this section of the interview. It is often helpful to draw pedigrees in complicated cases.

Social History

This section of the history contains a summary of the patient's current social situation. It summarizes marital status, occupation, and income. The location of his residence should be described, as well as the specific family members who live with the patient. This section of the history should provide information about the various social supports currently available to the patient. Record habits as well (e.g, smoking, use of alcohol).

General Medical History

The patient's current and past state of health should be summarized. Any existing illness for which the patient is currently being treated should be noted, as well as the types of treatments, medications, and their doses. Allergies, past surgeries, traumatic injuries, or other serious medical illnesses should be summarized. Head injuries, headaches, seizures, and other problems involving the central nervous system are particularly relevant.

Mental Status Examination

The mental status examination is the psychiatric equivalent of the physical examination in medicine. It includes a comprehensive evaluation of the patient's appearance, thinking, speech patterns, and so forth. It is described in more detail below.

The components of the mental status examination are summarized in Table 3–2. Some portions of mental status are determined simply by observing the patient (e.g., appearance, affect). Others are determined by asking the patient relatively specific questions (e.g, mood, abnormalities in perception). Still others are assessed through asking the patient a specified set of questions (e.g., memory, general information). To evaluate functions such as memory, general information, and calculation, the interviewer should develop his or her own repertoire of techniques for assessment. The interviewer should consistently use this same repertoire for all patients in order to develop a good sense of the range of normal and abnormal responses in individuals of various ages, educational levels, and psychopathological states.

Table 3–2. Mental status examination

Appearance and attitude	General information
Motor activity	Calculations
Thought and speech	Capacity to read and write
Mood and affect	Visuospatial ability
Perception	Attention
Orientation	Abstraction
Memory	Judgment and insight

Appearance and attitude. Describe the patient's general appearance, including grooming, hygiene, and facial expression. Note whether the patient looks his stated age, younger, or older. Note type and appropriateness of dress. Describe whether the patient's attitude is cooperative, guarded, angry, or suspicious.

Motor activity. Note the patient's level of motor activity. Does he sit quietly, or is he physically agitated? Note any abnormal movements, tics, or mannerisms. If relevant, evaluate for and note any indications of catatonia such as waxy flexibility (see below). Determine whether any indications of tardive dyskinesia, or any other abnormal movements, are present.

Thought and speech. Psychiatrists often speak about "thought disorder" or "formal thought disorder." This concept refers to the patient's pattern of speech, from which abnormal patterns of thought are inferred. It is, of course, not possible to evaluate thought directly. Note the rate of the patient's speech—whether it is normal, slowed, or pressured. Indicate whether his speech indicates a pattern of thought that is logical and goal oriented, or whether any of a variety of abnormalities in thought is present (e.g., derailment, incoherence, poverty of content of speech). Summarize the content of the thought, noting in particular any delusional thinking that is currently observed. If delusions are present, they should be described in detail. (If this has already been done in the history of the present illness, that can be noted with a simple statement such as "Delusions were present as described above.")

Mood and affect. The term *mood* refers to an emotional attitude that is relatively sustained; it is typically determined through the patient's own self-report, although some inferences can be made from the patient's facial expression. Note whether the patient's mood is neutral, euphoric, depressed, anxious, or irritable.

Affect is inferred from emotional responses that are usually triggered by some stimulus. Affect refers to the way that a patient conveys his emotional state, as perceived by others. The examiner watches the response of the patient's face to a joke or a smile, determines whether the patient shows appropriate or inappropriate emotional reactions, and notes the degree of reactivity of emotion. Affect is typically described as full, flat, blunted, or inappropriate. Flat or blunted affect is inferred when the patient shows very little emotional response and seems emotionally dulled, whereas inappropriate affect refers to emotional responses that are not appropriate to the content of the discussion, such as silly laughter for no apparent reason.

Perception.   Note any abnormalities in perception. The most common perceptual abnormalities are hallucinations: abnormal sensory perceptions in the absence of an actual stimulus. Hallucinations may be auditory, visual, tactile, or olfactory. Sometimes hypnagogic or hypnopompic hallucinations occur when the patient is falling asleep or waking from sleep; these are not considered true hallucinations.

Orientation.   Describe the patient's level of orientation. Normally, this includes orientation to time, place, and person. Orientation is assessed by asking the patient to describe the day, date, year, time, place where he is currently residing, and his name and identity.

Memory.   Memory is divided into very short term, short term, and long term. All three should be described. Very short term memory involves the immediate registration of information, usually assessed by having the patient repeat back immediately a series of digits or three pieces of information (e.g., the color green, the name Mr. Williams, and the address 1915 High Street). The examiner determines whether the patient can recall these items immediately after he is told them. If the patient has difficulty, he should be given the items repeatedly until he is able to register them. If he is unable to register the items after three or four trials, this should be noted. The patient should then be warned that he will be asked to recall these items in 3–5 minutes. His ability to remember them after that time interval is an indication of his short-term memory. Remote memory is assessed by asking the patient to recall events that occurred in the past several days, as well as events occurring in the more remote past, such as months or years ago.

General information.   General information is assessed by asking the patient a specific set of questions covering topics such as the names of the last five presidents, current events, or information about history or geography. The patient's fund of general information should be noted in relation to his level of educational achievement. This is particularly important in assessing the possibility of dementia.

Calculations. The standard test is serial 7s. This test involves having the patient subtract 7 from 100, then 7 from that product, and so on for at least five subtractions. Some chronic patients become relatively well trained on this exercise, so it is a good idea to have other tools in one's repertoire. One that is quite useful involves asking the patient to make calculations necessary in daily living (e.g., "If I went to the store and bought six oranges, priced at three for a dollar, and gave the clerk a $10 bill, how much change would I get back?"). Calculations can be modified for the patient's educational level: Poorly educated patients may need to calculate serial 3s. Likewise, real-life calculations can be simplified or made more complicated.

Capacity to read and write. The patient should be given a simple text and asked to read it aloud. He should also be asked to write down some specific sentence, either of the examiner's choice or his own. The patient's ability to read and write should be assessed relative to his level of education.

Visuospatial ability. The patient should be asked to copy a figure. This figure can be quite simple, such as a square inside a circle. An alternate task is to ask the patient to draw a clock face and set the hands at some specified time, such as twenty minutes to three.

Attention. Attention is assessed in part by a number of the tasks above, such as calculations or clock setting. Additional tests of attention can be used, such as asking the patient to spell a word backwards (e.g., world). The patient can also be asked to name five things that start with some specific letter, such as the letter d. The latter is also a good test of cognitive and verbal fluency.

Abstraction. The patient's capacity to think abstractly can be assessed in a variety of ways. One favorite method is asking the patient to interpret proverbs, such as "A rolling stone gathers no moss" or "Don't cry over spilt milk." Alternatively, the patient can be asked to identify commonalities between two items (e.g., How are an apple and an orange alike? How are a fly and a tree alike?).

Judgment and insight. Assess the patient's overall judgment and insight by noting how realistically he has assessed his illness and his various life problems. Insight can be ascertained relatively directly. Does the patient understand that he is ill? Does the patient express a need for treatment? Judgment may not be as easily assessed, but the patient's recent choices and decisions will help in its determination. Sometimes simple questions may be helpful. The following are frequently used: "If you found a stamped, addressed envelope, what would you do?" or "If you were in a movie theater and smelled smoke, what would you do?"

General Physical Examination

This examination should follow the standard format used in the rest of medicine, covering organ systems of the body from head to foot. Examinations of patients of the opposite sex (e.g., male physician examining a female patient) should be chaperoned.

Neurological Examination

Likewise, a standard neurological examination should be done. A detailed neurological evaluation is particularly important in psychiatric patients to rule out focal signs that might explain the patient's symptoms.

Diagnostic Impression

This section of the history indicates the clinician's diagnostic impression. Whenever possible, diagnoses should be made using all five DSM-IV axes. When appropriate, more than one diagnosis should be made. When the diagnosis is uncertain, the qualifier *provisional* should be added. Not infrequently, it will be difficult to make a definitive diagnosis at the time of the index evaluation. When this situation occurs, a listing of differential diagnostic possibilities should be made.

Treatment and Management Plan

This section will vary depending on the level of diagnostic certainty. If the diagnosis is quite uncertain, the first step in treatment and management will involve additional assessments to determine the diagnosis with more certainty. Thus, the treatment and management plan may include a list of laboratory tests appropriate to assist in the differential diagnosis listed above. Alternatively, when the diagnosis is straightforward, it will be possible to outline a specific treatment plan, including a proposed medication regimen, plans for vocational rehabilitation, a program for social skills training, marital counseling, or other ancillary treatments appropriate to the patient's specific problems.

Definitions of Common Signs and Symptoms and Methods for Eliciting Them

A vast panoply of signs and symptoms can characterize major mental illnesses. The following are some of the more common signs and symptoms seen in relatively severe psychopathology. They include symptoms seen in psychotic states, affective syndromes, and anxiety states. Where appropriate, some suggested questions are provided that can be used to probe for these symptoms. Those in parentheses are follow-up questions.

Symptoms That Frequently Occur in Psychotic Illnesses

The term *psychosis* has several different meanings, which may be especially confusing to beginning students. In the broadest sense, the term refers to the group of symptoms that characterize the most severe mental illnesses, such as schizophrenia or mania, and that involve an impairment in the ability to make judgments about the boundaries between what is real and unreal (sometimes called "an impairment in reality testing"). In a more operational sense, psychosis refers to a specific group of symptoms that are common in these severe disorders. In the narrowest sense, psychosis is synonymous with having delusions and hallucinations. A somewhat broader operational definition also includes bizarre behavior, disorganized speech ("positive formal thought disorder"), and inappropriate affect.

Another way to classify some of the major symptoms of severe mental illnesses is to divide them into two broad groups: positive and negative. *Positive symptoms* represent an exaggeration or distortion of functions that are normally present (e.g., perception, inferential thinking). They include delusions, hallucinations, disorganized speech, bizarre or disorganized behavior, and inappropriate affect. The first two are evaluated by questioning and the final three by observation. Sometimes this group of positive symptoms is further subdivided into two dimensions. The *psychotic dimension* includes delusions and hallucinations, whereas the *disorganized dimension* includes disorganized speech and behavior and inappropriate affect. *Negative symptoms* are characterized by a diminution or loss of functions that are normally present, such as fluency of speech or emotional expression. Negative symptoms are common in psychosis, but they may also occur in nonpsychotic illnesses such as depression. They include alogia, affective blunting, avolition-apathy, anhedonia-asociality, and attentional impairment. The first two of these are evaluated primarily by observation and the last three by interviewing.

Some of the negative symptoms may be difficult to distinguish from the effects of neuroleptic medications used to treat psychotic illnesses. These medications often produce parkinsonian side effects and akinesia, which look quite similar to some of the common negative symptoms such as affective blunting or avolition. Sometimes negative symptoms are also difficult to distinguish from depressive symptoms, particularly anhedonia. It has been suggested that clinicians should attempt to determine whether negative symptoms are *secondary* (i.e., due to neuroleptics or depression) or *primary* (i.e., intrinsic to the illness). As is discussed in the chapter on schizophrenia (Chapter 7), negative symptoms are thought to reflect some type of fundamental neural abnormality occurring in schizophrenia; disentangling primary from secondary negative symptoms could be important in the search for this abnormality. At a practical clinical level, however, this distinction may be difficult to make reliably.

Delusions

Delusions represent an abnormality in content of thought. They are false beliefs that cannot be explained on the basis of the subject's cultural background. Although delusions are sometimes defined as *fixed false beliefs*, in their mildest form delusions may persist only for weeks to months, and the subject may question her beliefs or doubt them. The subject's behavior may or may not be influenced by her delusions. The assessment of the severity of individual delusions and of the global severity of delusional thinking should take into account their persistence, their complexity, the extent to which the subject acts on them, the extent to which the subject doubts them, and the extent to which the beliefs deviate from the ones that psychiatrically normal people might have.

Persecutory delusions. People with persecutory delusions believe that they are being conspired against or persecuted in some way. Common manifestations include the belief that one is being followed, that one's mail is being opened, that one's room or office is bugged, that the telephone is tapped, or that police, government officials, neighbors, or fellow workers are harassing the subject. Persecutory delusions are sometimes relatively isolated or fragmented, but sometimes the person has a complex system of delusions involving both a wide range of forms of persecution and a belief that there is a well-designed conspiracy behind them: for example, that the patient's house is bugged and that she is being followed because the government wrongly considers her a se-

Have you had trouble getting along with people?

Have you felt that people are against you?

Has anyone been trying to harm you in any way?

(Do you think people have been plotting against you?)

cret agent of a foreign government. This delusion may be so complex that it explains almost everything that happens to her.

Delusions of jealousy. The patient believes that his mate is having an affair with someone. Miscellaneous bits of information are construed as "evidence." The person usually goes to great effort to prove the existence of the affair, searching for hair in the bedclothes, the odor of shaving lotion or smoke on clothing, or receipts or checks indicating a gift has been bought for the lover. Elaborate plans are often made to trap the two together.

Have you worried that your (husband, wife, boyfriend, girlfriend) might be unfaithful to you?

(What evidence do you have?)

Delusions of sin or guilt. The patient believes that she has committed some terrible sin or done something unforgivable. Sometimes the patient is excessively or inappropriately preoccupied with things she did wrong as a child, such as masturbating. Sometimes the patient feels responsible for causing some disastrous event, such as a fire or accident, with which she in fact has no connection. Sometimes these delusions have a religious flavor, involving the belief that the sin is unpardonable and that the subject will suffer eternal punishment from God. Sometimes the patient simply believes that she deserves punishment by society. The patient may spend a good deal of time confessing these sins to whoever will listen.

Have you felt that you have done some terrible thing?

Is there anything that's bothering your conscience?

(What is it?)

(Do you feel you deserve to be punished for it?)

Grandiose delusions. The patient believes that he has special powers or abilities. He may think he is actually some famous person, such as a rock star, Napoleon, or Christ. He may believe he is writing some definitive book, composing a great piece of music, or developing some wonderful new invention. The patient is often suspicious that someone is trying to steal his ideas, and he may become quite irritated if his abilities are doubted.

Do you have any special powers, talents, or abilities?

Do you feel you are going to achieve great things?

Religious delusions. The patient is preoccupied with false beliefs of a religious nature. Sometimes these exist within the context of a conventional religious system, such as beliefs about the Second Coming, the Anti-Christ, or possession by the Devil. At other times, they may involve an entirely new religious system or a pastiche of beliefs from a variety of religions, particularly Eastern religions, such as ideas about reincarnation or Nirvana. Religious delusions may be combined with grandiose delusions (if the subject considers herself a religious leader), delusions of guilt, or delusions of being controlled. Religious delusions must be outside the range of beliefs considered normal for the patient's cultural and religious background.

Are you a religious person?

Have you had any unusual religious experiences?

(What was your religious training as a child?)

Somatic delusions. The patient believes that somehow his body is diseased, abnormal, or changed. For example, he may believe that his

Is there anything wrong with the way your body is working?

stomach or brain is rotting, that his hands have become enlarged, or that his facial features are unusual (dysmorphophobia). Sometimes somatic delusions are accompanied by tactile or other hallucinations, and when this occurs, both should be considered to be present. (For example, the patient believes that he has ball bearings rolling about in his head, placed there by a dentist who filled his teeth, and can actually hear them clanking against one another.)

Have you noticed any change in your appearance?

Ideas and delusions of reference. The patient believes that insignificant remarks, statements, or events refer to her or have some special meaning for her. For example, the patient walks into a room, sees people laughing, and suspects that they were just talking about her and laughing at her. Sometimes items read in the paper, heard on the radio, or seen on TV are considered to be special messages to the subject. In the case of ideas of reference, the patient is suspicious, but recognizes that her idea may be erroneous. When the patient actually believes that the statements or events refer to her, this is considered a delusion of reference.

Have you walked into a room and thought people were talking about you or laughing at you?

Have you seen things in magazines or on TV that seem to refer to you or contain a special message for you?

Have you received special messages in any other ways?

Delusions of being controlled. The patient has a subjective experience that his feelings or actions are controlled by some outside force. The central requirement for this type of delusion is an actual strong subjective experience of being controlled. It does

Have you felt that you were being controlled by some outside force?

Do you feel that any person is controlling you?

not include simple beliefs or ideas, such as that the subject is acting as an agent of God or that friends or parents are trying to coerce him into something. Rather, the patient must describe, for example, that his body has been occupied by some alien force that is making it move in peculiar ways, or that messages are being sent to his brain by radio waves and causing him to experience particular feelings that he recognizes are not his own.

Delusions of mind reading.   The patient believes that people can read her mind or know her thoughts. This is different from thought broadcasting (see below) in that it is a belief without a percept. That is, the patient subjectively experiences and recognizes that others know her thoughts, but she does not think that they can be heard out loud.

Have you had the feeling that people could read your mind or know what you are thinking?

Thought broadcasting/audible thoughts.   The patient believes that his thoughts are broadcast so that he or others can hear them. Sometimes the patient experiences his thoughts as a voice outside his head; this is an auditory hallucination as well as a delusion. Sometimes the subject feels his thoughts are being broadcast, although he cannot hear them himself. Sometimes he believes that his thoughts are picked up by a microphone and broadcast on the radio or television.

Have you heard your own thoughts out loud, as if they were a voice outside your head?

Have you felt your thoughts were broadcast so other people could hear them?

Thought insertion. The patient believes that thoughts that are not her own have been inserted into her mind. For example, the patient may believe that a neighbor is practicing voodoo and planting alien sexual thoughts in her mind. This symptom should not be confused with experiencing unpleasant thoughts that the patient recognizes as her own, such as delusions of persecution or guilt.

Have you felt that thoughts were being put into your head by some outside force or person?

Thought withdrawal. The patient believes that thoughts have been taken away from his mind. He is able to describe a subjective experience of beginning a thought and then suddenly having it removed by some outside force. This symptom does not include the mere subjective recognition of alogia.

Have you felt your thoughts were taken away by some outside force or person?

Hallucinations

Hallucinations represent an abnormality in perception. They are false perceptions occurring in the absence of some identifiable external stimulus. They may be experienced in any of the sensory modalities, including hearing, touch, taste, smell, and vision. True hallucinations should be distinguished from illusions (which involve a misperception of an external stimulus), hypnagogic and hypnopompic experiences (which occur when a patient is falling asleep and waking up, respectively), or normal thought processes that are exceptionally vivid. If the hallucinations have a religious quality, they should be judged within the context of what is normal for the patient's social and cultural background. The patient should always be requested to describe the hallucination in detail. The term *pseudohallucinations* refers to hallucinations that the patient reports but that have no identifiable percept (e.g., the patient "sees things that aren't there," but is unable to describe any actual specific perceptions). Pseudohallucinations are more fully discussed in Chapter 13.

Auditory hallucinations. The patient has reported voices, noises, or sounds. The most common auditory hallucinations involve hearing voices speaking to the patient or calling her names. The voices may be male or female, familiar or unfamiliar, and critical or complimentary. Typically, patients with schizophrenia experience the voices as unpleasant and negative. Hallucinations involving sounds other than voices, such as noises or music, should be considered less characteristic and less severe.

Have you heard voices or other sounds when no one is around, or when you couldn't account for them?

(What did they say?)

Voices commenting. These hallucinations involve hearing a voice that makes a running commentary on the patient's behavior or thought as it occurs.

Have you heard voices commenting on what you are thinking or doing?

(What do they say?)

Voices conversing. These hallucinations involve hearing two or more voices talking with one another, usually discussing something about the patient.

Have you heard two or more voices talking with each other?

(What do they say?)

Somatic or tactile hallucinations. These hallucinations involve experiencing peculiar physical sensations in the body. They include burning sensations, tingling, and perceptions that the body has changed in shape or size.

Have you had burning sensations or other strange feelings in your body?

(What were they?)

Olfactory hallucinations. The patient experiences unusual smells that are typically quite unpleasant. Sometimes the patient may believe that he himself smells. This belief should be considered a hallucination if the pa-

Have you experienced any unusual smells or smells that others don't notice?

(What were they?)

tient can actually smell the odor himself, but should be considered a delusion if he believes that only others can smell the odor.

Visual hallucinations. The patient sees shapes or people that are not actually present. Sometimes these are shapes or colors, but most typically they are figures of people or humanlike objects. They may also be characters of a religious nature, such as the Devil or Christ. As always, visual hallucinations involving religious themes should be judged within the context of the patient's cultural background.

Have you had visions or seen things that other people cannot?

(What did you see?)

(Did this occur when you were falling asleep or waking up?)

Bizarre or Disorganized Behavior

The patient's behavior is unusual, bizarre, or fantastic. The information for this symptom will sometimes come from the patient, sometimes from other sources, and sometimes from direct observation. Bizarre behavior due to the immediate effects of intoxication with alcohol or drugs should not be considered a symptom of psychosis. Social and cultural norms must be considered in making the determination of bizarre behavior, and detailed examples should be elicited and noted.

Clothing and appearance. The patient dresses in an unusual manner or does other strange things to alter his appearance. For example, he may shave off all his hair or paint parts of his body different colors. His clothing may be quite unusual; for example, he may choose to wear some outfit that appears generally inappropriate and unacceptable, such as a baseball cap backwards with rubber galoshes and long underwear covered by denim overalls. He may dress in a fantastic

Has anyone made comments about the way you look?

(What did they say?)

costume representing some historical personage or a man from outer space. He may wear clothing completely inappropriate to the climatic conditions, such as heavy wools in the midst of summer.

Social and sexual behavior. The patient may do things that are considered inappropriate according to usual social norms. For example, she may masturbate in public, urinate or defecate in inappropriate receptacles, walk along the street muttering to herself, or begin talking to people whom she has never before met about her personal life (as when riding on a subway or standing in some public place). She may drop to her knees praying and shouting or suddenly sit in an unusual position when in the midst of a crowd. She may make inappropriate sexual overtures or remarks to strangers.

Have you done anything that others might think unusual or that has called attention to yourself?

(What did you do?)

Has anyone complained or commented about your behavior?

(Why did they complain or comment?)

Aggressive and agitated behavior. The patient may behave in an aggressive, agitated manner, often quite unpredictably. He may start arguments inappropriately with friends or members of his family, or he may accost strangers on the street and begin haranguing them angrily. He may write letters of a threatening or angry nature to government officials or others with whom he has some quarrel. Occasionally, patients may perform violent acts such as injuring or tormenting animals or attempting to injure or kill human beings.

Have you been unusually angry or irritable with anyone?

(How did you express your anger?)

(Have you done anything to try to harm animals or people?)

Ritualistic or stereotyped behavior. The patient may develop a set of repetitive actions or rituals that she must perform over and over. Sometimes she will attribute some symbolic significance to these actions and believe that they are either influencing others or preventing the patient herself from being influenced. For example, she may eat jelly beans every night for dessert, assuming that different consequences will occur depending on the color of the jelly beans. She may have to eat foods in a particular order, wear particular clothes, or put them on in a certain order. She may have to write messages to herself or to others over and over, sometimes in an unusual or occult language.

Are there any things you do over and over?

Are there any things that you have to do in a certain way or in a particular order?

(Why do you do it?)

(Does it have any special meaning or significance?)

Disorganized Speech (*Positive Formal Thought Disorder*)

Disorganized speech, which is also referred to as positive formal thought disorder, is fluent speech that tends to communicate poorly for a variety of reasons. The patient tends to skip from topic to topic without warning; to be distracted by events in the nearby environment; to join words together because they are semantically or phonologically alike, even though they make no sense; or to ignore the question asked and answer another. This type of speech may be rapid, and it frequently seems quite disjointed. It has sometimes been referred to as *loose associations.* Unlike alogia (negative formal thought disorder) (see below), a wealth of detail is provided, and the flow of speech tends to have an energetic rather than an apathetic quality to it.

To evaluate thought disorder, the patient should be permitted to talk without interruption for as long as 5 minutes. The interviewer should observe closely the extent to which the patient's sequencing of ideas is well connected. He or she should also pay close attention to how well the patient can reply to a variety of different questions, ranging from simple (when were you born?) to more complicated (why did you come to the hospital?). If the ideas seem vague or incomprehensible, the interviewer should prompt the patient to clarify or elaborate.

Derailment (loose associations). A pattern of spontaneous speech in which the ideas slip off the track onto another that is clearly but obliquely related, or onto one completely unrelated. Things may be said in juxtaposition that lack a meaningful relationship, or the patient may shift idiosyncratically from one frame of reference to another. At times there may be a vague connection between the ideas, and at other times none will be apparent. This pattern of speech is often characterized as sounding "disjointed." Perhaps the most common manifestation of this disorder is a slow, steady slippage, with no single derailment being particularly severe, so that the speaker gets farther and farther off the track with each derailment without showing any awareness that his reply no longer has any connection with the question that was asked. This abnormality is often characterized by lack of cohesion between clauses and sentences and by unclear pronoun references.

Example: *Interviewer: Did you enjoy college? Subject: Um-hm. Oh hey well I, I, oh, I really enjoyed some communities. I tried it, and the, and the next day when I'd be going out, you know, um, I took control like uh, I put, um, bleach on my hair in, in California. My roommate was from Chicago and she was going to the junior college. And we lived in the Y.W.C.A., so she wanted to put it, um, peroxide on my hair, and she did, and I got up and I looked at the mirror and tears came to my eyes. Now do you understand it—I was fully aware of what was going on but why couldn't I, I . . . why the tears? I can't understand that, can you?*

Tangentiality. Replying to a question in an oblique, tangential, or even irrelevant manner. The reply may be related to the question in some distant way, or the reply may be unrelated and seem totally irrelevant.

Example: *Interviewer: What city are you from? Subject: Well, that's a hard question to answer because my parents . . . I was born in Iowa, but I know that I'm white instead of black, so apparently I came from the North somewhere and I don't know where, you know, I really don't know whether I'm Irish or Scandinavian, or I don't, I don't believe I'm Polish, but I think I'm, I think I might be German or Welsh.*

Incoherence (word salad, schizophasia). A pattern of speech that is essentially incomprehensible at times. Incoherence is often accompanied by derailment. It differs from derailment in that in incoherence the abnormality occurs within the level of the sentence or clause, which contains words or phrases that are joined incoherently. The abnormality in derailment involves unclear or confusing connections between larger units, such as sentences or clauses. This type of language disorder is relatively rare. When it occurs, it tends to be severe or extreme, and mild forms are quite uncommon. It may sound quite similar to Wernicke's aphasia or jargon aphasia, and in these cases the disorder should only be called incoherence definitively when history and laboratory data exclude the possibility of a past stroke, and clinical testing for aphasia is negative.

Example: *Interviewer: What do you think about current political issues like the energy crisis? Subject: They're destroying too many cattle and oil just to make soap. If we need soap when you can jump into a pool of water, and then when you go to buy your gasoline, my folks always thought they should, get pop but the best thing to get, is motor oil, and, money. May, may as, well go there and, trade in some, pop caps and, uh, tires, and tractors to grup, car garages, so they can pull cars away from wrecks, is what I believed in.*

Illogicality. A pattern of speech in which conclusions are reached that do not follow logically. Illogicality may take the form of non sequiturs (meaning "it does not follow"), in which the patient makes a logical inference between two clauses that is unwarranted or illogical. It may take the form of faulty inductive inferences. It may also take the form of reaching conclusions based on faulty premises without any actual delusional thinking.

Example: *Parents are the people that raise you. Anything that raises you can be a parent. Parents can be anything—material, vegetable, or mineral—that has taught you something. Parents would be the world of things that are alive, that are there. Rocks—a person can look at a rock and learn something from it, so that would be a parent.*

Circumstantiality. A pattern of speech that is very indirect and delayed in reaching its goal ideas. In the process of explaining something, the speaker brings in many tedious details and sometimes makes parenthetical remarks. Circumstantial replies or statements may last for many minutes if the speaker is not interrupted and urged to get to the point. Interviewers will often recognize circumstantiality on the basis of needing to interrupt the speaker to complete the process of history taking within an allotted time. When not called circumstantial, these people are often referred to as long-winded.

Although it may coexist with instances of poverty of content of speech or loss of goal, circumstantiality differs from poverty of content of speech in containing excessive amplifying or illustrative detail and from loss of goal in that the goal is eventually reached if the person is allowed to talk long enough. It differs from derailment in that the details presented are closely related to some particular goal or idea and that the particular goal or idea must, by definition, eventually be reached (unless the patient is interrupted by an impatient interviewer).

No example is provided because it would require too much space!

Pressure of speech. An increase in the amount of spontaneous speech compared with what is considered ordinary or socially customary. The patient talks rapidly and is difficult to interrupt. Some sentences may be left

No example is provided because the abnormality is manifested by rate, loudness, and amount of speech.

uncompleted because of eagerness to get on to a new idea. Simple questions that could be answered in only a few words or sentences are answered at great length so that the answer takes minutes rather than seconds, and indeed may not stop at all if the speaker is not interrupted. Even when interrupted, the speaker often continues to talk. Speech tends to be loud and emphatic. Sometimes speakers with severe pressure will talk without any social stimulation and talk even though no one is listening. When patients are receiving neuroleptics or lithium, their speech is often slowed down by medication, and then it can be judged only on the basis of amount, volume, and social appropriateness. If a quantitative measure is applied to the rate of speech, then a rate greater than 150 words per minute is usually considered rapid or pressured. This disorder may be accompanied by derailment, tangentiality, or incoherence, but it is distinct from them.

Distractible speech. During the course of a discussion or interview, the patient stops talking in the middle of a sentence or idea and changes the subject in response to a nearby stimulus, such as an object on a desk, the interviewer's clothing or appearance, and so forth.

Example: *Then I left San Francisco and moved to . . . where did you get that tie? It looks like it's left over from the '50s. I like the warm weather in San Diego. Is that a conch shell on your desk? Have you ever gone scuba diving?*

Clanging. A pattern of speech in which sounds rather than meaningful relationships appear to govern word choice, so that the intelligibility of

Example: *I'm not trying to make a noise. I'm trying to make sense. If you can make sense out of nonsense, well, have fun. I'm trying to make sense out of* the speech is impaired and redundant words are introduced in addition to rhyming relationships. This pattern of speech may also include punning associations, so that a word similar in sound brings in a new thought.

sense. I'm not making sense [cents] any more. I have to make dollars.

Catatonic Motor Behavior

These symptoms are not common and should only be considered present when they are obvious and have been directly observed by the clinician or some other professional.

Stupor. There is a marked decrease in reactivity to the environment and reduction of spontaneous movements and activity. The patient may appear to be aware of the nature of her surroundings.

Rigidity. The patient exhibits signs of motor rigidity, such as resistance to passive movement.

Waxy flexibility. The patient maintains postures into which he is placed for at least 15 seconds.

Excitement. There is apparently purposeless and stereotyped excited motor activity not influenced by external stimuli.

Posturing and mannerisms. The patient voluntarily assumes an inappropriate or bizarre posture. Manneristic gestures or tics may also be observed. These involve movements or gestures that appear artificial or contrived, are not appropriate to the situation, or are stereotyped and repetitive. (Patients with tardive dyskinesia may have manneristic gestures or tics, but these should not be considered manifestations of catatonia.)

Alogia

Alogia is a general term coined to refer to the impoverished thinking and cognition that often occur in patients with schizophrenia (Greek *a*, "no"; *logos*, "mind, thought"). Subjects with alogia have thinking processes that seem empty, turgid, or slow. Because thinking cannot be observed directly, it is inferred from the patient's speech. The two major manifestations of alogia are nonfluent empty speech (poverty of speech) and fluent empty speech (poverty of content of speech). Blocking and increased latency of response may also reflect alogia.

Poverty of speech. Poverty of speech is restriction in the amount of spontaneous speech, so that replies to questions tend to be brief, concrete, and unelaborated. Unprompted additional information is rarely provided. Replies may be monosyllabic, and some questions may be left unanswered altogether. When confronted with this speech pattern, the interviewer may find that he or she frequently prompts the patient to encourage elaboration of replies. To elicit this finding, the interviewer must allow the patient adequate time to answer and to elaborate her answer.

Example: *Interviewer: Can you tell me something about what brought you to the hospital? Patient: A car.*

Interviewer: I was wondering about what kinds of problems you've been having. Can you tell me something about them? Patient: I dunno.

Poverty of content of speech. Although the replies are long enough so that speech is adequate in amount, it conveys little information. Language tends to be vague, often overabstract or overconcrete, repetitive, and stereotyped. The interviewer may recognize this finding by observing that the patient has spoken at some length but has not given adequate information to answer the question. Alternatively, the patient may provide enough information but require many words to do so, so that a lengthy reply can be summarized in a sentence or two.

This abnormality differs from circumstantiality in that the circumstantial patient tends to provide a wealth of detail.

Example: *Interviewer: Why is it, do you think, that people believe in God? Patient: Well, first of all because he, uh, he are the person that is their personal savior. He walks with me and talks with me. And uh, the understanding that I have, um, a lot of people, they don't readily, uh, know their own personal self. Because, uh, they ain't, they all, just don't know their personal self. They don't, know that he uh—seemed like to me, a lot of 'em don't understand that he walks and talks with 'em.*

Blocking. Blocking is interruption of a train of speech before a thought or idea has been completed. After a pe-

Example: *Patient: So I didn't want to go back to school so I . . . (1-minute silence while the patient stares blankly).*

riod of silence, which may last from a few seconds to minutes, the person indicates that he cannot recall what he has been saying or meant to say. Blocking should only be judged to be present if a person voluntarily describes losing his thought or if, on questioning by the interviewer, the person indicates that that was his reason for pausing.

Interviewer: What about going back to school? What happened? Patient: I dunno. I forgot what I was going to say.

Increased latency of response. The patient takes a longer time to reply to questions than is usually considered normal. She may seem distant, and sometimes the examiner may wonder whether she has heard the question. Prompting usually indicates that the patient is aware of the question, but she has been having difficulty in formulating her thoughts to make an appropriate reply.

Example: *Interviewer: When were you last in the hospital? Patient: (30-second pause) A year ago.*

Interviewer: Which hospital was it? Patient: (30-second pause) This one.

Perseveration. Perseveration is persistent repetition of words, ideas, or phrases so that once a patient begins to use a particular word, he continually returns to it in the process of speaking.

Exclusions: Perseveration differs from "stock words" in that the repeated words are used in ways inappropriate to their usual meaning. Some words or phrases are commonly used as pause fillers, such as "you know" or "like." These should not be considered perseverations.

Example: *Interviewer: "Tell me what you are like—what kind of person you are." Patient: "I'm from Marshalltown, Iowa. That's 60 miles northwest, northeast of Des Moines, Iowa. And I'm married at the present time. I'm 36 years old, my wife is 35. She lives in Garwin, Iowa. That's 15 miles southeast of Marshalltown, Iowa. I'm getting a divorce at the present time. And I am at present in a mental institution in Iowa City, Iowa, which is 100 miles southeast of Marshalltown, Iowa.*

Affective Flattening or Blunting

Affective flattening or blunting manifests itself as a characteristic impoverishment of emotional expression, reactivity, and feeling. Affective flattening can be evaluated by observation of the patient's behavior and responsiveness during a routine interview. The evaluation of affective expression may be influenced by the patient's use of prescription drugs, because the parkinsonian side effects of neuroleptics may lead to masklike facies and diminished associated movements. Other aspects of affect, such as responsivity or appropriateness, will not be affected, however.

Unchanging facial expression.   The patient's face does not change expression, or changes less than normally expected, as the emotional content of the discourse changes. It appears wooden, mechanical, and frozen. Because neuroleptics may partially mimic this effect, the interviewer should be careful to note whether the patient is on medication.

Decreased spontaneous movements.   The patient sits quietly throughout the interview and shows few or no spontaneous movements. She does not shift position, move her legs, or move her hands, or does so less than normally expected.

Paucity of expressive gestures.   The patient does not use his body as an aid in expressing his ideas through such means as hand gestures, sitting forward in his chair when intent on a subject, or leaning back when relaxed. Paucity of expressive gestures may occur in addition to decreased spontaneous movements.

Poor eye contact.   The patient avoids looking at others or using her eyes as an aid in expression. She appears to be staring into space even when she is talking. Consider the quality of eye contact as well as the quantity.

Affective nonresponsivity.   Failure to smile or laugh when prompted may be tested by smiling or joking in a way that would usually elicit a smile from a psychiatrically normal individual.

Lack of vocal inflections.   While speaking, the patient fails to show normal vocal emphasis patterns. Speech has a monotonic quality, and important words are not emphasized through changes in pitch or volume. The patient also may fail to change volume with changes of content, so that he does not drop his voice when discussing private topics or raise it as he discusses things that are exciting or for which louder speech might be appropriate.

Inappropriate Affect

The affect expressed is inappropriate or incongruous, not simply flat or blunted. Most typically, this manifestation of affective disturbance takes the form of smiling or assuming a silly facial expression while talking about a serious or sad subject. For example, the patient may laugh inappropriately when talking about thoughts of harming another person. (Occasionally, patients may smile or laugh when talking about a serious subject that they find uncomfortable or embarrassing. Although their smiling may seem inappropriate, it is due to anxiety and therefore should not be rated as inappropriate affect.)

Avolition-Apathy

Avolition manifests itself as a characteristic lack of energy and drive. Patients become inert and are unable to mobilize themselves to initiate or persist in completing many different kinds of tasks. Unlike the diminished energy or interest of depression, the avolitional symptom complex in schizophrenia is usually not accompanied by saddened or depressed affect. The avolitional symptom complex often leads to severe social and economic impairment.

Grooming and hygiene. The patient displays less attention to grooming and hygiene than is normal. Clothing may appear sloppy, outdated, or soiled. Subject may bathe infrequently and not care for hair, nails, or teeth—leading to such manifestations as greasy or uncombed hair, dirty hands, body odor, or unclean teeth and bad breath. Overall, the appearance is dilapidated and disheveled. In extreme cases, the patient may even have poor toilet habits.

Impersistence at work or school. The patient has difficulty in seeking or maintaining employment (or doing schoolwork) as appropriate for her age. If a student, she does not do homework and may even fail to attend class. Grades will tend to reflect this. If a college student, she may have

Have you been able to (work, go to school) during the past month?

Have you been attending vocational rehabilitation or occupational therapy sessions (in the hospital)?

registered for courses, but dropped several or all of them. If of working age, the patient may have found it difficult to work at a job because of her inability to persist in completing tasks and apparent irresponsibility. She may go to work irregularly, wander away early, fail to complete expected assignments, and/or complete them in a disorganized manner. She may simply sit around the house and not seek any employment or seek it only in an infrequent or desultory manner. If a homemaker or a retired person, the patient may fail to complete chores, such as shopping or cleaning, or complete them in an apparently careless and half-hearted way. If in a hospital or institution, she does not attend or persist in vocational or rehabilitative programs effectively.

What have you been able to do?

(Do you have trouble finishing what you start?)

(What kinds of problems have you had?)

Physical anergia. The patient tends to be physically inert; he may sit in a chair for hours at a time and not initiate any spontaneous activity. If encouraged to become involved in an activity, he may participate only briefly and then wander away or disengage himself and return to sitting alone. He may spend large amounts of time in some relatively mindless and physically inactive task such as watching TV or playing solitaire. His family may report that he spends most of his time at home "doing nothing except sitting around." Either at home or in an inpatient setting, he may spend much of his time sitting in his room.

How have you been spending your time?

Do you have any trouble getting yourself going?

Anhedonia-Asociality

This symptom complex encompasses the patient's difficulties in experiencing interest or pleasure. It may express itself as a loss of interest in pleasurable activities, an inability to experience pleasure when participating in activities normally considered pleasurable, or a lack of involvement in social relationships of various kinds.

Recreational interests and activities. The patient may have few or no interests, activities, or hobbies. Although this symptom may begin insidiously or slowly, there will usually be some obvious decline from an earlier level of interest and activity. Patients with relatively milder loss of interest will engage in some activities that are passive or nondemanding, such as watching TV, or will show only occasional or sporadic interests. Patients with the most extreme loss will appear to have a complete and intractable inability to become involved in or enjoy activities. The evaluation in this area should take both the quality and quantity of recreational interests into account.

What do you do for enjoyment?

How often do you do that (those things)?

Have you been attending recreational therapy?

(What have you been doing?)

(Do you enjoy it?)

Sexual interest and activity. The patient may show a decrement in sexual interest and activity or enjoyment that would be judged normal for the patient's age and marital status. Individuals who are married may manifest disinterest in sex or may engage in intercourse only at the partner's request. In extreme cases the patient may not engage in sex at all. Single patients may go for long periods of time without sexual involvement and make no effort to satisfy this drive. Whether

What has your sex drive been like?

Have you been able to enjoy sex lately?

(What is your usual sexual outlet?)

(When was the last time?)

married or single, they may report that they subjectively feel only minimal sex drive, or they take little enjoyment in sexual intercourse or in masturbatory activity even when they engage in it.

Ability to feel intimacy and closeness. The patient may display an inability to form close and intimate relationships of a type appropriate for her age, gender, and family status. In the case of a younger person, this area should be evaluated in terms of relationships with the opposite sex, as well as with parents and siblings. In the case of an older person who is married, the relationship with spouse and with children should be evaluated, whereas older unmarried individuals should be judged in terms of relationships with the opposite sex and any family members who live nearby. Patients may display few or no feelings of affection to available family members, or they may have arranged their lives so that they are completely isolated from any intimate relationships, living alone and making no effort to initiate contacts with family or members of the opposite sex. If the patient is homosexual, relationships with members of the same sex may be evaluated as indications of ability to feel intimacy and closeness.

Do you feel close to your family (husband, wife, children)?

Is there anyone outside your family that you feel especially close to?

(How often do you see [them, him, her]?)

Relationships with friends and peers. Patients may also be relatively restricted in their relationships with friends and peers of either sex.

Do you have many friends?

(Are you very close to them?)

They may have few or no friends, make little or no effort to develop such relationships, and choose to spend all or most of their time alone.

(How often do you see them?)

(What do you do together?)

Have you gotten to know any patients in the hospital?

Attention

Attention is often poor in patients who have severe mental illnesses. The patient may have trouble focusing his attention, or he may only be able to focus sporadically and erratically. The patient may ignore attempts to converse with him, wander away while in the middle of an activity or task, or appear to be inattentive when engaged in formal testing or interviewing. He may or may not be aware of his difficulty in focusing his attention.

Social inattentiveness. While involved in social situations or activities, the patient appears inattentive. She looks away during conversations, does not pick up the topic during a discussion, or appears uninvolved or disengaged. She may abruptly terminate a discussion or a task without any apparent reason. She may seem "spacey" or "out of it." She may seem to have poor concentration when playing games, reading, or watching TV.

Inattentiveness during mental status testing. The patient may perform poorly on simple tests of intellectual functioning in spite of adequate education and intellectual ability. This should be assessed by having the patient spell *world* (or some equivalent five-letter word) backward and by testing him on serial 7s (at least a 10th-grade education) or serial 3s (at least a 6th-grade education) for a series of five subtractions.

Manic Symptoms

Euphoric mood. The patient has had one or more distinct periods of euphoric, irritable, or expansive mood, not due to alcohol or drug intoxication.

Have you been feeling extremely good or high—clearly different from your normal self?

Do your friends or family think this is more than just feeling good?

Have you felt irritable and easily annoyed?

How long has this mood lasted?

Increase in activity. The patient shows an increase in involvement or activity level associated with work, family, friends, sex drive, new projects, interests, or activities (e.g., telephone calls, letter writing).

Are you more active or involved in things compared with the way you usually are?

(How about at work, at home, with your friends, or with your family?)

(What about your involvement in hobbies or other interests?)

Have you been unable to sit still, or have you had to be moving or pacing up and down?

Racing thoughts/flight of ideas. The patient has the subjective experience that thinking is markedly accelerated. Example: "My thoughts are ahead of my speech."

Have your thoughts been racing through your mind?

(Do you have more ideas than usual?)

Inflated self-esteem. The patient displays increased self-esteem and appraisal of his worth, contacts, influence, power, or knowledge (may be delusional) compared with his usual level. Persecutory delusions should not be considered evidence of grandiosity unless the patient feels persecution is due to some special attributes (e.g., power, knowledge, or contacts).

Do you feel more self-confident than usual?

(What about special plans?)

Do you feel that you are a particularly important person or that you have special talents or abilities?

Decreased need for sleep. The patient needs less sleep than usual to feel rested. (This rating should be based

Do you need less sleep than usual to feel rested?

on the average of several days rather than a single severe night.)

(How much sleep do you ordinarily need?)

(How much sleep do you need now?)

Distractibility. The patient's attention is too easily drawn to unimportant or irrelevant external stimuli. For example, the patient gets up and inspects some item in the room while talking or listening, shifts his topic of speech, and so forth.

Are you easily distracted by things around you?

Poor judgment. The patient shows excessive involvement in activities that have a high potential for painful consequences that are not recognized—for example, buying sprees, sexual indiscretions, foolish business investments, reckless giving.

Have you done anything to cause trouble for you or your family or friends?

Looking back now, have you done anything that showed poor judgment?

Have you done anything foolish with money?

Have you done anything sexually that was unusual for you?

Depressive Symptoms

Dysphoric mood. The patient feels sad, despondent, discouraged, or unhappy; significant anxiety or tense irritability should also be rated as a dysphoric mood. The evaluation should be made irrespective of length of mood.

Have you been having periods of feeling depressed, sad, or hopeless? When you didn't care about anything or couldn't enjoy anything?

Have you felt tense, anxious, or irritable?

(How long did this last?)

(Was the mood . . . ?)

Change in appetite or weight. The patient has had significant weight loss. This should not include dieting, unless the dieting is associated with some depressive belief that approaches delusional proportions.

Did you have any changes in your appetite—either increase or decrease?

Did you lose or gain much more weight than is usual for you?

Insomnia or hypersomnia. Insomnia may include waking up after only a few hours of sleep, as well as difficulty in getting to sleep. Patterns of insomnia include **middle** (waking in the middle of the night, but eventually falling asleep again), **initial** (trouble going to sleep), and **terminal** (waking early, e.g., 2:00–5:00 A.M., and remaining awake).

Have you had trouble sleeping?

(What was it like?)

(Do you have trouble falling asleep?)

(Do you wake up too early in the morning?)

Have you been sleeping more than usual?

How much sleep do you get in a typical 24-hour period?

Psychomotor agitation. The patient is unable to sit still, with a need to keep moving. Do not include mere subjective feelings of restlessness. Objective evidence should be present (e.g., hand-wringing, fidgeting, pacing).

Have you felt restless or agitated? Do you have trouble sitting still?

Psychomotor retardation. The patient feels slowed down and experiences great difficulty moving. Do not include mere subjective feelings of being slowed down. Objective evidence (e.g., slowed speech) should be present.

Have you been slowed down?

Loss of interest or pleasure. The patient has loss of interest or pleasure in usual activities, or a decrease in sexual drive. This may be similar to the anhedonia seen in psychosis. In the depressive syndrome, however, loss of interest or pleasure is invariably accompanied by intense, painful affect, whereas in psychosis the affect is often blunted.

Have you noticed a change in your interest in things?

What kinds of things do you normally enjoy?

Loss of energy. This symptom includes loss of energy, becoming easily fatigued, or feeling tired. These energy comparisons should be based on the person's usual activity level whenever possible.

Have you had a tendency to feel more tired than usual?

(Have you been feeling as if all your energy is drained?)

Feelings of worthlessness. In addition to feelings of worthlessness, the patient may report feeling self-reproach or excessive or inappropriate guilt. (Either may be delusional.)

Have you been feeling down on yourself?

Have you been feeling guilty about anything?

(Could you tell me about some of the things for which you feel guilty?)

Diminished ability to think or concentrate. The patient complains of diminished ability to think or concentrate, such as slowed thinking or indecisiveness; not associated with marked derailment or incoherence.

Have you had trouble thinking?

What about your concentration?

Have you had trouble making decisions?

Recurrent thoughts of death/suicide. The patient has thoughts about death and suicide, plus possible wishes to be dead and/or suicide attempts.

Have you been thinking about death, or about taking your own life?

(How often have these thoughts occurred?)

If yes, inquire for more details.

Distinct quality to mood. The patient's depressed mood is experienced as distinctly different from the kind of feelings experienced after the death of a loved one. If the patient has not lost a loved one, ask her to compare the feelings with those after some significant personal loss appropriate to her age and experience.

The feelings of (sadness) you are having now—are they the same as the feelings you would have had when someone close to you died, or are they different?

(How are they similar or different?)

Nonreactivity of mood. The patient does not feel much better, even temporarily, when something good happens.

Do your feelings of depression go away or get better when you do something you enjoy—like talking with friends, visiting your family, or (mention some favorite recreation)?

Diurnal variation. The patient's mood shifts during the course of the day. Some patients feel terrible in the morning, but feel steadily better as the day goes on, and even near normal in the evening. Others feel good in the morning and worse as the day progresses.

Is there any time of the day that is especially bad for you?

(Do you feel worse in the morning?) (In the evening?)

(Or is it about the same all the time?)

Anxiety Symptoms

Panic attacks. These are discrete episodes of intense fear or discomfort, in which a variety of symptoms occur such as shortness of breath, dizziness, palpitations, or shaking.

Have you ever experienced a sudden attack of panic or fear, in which you felt extremely uncomfortable?

(How long did it last?)

(Did you notice any other symptoms occurring at the same time?)

(Did you feel as if you were going to die?)

Agoraphobia. This is a fear of going outside (literally "a fear of the marketplace"). In many patients, however, the fear is more generalized and involves being afraid of being in a place or situation from which escape might be difficult.

Have you ever been afraid of going outside, so that you tended to just stay home all the time?

Have you been afraid of getting caught or trapped somewhere, so that you would be unable to escape?

Social phobia. The patient has a fear of being in some social situation where he will be seen by others and may do something that he might find to be humiliating or embarrassing. Some common social phobias include fear of public speaking, fear of eating in front of others, or fear of using public bathrooms.

Do you have any specific fears, such as a fear of public speaking?

Of eating in front of others?

Specific phobia. The patient is afraid of some specific circumscribed stimulus. Specific phobias often involve animals, such as snakes or insects; they also involve seeing blood, being in high places, or fear of flying on airplanes.

Do you have any other specific fears?

Are you afraid of snakes?

The sight of blood?

Air travel?

Obsessions. The patient experiences persistent ideas, thoughts, or impulses that are unwanted and experienced as unpleasant. The patient tends to ruminate and worry about them. The patient may try to ignore or suppress them, but she typically finds this difficult. Some common obsessions include repetitive thoughts of performing some violent act or becoming contaminated by

Are you ever bothered by persistent ideas that you can't get out of your head?

(Can you give me some specific example)?

touching other people or public objects.

Compulsions. The patient has to perform specific acts over and over in a way that he recognizes to be senseless or inappropriate. Usually, the compulsive acts are performed to ease some worry or obsession or to prevent some feared event from occurring. For example, a patient may have the worry that he has left the door unlocked and have to return over and over to check it. Obsessions about contamination may lead to repetitive hand washing. Obsessions about thoughts of violence may lead to ritualistic behavior designed to prevent injury to the person about whom violence has been imagined.

Do you have any acts you have to perform over and over?

(Can you give me some examples?)

Interviews and Rating Scales for Research

To standardize research assessments, a variety of interviews and rating scales have been developed. Typically, these interviews and rating scales have been rigorously evaluated to document that they have excellent reliability, making them relatively precise instruments for measurement and assessment.

Structured Interviews

Eight major structured interviews are currently available for psychiatric research. They are listed in Table 3–3. Each of these has various strengths and weaknesses. All use a structured or systematic approach to eliciting information about the patient's current and past history.

The *Present State Examination (PSE)*, developed by John Wing in England in the 1960s, is the oldest of the structured psychiatric interviews. Its time frame is limited to symptoms present during the past month, making it unsatisfactory for lifetime diagnoses. It cannot be used to make DSM-IV diagnoses without substantial adaptations and additions. Consequently, it is used infrequently in American research.

The *Schedule for Affective Disorders in Schizophrenia (SADS)*, which became available in the 1970s, was the first well-developed American structured interview. It includes two sections, one evaluating the current condition and a second evaluating symptoms occurring during the patient's lifetime. Thus, it gives broader coverage of symptoms and past history. It was developed before DSM-III, however, and cannot be used to make DSM-IV diagnoses. It has its own set of diagnostic criteria, the Research Diagnostic Criteria (RDC).

The *Diagnostic Interview Schedule (DIS)* was designed largely to do epidemiological field studies of large samples of patients. Unlike the PSE and the SADS, it does not require interviewers with prior experience in working with psychiatric patients. It can be used to make DSM-III diagnoses. Although it is well suited for large-scale epidemiological studies, its coverage is relatively sparse for working with actual patients who have relatively severe psychiatric syndromes.

The *Structured Clinical Interview for Diagnosis (SCID)* was the first interview designed specifically to apply DSM criteria to psychiatrically ill patients. Its focus is largely on making diagnoses, and it therefore primarily includes information listed in the DSM diagnostic criteria. It is concise and user friendly, but incomplete in its coverage. Several versions of the SCID are available, which focus on different aspects of psychopathology (e.g., psychoses, anxiety disorders, personality disorders). The specific version chosen will depend on the interests of the investigator.

The *Comprehensive Assessment of Symptoms and History (CASH)* was developed in the 1980s. Because diagnostic criteria have been changing rapidly during the past few years, the CASH was designed to provide a broad coverage of symptoms so that investigators would have a comprehensive database that could be adapted to a variety of different diagnostic systems. It includes a current and a past section. It also includes structured sections to assess sociodemographic

Table 3–3.   Structured interviews

Present State Examination
Schedule for Affective Disorders in Schizophrenia (SADS)
Diagnostic Interview Schedule (DIS)
Structured Clinical Interview for Diagnosis (SCID)
Comprehensive Assessment of Symptoms and History (CASH)
Structured Interview for the Diagnosis of DSM-IV Personality Disorders (SIDP-IV)
Composite International Diagnostic Interview (CIDI)
Personality Disorders Examination (PDE)

---

history, handedness, memory impairment, negative symptoms, and a variety of other aspects of clinical descriptions that are not included in the structured interviews listed above.

The *Structured Interview for the Diagnosis of DSM-IV Personality Disorders (SIDP-IV)* was developed as a complement to the other structured interviews designed to make Axis I diagnoses. It provides a structured interview that permits clinicians and investigators to make assessments for diagnosis of personality syndromes according to DSM-IV criteria.

The *Composite International Diagnostic Interview (CIDI)*, based on the DIS, was developed for use in cross-sectional epidemiological research by the World Health Organization. The questions are modular in design, so researchers can choose diagnostic categories of interest to them. It is designed to be used by lay interviewers.

The *Personality Disorders Examination (PDE)* was also developed by the World Health Organization; it is designed for cross-sectional research on personality disorders. Unlike the CIDI and the DIS, it is intended for use by experienced clinicians.

Rating Scales

Rating scales typically are designed to provide a rapid and concise assessment of a specific aspect of psychopathology. Most rating scales have been developed for use in clinical drug trials or other situations in which investigators want to assess a change in the patient's status by taking repeated measurements over time (usually at weekly intervals). Table 3–4 summarizes some of the rating scales that are commonly used in psychiatric research of this type. Copies of each of these scales appear in the Appendix (except for the Beck Depression Inventory).

Table 3–4. Rating scales

Brief Psychiatric Rating Scale (BPRS)
Scale for the Assessment of Negative Symptoms (SANS)
Scale for the Assessment of Positive Symptoms (SAPS)
Hamilton Rating Scale for Depression
Beck Depression Inventory (BDI)
Hamilton Anxiety Scale
Yale-Brown Obsessive-Compulsive Disorder Scale (YBOCS)
Abnormal Involuntary Movement Scale (AIMS)
Simpson-Angus Scale
Mini-Mental State Examination (MMSE)
Global Assessment Scale (GAS)

The *Brief Psychiatric Rating Scale (BPRS)* is the oldest of the rating scales. Developed in the 1960s, it used factor analysis to sift through a broad array of symptoms seen in psychiatric patients and generate a relatively small number of factors. These include things such as conceptual disorganization, hostility, and social withdrawal. The BPRS is still widely used, although most of the items rated are relatively abstract compared with the specific symptoms currently used to assess psychopathology.

The *Scale for the Assessment of Negative Symptoms (SANS)* and the *Scale for the Assessment of Positive Symptoms (SAPS)* were designed to provide more complete coverage of the symptoms of psychosis than is provided by the BPRS. The SANS is the only scale currently in wide use that assesses negative symptoms. These scales rate the phenomena that clinicians are accustomed to assessing, such as delusions, hallucinations, and positive formal thought disorder.

The *Hamilton Rating Scale for Depression (HRSD)* is also among the oldest rating scales. It was specifically designed to provide a quantitative measurement of symptoms of depression that would be sensitive to change. Like the BPRS, it was developed shortly after the discovery of psychoactive drugs and was a standard instrument used to assess the efficacy of new antidepressants as they were developed. Although a number of other rating scales for depression have been developed, none has supplanted the HRSD in general use.

The *Beck Depression Inventory (BDI)* is also very commonly used. Unlike the HRSD, the BDI focuses on cognitive symptoms of depression.

The *Hamilton Anxiety Scale* performs a function similar to that of the HRSD for assessing anxiety. It is also widely used in clinical drug trials and as an overall assessment instrument.

The *Yale-Brown Obsessive-Compulsive Scale (YBOCS)* is commonly used to assess obsessive-compulsive symptoms. Its sensitivity to change makes it particularly useful for clinical treatment studies.

The *Abnormal Involuntary Movement Scale (AIMS)* was developed to determine whether patients had developed abnormal movements characteristic of tardive dyskinesia. It is currently widely used in neuroleptic trials.

The *Simpson-Angus Scale* is also widely used and is similar to the AIMS, but it focuses more specifically on the side effects of neuroleptics, such as parkinsonian symptoms or akathisia.

The *Mini-Mental State Examination (MMSE)* is a brief structured interview designed to assess cognitive status. It provides quantitative measurements of orientation, memory, calculations, and other aspects of the systematic mental status examination. It is a quantitative scale with a perfect score of 30 points. It is now widely used as a simple, rapid method for assessing abnormalities in mental status.

The *Global Assessment Scale (GAS)* is a 100-point scale (0 = extremely poor, 100 = superior) that is included in a variety of structured interviews, such as the SADS or the CASH. It is very similar to the Global Assessment of Functioning (GAF) Scale (described in Chapter 2), which was derived from the GAS. This scale provides a brief, simple way of assessing the patient's level of functioning and severity of psychopathology. Because the GAS is quite sensitive to change, it is frequently used as an overall index of the patient's improvement over time.

Bibliography

Andreasen NC: Thought, language, and communication disorders, I: clinical assessment, definition of terms, and evaluation of their reliability. Arch Gen Psychiatry 36:1315–1321, 1979

Andreasen NC: Thought, language, and communication disorders, II: diagnostic significance. Arch Gen Psychiatry 36:1325–1330, 1979

Andreasen NC: Negative symptoms in schizophrenia: definition and reliability. Arch Gen Psychiatry 39:784–788, 1982

Andreasen NC: The Scale for the Assessment of Negative Symptoms (SANS). Iowa City, IA, The University of Iowa, 1983

Andreasen NC: The Scale for the Assessment of Positive Symptoms (SAPS). Iowa City, IA, The University of Iowa, 1984

Andreasen NC: Comprehensive Assessment of Symptoms and History (CASH). Iowa City, IA, The University of Iowa, 1985

Andreasen NC, Flaum M, Arndt S: The Comprehensive Assessment of Symptoms and History (CASH): an instrument for assessing psychopathology and diagnosis. Arch Gen Psychiatry 49:615–623, 1992

Arndt S, Alliger RJ, Andreasen NC: The distinction of positive and negative symptoms: the failure of a two-dimensional model. Br J Psychiatry 158:317–322, 1991

Beck AT, Ward CH, Mendelson M, et al: An inventory for measuring depression. Arch Gen Psychiatry 4:561–571, 1961

Department of Health, Education, and Welfare: Abnormal Involuntary Movement Scale. Washington, DC, Alcohol, Drug Abuse and Mental Health Administration, 1974

Endicott J, Spitzer RL: A diagnostic interview: The Schedule for Affective Disorders and Schizophrenia (SADS). Arch Gen Psychiatry 35:837–844, 1978

Endicott J, Spitzer RL, Fleiss JL, et al: The Global Assessment Scale: a procedure for measuring overall severity of psychiatric disturbance. Arch Gen Psychiatry 33:766–771, 1976

Folstein MF, Folstein SE, McHugh P: Mini-Mental State: a practical method for grading the cognitive state of patients for the clinician. J Psychiatr Res 12:189–198, 1975

Goodman WK, Price LH, Rasmussen SA, et al: The Yale-Brown Obsessive-Compulsive Scale, I: development, use, and reliability. Arch Gen Psychiatry 46:1006–1011, 1989

Hamilton M: The assessment of anxiety states by rating. Br J Med Psychol 32:50–55, 1959

Hamilton M: A rating scale for depression. J Neurol Neurosurg Psychiatry 23:56–62, 1960

Miller DD, Arndt S, Andreasen NC: Alogia, attentional impairment, and inappropriate affect: their status in the dimensions of schizophrenia. Compr Psychiatry 34:221–226, 1993

Overall J, Gorham D: Brief Psychiatric Rating Scale. Psychol Rep 10:799–812, 1962

Robins LN, Helzer JE, Croughan J, et al: National Institute of Mental Health Diagnostic Interview Schedule: its history, characteristics, and validity. Arch Gen Psychiatry 38:381–389, 1981

Robins LN, Wing J, Wittchen HV, et al: The Composite International Diagnostic Interview—an epidemiological instrument for use in conjunction with different diagnostic systems and in different cultures. Arch Gen Psychiatry 45:1069–1077, 1988

Simpson GM, Angus JWS: A rating scale for extrapyramidal side effects. Acta Psychiatr Scand Suppl 212:11–19, 1970

Stangl D, Pfohl B, Zimmerman M et al: A structured interview for DSM-III personality disorders: a preliminary report. Arch Gen Psychiatry 42:591–596, 1985

Wing JK: A standard form of psychiatric Present State Examinations (PSE) and a method for standardizing the classification of symptoms, in Psychiatric Epidemiology. Edited by Hare EH, Wing JK. London, Oxford University Press, 1970, pp 93–108

Self-Assessment Questions

1. Describe the way in which the patient's chief complaint can be used to take a history and to develop a differential diagnosis.
2. Describe several techniques that are important for concluding the initial interview with a patient.
3. Enumerate the components of a standard psychiatric history, giving each of the main headings of the overall outline.
4. Summarize the major components of the mental status examination.

5. Enumerate the five positive symptoms of psychosis. Give examples of some typical kinds of delusions and hallucinations.
6. List the five common negative symptoms.
7. Enumerate and define some of the symptoms observed in depression.
8. Enumerate and define some of the symptoms observed in mania.
9. Enumerate and define some of the symptoms observed in anxiety disorders.

Chapter 4

Laboratory Tests

There is no observer outside the experiment.

Heisenberg

Although psychiatry places a greater emphasis on careful history taking and assessment than do most other medical specialties, laboratory tests are also growing in importance. Because so much has been discovered about the neural substrates of mental illnesses during the past several decades, psychiatrists have begun to identify tests of brain structure and function that may provide useful information to help guide diagnosis and treatment. Currently there are few laboratory tests that have a sensitivity and specificity equivalent to the glucose tolerance test for diabetes or a serum thyroxin test for myxedema or thyrotoxicosis. Tests of this type are only available for a few disorders (e.g., Alzheimer's disease), and even in these few instances their diagnostic validity is still not firmly established. Nevertheless, some type of laboratory workup will be appropriate for many psychiatric patients to establish baseline levels of function, to rule out confounding medical conditions, or to evaluate the presence of toxins that may cause symptoms of mental illness.

In the current era of cost-consciousness, laboratory tests should not be ordered unnecessarily, but they also should not be avoided if needed. Psychiatric patients require the same type of careful and high-quality workup as patients who are evaluated for cardiac, pulmonary, or renal symptoms. Although their symptoms may appear to be "in their minds," these symptoms may actually be mediated by processes affecting their brains or arising from other bodily organs. The

91

rationale for obtaining laboratory tests will depend on the clinical presentation and should be tailored to the needs of the individual patient and the setting in which he or she is seen.

Some laboratory tests should usually be ordered for patients admitted to a psychiatric unit, although the laboratory workup may be quite simple. The need for laboratory evaluations among outpatients will vary, depending on the age of the patient, the type of symptoms with which he or she presents, and the type of treatment plan. Young healthy individuals who have received a medical evaluation within the past few years, and who have relatively mild psychiatric symptoms, will probably need nothing. On the other hand, even among outpatients some laboratory assessments may be necessary in patients who are elderly or who present with severe or complex problems, particularly when there is a differential diagnosis that suggests some medical cause for the presenting symptoms.

Most laboratory procedures conducted for psychiatric patients are done for one of five purposes:

1. To complete a general medical workup of the sort done routinely for any hospital admission
2. To rule out some nonpsychiatric cause of the presenting symptoms
3. To conduct a specific workup appropriate for a specific treatment that has been planned (e.g., a workup before conducting electroconvulsive therapy [ECT])
4. To obtain information that will assist in making a differential diagnosis among several different mental illnesses
5. To assist in determining pathophysiology, estimating prognosis, and formulating a treatment plan

Each of these purposes, and the relevant laboratory procedures, is discussed in more detail below.

The General Medical Workup

Standards as to what is considered an appropriate general medical workup may vary in different hospital settings. In general, however, most patients admitted to a hospital receive a set of screening laboratory evaluations. Typically, these consist of a complete blood count, urinalysis, serum electrolytes, liver enzymes (i.e., serum glutamic-oxaloacetic transaminase [SGOT], serum glutamic-pyruvic transaminase [SGPT]), serum creatinine, blood urea nitrogen (BUN), and sometimes a chest film or electrocardiogram (ECG). The relevance of the latter two depend in part on the patient's age, smoking history, and overall physical condition. Given that many patients with mental illnesses have a history of heavy smoking, an evaluation of pulmonary and cardiac status may be very appropriate. Female patients need a Pap test, and women over age 45 years should be evaluated with mammography at periodic intervals. The inpatient psychiatrist should assume responsibility for ensuring that appropriate laboratory screens are obtained, taking into account whether the patient has had any of these evaluations recently.

A psychiatrist who is seeing outpatients at regular intervals should also assume responsibility for ensuring that his or her patients receive annual general medical workups, including appropriate histories, physicals, and laboratory tests. In many cases, the psychiatrist assumes the role of a primary care physician, because he or she is the physician whom the patient sees most frequently. The psychiatrist will always assume primary responsibility for conducting a physical and neurological examination in an inpatient setting and obtaining referrals to a specialist if questions arise. In an outpatient setting the responsibility will vary, depending on the working environment and regional mores. If working in a general medical clinic or health maintenance organization (HMO), the psychiatrist will share the responsibility, whereas psychiatrists in solo practice or a specialty group will usually conduct a physical and neurological examination, order appropriate tests, and interpret them. (Some psychiatrists who do only psychotherapy may, however, prefer to refer their patients to an internist or family practitioner because of concerns that the physical contact may interfere with the process of psychotherapy.) Overall, the rule that fragmenting care across multiple specialists gives patients poor service holds as much for patients with mental illnesses as it does for patients with other types of illness. Consequently, the psychiatrist should maintain good general medical skills and be prepared to handle simple and routine medical problems.

Laboratory Tests to Rule Out Nonpsychiatric Causes of Symptoms

Many diagnoses in psychiatry are diagnoses of exclusion. That is, they are typically made after it has been determined that the symptoms the patient manifests are not due to some other specific medical or neurological disorder. Historically, psychiatrists used to say that they were ruling out "organic" causes of the symptoms. In fact, disorders were divided into those that were "organic" (i.e., physically based) and those that were "functional" (i.e., mentally based). This phraseology has clearly become outdated, however, because diseases such as schizophrenia or manic-depressive illness (i.e., bipolar disorder) almost certainly have a specific organic cause, rooted in aberrations in brain chemistry or circuitry. Consequently, this outmoded distinction has been abandoned in DSM-IV.

Table 4–1 lists a variety of conditions commonly considered in the differential diagnosis of serious mental illnesses such as the dementias, schizophrenia, bipolar disorder, or the various anxiety disorders. In general, when DSM-IV states that "the disturbance is not due to a general medical condition," one of the group of disorders in Table 4–1 is to be ruled out. These various disorders are discussed in more detail under the differential diagnosis of the various conditions presented in Section II of this volume ("Psychiatric Disorders"). If one of these conditions is being given serious consideration, the psychiatrist will often order a screening test. If the results are suggestive of a neurological or general medical diagnosis, the clinician will then usually consult with another medical specialist to select additional laboratory tests and interpret them.

Patients with multi-infarct dementia, subdural hematoma, normal-pressure hydrocephalus, tumors, and human immunodeficiency virus (HIV)-related dementia may all present with confusion, memory impairment, personality change, poor attention and drive, tearfulness and depression, or suspiciousness and even frank psychosis. The most common psychiatric illnesses that must be differentiated from these conditions include Alzheimer's disease, schizophrenia and related psychotic conditions (e.g., schizophreniform disorder, delusional disorder), and the various mood disorders.

Neuroimaging provides the most efficient method for ruling out the majority of these conditions. A simple computed tomography (CT) scan may be sufficient. Magnetic resonance imaging (MRI) is more effective, because it permits the identification of small focal lesions, which may represent old infarcts and which typically appear as areas of increased signal intensity. The white-matter lesions of multiple sclerosis are also readily seen with MRI, and patients with HIV-related dementia may show similar small focal lesions. Because of its excellent resolution and three-dimensional capacity, MRI is particularly useful for

Table 4–1. Conditions commonly considered in the differential diagnosis of major mental illnesses

Multi-infarct dementia	Vitamin deficiency syndromes (e.g., pernicious anemia)
Subdural hematoma	
Normal-pressure hydrocephalus	Other central nervous system infections (e.g., syphilis)
Tumors	
Acquired immunodeficiency syndrome (AIDS) dementia	Substance-induced symptoms
	Neuropsychiatric effects of medical treatment (e.g., potassium deficiency from diuretics, fatigue from propranolol, digitalis toxicity, phenytoin [Dilantin] toxicity)
Temporal lobe epilepsy	
Endocrine/metabolic disorders	
Exposure to toxins	

identifying tumors. Tumors typically appear bright on MRI when T2-weighted sequences (specific scanning sequences that are especially sensitive for detecting abnormal tissue, but are poorer for seeing structure) are used.

As is described in more detail below, Alzheimer's disease represents a special case in neuroimaging evaluations. With functional imaging techniques such as single photon emission computed tomography (SPECT) or positron-emission tomography (PET), 70%–80% of patients with Alzheimer's disease show a characteristic decrease in metabolic function or cerebral blood flow in posterior temporoparietal regions. Alzheimer's disease appears at present to be the only major mental illness that shows this characteristic pattern of hypometabolic function; thus, functional imaging techniques such as SPECT or PET may be particularly useful in differentiating Alzheimer's disease from other disorders that present with confusion and intellectual deterioration. Other laboratory tests, such as electroencephalography (EEG) or neuropsychological assessment, may also be useful in evaluating this particular group of "rule outs."

Patients with temporal lobe epilepsy (TLE) typically present with dissociative-like episodes or personality changes such as hyperreligiosity, hypergraphia (writing prolifically), hyposexuality, temper outbursts, and occasionally mood or psychotic-like symptoms. Thus, its differential diagnosis includes the various dissociative disorders, obsessive-compulsive personality disorder, antisocial personality, conduct disorders, and the mood and psychotic disorders. Because TLE is due to an electrical and functional disturbance in the brain, it is best evaluated by the laboratory tests that use the methods of neurophysiology or functional neuroimaging. EEG is the test of choice because of its noninvasive nature, inexpensiveness, and ease of administration. Nevertheless, the focal lesion in TLE may be deeply embedded inside the brain in the anterior poles of the temporal lobes or even the medial aspects of the temporal lobes. Because EEG uses surface electrodes, it may not pick up seizure foci in these deep brain regions. Consequently, the assessment of TLE may require additional techniques, even when EEG is used. Sleep deprivation may bring out focal abnormalities not noticed with routine EEG, and nasopharyngeal leads are particularly appropriate if a diagnosis of TLE is being considered. PET scanning may also pick up focal regions of hypometabolic function, but this neuroimaging technique is not widely available and is much more costly.

Patients with endocrine disorders, exposure to toxins, vitamin deficiency syndromes (e.g., pernicious anemia), and other central nervous system (CNS) infections apart from the acquired immunodeficiency syndrome (AIDS) (e.g., syphilis) may present with fatigue, weakness, decreased drive, memory impairment, intellectual confusion, and personality change. Again, the most common psychiatric differential diagnoses are the various dementias, psychotic conditions, mood disorders, and a few anxiety or personality disorders. Hyperthyroidism is a common mimic of anxiety conditions, whereas myxedema is a common mimic of mood disorders. The other rule outs are considerably less common. These conditions are evaluated by a variety of specific assessment techniques, including serum T_3 and T_4, a complete blood count, serum assays for toxins, or a Venereal Disease Research Laboratory test for syphilis.

Finally, the clinician must attempt to determine whether a patient's presenting symptoms are due to a variety of street drugs that are all too readily available or to a variety of medications prescribed by physicians, which also are often all too readily available. Street drugs such as amphetamines, cocaine, and phencyclidine are special culprits in producing psychotic-like syndromes that resemble schizophrenia. Marijuana abuse leads to lethargy and withdrawal that may mimic depression, the negative symptoms of schizophrenia, or personality syndromes such as schizoid or schizotypal personality. These drugs may also produce periods of feeling high that may mimic mood disorders. Use of street drugs, which is often denied by patients on interview, can be assessed through routine urine drug screens. Because of the substantial prevalence of substance abuse in contemporary American society, a urine drug screen should be virtually a routine diagnostic test for patients admitted as inpatients to psychiatric facilities.

Iatrogenic psychiatric disorders are also not uncommon. Patients who have received large quantities of prescribed drugs may also present with a variety of symptoms that mimic psychiatric disorders. Patients being treated with diuretics for hypertension may have a potassium deficiency that produces fatigue and that mimics depression. Propranolol may have similar effects. Digitalis toxicity and phenytoin (Dilantin) toxicity can produce fatigue and intellectual confusion that may mimic depression, psychosis, or dementia. Particularly in elderly patients, the clinician should maintain a high index of suspicion that symptoms that present as possible psychiatric disorders are in fact due to prescribed medications. Anxiolytics and hypnotics, which are frequently prescribed by nonpsychiatric physicians, can also produce a variety of symptoms that mimic classic psychiatric disorders, such as confusion, lethargy, or withdrawal. Frequently, the diagnosis of a psychiatric condition due to prescribed drugs can be made simply from the history. Sometimes, however, laboratory tests are also needed, for example, to establish low serum potassium levels or to obtain quantitative blood levels for prescribed medications such as digitalis.

Workups Pertaining to Specific Types of Psychiatric Treatments

In addition to laboratory evaluations to assist in diagnosis and differential diagnosis, some laboratory procedures may be necessary before instituting a particular treatment. Some treatments, such as ECT, have a modest risk associated with them. Therefore, it is desirable to obtain laboratory assessments to determine and document the patient's physical condition before the treatment, to rule out conditions that might be adversely affected by the treatment, and to establish baseline values for the patient before instituting treatment.

Electroconvulsive therapy. As is discussed in more detail in the chapter on somatic therapies (Chapter 26), ECT is a relatively safe and highly effective treatment for some psychiatric disorders, such as severe depression. The physical convulsion involved is typically attenuated by using succinylcholine, but there is nevertheless a very modest risk for fractures if the initial dose of succinylcholine is not correctly established. Spine films may be indicated in elderly or arthritic patients before instituting ECT. Noticing signs of osteoporosis on spine films does not necessarily rule out the use of ECT, if it is clinically appropriate, but it may suggest that a higher dose of succinylcholine is desirable. An ECG is usually obtained to determine baseline cardiac status, because arrhythmias may occur during or after a treatment. Some clinicians also like to obtain an EEG on patients before ECT: EEG obtained after ECT has been begun is uninterpretable, because ECT can produce EEG changes that may last for months. Thus, if an elderly, depressed patient has questionable signs of dementia before ECT, it is best to obtain a full dementia workup before ECT, because ECT may produce some memory impairment. Neuropsychological tests obtained after ECT may also be uninterpretable for several months.

Lithium treatment. Lithium carbonate (used for the treatment of bipolar disorder) occasionally has adverse effects on both the thyroid gland and the kidney. Thus, it is desirable to obtain a urinalysis, serum electrolytes, BUN, serum creatinine, and serum T_3 and T_4 before instituting lithium treatment. Because lithium produces ECG changes, which are nonspecific in nature and do not reflect cardiotoxicity, many clinicians often consider it worthwhile to obtain an ECG before prescribing lithium. This decision will be heavily dependent on the age and general health of the patient.

Whether the patient is receiving a therapeutic level of lithium is also determined through a simple laboratory test to measure blood lithium levels. These are usually obtained twice weekly during the first few weeks of lithium treatment. Thereafter, they are typically obtained at regular intervals, such as every 6 months or every year, on an outpatient basis as long as the patient remains on lithium. Serum electrolytes, BUN, serum creatinine, and serum T_3 and T_4 are also typically rechecked at similar intervals. An elevated serum creatinine level should be followed up with a 24-hour creatinine clearance test.

Tricyclic and other antidepressants.   Tricyclics do not necessarily require any specific laboratory workup before instituting treatment. The decision about this will depend on the age and physical condition of the patient. Typically, no tests are needed for healthy young adults. Because tricyclics also produce ECG changes, however, an ECG should be obtained before prescribing tricyclics if there is any question that it may be needed later on. Older patients or patients in whom there is any possible cardiac abnormality should definitely be evaluated with an ECG before prescribing tricyclics, because the major adverse effects of tricyclics involve the cardiac conduction system.

Blood levels may be monitored for tricyclics. Use of blood levels to monitor treatment may serve several purposes. A few tricyclics, such as nortriptyline, have a therapeutic window. Blood levels may also be ordered when the clinician is wondering whether the patient is taking the medication at all (to determine the presence of some blood level), when the clinician is concerned that the patient might be experiencing toxic effects, or when the patient is failing to respond to established therapeutic doses. (See Chapter 26, "Somatic Treatments," for a more complete discussion of management of dosages of psychoactive medications.)

All patients treated with tricyclics should receive an annual physical examination with close attention to cardiac function, as well as evaluation of blood pressure every 3–6 months, because the primary adverse effects of tricyclics are on cardiac conduction and baroreceptors. Tricyclics can also produce changes in liver enzymes, which should be checked annually.

Antipsychotic treatments.   Antipsychotics, like tricyclics, may need no special workup before prescription. Typically, no tests are needed. Blood levels are more difficult to monitor for neuroleptics because many produce active metabolites. Assays are currently available for several antipsychotics, but they are of questionable value, because research has not definitely shown a relationship between blood level and clinical response. Only haloperidol and clozapine blood levels are clinically meaningful. (See Chapter 26 for additional information.) The main reasons for ordering blood levels of neuroleptic drugs are similar to those described above for tricyclics.

The major adverse effects of neuroleptics appear to be on the extrapyramidal system in the brain. The development of tardive dyskinesia is the single most important serious long-term side effect. No laboratory tests are available to test for this side effect at present, and its emergence is best monitored through regular physical examinations with careful attention to the development of abnormal movements using the Abnormal Involuntary Movement Scale (described in Chapter 3).

Laboratory Procedures Used to Assist in Psychiatric Differential Diagnosis and Treatment Planning

In addition to the above highly specific indications for laboratory tests, a variety of tests may be obtained in psychiatric patients to assist in differential diagnosis or to assist in understanding the nature and severity or the pathophysiology of the illness. Information about the pathophysiology can be helpful in counseling the patient and family about prognosis and in treatment planning. Some tests that are especially useful in this regard include the various neuroimaging procedures and various types of psychological tests. These may assist in determining the overall integrity of brain function, the presence of structural abnormalities, or the presence of generalized intellectual deficits or specific learning disabilities. Although very few of these tests give highly specific diagnostic information, they can sometimes assist in making a diagnosis and can be quite useful in treatment planning. As discussed above, a normal EEG may rule out a condition such as TLE, whereas a SPECT scan will sharpen the differential diagnosis between depression and dementia. Nonspecific neural abnormalities are sometimes observed in patients with schizophrenia or manic-depressive illness; when present, these suggest that the patient may be more sensitive to medication side effects and may be more refractory to treatment. Some of the laboratory tests that are especially useful for psychiatric differential diagnosis and treatment planning are described in detail below.

Overview of Laboratory Tests Frequently Used in Psychiatry

Neurophysiological Techniques

Electroencephalogram (EEG).   The EEG is one of the oldest laboratory tests available to psychiatrists. Hans Berger, a psychiatrist who pioneered the development of EEG, was the first person to record the electrical activity of the brain. Until the advent of structural imaging techniques such as CT and MRI, EEG was the major method for evaluating abnormalities in brain activity produced by abnormalities such as tumors, head injuries, or seizures. CT and MRI now offer relatively benign methods for studying the brain in vivo to rule out the presence of diseased regions of tissue, but the EEG remains the simplest, most noninvasive method for evaluating seizures and metabolic dysfunctions.

EEG measures electrical activity with a montage of electrodes scattered over the surface of the brain. An example of a typical montage appears in Figure 4–1.

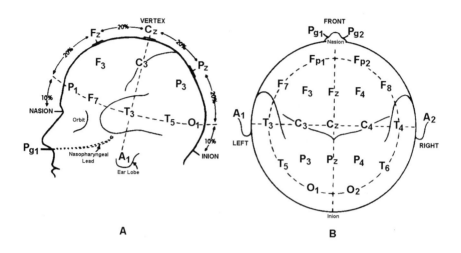

Figure 4–1. A typical electroencephalogram montage. Leads are arrayed in order to cover the entire brain, ranging from frontal to occipital.

Electrical activity is recorded from leads connected to these surface electrodes; a typical modern EEG uses 16 leads. The electrical activity is then recorded on a polygraph, much like an ECG, and the pattern of activity is evaluated. Although computerized methods have been developed for reading EEGs, the best computer continues to be the human brain connected to the human eye.

EEG characteristics are described in terms of the frequency of the waveforms observed (measured in cycles per second [cps]). The normal human brain typically shows activity in either the beta (>12 cps) or alpha (8–12 cps) range during the waking state. As individuals become drowsy, theta (4–8 cps) and delta (<4 cps) activity is observed. In the waking state, both theta and delta activity are considered to be abnormal in the healthy human brain. (Diffuse theta activity is sometimes seen in elderly individuals while awake, however.) Delta activity is clearly abnormal and represents sick or dying tissue.

Abnormalities observed on EEG include spike and wave patterns, focal slowing, and diffuse slowing. Spike and wave patterns are typically seen in brains susceptible to seizures. The location of the spike may indicate the primary focus from which the seizure derives. The spikes of a brain predisposed to produce epileptic attacks are less often seen during the waking state. Consequently, EEGs are best obtained while the patient is asleep; sedation is often prescribed to induce sleep during EEG, so that abnormal seizure foci can be observed.

Encephalographers believe that a seizure disorder cannot be ruled out through a simple waking EEG. In addition, nasopharyngeal leads may be needed to identify a deep seizure focus. The tendency to manifest spike activities is suppressed by anticonvulsant medications, such as phenytoin. Thus, a patient with epilepsy may have a normal EEG if he or she is appropriately medicated, particularly if only a waking EEG is obtained. A normal EEG does not rule out the existence of a seizure disorder, because the identification of spike and wave activity requires catching the brain during the elusive moments when spikes are occurring. Nevertheless, serial normal EEGs obtained in sleeping, unmedicated individuals do make the diagnosis of a seizure disorder unlikely.

EEG is very sensitive to metabolic dysfunctions and to the effects of a variety of drugs. In the case of metabolic dysfunctions, EEG may be the simplest method for determining that the patient's cognitive symptoms are due to some type of metabolic disorder. A variety of psychoactive drugs affect the EEG: lithium, for example, produces an increase in theta activity, whereas benzodiazepines produce rapid, fast activity (i.e., beta activity). Sometimes EEG provides a clinician with the first clue that a patient has been taking unprescribed medications or even medications prescribed by another physician. In a few rare instances, EEG can serve as a useful test for ruling out psychiatric disorders that represent conversion phenomena or malingering. For example, the presence of photic driving (produced by visual stimulation with flashes of bright lights) on EEG will rule out hysterical (i.e., conversion) blindness.

Sleep EEG (polysomnography) is a special type of electroencephalography involving the collection of electrical brain activity data during all-night sleep. During a normal full night's sleep, individuals go through a sleep cycle characterized by drowsiness (indicated with theta activity on the EEG), leading into alternating periods of rapid eye movement (REM) sleep and deep dreamless sleep (delta sleep). The healthy individual passes through approximately five such cycles during the course of a night's sleep. Polysomnography can be used to monitor a variety of sleep disorders that are often characterized by abnormal sleep patterns, such as those associated with depression. A short REM latency and reduced delta sleep are frequently observed in depressed patients. This abnormality occurs so frequently in depression that some investigators consider it a biological marker, but polysomnography is too time consuming and expensive to be widely used to screen for this abnormality. Additional information about polysomnography and sleep disorders is found in Chapter 23 ("Sleep Disorders").

Brain electrical activity mapping.　　Brain electrical activity mapping (BEAM) extends the capacity of EEG by generating computerized maps of brain electrical activity to produce images or pictures of it. The brain electrical mapping techniques start from the basic 20-lead montage of electrodes. Clinicians and investigators can work with the basic EEG information, or they can study evoked potentials (large waveforms that stand out from the background of the EEG and are produced by giving the individual a specific stimulus to evoke a large burst of activity, such as is produced by an auditory click). A computer is used to average electrical activity over some specified period. Information about electrical activity can be summarized by superimposing a grid matrix (typically 64×64) over the summarized numerical data generated by a computer (using a fast Fourier transformation). The numerical values contained in the matrix can then be converted to a color scale, with red typically representing high activity and blue low activity (or fast versus slow), and a picture of the brain's electrical activity can thereby generated. Brain electrical mapping techniques have no established clinical diagnostic utility in psychiatry. Abnormal electrical patterns have been reported in some mental illnesses, such as increased frontal delta activity in schizophrenia, but these findings have not been consistently replicated and are not diagnostic of the disorder. BEAM may provide some useful information in specific individuals, however, by extending the basic information inherent in EEG evaluations.

Evoked potentials of various kinds also provide ancillary information. Evoked potentials are changes in brain electrical activity that are usually seen in specific regions in response to a stimulus, such as a particular kind of sound, instructions to monitor for a target displayed on a video screen, or some other type of cognitive or perceptual task. In contrast to a simple EEG, which is a general indicator of overall brain electrical activity, evoked potentials (also called *event-related potentials*) reflect the behavior of the brain while it is performing higher cognitive tasks. The most commonly used is the P300. This is a large positive wave usually seen 300 milliseconds after the stimulus that was used to evoke it. The P300 is thought to reflect some aspect of the ability to focus attention. It appears to be decreased in patients with schizophrenia, and abnormalities also have been reported in patients with other disorders that involve cognitive dysfunctions.

All these neurophysiological techniques are relatively crude compared with neuroimaging techniques such as CT, SPECT, and PET. Nevertheless, they may have clinical utility for several different reasons. First, they do not involve any radiation exposure and are noninvasive. Therefore, they may be particularly valuable for studying brain activity in special populations, such as children. Second, they represent the only functional imaging technique (i.e., a technique that permits visualization of the brain performing particular functions or tasks) that has very fine temporal resolution. They can record events that occur in milliseconds, whereas the time window for SPECT and PET studies is seconds to hours. Third, they are simple to perform and therefore are inexpensive and accessible. As a result, they may be used as a first-line assessment technique in some situations.

Structural Neuroimaging Techniques

Structural neuroimaging techniques include CT and MRI.

Computed tomography.   CT scanning has been available since the early 1970s and was the first in vivo brain imaging technique to become widely used. Before CT, brain structure could be visualized only through the use of crude and invasive techniques such as pneumoencephalography.

The development of CT only became possible after the invention of efficient, high-speed computers. CT provides the prototype for most of the other neuroimaging techniques currently in use. In CT, an X-ray beam is passed through serial slices of the brain, and the degree of attenuation is measured when it emerges on the other side. The brain slice is divided into a series of tiny cubes (voxels or volume elements), and a number reflecting the degree of attenuation can be assigned to each of the voxels. These numerical codes are then assigned a shade of gray, reflecting the degree of X-ray attenuation, which gives a visual picture of brain structure. Cerebrospinal fluid, which attenuates least, appears darkest, whereas white matter, which attenuates most, appears lightest.

Research studies using CT on a wide range of psychiatric populations have shown detectable abnormalities, and CT scanning is now used to assess a wide variety of psychiatric conditions. CT abnormalities may be seen in many mental disorders, including dementia, schizophrenia, alcoholism, anorexia nervosa, and perhaps some mood disorders. The types of abnormalities observed are nonspecific in terms of both pathophysiology and diagnosis. The most typical findings are ventricular enlargement or cortical atrophy. A CT scan showing these types of abnormalities is seen in Figure 4–2. In general, these findings, when present, do not confirm a specific diagnosis because the same types of abnormalities may be present in many different disorders. Further, in interpreting CT scans, the age of the individual must be taken into consideration. Neuronal loss and the development of ventricular enlargement and cortical atrophy appear to occur in healthy individuals as part of the aging process. Thus, in interpreting CT scans in elderly individuals to make a diagnosis of dementia, it can often be difficult to decide whether the atrophy and ventricular enlargement seen on CT are within normal limits for an individual's age or whether they represent a pathological process. These same concerns about evaluating the effects of aging pertain to the interpretation of MRI scans as well. In spite of these problems, assessment with CT scanning can be useful in a variety of ways.

Schizophrenia is the psychiatric illness that has been most extensively studied with CT scanning. By now, more than 50 controlled CT studies have been conducted. As the summary of studies in Figure 4–3 indicates, the vast majority

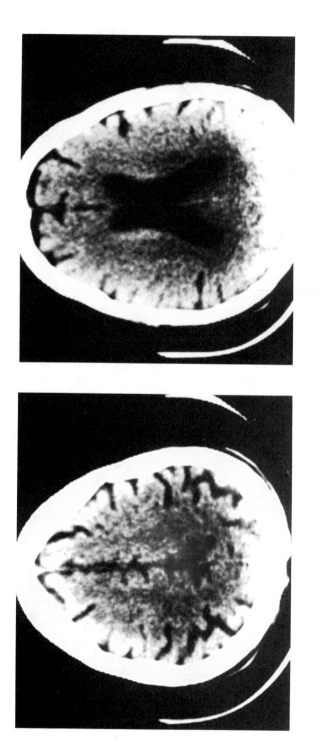

Figure 4–2. Computed tomography scan from an individual with schizophrenia. The slice on the *bottom* passes through the body of the ventricles and shows ventricular enlargement. Sulcal prominence is noted as well. The slice on the *top* is obtained from a higher level in the same individual brain and also shows prominent cortical sulci.

of these studies have shown that schizophrenic patients as a group tend to have an increase in ventricular size compared with healthy control subjects. Among the positive studies, the prevalence of extreme degrees of abnormality varies from study to study, ranging from as low as 5% to as high as 40%.

It is quite clear that ventricular enlargement is not seen in all schizophrenic patients. When present, ventricular enlargement appears to be correlated with a variety of other characteristics. Thus, a CT scan may provide the clinician with some information about long-term clinical course and prognosis. Schizophrenic patients with ventricular enlargement tend to have a lower level of educational achievement, often a more insidious onset, and indications of cognitive impairment when assessed neuropsychologically. They may also respond less well to

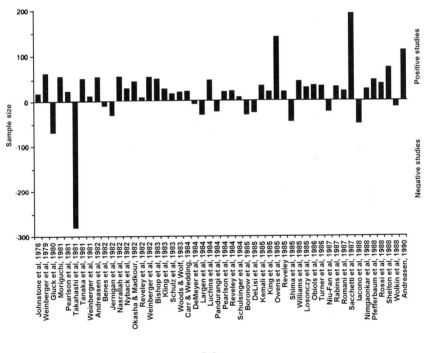

Figure 4–3. Summary of 50 controlled computed tomography studies evaluating the presence of ventricular enlargement in schizophrenia. The majority of the studies demonstrated ventricular enlargement. Reprinted with permission from Andreasen NC, Swayze VW II, Flaum M, et al: Ventricular enlargement in schizophrenia evaluated with computed tomographic scanning—effects of gender, age, and stage of illness. Arch Gen Psychiatry 47:1008–1015, 1990

neuroleptic medication, and some even appear to be worsened by it. Thus, their treatment should be managed somewhat more cautiously than that of patients whose CT scans indicate normal brain structure.

It has recently been observed that ventricular enlargement in schizophrenic patients probably does not represent a progressive neuronal loss, as occurs in patients with Alzheimer's disease. Although very few studies as yet have examined a single cohort of patients with serial scans over a 5- to 10-year period, ventricular size has been observed in a large group of schizophrenic patients with a broad range of ages. The results suggest that, unlike the changes associated with degenerative dementia, the brain changes in schizophrenic patients are not progressive over time, and in fact ventricular enlargement and prominent sulci are present early in the illness (i.e., at the time of first evaluation for symptoms). Further, these brain abnormalities tend to be more prominent and severe in male patients. Because males are known to be much more vulnerable to birth injuries and developmental defects (e.g., males have a higher rate of learning disability, hyperactivity, and being spontaneously aborted), it seems likely that the finding of ventricular enlargement in young male schizophrenic patients presenting with their first episode reflects some type of cerebral injury that occurred relatively early in life and created a cerebral substrate that was more vulnerable to the development of schizophrenia in later years.

Studies of mood disorders have been more equivocal. Unlike schizophrenia, where the preponderance of studies have indicated that the disorder is characterized by structural abnormalities, only about half of the studies of mood disorders have found abnormalities to be present. In general, sample sizes have been too small to evaluate age and gender effects. The existing data appear to suggest that there is also a gender effect in the presence of ventricular enlargement in bipolar patients, with males being more vulnerable. The ventricular enlargement seen in depressed patients may not exceed that which is normal for the aging process, making it appear that ventricular enlargement is not statistically increased in patients with depression when age is controlled for. This does not mean, of course, that ordering a CT scan is inappropriate in an elderly depressed patient, because the differential diagnosis of dementia and depression is often a difficult one in this age group; a finding of substantial cortical atrophy and ventricular enlargement would definitely tip the balance in the direction of diagnosing dementia.

Magnetic resonance imaging.   MRI has a substantial number of advantages over CT. The images produced through MRI are developed through placing the patient's brain or body in a magnetic field, which causes the hydrogen protons to be aligned and concentrates the force of the magnetic moment produced so that it is large enough to be measurable. Thereafter, the protons can be raised to a higher energy level through stimulation with a radiofrequency signal targeted to their own Larmor frequency; the relaxation, or decay, to the original energy state can then be measured as a signal that is produced from tissue voxels, much as in the case of CT.

Only a few risks are involved in the use of MRI scanning. Because of the presence of the magnetic field, patients whose bodies contain metal objects, such as aneurysm clips or metal plates in their skulls, cannot be imaged. Patients with pacemakers must also be excluded. Because patients must be placed inside a tube-like metal cavity to be scanned, there is some risk of experiencing claustrophobia. This can usually be minimized or eliminated with adequate patient preparation, however.

In addition to being relatively risk free, MRI has a number of other advantages. Unlike CT, whose images are limited to the transverse or transaxial plane, MRI permits reconstruction and visualization of images from the brain in all planes. Because of the brain's complex three-dimensional structure, multiple perspectives are very useful. Coronal cuts, in particular, are especially valuable for visualizing small subcortical structures of great interest to psychiatry, such as the caudate, the putamen, the amygdala, and the hippocampus. Resolution is superb with MRI, producing "slices" of brain that look as if they were obtained in a pathology lab at postmortem. With CT scanning, it is difficult to see the posterior fossa because of the great density of bone in that region, but bony artifacts are not a problem with MRI, and posterior fossa structures are well visualized.

MRI is somewhat more difficult to use than CT, however. One major difficulty arises because many different imaging options are available. The technician can substantially change the type of pictures produced by altering imaging parameters such as repetition time or echo time. The actual image signal is a mixture of four components: flow velocity, proton density, and relaxation of the protons in different three-dimensional planes (T1 and T2 relaxation times). Depending on the scanning sequence used, images can be weighted by enhancing the proton density component, the T1 component, or the T2 component. A scanning sequence may be selected to produce impressive anatomical resolution (e.g., a proton density image or a T1-weighted image), or a sequence may be selected that shows very poor anatomical resolution, but displays clear, specific areas of tissue abnormality (e.g., T2-weighted images with a long echo time and repetition time). Examples of types of MRI scans appear in Figure 4–4.

Clinicians need to be aware of what they may be looking for when they decide to order an MRI scan. If they are looking for a tumor, multiple sclerosis plaques, or areas of microinfarction, they may prefer a T2-weighted image. If they are seeking a clear picture of the size and shape of the ventricles or the amygdala-

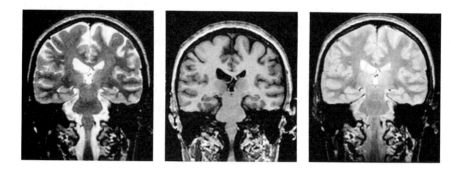

Figure 4–4. Magnetic resonance imaging scans from the same individual showing how the images appear different depending on the type of scanning sequence used. Proton density (*left*), T1-weighted (*center*), and T2-weighted (*right*) images were obtained and are shown for a coronal slice that passes through the hippocampus.

hippocampus, they will prefer a T1-weighted image. The question to be answered should therefore be clearly stated on the order form used to request an MRI scan, so that the radiologist and technicians can use the appropriate sequence.

Advances in MRI technology now also permit clinicians to acquire MRI data three-dimensionally and to obtain very thin slices. This has opened up the opportunity to develop software that allows visualization of the surface anatomy of the brain through methods known as surface/volume rendering. Because the slices contain voxels that are "cubic" (i.e., about 1 mm in all three dimensions), the brain can also be resliced or resampled after acquisition. Clinicians with access to such software can now identify major landmarks on the brain surface, such as the central sulcus or sylvian fissure; cleave through planes to visualize regions such as the planum temporale or Heschl's gyrus; and resample their images so that they can simultaneously visualize the brain in three orthogonal planes. Figure 4–5 shows the effects of decreasing slice thickness on the ability to resample. Figure 4–6 shows the ability to visualize brain surface anatomy and three orthogonal planes simultaneously, using image analysis software developed for this purpose in our Image Processing Laboratory. This software, BRAINS (Brain Research: Analysis of Images, Networks, and Systems), also permits automated measurements of subregions, measurement of surface features, and alignment of structural and functional images. Software of this type has essentially turned MRI into a tool that permits clinicians to do an anatomical postmortem in the antemortem state. Table 4–2 lists some of the basic problems inherent in the analysis and measurement of MRI images that are solved through the use of software such as BRAINS. Figure 4–7 illustrates its application to cleave along the sylvian fis-

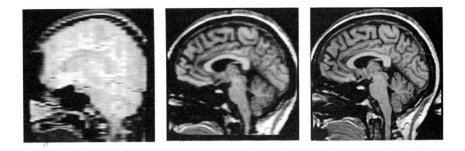

Figure 4–5. Three resampled images, using a sagittal plane, are shown. In each case the image was originally acquired in the coronal plane. After acquisition, the information was assembled as a three-dimensional image of the entire brain, which was subsequently resampled (resliced) in the sagittal plane. Slice thickness, from *left,* is 5 mm, 3 mm, and 1.5 mm. Note how the quality of the resampled images improves substantially as slice thickness decreases.

sure and to visualize the planum temporale in vivo.

Because MRI is still a relatively new technique, generalizations about its clinical usefulness are in a continual state of evolution as new information is acquired. As might be expected, the presence of ventricular enlargement in schizophrenic patients has already been repeatedly confirmed with MRI. A variety of other specific anomalies have also been reported, such as partial agenesis of the callosum and decreased temporal lobe size. A summary of the types of abnormalities that have been observed in schizophrenic patients appears in Table 4–3. Figure 4–8 shows an image of a patient with schizophrenia who has agenesis of the corpus callosum. This is one of many different types of midline abnormalities or developmental anomalies that have an increased incidence in schizophrenic patients. Others include cavum septi pellucidi, ectopic gray matter, and changes in gray-matter structures such as the thalamus or hippocampus. Many of these anomalies that have been seen with MRI are supported through independent observation using postmortem tissue and doing analyses of cell counts or cellular alignment.

Some patients with a bipolar disorder have been reported to have an increased number of small regions of high signal intensity (referred to colloquially as *unidentified bright objects* [UBOs]). The clinical significance of UBOs is uncertain, both in bipolar illness and in other disorders in which they are seen, such as the dementias; however, it is almost certain that they represent tiny areas of tissue loss, which result from microinfarctions in at least some cases.

Starvation, as occurs in anorexia nervosa and alcoholism, also can result in characteristic abnormalities on MRI scan. Anorectic patients who have fallen

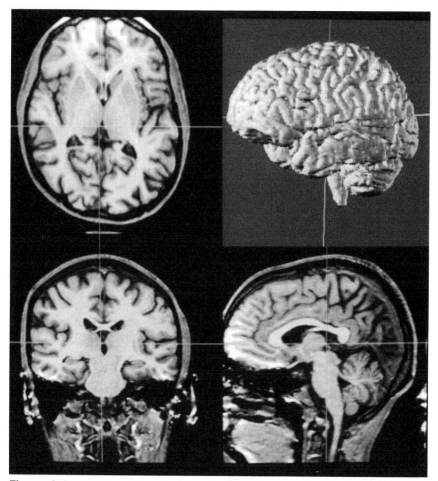

Figure 4–6.   A view of the brain surface, with resampling in three orthogonal planes, as produced by the software program BRAINS. The capacity to simultaneously visualize anatomy in three planes and on the brain surface is extremely useful for understanding the interrelationships between structures and their circuitry.

Table 4–2.   Basic problems in image analysis

Defining boundaries of structures	Three-dimensional visualization
Measuring volumes	Integrating data from multiple modalities
Measuring physiological parameters (e.g., blood flow, receptor density)	(e.g., magnetic resonance imaging, positron-emission tomography)

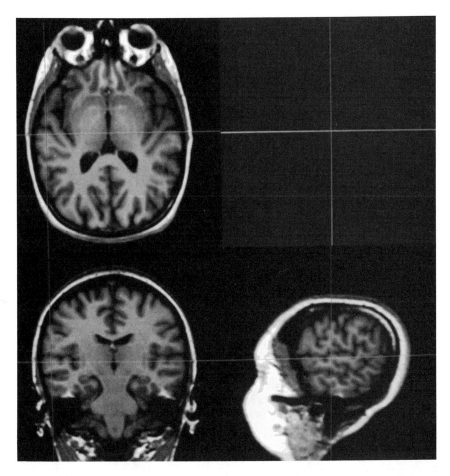

Figure 4–7. A view of the planum temporale, produced by using the resampling feature of the software program BRAINS. A plane has been drawn parallel to the sylvian fissure and the overlying parietal regions lifted off, much as would be done with a postmortem dissection.

Table 4–3. Abnormalities commonly seen in schizophrenia

Ventricular enlargement	Decreased hippocampal size
Prominent cortical sulci	Decreased size of superior temporal gyrus
Decreased cerebral size	Decreased thalamic size
Decreased frontal size	Increased caudate/putamen size
Decreased temporal size	Midline developmental abnormalities

substantially below their normal weight typically have cortical atrophy, which reverses with adequate nutrition. An example of this process is shown in Figure 4–9. Younger alcoholic patients with malnutrition and dehydration may also have reversible MRI abnormalities. On the other hand, long-term severe alcohol abuse is likely to produce irreversible abnormalities. Maternal consumption of large quantities of alcohol during pregnancy may produce the fetal alcohol syndrome, which is characterized by craniofacial anomalies, decreased cerebral size, and sulcal/gyral anomalies such as pachygyria. A brain from a person with fetal alcohol syndrome is shown in Figure 4–10, along with a surface rendered brain from a healthy individual of similar age and sex for comparison. A variety of developmental anomalies may also be seen in individuals with autism.

Recent developments in MRI acquisition and analysis are also pushing this

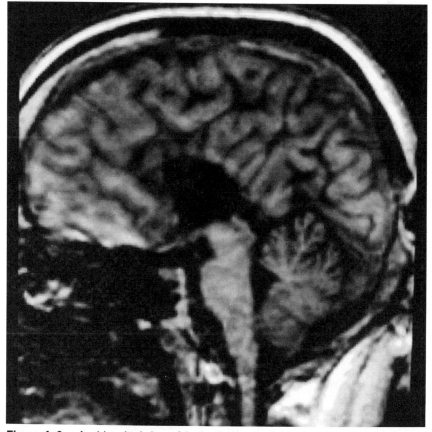

Figure 4–8.   A midsagittal view of the brain of an individual with schizophrenia who has nearly complete agenesis of the corpus callosum.

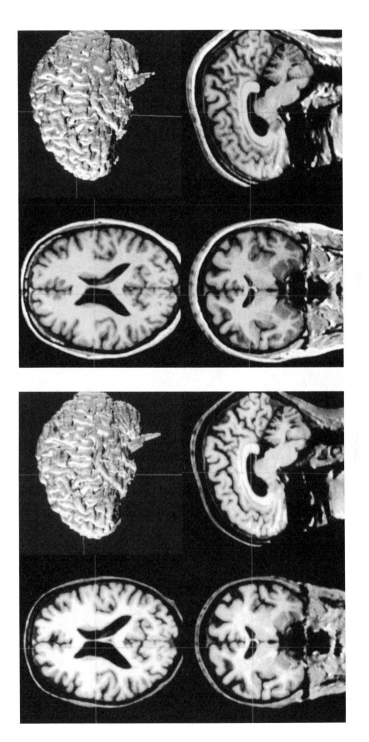

Figure 4–9. A view of the brain surface and its internal contents shown in three orthogonal planes in an individual with anorexia nervosa. The *left* image shows the brain during starvation, whereas the *right* image shows the individual's brain after her weight had returned to normal. Note the reversal of brain shrinkage that occurs with weight normalization.

technology into the realm of functional imaging. Through the use of echo planar imaging and other types of pulse sequences, it is now possible to use MRI to visualize changes in cerebral blood flow in response to various types of perceptual or cognitive challenges. Likewise, MRI spectroscopy is being applied to measure phosphorus, hydrogen, and fluorine spectra, which may provide information about the integrity of membranes or concentrations of drugs in the brain. These functional applications of MRI are currently used solely for research into the pathophysiology of mental illnesses, but clinical applications may eventually be developed.

The indications for ordering a structural imaging technique such as CT or MRI are summarized in Table 4–4. In general, clinicians will want to order one of these procedures when they need to rule out physical causes for the patient's symptoms, such as a tumor or multiple sclerosis. Because of the rather substantial literature supporting the presence of structural abnormalities in schizophrenia, as well as their prognostic significance, it is probably appropriate to obtain a CT or MRI scan in a young individual presenting with his or her first episode of psychosis. These techniques may also be used to monitor progressive loss of tissue in the

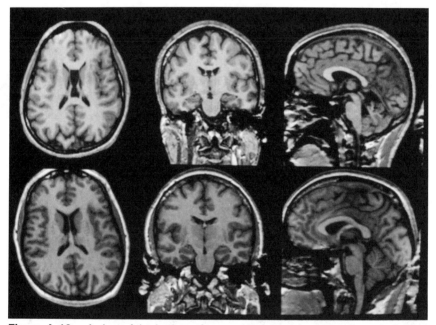

Figure 4–10. A view of the brain surface and its internal contents in an individual with fetal alcohol syndrome *(top)* and in a person of comparable age and gender who did not experience in utero exposure to alcohol *(bottom)*. Note the marked decrease in cerebral size in the person suffering from fetal alcohol syndrome.

Table 4–4. Indications for ordering a computed tomography or magnetic resonance imaging scan

Confusion and/or dementia of unknown cause	History of recent head trauma
	Anorexia nervosa with marked weight loss
First episode of a psychotic disorder of unknown etiology	Alcoholism or other substance abuse disorder with signs or symptoms of cognitive deterioration
First episode of a major affective disorder after age 50 years	
Marked personality change after age 50 years	

dementias, as well as to observe the reversibility of structural changes in conditions such as anorexia nervosa or alcoholism.

As MRI has become increasingly available, physicians are faced with a decision as to whether to order a CT or MRI first. Until recently, the choice was almost invariably CT, largely because of its wide availability and inexpensiveness. Because MRI is a much superior imaging technique, however, it is has begun to supplant CT, particularly for the evaluation of psychiatric populations, in whom a detailed view of brain surface and subcortical regions may be very useful.

Functional Neuroimaging

Functional neuroimaging includes two major modalities: SPECT and PET. Both of these techniques are used to observe regional metabolic functions and dysfunctions in the brain. Currently, SPECT is used primarily to measure regional cerebral blood flow, although applications have also recently been developed to visualize and measure densities of neuroreceptors. PET can currently be used to measure regional blood flow, glucose utilization, and density of neuroreceptors.

The characteristics, strengths, and limitation of these two functional imaging techniques are summarized in Table 4–5. The basic principles of both techniques are the same, in that they involve imaging the regional localization of radioactive isotopes that localize in an area of high functional activity in the brain. In the case of SPECT, the isotopes are single-photon emitters, whereas in the case of PET, the isotopes are positron emitters. The isotopes used in SPECT, such as technetium-99 and iodine-123, are stable and have a relatively long high-life, making them convenient for long-term storage and relatively handy to use. On the other hand, these molecules are not normally present in the human body, and they are relatively difficult to attach to informative compounds to make them suitable as imaging agents. When they are attached, there is some risk that the biological activity of the compound will be changed because of the introduction of the foreign isotope.

Table 4–5.   Comparison of strengths and weaknesses of single photon emission computer tomography (SPECT) versus positron-emission tomography (PET)

	SPECT	PET
Resolution	0.8–2.0 cm	0.3–1.2 cm
Imaging time	10–60 minutes	10–60 minutes
Contraindications	None apart from those associated with radiation exposure	None apart from those associated with radiation exposure
Special strengths	Uses commercially available tracers, low in cost, widely available	Superior resolution, very flexible in applications (e.g., blood flow, glucose metabolism, neuroreceptors)
Special weaknesses	Generally poor resolution, difficult to quantify	Technically very difficult, very expensive
Cost	$300–$500	$1000–$5000

Single photon emission computed tomography.   SPECT studies most typically are done by using a triple-headed or single-headed rotating gamma camera of the sort available in most nuclear medicine departments. Some cameras for dedicated head imaging are currently in development. The dedicated head units tend to give either greater flexibility or improved resolution. Because the blood flow agents such as HMPAO (Ceretec) are commercially available and because the imaging equipment is available in most hospitals, SPECT is an imaging technique that is currently appropriate for evaluating psychiatric patients as needed.

At present, the clinical applications of SPECT as a laboratory test are limited to several areas. SPECT is well suited for documenting the occurrence of stroke, because it provides a direct measure of cerebral blood flow. In addition, SPECT is often diagnostically useful in the differential diagnosis of depression versus dementia in elderly patients. Patients with Alzheimer's disease have a relatively characteristic decrease in cerebral blood flow in posterior temporoparietal regions; this abnormality occurs in 70%–80% of patients with Alzheimer's disease. No specific blood flow abnormality has been observed consistently in depressed patients, although some patients display a generalized decrease in flow, whereas others show more focal right anterior decreases. In any case, however, the flow patterns observed in Alzheimer's disease are relatively distinctive. Thus, when making this particular differential diagnosis, a SPECT scan may provide useful information that is more specific than that obtained from structural images (CT or MRI), because ventricular enlargement and cortical atrophy occur relatively often in elderly healthy individuals as part of the aging process.

Other types of abnormalities occurring in other mental illnesses are currently under study. Patients with HIV-related dementia appear to begin to develop patchy areas of decreased perfusion as the symptoms of dementia begin. Caffeine and nicotine produce generalized decreases in cerebral perfusion, whereas anxiety appears to produce a generalized increase. Receptor blockage with neuroleptics appears to produce increased blood flow in the basal ganglia. A variety of strategies are also being developed to adapt static tracers to the study of cognitive activation; these typically use two sequential injections during a resting or control state and an activated state. The two conditions can be separated from one another either by subtraction or by some other type of postacquisition processing.

Recently new agents have been developed to visualize neuroreceptors such as the D_2 receptor or benzodiazepine receptors. As they are developed further during the coming years, these agents may permit clinicians to monitor the effects of treatment (i.e., the degree of receptor blockade produced by various specific neuroleptics and other drugs) or to determine whether a high degree of receptor upregulation heralds the development of tardive dyskinesia.

Positron-emission tomography.   PET scanning is the second major functional imaging technique. Because of the great expense involved in conducting PET studies, it is less widely available as either a clinical or a research tool. Its cost is based on the fact that the tracers used consist of positrons (positively charged electrons), which must be generated in an on-site cyclotron and which tend to have short half-lives (2 minutes for oxygen-15, 30 minutes for carbon-11, approximately 2 hours for fluorine-18). Nevertheless, because the nonradioactive forms of these tracers are widely present in biological substances, they can more readily be attached to informative molecules and used to study a variety of metabolic, neurochemical, and physiological processes, making PET an extremely powerful research tool and perhaps ultimately a powerful clinical tool as well.

PET scanning became available in a few centers in the middle to late 1970s. Its first applications were to the study of glucose utilization in the brain. Many of the early years of PET work were devoted to developing models for quantitatively measuring glucose utilization with fluorodeoxyglucose (FDG), which is trapped in the brain in the midst of its metabolic pathway, thereby permitting efficient study. Abnormal metabolic patterns of glucose utilization have been observed in a variety of disorders, such as seizures, tumors, stroke, Alzheimer's disease, schizophrenia, bipolar disorder, and obsessive-compulsive disorder. In addition, FDG has been used to map cognitive function and cognitive activation. FDG already has clear clinical applications in the presurgical evaluation of intractable seizures, because it provides more specific focal localization than EEG. The decreased cerebral blood flow in posterior temporoparietal regions observed in Alzheimer's disease with SPECT can also be seen as decreased glucose utilization with PET, making this another current clinical application of PET. Because of the expense involved in doing PET studies, as well as their limited availability, SPECT is likely to be used more frequently for this differential diagnosis.

Other abnormalities have also been observed with PET, using either FDG or other ligands and tracers. As in the case of SPECT, these findings are promising but not definitive. Schizophrenic patients show difficulty activating their frontal lobes, bipolar patients show switches from high glucose utilization during mania to low glucose utilization during depression, and obsessive-compulsive patients have hypermetabolic activity in both their prefrontal cortex and their basal ganglia. Increased areas of cerebral blood flow have been observed in the hippocampal regions in individuals with panic attacks. Schizophrenic patients with tardive dyskinesia may have hypermetabolic activity in their basal ganglia, whereas patients with Parkinson's disease show decreased activity. When these various findings, now typically reported from a single research center, have been consistently replicated, PET may also move into the diagnostic arena in psychiatry.

Studies using ^{15}O-labeled H_2O, a tracer with a very short half-life, have also been used to examine the components of mental activities such as learning and memory, language, and attention. Because oxygen-15 has a half-life of approximately 2 minutes, it can be used to measure cerebral blood flow in repeated back-to-back studies. As many as 8–10 studies can be completed in a single individual within a 2-hour period. Because each person is his or her own control, experimental noise due to individual variation is reduced. A mental activity can be divided into component parts, such as long-term versus short-term memory or memory for words versus memory for faces. This technology is currently being used to map cognitive processes in healthy individuals and to determine the extent to which cognitive processing is disturbed in patients who have mental illnesses. Evidence to date most strongly supports disruptions in frontal circuitry in schizophrenia and perhaps in mood disorders as well.

Another major application of PET is to the study of the neurochemical systems within the brain. To date, this study has involved the labeling of neuroreceptors. Because this application of PET is somewhat more technically difficult, most of the developmental work in this area occurred after the FDG model had been well established. Thus, the study of neurotransmitter systems in the human brain with PET is a young but rapidly growing field. This application of PET can be used both to study the distribution of neurochemical systems in the human brain and to seek specific abnormalities (either increases or decreases in function) in specific disorders. Quantitative models have been developed to measure receptor density. For example, methods have already been developed to measure the receptor density (B_{max}) of D_2 receptors by using either raclopride or spiperone. These techniques have been used to demonstrate the differences in binding affinity (K_d) for different classes of neuroleptics and have also shown that nearly complete receptor occupancy occurs within hours after neuroleptic administration, indicating that the therapeutic effect (which typically lags by several weeks) involves a downstream neurochemical process.

Although methods for studying transmitter synthesis and metabolism are technically more difficult, these too are in the process of development. Thus, during the next decade, PET will almost certainly be applied extensively to the visualization and measurement of neurochemical systems in the healthy human brain and in the brains of patients who have major mental illness and neurological diseases.

Neuroendocrine Techniques

Some mental illnesses, such as depression or the anxiety disorders, have a variety of symptoms that suggest some type of neuroendocrinological abnormality. Just as frontal lobe tumor or TLE is important in the differential diagnosis of schizophrenia (thereby suggesting the importance of frontal and temporal abnormalities in that illness), so too adrenal and thyroid diseases provide important differential diagnoses for depression and anxiety disorders. Depression, in particular, has many symptoms suggestive of chronobiological dysregulation: insomnia, anorexia, and disrupted diurnal variation.

This recognition has been supported by nearly three decades of research in neuropsychoendocrinology. This research necessarily confronted many difficult methodological problems, because of the well-recognized effects of stress on the endocrine system and the resultant difficulty in separating cause from effect. Nevertheless, a picture has emerged suggesting that some patients with major mental illnesses show clear neuroendocrine abnormalities.

One specific laboratory test that developed out of this research is the dexamethasone suppression test (DST) to assist in the diagnosis of depression. When the DST is used as a laboratory test, typically 1 mg of dexamethasone is given at 11 P.M., and blood samples are drawn the next day at 8 A.M., 4 P.M., and 11 P.M. If the patient breaks through the dexamethasone suppression, displaying a serum cortisol level above 5 μg/dl, the test is considered to be positive. Approximately 40% of depressed patients have a positive ("abnormal") DST; unfortunately, positive DSTs are seen in a variety of other conditions, such as anorexia nervosa or other disorders characterized by weight loss. Thus, although psychiatrists for a time hoped that they might have a relatively sensitive and specific laboratory test for severe depression, this is clearly not the case. Nevertheless, a DST may at times be useful to the psychiatrist confronting a difficult differential diagnosis, particularly when other causes of an abnormal DST, such as weight loss, have been excluded. The DST may also sometimes be useful as a prognostic indicator; depressed patients who have an abnormal DST at the onset of treatment and who fail to convert to a normal test after responding to treatment are more likely to relapse quickly.

IQ Testing

IQ testing is a relatively simple "laboratory test" that has been used in psychiatry for many years. Generally, IQ testing is done with one of two standard tests: the Wechsler Adult Intelligence Scale—Revised (WAIS-R) and the Wechsler Intelligence Scale for Children—Revised (WISC-R). Both of these tests are revisions developed in 1981 and 1974, respectively, based on earlier tests developed by David Wechsler in the 1940s and 1950s.

These tests consist of 11 subscales, summarized in Table 4–6. Six of these tests measure verbal abilities, whereas five are considered to be performance tests. These tests are well normed, and the scoring has been devised so that the average individual will achieve a score of 100.

Although the WAIS-R and the WISC-R are frequently referred to as intelligence tests, and are indeed used to generate verbal, performance, and full-scale IQs, their most powerful application is to observe the patterning of intellectual abilities that is reflected by the 11 subtests. Most psychiatrically normal individuals tend to have similar scores on all tests. Individuals who have various psychopathological conditions can show a variety of deviations from this pattern. For example, with normal aging, scores on the verbal items tend to remain relatively high, whereas scores on the performance items tend to decline; these are sometimes referred to as "hold" and "don't hold" tests because of their characteristic changes with aging. If an elderly individual shows poor performance on both the verbal and the performance tests to a degree inconsistent with his or her past education, this pattern of findings is consistent with the diagnosis of dementia.

Table 4–6.   Subscales of the Wechsler Adult Intelligence Scale—Revised

Verbal tests	Performance tests
Information	Picture completion
Digit span	Picture arrangement
Vocabulary	Block design
Arithmetic	Object assembly
Comprehension	Digit symbol
Similarities	

Because motivation, attention, and effort are an important part of IQ testing, however, poor performance may be relatively nonspecific. A depressed individual may also perform poorly on the verbal tests due to disinterest and apathy, although typically these tests are affected less by depression than the performance tests.

IQ testing can also be quite helpful in evaluating children and adolescents. It may provide some index to specific intellectual deficits that may be interfering with the child's capacity to perform well in school. Again, erratic patterns are particularly helpful in assessment. For example, children with specific learning disabilities may be performing very poorly in school and yet have normal or even high intelligence, indicating that they have the basic intellectual capacity to perform at a normal or high level if the specific learning handicaps can be minimized (e.g., reading disability, mathematics disability). Children with conduct disorders typically have higher scores on the performance tests than on the verbal tests.

Personality Testing

The most widely used personality test is the Minnesota Multiphasic Personality Inventory (MMPI), developed in the 1940s. The MMPI generates scores on nine scales: hypochondriasis, depression, hysteria, psychopathic deviance, masculinity/femininity, paranoia, psychasthenia (or anxiety), schizophrenia, and mania.

This test was developed empirically, with the original intent of creating a measure of psychopathology. A list of symptom items was generated and then given to individuals diagnosed with the various conditions that the scales measure. Psychiatrically normal individuals were also assessed. If groups of patients with a specific condition such as paranoia assented to specific items to a degree that differentiated them significantly from psychiatrically normal individuals, those items were considered to be markers for that diagnosis. For example, patients diagnosed as having schizophrenia often answered "yes" on the item "I sometimes think about things too terrible to mention."

Although the MMPI was originally developed to aid in diagnosis, its widest use at present is more descriptive than diagnostic. As in the case of the WAIS, clinicians can learn much more by looking at profiles and patterns than they can by looking at a single peak. Thus, for example, a patient who is depressed may indeed score high on the depression scale, but a high score on the psychasthenia scale may suggest that the patient's depressive symptoms are largely neurotic and likely to be chronic. High scores on scales 1 and 3 (hypochondriasis and hysteria) coupled with a low score on scale 2 (depression) are consistent with acting-out personality disorders that are likely to be difficult to treat psychotherapeutically because the patient lacks the capacity to feel depression. Patients who score high on the hysteria, psychopathic deviance, and mania scales are also likely to have difficult personality problems that may be consistent with borderline personality disorder.

Although the MMPI is the most widely used personality inventory, several others have also been developed. The Cattell-16 PF was developed as a more pure personality test, because it did not attempt to base its profiles on individuals with diagnosed psychopathology. Rather, a variety of psychiatrically normal individuals were evaluated by using a preselected set of items. Subsequently, the items were subjected to factor analysis, yielding a profile consisting of 16 personality factors. The Eysenck Personality Inventory, a more modest instrument, was also developed through factor analysis. It measures the dimensions of introversion, extraversion, and neuroticism. Although the Cattell-16 PF and the Eysenck Personality Inventory are sometimes used in personality research, the MMPI remains the most widely used instrument in clinical settings.

Neuropsychological Testing

Neuropsychological testing was developed as a method for assessing cognitive deficits believed to be neurally based. Originally, as was the case for the MMPI and the WAIS, batteries were developed in the hope that they would assist in making a specific diagnosis. The premier example is the Halstead-Reitan Neuropsychological Test Battery, originally developed to assist in the differential diagnosis of dementia and specific neurological conditions. Again, it has become increasingly clear that no single test can bear the burden of making specific diagnoses that clinicians themselves find difficult to make. Thus, the area of neuropsychology has also turned recently toward the goal of examining profiles and patterns and attempting to identify specific kinds of abnormality.

Increasingly, neuropsychology attempts to assess a variety of specific cognitive functions, such as memory, attention, and fluency of thinking. A clinician assessing patients neuropsychologically will tailor the assessment to the types of problems that the specific patient is having to try to identify whether a specific area of deficit is present.

For example, a group of tests is available to assess aphasia. These evaluate the patient's capacity to comprehend verbal and written information, to follow commands, to process syntactically versus semantically, and to speak fluently. When a comprehensive assessment for aphasia is completed, the clinician can define the patient's specific areas of deficit. For example, he or she will be able to indicate that the patient has impaired fluency of expression and poor syntactic expression, but with intact syntactic comprehension, a pattern consistent with a posterior frontal lesion.

In addition, a variety of specific neuropsychological tests are often used to assess other specific aspects of mental functions. Some of the most common, categorized according to the function they are thought to assess most prominently, are described below.

Attention
Attention may be impaired in dementia, psychotic disorders, or a variety of other mental illnesses, including mood disorders.

Continuous Performance Test.   The Continuous Performance Test (CPT) is perhaps the most widely used test of attention currently available. The CPT was originally developed to detect deficits in sustained alertness in patients with brain damage. A number of different versions of this test are available, but most involve attentional tasks in which patients observe series of letters or numbers that are presented very briefly one at a time with a relatively short interval in between, and the subject is asked to press a button each time a predesignated target stimulus appears in a random series.

Trails A and B.   These tests are widely used components of the Halstead-Reitan Neuropsychological Test Battery used to assess attention and sequencing. The individual is asked to connect items in a series (e.g., A to 1, B to 2) from among items randomly selected on a page.

Executive Functions
These functions are considered to be "higher cortical functions" and involve decision making, planning, and changing strategies for abstraction or conceptualizing. They are particularly likely to be impaired in patients with dementia, but they may also be impaired in schizophrenic patients. Although abnormalities may be noted in the mood disorders, they are likely to be reversible.

Wisconsin Card Sorting Test.   This test is widely regarded as an important test for assessing problem-solving abilities and the capacity to alter response set. The test involves sorting cards according to color, shape, or number. Intermittently, the individual is corrected while using a sorting strategy and at that point must recognize that he or she needs to shift response set.

Stroop Test.   This test also assesses the individual's capacity to shift response set, as well as testing his or her attention and mental control.

Porteus Mazes.   This is a standard maze test, in which the ability of the subject to plan is challenged by the task of figuring out a path between the entrance and exit of a maze.

Tower of London.   This is a planning task, which requires the subject to develop a strategy for moving balls lined up on sticks from an initial position to a final goal position.

Fluency

Many patients with schizophrenia or depression have an impairment in their ability to generate spontaneous ideas or activities. Important clinical correlates are symptoms such as alogia and avolition. Several tests are used to assess fluency, which is also often considered to be a "frontal" function.

Controlled Oral Word Association Test.   This test assesses the subject's verbal fluency by providing probes, such as asking the subject to name as many words as possible that start with the letter D. This test has been widely used as part of the Multilingual Aphasia Examination.

Category Fluency Test.   This task assesses the subject's fluency by asking him or her to name as many words as possible that belong to a specific semantic category (e.g., animals, fruits, vegetables). One minute is allowed for each category.

Verbal Memory

Because verbal memory is an important temporolimbic function, it may be important to assess its dimensions in patients with a variety of mental illnesses, especially dementia.

Logical Memory (Wechsler Memory Scale).   This memory task involves having the subject listen to a coherent story and then recall as many details of the story as possible. Both immediate and delayed recall is assessed.

Rey Auditory Verbal Learning Test.   This test involves determining the subject's capacity to learn a list of words by rote. Both immediate memory and delayed recall are assessed. A learning curve is also established.

Paired Associate Learning.   This somewhat more complicated memory task asks the subject to learn a list of words that are associated with a cue set of words (e.g., metal-iron, baby-cries).

Visual Reconstructive Memory

The following tests of visual reconstructive memory are frequently considered to assess right-hemisphere function.

Rey-Osterreith Complex Figure.   This task involves showing a complex figure to the subject, having him or her copy it, and having him or her draw it again from memory immediately and after a delay. Although this task is somewhat difficult to administer, it can be given in a reliable and standardized way by giving the subject colored pencils in a set sequence.

Benton Visual Retention Test.   This widely used test examines the ability to copy and recall a variety of figures and shapes. (See Figure 4–11 for an illustration of one of the figures that the subject is asked to remember and draw.)

Motor Function

It may be important to assess motor function in patients with mental illnesses, both because motor slowness may be a correlate of some diagnoses such as depression and because of the motor side effects of neuroleptic medications.

The Finger Oscillation Test.   This test measures tapping speed with the left and right hands. It gives a measure of overall motor speed as well as an assessment of lateral asymmetries in motor performance.

Purdue Pegboard.   This test was developed to assess manual dexterity. Fine motor performance is assessed with the right hand, the left hand, and then both hands simultaneously. It provides a useful measure of lateralization.

Clinical Utility of Neuropsychological Tests

When a grouping of neuropsychological tests such as those described above is administered to an individual, the clinician obtains some sense of the person's overall patterns of abilities and deficits. Patients who have psychosis or depression often have a generalized impairment on all tests, although patients with schizophrenia may have specific regional deficits (e.g., frontal lobe deficits) depending on their symptoms. Tests of verbal versus visual memory can be used to compare left-hemisphere versus right-hemisphere function and to isolate patterns of abnormality within a single hemisphere. Tests of memory are particularly useful in evaluating dementia versus depression. Although depressed patients may score somewhat poorly on all tests due to a lack of interest and motivation, they typically do not have highly selective memory deficits. Following a patient's performance on these tests over time may also assist in diagnosis, because an improvement in performance accompanied by a clinical improve-

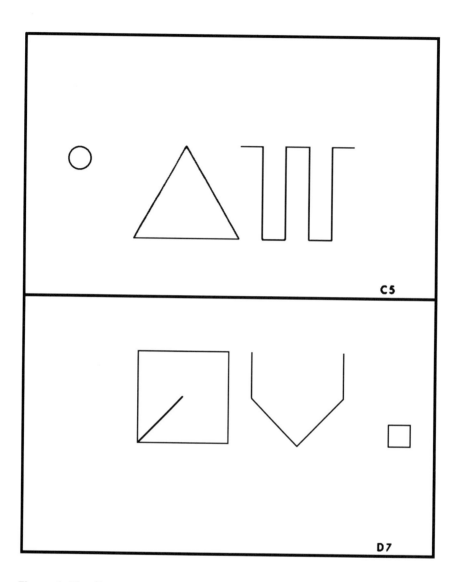

Figure 4–11.   Examples of figures that patients are asked to copy and recall using the Benton Visual Retention Test.

ment in symptoms is supportive of the diagnosis of a reversible mental disorder, such as depression (as opposed to a dementia, where a progressive course would be expected).

Bibliography

American Psychiatric Association Task Force on Laboratory Tests in Psychiatry: The dexamethasone suppression test: an overview of its current status in psychiatry. Am J Psychiatry 144:1253–1262, 1987

Anastasi A: Psychological Testing. London, Macmillan, 1968

Andreasen NC: Brain imaging: applications in psychiatry. Science 239:1381–1388, 1988

Andreasen NC (ed): Brain Imaging: Applications in Psychiatry. Washington, DC, American Psychiatric Press, 1989

Andreasen NC: Brain imaging, in American Psychiatric Press Review of Psychiatry, Vol 12. Edited by Oldham JM, Riba MB, Tasman A. Washington DC: American Psychiatric Press, 1993, pp 309–511

Carroll BJ: The dexamethasone suppression test for melancholia. Br J Psychiatry 140:292–304, 1982

Elster AD (ed): Magnetic Resonance Imaging: A Reference Guide and Atlas. Philadelphia, PA, JB Lippincott, 1986

Gold PW, Goodwin FK, Chrousos GP: Clinical and biochemical manifestations of depression: relation to the neurobiology of stress, Part 1. N Engl J Med 319:348–353, 1988

Gold PW, Goodwin FK, Chrousos GP: Clinical and biochemical manifestations of depression: relation to the neurobiology of stress, Part 2. N Engl J Med 319:413–420, 1988

Heilman KM, Valenstein E: Clinical Neuropsychology. New York, Oxford University Press, 1979

Kooi KA: Fundamentals of Electroencephalography. New York, Harper & Row, 1971

Krishnan KRR, Manepalli AN, Ritchie JC, et al: Growth hormone-releasing factor stimulation test in depression. Am J Psychiatry 145:90–92, 1988

Kupfer DJ, Thase ME: The use of the sleep laboratory in the diagnosis of affective disorders. Psychiatr Clin North Am 5:3–25, 1983

Lavine RA: Neurophysiology: The Fundamentals. Lexington, MA, DC Heath, 1983

Lezak MD: Neuropsychological Assessment. New York, Oxford University Press, 1983

Nemeroff CB: The role of corticotropin-releasing factor in the pathogenesis of major depression. Pharmacopsychiatry 21:76–82, 1988

Phelps ME, Mazziotta JC, Schelbert HR: Positron Emission Tomography and Autoradiography Principles and Applications for the Brain and Heart. New York, Raven, 1986

Reynolds CF, Kupfer DJ: Sleep research in affective illness: state of the art circa 1987. Sleep 10:199–215, 1987

Ribeiro SCM, Tandon R, Gruenhaus L, et al: The DST as a predictor of outcome in depression: a meta-analysis. Am J Psychiatry 150:1618–1629, 1993

Salamon G, Huang YP: Computed Tomography of the Brain. Berlin, Springer-Verlag, 1980

Self-Assessment Questions

1. What are some of the conditions that must be considered in the differential diagnosis of serious mental illnesses? Describe ways in which laboratory tests can be used in ruling out these disorders.

2. Describe the workup usually required before ECT.

3. Describe some special techniques that may be necessary to enhance the power of EEG, particularly to detect seizure foci deep within the brain. What is polysomnography? What is BEAM?

4. Describe some applications of structural imaging techniques such as CT scanning or MRI to the study of mental illnesses such as schizophrenia. Why must the clinician carefully specify the question that he or she is asking before ordering an MRI scan?

5. What is *functional neuroimaging?* Describe some applications of functional neuroimaging to the evaluation of psychiatric patients.

6. What is the most widely used test to assess personality? What are its major clinical applications?

7. What is *neuropsychological testing?* Enumerate four different neuropsychological tests, and describe the cognitive functions that they are designed to evaluate.

Chapter 5

The Neurobiology of Mental Illness

Men ought to know that from the brain, and from the brain only, arise our pleasures, joys, laughter, and jests, as well as our sorrows, pains, griefs, and fears. Through it, in particular, we think, see, hear . . .

Hippocrates

Both historically and conceptually, psychiatry grows from the soil of neurobiology. Its fruits are the improved understanding and treatment of the aberrations in thinking, behavior, and emotions that characterize mental illnesses. These fruits are only able to mature, however, as they reach back to their roots in neuroscience. We will only be able to understand how and why we think, hear, and feel if we understand how our brains work.

Psychiatry as a discipline begins with abnormal behavior. Its understanding of abnormal behavior is dependent on the understanding of the mechanisms of normal behavior. Normal behavior must be understood in turn as a consequence of functional brain systems that mediate language, perception, memory, attention, and other cognitive systems. These functional brain systems are more or less "hardwired" in the normal adult brain, although they are plastic and dynamic in the young developing brain.

The functional systems are the product of a set of neural systems or networks that communicate with one another electrically and chemically. Although the circuits within these neural networks may also be more or less hardwired in the mature adult brain, in that long tracts and connections are established, the neurochemical circuits of the brain appear to be highly adaptable and subject to multiple modulatory influences and feedback loops. These neural circuits are in turn composed of cells, and the cells communicate with one another through chemical messengers such as dopamine, which in turn communicate through second-messenger systems. Instructions for synthesizing and metabolizing the molecular messengers of the mind are coded in the neuron's DNA within its nucleus, as are instructions for synthesizing the complex proteins that form the receptors embedded in cell membranes that serve as transducers for the molecular messengers. During the past several years, many of these receptors have been cloned, opening up the possibility that we can improve the medications that modulate brain chemistry.

Thus, psychiatry stretches from mind to molecule and from clinical neurobiology to molecular neurobiology as it attempts to understand how aberrations in behavior are rooted in underlying biological mechanisms. Abnormalities in DNA can be studied directly through the developing techniques of molecular biology and molecular genetics, whereas the genetic transmission of illnesses within families must be determined through clinical assessment of affected and unaffected individuals. This process brings us back full circle from the molecule to the mind and from the laboratory to the clinic.

This chapter provides a selective overview of a few topics from neurobiology that are relevant to the study of mental illnesses. During the past several decades, neuroscience has grown to become one of the largest domains of contemporary scientific research. Many aspects of neuroscience are relevant to the study of psychiatry. This chapter highlights a few aspects that are relevant to understanding either symptoms or treatment.

Anatomical and Functional Brain Systems

The human brain can be divided into various systems that mediate many different cognitive, emotional, and perceptual functions, such as the motor system, the visual system, the auditory system, and the somatosensory cortical system. The systems of special interest to psychiatry are those representing circuitry or functions that are particularly disturbed in mental illnesses. These systems represent some of the last frontiers in the study of the human brain. Three important anatomical systems are the prefrontal system, the limbic system, and the basal ganglia system. Important functional systems include memory, language, attention, and "executive functions."

Any method for dividing the brain into parts or systems is somewhat arbitrary. The three anatomical systems are all interconnected and work interactively. The functional systems are also highly interdependent with one another and with the prefrontal, limbic, and basal ganglia systems as well. Further, the division of the brain into functional and anatomical systems and neurochemical systems is also arbitrary. These oversimplifications are introduced purely for conceptual convenience, providing a strategy for reducing the overwhelming complexity of the central nervous system to a level that permits discussion and analysis. Ultimately, however, a full understanding of the brain can only be gained by an ongoing process of analysis (or breakdown and simplification) and synthesis (or rebuilding and unifying).

In addition to the above words of caution about the temptations of oversimplification, a word of caution about our existing level of ignorance must be added. We do not yet have a complete map of the human brain, summarizing accurately its various neural circuits, chemical anatomy, and functional specialization and interaction. Just as molecular biologists are striving to map the human genome, neuroscientists are working to map the human brain. This process is ongoing and not likely to be complete for many years. The process is, however, becoming much more sophisticated, particularly with the aid of neuroimaging techniques such as magnetic resonance imaging (MRI) and positron-emission tomography (PET), which permit in vivo study of the anatomy and physiology of the human brain in ways that were previously impossible. Before the availability of neuroimaging, our knowledge about circuitry and functional systems was based primarily on lesion and postmortem studies. Directly visualizing how the brain performs mental work during a PET imaging procedure is clearly more accurate than trying to infer indirectly how it works by observing what it cannot do when parts are missing.

The Prefrontal System and "Executive Functions"

The prefrontal system, or prefrontal cortex, is one of the largest cortical subregions in the human brain. Brodmann estimated that it constitutes 29% of the cortex in humans, compared to 17% in chimpanzees, 7% in dogs, and 3.5% in cats. The relative development of the prefrontal cortex in various animal species is shown in Figure 5–1.

Because of the extraordinary development of the prefrontal cortex in humans, its function has been a focus of both speculation and investigation for many years. The lesion method provided an early landmark in our understanding of the prefrontal cortex through the case of Phineas Gage, a quarry worker who was accidentally injured by an explosion that drove an iron bar through his left frontal lobe. Gage survived the bizarre accident, but he sustained major personality changes, which were originally described by Harlow. Before the accident,

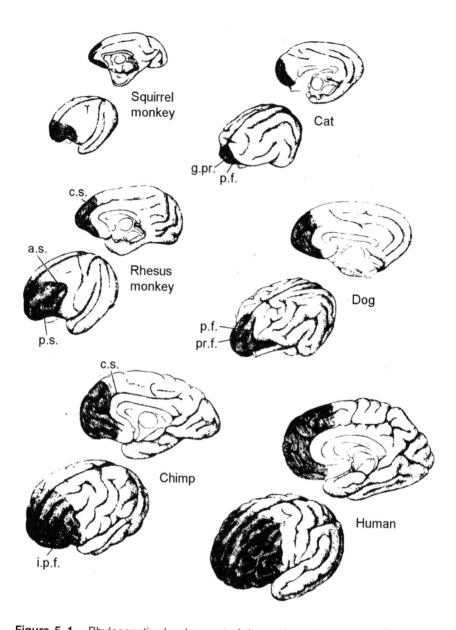

Figure 5–1. Phylogenetic development of the prefrontal cortex. a.s. = arcuate sulcus. c.s. = cingulate sulcus. g.pr. = gyrus proreus. i.p.f. = inferior precentral fissure. p.f. = presylvian fissure. pr.f. = proreal fissure. p.s. = principal sulcus. Reprinted with permission from Fuster JM (ed): *The Prefrontal Cortex: Anatomy, Physiology, and Neuropsychology of the Frontal Lobes,* 2nd Edition. New York, Raven, 1989.

Gage was conscientious, serious, and hardworking, but after the accident, he became immature, childlike, socially inappropriate, and irresponsible. This early initial report has been supplemented by a substantial literature based on studies of patients with frontal lobe tumors, traumatic injuries to the frontal lobes, and surgical treatments for epilepsy, psychosis, and obsessive-compulsive disorder. This work clearly indicates that substantial damage to the prefrontal cortex typically produces a syndrome quite similar to that of Gage. Although gross intelligence is not necessarily impaired by frontal lobe lesions (and actually may be improved in patients with severe psychosis), individuals with substantial frontal lobe injury lose other capacities such as volition, the ability to plan, and social judgment.

These clinical studies of humans have been supplemented during recent years by substantial neurophysiological studies of nonhuman primates, using techniques of neurophysiology, neuroanatomy, and neurochemistry. Primate studies have reinforced the conclusions from the earlier clinical work, indicating that the prefrontal cortex subserves a variety of major functions that permit us to integrate information from a variety of sources, to plan and make decisions, and to generate new thoughts and ideas.

The prefrontal cortex is a massive association cortex receiving connections from all over the brain. An oversimplified schematic "wiring diagram" of its multiple connections is shown in Figure 5–2. Although the prefrontal cortex has been defined in a variety of ways, perhaps the most widely accepted definition is based on its thalamic connections. According to this definition, the *prefrontal cortex* is defined as the anterior (or rostral) brain region that receives projections from the medial dorsal nucleus of the thalamus. This definition identifies more or less homologous brain regions across a variety of species. In primates, the morphological boundaries are the arcuate sulcus, the inferior precentral sulcus, and the anterior cingulate gyrus. The cortical region thus defined typically has six layers, with pyramidal cells in layers three and five and granular cortex in layer four. In the more posterior (or caudal) portions of the prefrontal cortex, however, layer four becomes transitional.

The interconnections of the prefrontal cortex provide some clues about its functions. The medial dorsal thalamic projections have two components: magnocellular and parvicellular. The magnocellular component projects principally to the orbital and medial portions of the prefrontal cortex, and the parvicellular component projects to the dorsolateral portion of the prefrontal cortex. These different projections appear to be related to differences in function in these two parts of the prefrontal cortex. Two quite different types of frontal syndromes have been observed. Lesions to the orbital region of the prefrontal cortex tend to produce euphoria, hyperkinesis, and inappropriate social behavior, whereas lesions

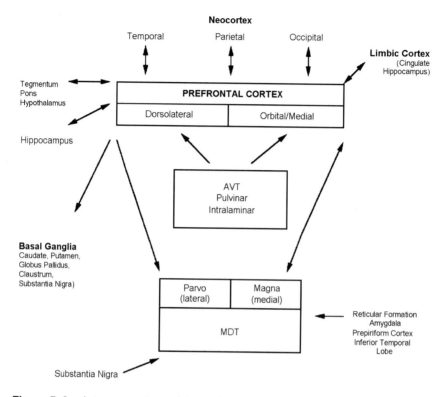

Figure 5–2. Interconnections of the prefrontal cortex. AVT = anterior ventral thalamus. MDT = medial dorsal thalamus. Copyright 1986 Nancy C. Andreasen.

to the dorsolateral portion produce apathy, hypokinesis, and impairment in cognitive performance.

The prefrontal cortex has reciprocal connections with most other parts of the neocortex, including somatic, auditory, and visual regions, suggesting that the prefrontal cortex is responsible for integrating information from a variety of sensory modalities. It also has direct reciprocal connections with the hippocampus and amygdala, indicating that it may play some role in integrating learning and memory. In addition, it has reciprocal connections with three other thalamic nuclei (anterior ventral, intralaminar, and pulvinar) and to the tegmentum, pons, substantia nigra, and septal area. Although these connections are reciprocal, the prefrontal cortex is the only cortical region that sends direct projections to the hypothalamus and septal regions, suggesting a major role for the prefrontal cortex in the regulation of limbic functions (whatever they may be!). In addition, the orbitomedial portion of the prefrontal cortex sends direct, and unreciprocated, projections to the basal ganglia (caudate, putamen, globus pallidus, claustrum, and substantia nigra). These projections appear to be excitatory (i.e., glutaminergic); because of the possible importance of the dopamine-rich basal ganglia in mediating the symptoms of psychosis, as well as in the development of side effects to long-term neuroleptic treatment such as tardive dyskinesia, this particular set of efferent fibers may suggest the mechanism by which the prefrontal cortex could interact with the basal ganglia to produce psychotic symptoms.

The above survey of anatomical connections suggests some of the functions of the prefrontal cortex. It is clearly a huge association region in the brain that integrates input from much of the neocortex, limbic regions, hypothalamic and brain stem regions, and (via the thalamus) most of the rest of the brain. Its high degree of development in humans suggests that it may mediate a variety of specifically human functions often referred to as executive functions, such as high-order abstract thought, creative problem solving, and the temporal sequencing of behavior.

Lesion and trauma studies, supplemented by experimental studies in nonhuman primates, have substantially added to this view of the functions of the prefrontal cortex. It is now clear that the prefrontal cortex mediates a large variety of functions, including attention and perception, motility, temporal integration, and affect and emotion. Lesions to the prefrontal cortex can produce lowering of awareness, sensory neglect, distractibility, disorders of visual search and gaze control, difficulty in concentrating, hyperkinesis or hypokinesis (depending on the site of the lesion), difficulty in planning and completing sequential acts, difficulty in organizing speech, defective memory, defective control of interference, defective planning, and abnormalities in affect (apathy or euphoria).

Depending on the site of the lesion, some features may predominate, suggesting some specialization in the organization of the prefrontal cortex. Orbital medial lesions produce the "euphoric syndrome," characterized by sporadically hypomanic affect, hyperactivity, distractibility, emotional shallowness, childish humor, antisocial behavior, and disinhibition of sexual drive and other basic instinctual drives. Dorsolateral lesions, on the other hand, tend to produce an "apathetic syndrome" characterized by impoverished affect, hypokinesis, inattentiveness, decreased drive and initiative, impoverished speech, "pseudodepression," and impaired capacity to generate abstract concepts. Within both of these syndromes, however, lies a common core: impairment in the capacity to pursue goal-directed behavior based on the integration of environmental and internal cues. Most investigators believe that this function is the basic one pursued in the prefrontal cortex.

The intactness of the prefrontal cortex can be assessed by a variety of cognitive tasks, and it has been explored through neuroimaging as well. The Wisconsin Card Sorting Test, which assesses the capacity to think abstractly and to shift response set, and the Tower of London or Porteus Mazes, which assess the capacity to plan ahead, are three standard frontal lobe tests in neuropsychology. The Continuous Performance Test (CPT) is a measure of attention that is also thought to tap prefrontal cortical functioning.

Several of these tests have been explored with neuroimaging and shown (at least in some individuals) to produce frontal lobe activation. Because of the close resemblance between the apathetic syndrome and the negative symptoms of schizophrenia, investigators have proposed that some patients with schizophrenia might show "hypofrontality," a finding that has been supported in some (but not all) studies with both single photon emission computed tomography (SPECT) and PET. Patients with obsessive-compulsive disorder, which is characterized by excessive planning and overabstractness of thought, have been shown in PET studies to be hyperfrontal.

The Limbic System

The word *limbic* comes from the Latin *limbus* (border). This term was first used by Broca to refer to the circular ring of tissue that appears to "hem" the prefrontal, parietal, and occipital neocortex when the brain is viewed from a midsagittal perspective. (He also called it the "great lobe of the hem.") Because the olfactory nerve is connected to both the superior (septal region) and inferior (uncus, amygdala) portions of this reverse-**C**–shaped group of structures in the center of the brain, it was also known for a time as the *rhinencephalon* (nose brain). Cytoarchitectonic maps also revealed that the cellular structure in these regions was paleocortex rather than neocortex.

The function of this "primitive" central brain region was assumed to be related to olfaction until the 1930s, when James Papez proposed another alternative. He introduced the idea of the *Papez circuit,* which is illustrated in Figure 5–3. He suggested that the major input to this circuit was not the olfactory portion of the brain, but rather a group of association cortices that collected information from a variety of neocortical regions and then relayed this information to the Papez circuit in the limbic system. Papez suggested that the major function of this brain region was to experience and regulate emotion. Within the circuit, messages would flow from higher cortical regions to the cingulate gyrus, hippocampus, amygdala, mamillary bodies, and anterior thalamus. Papez suggested that emotions were concentrated in deeper structures such as the hippocampus, whereas awareness of them occurred in the cingulate gyrus.

The work of Papez was subsequently supplemented by that of Paul MacLean, Walle Nauta, and many others. There is still no consensus as to what constitutes a clear definition of the limbic system or of its components. As in other brain

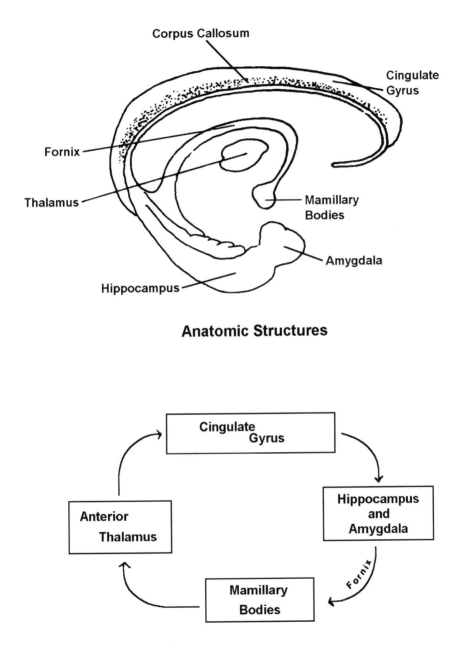

Anatomic Structures

The Papez Circuit

Figure 5-3. The limbic system as conceptualized by Papez. Copyright 1984 Nancy C. Andreasen.

systems, boundaries can be defined on the basis of cytoarchitectonics, inter-connections, or inputs. Nauta proposed, as a unifying concept, that the various structures in the limbic system share circuitry that connects them to the hypo-thalamus. He pointed out that the interconnections between the hypothalamus (via the mammillary bodies), the amygdala, the hippocampus, and the cingulate gyrus are reciprocal. The hypothalamus collects visceral sensory signals from the spinal cord and brain stem; input also comes to this circuit through two major neocortical association regions, the prefrontal cortex and the inferior temporal association cortex.

The functions of the limbic system are also uncertain, although clearly of great importance to the understanding of human emotion and psychological ex-perience. The various interconnections suggest functions related to integrating visceral sensation and the experience of the external environment through mul-tiple modalities (e.g., visual, sensory, auditory). On the basis of lesion studies (described below in the section entitled "The Memory System"), it has been believed for many years that the amygdala and the hippocampus mediate aspects of learning and memory. Thus, references to past experiences may also occur within the limbic system. Amygdala lesions in particular appear to lead to fear-fulness and suspiciousness, suggesting that this region may play some role in the development of paranoia.

The symptoms and subjective experiences of patients with temporal lobe epilepsy may also provide some clues to the functions of this region. Such pa-tients experience a variety of phenomena, including olfactory or gustatory hallu-cinations, déjà vu, derealization, and depersonalization. They also perform repetitive motoric acts that may be highly complex and that appear to rely on procedural memory. Patients with temporal lobe epilepsy have an increased rate of psychosis, and temporal lobe epilepsy is often considered to be a crude neuro-logical model for the psychotic syndromes.

The Basal Ganglia

At first impression it might seem that the basal ganglia have no relevance to psychiatry. The usual concept of the basal ganglia is that they primarily regulate and mediate motor activity. For a variety of reasons, however, it appears likely that the basal ganglia may also play a major role in the expression and regulation of emotion and cognition.

The major structures of the basal ganglia include the caudate, putamen, and globus pallidus, which are shown schematically in Figure 5–4. A triplanar view of the caudate and other basal ganglia structures, as seen on MRI scan, is shown in Figure 5–5. The substantia nigra, located in the midbrain, is not visualized.

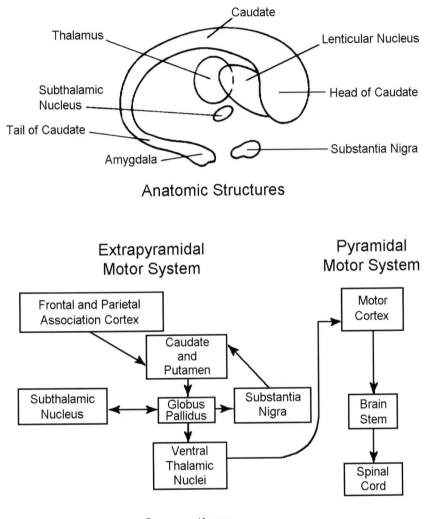

Anatomic Structures

Connections

Figure 5–4. Interconnections of the basal ganglia. Reprinted with permission from Andreasen NC: The Broken Brain: The Biological Revolution in Psychiatry. New York, Harper & Row, 1984, p 105. Copyright 1984 Nancy C. Andreasen.

The caudate is a C-shaped mass of gray matter tissue that has its head at the lateral anterior borders of the frontal horns of the ventricles. It arches back posteriorly in a circular fashion and then curls forward again, ending in the amygdala bilaterally. Separated from it, and lateral to it, is the lentiform nucleus, so called because it is shaped like a lens. The medial portion of the lentiform nucleus,

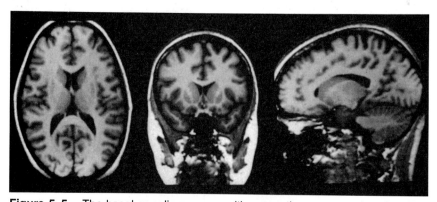

Figure 5–5.   The basal ganglia as seen with magnetic resonance imaging. The triplanar resampling and visualization, achieved through locally developed software for image analysis (BRAINS, or Brain Research: Analysis of Images, Networks, and Systems), permits viewing of structures with a complex shape such as the caudate from three different angles, thus enhancing our capacity to understand brain anatomy three-dimensionally. Copyright 1993 Nancy C. Andreasen.

which is darker and more densely full of gray matter, is the putamen; the globus pallidus is lateral to it. The caudate is separated from the lentiform nucleus by the anterior limb of the internal capsule, but the MRI scan shows clearly that bands of gray matter interconnect these two nuclei; posteriorly the lentiform nucleus is separated from the thalamus by the posterior limb of the internal capsule. Because these structures contain an intermixture of gray and white matter, they have a striped appearance in postmortem brains and on MRI scan, causing them to be referred to as the *corpus striatum* (striped body).

This brain region may be important to the understanding of mental illness, for several reasons. First, several major syndromes involving abnormalities in these regions manifest psychiatric symptoms. Patients with Huntington's chorea, characterized by severe atrophy in the caudate nucleus, typically present with a variety of mental symptoms that are similar to those seen in patients with psychosis. Patients with Huntington's disease often develop delusional thinking, depression, and/or inappropriate impulsive behavior. Of course, they also develop severe dementia, occurring in the context of a previously normal personality. Parkinson's disease is another syndrome affecting the basal ganglia; it is due to neuronal loss in the substantia nigra, the midbrain region of the basal ganglia that sends projections to the caudate, using dopamine as its primary neurotransmitter. MRI resolution is now sufficiently good that we can directly visualize the substantia nigra; a triplanar view appears in Figure 5–6. Unfortunately, this ability is not of great utility in monitoring the development of Parkinson's disease in predisposed individuals, because symptoms do not begin to appear until the ma-

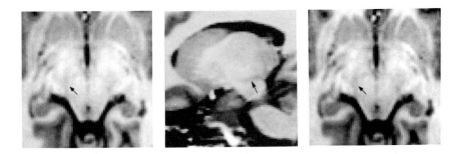

Figure 5–6.   A triplanar view of the substantia nigra. The dark-pigmented neurons show up as a subtle dark shading *(arrows)*. Copyright 1993 Nancy C. Andreasen.

jority of the pigmented neurons have been lost. In patients with Parkinson's disease, loss of pigmented neurons—and the associated loss of dopaminergic activity—produce a variety of symptoms similar to the negative symptoms of schizophrenia, including affective blunting and loss of volition. Mild dementia may also occur.

A second reason for thinking that the basal ganglia may be of some relevance to the development of symptoms of major mental illnesses derives from their chemical anatomy. One set of cell bodies within the cerebral dopamine system resides in this system, within the pigmented neurons of the substantia nigra. The caudate and putamen contain a very high concentration of dopamine receptors, particularly D_2 receptors. The efficacy of antipsychotic medications has been shown to be highly correlated with their ability to block D_2 receptors (see "Neurochemical Systems," below). Because D_2 receptors have a very high density in these regions, the caudate and putamen may be important sites for antipsychotic drug action and may play a role in generating psychotic symptoms such as delusions and hallucinations.

The Memory System

The memory system is a major functional brain system that may be impaired in some patients who have major mental illnesses. Deficits in learning and memory are the hallmark of the dementias. Although patients with psychoses do not typically have severe memory deficits, some investigators have speculated that the neural mechanisms of psychotic phenomena such as delusions and hallucinations might be based, at least in part, on either abnormal excitability or abnormal "wiring" in the neural circuitry involved in encoding, retrieval, and interpretation of memories. Within psychoanalytic theory, it has long been believed that the various neuroses, such as anxiety disorders and hysteria (i.e., somatization disorder), might represent the painful stimulus of repressed memories that have not been psychologically integrated. The process of psychotherapy certainly involves the process of learning, which is based in turn on memory; patients who successfully complete a course of psychotherapy have learned new ways of thinking about themselves, understanding their past experiences, and relating to other people. Thus, the psychosocial treatment of mental illnesses probably also involves the memory system in the brain.

It is a truism that we still have a great deal to learn about learning and memory. Nevertheless, we have also learned a great deal during recent decades. For many years, cognitive psychologists have dedicated themselves to identifying the site or sites where memories are encoded, sometimes referred to as the "search for the engram." For example, Karl Lashley of Harvard spent much of his career placing lesions in various parts of the brain in experimental animals, demonstrating that no specific lesion could produce memory deficits and thereby suggesting that the brain was equipotential in its capacity for learning and memory. This situation changed radically, however, as the result of a single informative and very famous case, that of H.M. He was treated surgically for intractable epilepsy by removal of the anterior temporal poles bilaterally. Afterward, he was observed to have totally lost the capacity to remember any new information he was given, although his memory for information learned before the surgery was completely intact. This famous case focused attention on the gray matter structures located in the anterior poles of the temporal lobes, the amygdala and hippocampus, and on the possible importance of bilateral as opposed to unilateral lesions.

We now know, on the basis of the case of H.M. as well as a large quantity of other human and animal evidence, that unilateral lesions do not typically produce memory deficits, but that bilateral lesions in certain specific locations can completely destroy learning and memory. We now suspect that some aspects of learning and memory are mediated in two brain regions, the hippocampus and the amygdala. A triplanar view of the hippocampus, as visualized with MRI, appears in Figure 5–7; as that figure indicates, the hippocampus is a large elongated structure that reaches from the anterior temporal pole far back into more posterior brain regions.

Because the memory system appears to depend on the presence of multiple "backup files," identifying the circuitry involved has not been simple. For example, it was thought for a number of years that the hippocampus was a primary site for encoding memory and that the amygdala served very little function, based on evidence that bilateral removal of the amygdala alone did not impair learning and memory. Later, however, it was observed by Mishkin that similar bilateral lesions to the hippocampus also did not impair the performance of macaques on visual recognition memory tasks. Thus, most recently it has been concluded that

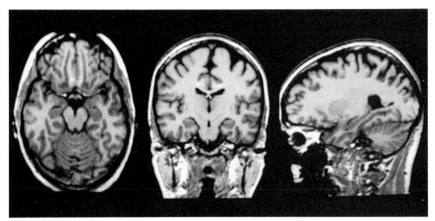

Figure 5–7. A triplanar view of the hippocampus. Note its long posterior section as seen in the less familiar sagittal view. Copyright 1991 Nancy C. Andreasen.

both of these brain regions work together to store memories. Loss of both produces massive memory defects, whereas loss of one or the other produces relatively restricted abnormalities or even none.

It is very likely, however, that the functions of these two nuclei are not simply duplicative. Current evidence suggests that the amygdala may work primarily to integrate memories learned from different modalities. For example, monkeys who have lesions in the amygdala cannot visually recognize objects that they have examined only by touch, whereas animals with lesions in the hippocampus can do so. The amygdala also plays an important role in social behavior, at least in nonhuman primates, because animals with lesions in the amygdala have difficulty recognizing social hierarchies, expressing aggression, experiencing fear, or demonstrating normal maternal behavior. It seems likely that the amygdala plays an important role in facial recognition and facial perception.

These lesion studies were recently supplemented by studies of memory with PET scanning. With this in vivo method, the hippocampus and amygdala have been surprisingly difficult to activate by using memory paradigms. The primary method for studying higher cortical functions with PET involves the use of $[^{15}O]$ H_2O, a tracer with a short half-life (2 minutes), that provides a measure of cerebral blood flow and that can be used in multiple back-to-back studies (usually eight) in a single individual. Thus, the person can be given multiple kinds of tasks that engage memory (e.g, verbal, visual, short-term, long-term), and the brain regions involved can be identified by measuring brain blood flow while the brain is being scanned as the individual performs the memory task. Each specific task is usually observed by using image subtraction (i.e., a baseline or control task is subtracted from the experimental task), and results from groups of individuals are usually averaged together to produce a generalizable result and to improve the signal-to-noise ratio. This method permits the direct observation of brain physiology during the performance of specific mental work; therefore, it is particularly powerful. Nevertheless, very few investigators have observed a high level of activity in the amygdala or hippocampus during memory tasks. Other brain regions that have an increased blood flow during memory tasks include the prefrontal and parietal cortices and the cerebellum. These results raise questions about the inferences concerning the mechanisms of memory that have been drawn from lesion studies. They suggest that learning and memory may be distributed and cortical—not unlike the early ideas of Lashley, which were roundly ridiculed during the era of localizationism that prevailed in psychiatry and neurology during the 1970s and 1980s.

Just as the brain regions that encode memories do not appear to be homogeneous or equipotential, so too memory itself is probably a diverse set of functions that are mediated in different ways. Typically, memory is now thought of as a two-stage process. The first stage involves short-term memory, or recognition and short-term recall memory. This type of memory is relatively brief. It is the form that we use when we "learn" a telephone number long enough to dial it or a driver's license number long enough to write it down. Sometimes this type of memory is also referred to as working memory, because it is accessible in some type of short-term storage. Long-term memory, on the other hand, consists of information that we have learned and retained for periods longer than a few minutes. This type of memory is sometimes referred to as consolidated memory. This type of memory is currently being used by the students reading this textbook.

Normal human experience, as well as research in neuroscience, indicates that a variety of techniques can be used to facilitate learning, or consolidation of memory. These techniques include such things as repetition, rehearsal, and mnemonic devices. This type of memory is probably mediated by a different set of mechanisms that lead to long-term storage of information. Once such information is stored, some of it may be slowly lost.

The mechanisms mediating short-term versus long-term memory are not clear, although an increasing consensus is developing that short-term memories and long-term memories are coded through different mechanisms. Current research suggests that short-term memory probably involves activating short synaptic circuits through neurochemical transmission; this type of neural activity is both rapidly implemented and rapidly reversed. On the other hand, long-term memory probably involves a more permanent process, most likely through the development of a sequence of molecules that encode information. Substantial work in this area has been conducted by Eric Kandel, using the gill withdrawal reflex in *Aplysia* as a model. Kandel suggested that long-term memory may depend on the synthesis of proteins and RNA in neurons that are synaptically connected during the time that short-term learning has been occurring; this type of process would represent a molecular consolidation of memory that could be permanently stored.

The Language System

As far as we know, the capacity to communicate in a highly developed and complex language is limited to humans. Although porpoises, dolphins, and a few other creatures are believed to communicate specific messages to one another, humans alone appear to have a syntactically complex language that exists in both oral and written forms. The ability to record our history and to communicate scientifically and culturally has permitted us to repeatedly build complex civilizations and social systems, and perhaps to destroy them as well.

The capacity to communicate in oral and written language is facilitated by dedicated brain regions that probably occur only in humans. These language systems are localized in the neocortex. A simplified schematic diagram of the human brain circuitry traditionally considered to mediate language functions appears in Figure 5–8. From lesion studies, this system appears to be located almost totally in the left hemisphere in most individuals, although about one-third of left-handed people use either their right hemisphere or both hemispheres to perform language functions.

Although the history of our understanding of the language system reaches back to the nineteenth century, and specifically to the work of Broca and Wernicke (each of whom has a neocortical region that bears his name), much of our early understanding of the specialized detail of the language system derives from the work of Norman Geschwind and his colleagues in Boston. Geschwind was one of the earliest neuroscientists to reawaken interest in hemispheric specialization and asymmetry, observing that the functional specialization of the brain is reflected at least partially in its anatomical structure. He observed that the planum temporale (the flat plane of the temporal lobe that is seen from the top when the cortex above is removed through dissection) is larger on the left side, reflecting the specialized development of the left hemisphere for language. (See Chapter 4 for a direct in vivo visualization of the planum temporale with MRI scanning.)

Within the left hemisphere are three major language regions, as well as some subsidiary ones. Broca's area is the region dedicated to the production of speech. It contains information about the syntactical structure of language, provides the

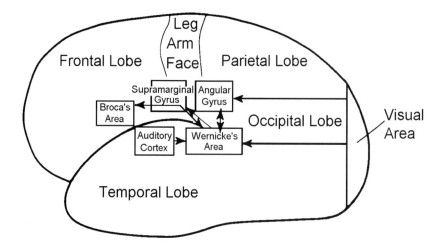

Figure 5–8. Interconnections of the language system. Reprinted with permission from Andreasen NC: The Broken Brain: The Biological Revolution in Psychiatry. New York, Harper & Row, 1984, p 113. Copyright 1984 Nancy C. Andreasen.

little words such as prepositions that tie the fabric of language together, and is the generator for fluent speech. Lesions to Broca's area, which occur in stroke victims (often with an accompanying right hemiparesis), lead to halting, stammering, ungrammatical speech. Wernicke's area is often referred to as the auditory association cortex. It encodes the information that permits us to understand or interpret information presented to us in auditory form. The perception of sound waves, which encode speech, occurs through transducers in the ear that convert the information to neural signals. The signals are received in the auditory cortex, but the meaning of the specific signals cannot be understood (i.e., perceived as constituting words with specific meanings—as opposed, for example, to the wordless music of a symphony) without being compared with "templates" in Wernicke's area. An analogous process occurs when we understand written language. In this case the information is collected through our eyes, relayed via the optic tracts back to the primary visual cortex in the occipital lobe, then forwarded on to the angular gyrus, a visual association cortex that contains the information or templates that permit us to recognize language presented in visual form.

A variety of stroke syndromes have been described that represent specific damage to these various specialized brain regions. For example, *Wernicke's aphasia* occurs as a result of damage to Wernicke's area and leaves individuals without the ability to understand what is said; this is a direct consequence of their loss of the auditory association cortex, which attributes meaning to the sound waves they hear. In addition, individuals with Wernicke's aphasia lose the ability to speak coherently because they have lost the meaning of language; individuals with this aphasia produce fluent, disorganized speech that is sometimes referred to as word salad or jargon aphasia. Wernicke's aphasia is sharply distinguished from *Broca's aphasia*; in the latter case, individuals can comprehend what is said to them, but they have a marked deficit in their ability to express themselves, a situation that typically leads to great frustration. Damage to the angular gyrus leads to loss of the ability to perform reading and writing—the two forms of language that are visually mediated—with no loss of auditory comprehension or spontaneous speech.

As in the case of memory, our understanding of the language system based on the study of stroke patients has been supplemented by studies using PET. Again, the results suggest that the intact, functioning brain appears to perform language functions in a more complex manner than was suggested by the lesion studies. Specifically, the strong left-hemisphere dominance for language is being called into question. PET studies indicate that auditory language perception appears to occur bihemispherically and that blood flow may also increase in both hemispheres during language generation. During the next decade the traditional maps of brain language regions, as shown in Figure 5–8, are likely to be redrawn, as more in vivo data are added to our knowledge of the human brain map.

Patients with major mental illnesses have a variety of disruptions in their capacity to communicate using language. Some of these incapacities are similar to those observed in patients with the aphasias produced by stroke, but none is identical. Some patients with schizophrenia have very impoverished speech that is reminiscent of Broca's aphasia but lacks its halting, agrammatical quality. Likewise, some patients with schizophrenic or manic psychosis produce very disorganized, abundant speech similar to that produced by patients with Wernicke's aphasia, but (unlike patients with Wernicke's aphasia) they appear to have intact comprehension. Auditory hallucinations (hearing voices) is abnormal auditory perceptions of language; that is, the individual perceives auditory speech when none is present. The reasons for these various disruptions and aberrations in language function in psychosis (and in many of the dementias as well) are still not clear. They may represent specific abnormalities in specialized language regions in the brain, but they more likely represent a disorganization at some "higher" or "lower" integrative level.

The Attention System

Attention is the cognitive process through which the brain identifies stimuli within the context of time and space and selects what is relevant for both input and output. We are bombarded continually with sensory information in multiple modalities, as well as with the information within our internal cognitive repertoire. A person driving a car on a busy highway is receiving information about other cars, the road, and the surrounding terrain from his or her visual system, as well as auditory input from the car motor or the rush of other vehicles as they pass, tactile input from hands on the steering wheel and the foot on the gas pedal, and the physical sensations experienced by the rest of the body as the car grips the road or bounces and sways. The person may also be talking on a cellular phone, listening to music, or thinking about a recent conversation. Attention is the cognitive process that permits the person to suppress irrelevant stimuli (e.g., to ignore most of the landscape), to notice important stimuli (e.g., that the car in front is putting on the brakes and slowing down suddenly), and to shift from one stimulus to another (e.g., from thoughts about the recent conversation to the traffic). If we lacked this capacity, we would be overwhelmed and bombarded with stimuli. Attention is sometimes compared to a spotlight, which the brain uses to highlight what is important to the survival, needs, or interests of the organism.

Attention may be the most "central" of the various cognitive systems; therefore, it is more difficult to study in isolation than the other systems described above. It is sometimes classified into different types. *Sustained attention* involves focusing for a prolonged period (as when studying for an examination); *directed attention* involves consciously selecting a particular feature or stimulus from the large array available (as when a professor instructs students to notice a particular lesion that they may not have recognized on an X ray); *selective attention* involves focusing attention on a stimulus that may have importance for personal or practical reasons (as when a person at a dinner party hears his or her name spoken in a nearby conversation); *divided attention* involves focusing attention on several things at the same time, or in rapidly shifting sequence (as when the person at the dinner party tries to listen to two conversations at once); *focused attention* involves directing attention to some particular stimulus or task (as when solving a mathematics problem or developing the outline for a paper to be written).

Attention appears to be mediated through multiple brain systems. Input to the brain is probably first provided by the *reticular activating system*, which arises in the brain stem. Midline circuitry passes this information through the thalamus, which appears to play a major role in gating or filtering. Many other brain regions also appear to play a major role in attention, including the cingulate gyrus, the hypothalamus, the hippocampus and amygdala, the prefrontal cortex, and the temporal, parietal, and occipital cortices. As Figure 5–2 indicates, these regions are all interconnected.

Lesion studies have emphasized the phenomenon of *sensory neglect* or *hemineglect*, first described by Hughlings-Jackson, who observed a patient who ignored sensory input as a result of a lesion in the right parietal lobe. More recent studies have examined this abnormality in a variety of patients. Although the classic case involves inability to focus spatial attention as a consequence of right-parietal injury, neglect may also occur after injury to the left hemisphere.

Neuroimaging studies using PET have shown that the cingulate gyrus shows increases in cerebral blood flow during tasks that place heavy demands on the attentional system, such as those that involve competition and interference between stimuli. They have also shown that blood flow can be shifted from one hemisphere to another as a consequence of directed attention; increased blood flow is seen in the right superior temporal gyrus as a consequence of instructions to listen to sounds in the left ear, and the increase shifts to the left superior temporal gyrus in response to instructions to attend to the right ear. Increasing the difficulty of the task through competing stimuli produces an increase in frontal flow as well.

Neurochemical Systems

In addition to the functional and anatomical systems described above, the brain also consists of a grouping of neurochemical systems. These systems provide the fuel that permits the functional and anatomical systems to run (or run poorly, when an abnormality occurs). The neurochemical systems are not isomorphic with the anatomical and functional systems. Rather, they are interwoven and interdependent. Any anatomical subsystem within the brain usually runs on multiple classes of neurotransmitters. Clearly, this complexity of anatomical and neurochemical organization permits much greater fine-tuning of the entire system.

Neuron, Synapse, Receptor, and Second Messenger

Neurons may have various structural configurations, depending on the function they perform. They all consist of a cell body containing the nucleus and at least one axon of variable length that transfers from the cell body the propagation of electrical excitation that ultimately leads to the release of neurotransmitters located in terminals at the synapses. The cell body is surrounded by dendrites that enlarge the capacity of the cell body to receive information through synaptic input from other neurons. Likewise, axons may branch as they terminate, and then produce multiple synaptic contacts.

Although the initial propagation of messages is electrical, communication at the synapse is chemical. It is mediated through a variety of substances recognized to be chemical messengers between neurons, or *neurotransmitters*. Neuroscientists have agreed for several decades on a set of criteria that define "classic" neurotransmitters (Table 5–1). For a substance to be accepted as a neurotransmitter, investigators must establish that it is contained within the neuron, synthesized by the neuron, and released at the synapse and that it causes a reproducible physiological response. The classic neurotransmitters that meet these criteria are principally catecholamines and amino acids, such as dopamine, serotonin, acetylcholine, γ-aminobutyric acid (GABA), and glutamate.

In addition to these classic neurotransmitters, chemical communication between regions also occurs through other neurotransmitters that have not yet been proved to meet all the above criteria. It has been recognized for nearly two decades that peptides are also synthesized in the central nervous system (CNS). Although the earliest peptides to be recognized were those that were clearly hormonal (e.g., corticotropin [ACTH]), the discovery of endogenous opioid peptide neurotransmitters (endorphins) substantially expanded interest in peptide transmitters within the CNS. Because they are proteins (i.e., have their synthesis directed by nuclear DNA), the peptide neurotransmitters must be synthesized in the neuronal cell body rather than in the synapse. They are carried down to the synapse through storage vesicles, where they can then be released. Although some peptide neurotransmitters function in much the same way as the classic neurotransmitters, others serve as cotransmitters.

Although the belief in a single neuron–single neurotransmitter used to be universal, it is now recognized that many neurons contain at least two neurotransmitters. Often a classic neurotransmitter and a neuropeptide are coupled. For example, cholecystokinin (CCK) serves as a cotransmitter with the dopamine neurons that project to the cortex and limbic system (but not those that project to the basal ganglia). The peptide cotransmitters are generally thought to be modulatory or regulatory.

A schematic representation of a synapse appears in Figure 5–9; an electron

Table 5–1.   Criteria for a "classic" neurotransmitter

1. It is synthesized in the neuron.
2. It is present in the presynaptic terminal and is released in an amount sufficient to exert a particular effect on a receptor neuron.
3. When applied exogenously (as drug) in reasonable concentrations, it mimics exactly the action of the endogenously released neurotransmitter.
4. A specific mechanism exists for removing it from its site of action, the synaptic cleft.

micrograph of an actual synapse is shown in Figure 5–10. The classic neurotransmitters are synthesized at the neuronal synapse from precursor molecules (e.g., tyrosine). The neurotransmitter molecules must be sequestered in vesicles to prevent breakdown by enzymes contained within the neuronal cytosol (e.g., by monoamine oxidase). Adequate quantities of neurotransmitter are maintained at the synapse through a variety of regulatory factors. Short-term monitoring to determine whether adequate quantities of the neurotransmitter are contained in vesicular storage is done through end-product inhibition. For example, tyrosine hydroxylase is the rate-limiting enzyme for the synthesis of dopamine and norepinephrine. If an adequate supply of norepinephrine is available at the terminal, it inhibits the activity of tyrosine hydroxylase, preventing further synthesis.

On the other hand, if the synapse is very active, leading to depletion of neurotransmitter, protein kinases stimulate phosphorylation of tyrosine hydroxylase, a process triggered by persistent membrane depolarization. Increased quantities of tyrosine hydroxylase can also be produced in the neuronal cell body under the supervision of nuclear DNA—a response that occurs as a result of long-term neuronal hyperactivity and synaptic depletion.

Finally, at least for neurons that possess presynaptic receptors, the release of neurotransmitter can also be downregulated through these presynaptic receptors. For example, noradrenergic neurons contain α_2 receptors at their terminals, which decrease the amount of norepinephrine released at the terminal when activated either by an increase in overall adrenergic activity or by exogenous

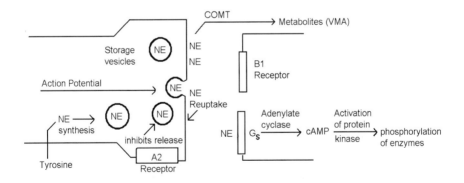

Figure 5–9. Schematic view of a synapse. This schematic drawing shows a simplified view of the cascade of events occurring during synaptic transmission, beginning with neurotransmitter release, stimulated through an action potential, and leading to occupation of a receptor and subsequent activation of second- messenger systems. cAMP = cyclic AMP. COMT = cathechol-*O*-methyl- transferase. NE = norepinephrine. VMA = vanillylmandelic acid. Copyright 1989 Nancy C. Andreasen.

α_2 agonists such as clonidine. The presynaptic receptors work principally to decrease the firing rate of the neuron and thereby the vesicular release of neurotransmitter. Thus, the regulation of neurotransmitter synthesis and release is governed by a complex set of interactive mechanisms that can adapt neuronal responsiveness to rapidly varying conditions.

After a neurotransmitter is released, it can experience a variety of fates. In the free-floating world of intersynaptic connections, enzymes such as catechol-O-methyltransferase (COMT) hover at the synapse and can lead to inactivation or breakdown of the neurotransmitter. It may saturate presynaptic receptors, thereby telling the transmitter neuron that it is time to slow down. It may cross

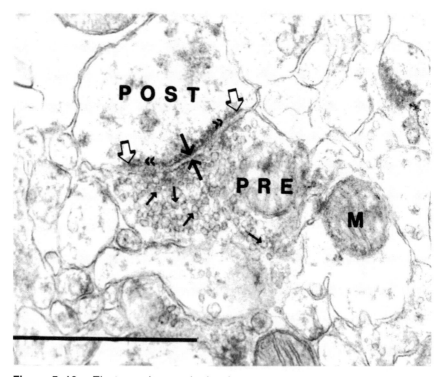

Figure 5–10.   Electron micrograph showing a synapse in the human brain. The presynaptic region (PRE) is an axon, which contains vesicles of neurotransmitters *(small arrows)*. It is adjacent to the postsynaptic region (POST) of another neuron. The receptors embedded in the postsynaptic membrane can be visualized. *Open arrows* delineate the extent of the synapse identified by parallel presynaptic and postsynaptic membranes *(medium arrows)*. Synaptic vesicles and a postsynaptic density are marked by *double brackets*. M indicates mitochondria in a nearby location. Courtesy of Carol Tamminga and Rosalinda C. Roberts.

the synapse and occupy a postsynaptic receptor, thereby actually succeeding in sending a message to another neuron. Finally, because nature often loves efficiency and abhors waste, it may be returned to the original transmitter neuron and again stored in the vesicles, eventually to be released again.

The receptor sites to which neurotransmitters complex are large protein molecules embedded in the neuronal membrane that recognize specific neurotransmitters in a highly selective way, which is related to the chemical structure of the receptor. There are two main superfamilies of receptors: G-protein coupled (metabotropic) and ion channel (ionotropic). The messages produced by G-protein receptors occur more slowly, whereas ion-channel receptors produce rapid changes in neuronal excitability. The G-protein receptors work principally by activating enzymes (e.g., adenylate cyclase, inositol phosphate, phospholipase A), which in turn aid in the amplification of the signal by a second messenger (e.g., cyclic AMP).

Knowledge concerning the structure and the working mechanisms of G-protein receptors has been increasing steadily. These receptors are of considerable interest in psychiatry, because many of the major neuroreceptors thought to be involved in mental illnesses and/or modulated by the drugs used to treat these illnesses are in this superfamily (e.g., serotonergic, dopaminergic, α- and β-adrenergic, and muscarinic cholinergic). GABAergic, nicotinic, and some glutamatergic receptors are ionotropic, however. Many of these receptors have now been cloned, providing us with information about their specific DNA-driven amino acid sequences and opening up the possibility that specific drugs can be designed to interact with receptors in key chemical systems or brain regions involved in specific illnesses.

All receptors in the G-protein superfamily have a similar structure. A schematic diagram of a G-protein receptor is shown in Figure 5–11. The receptor itself is composed of seven helical loops embedded in the membrane and composed of a specific sequence of amino acids. The various types of receptors—for example, D_1, D_2, D_3, D_4, D_5, serotonin type 2 (5-HT_2)— differ in amino acid sequence, which determines their affinity for specific drugs or neurotransmitters. Each receptor has a long tail on the extracellular side, which also determines drug affinity. Three loops of variable length are also present on the intracellular side, as well as an intracellular tail. These intracellular components provide the mechanism for passing the message on to the G-protein and the effector protein.

Among the second messengers, the one coupled with cyclic AMP is best understood; it appears to occur both at noradrenergic β receptors and at D_1 receptors. Within this system, the neurotransmitter-receptor interaction leads to a complexing of protein on the other side of the membrane, which then binds to adenylate cyclase and activates it, causing ATP to convert to cyclic AMP. Cyclic

AMP then activates protein kinases, which in turn promote phosphorylation of key enzymes. Other second-messenger systems, associated with α_1-adrenergic receptors and muscarinic M_1 receptors, stimulate the breakdown of phospholipids, thereby increasing intracellular concentrations of phosphoinositides and diacylglycerol, which in turn leads to enzyme phosphorylation and activation.

Medications used to treat mental illness often exert their primary effects through acting on one of these aspects of neural communication. For example, the monoamine oxidase inhibitors (MAOIs), which prevent the breakdown of norepinephrine, enhance noradrenergic transmission by blocking the action of monoamine oxidase. The classic antidepressants, such as imipramine, also facilitate noradrenergic transmission by blocking the uptake mechanisms. Clonidine decreases anxiety by blocking presynaptic α_2 receptors, thereby producing downregulation. For many years, classic antipsychotics were thought to decrease the symptoms of psychosis by diminishing hyperdopaminergic activity through blocking postsynaptic D_2 receptors, a view that has been revised in light of the documented efficacy of the new "atypical" neuroleptics, which have a different pharmacological profile. (See Chapter 26, "Somatic Treatments.")

The Dopamine System

Dopamine, a catecholamine neurotransmitter, is the first product synthesized from tyrosine through the enzymatic activity of tyrosine hydroxylase. Its syn-

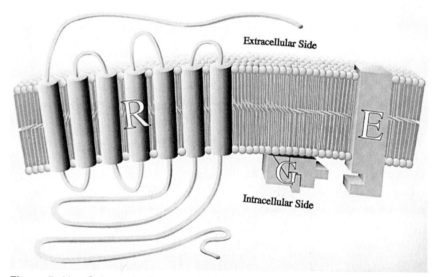

Figure 5–11. Schematic diagram of a G-protein receptor. R = receptor. G = G-protein. E = effector protein. Courtesy of Carol Tamminga.

thetic pathway, as well as the subsequent ones of norepinephrine and epineph-rine, is shown in Figure 5–12.

Three subsystems within the brain use dopamine as their primary neuro-transmitter. These all arise in the ventral tegmental area. One subsystem, arising in the substantia nigra, projects to the caudate and putamen and is referred to as the nigrostriatal pathway. Its terminations appear to be rich in both dopamine 1 (D_1) and dopamine 2 (D_2) receptors. A second major subsystem, called the mesocortical or mesolimbic (or mesocorticolimbic) tract, projects to the prefron-tal cortex and temporolimbic regions such as the amygdala and hippocampus. The concentration of D_2 receptors in these regions is minimal, and D_1 receptors predominate. The third component of the dopamine systems originates in the arcuate nucleus of the hypothalamus and projects to the pituitary. These various dopamine subsystems are summarized in Figure 5–13.

As Figure 5–12 indicates, the dopamine system is fairly specifically localized in the human brain. Because its projections include only a limited part of the cortex and focus primarily on brain regions important to cognition and emotion, it is considered one of the most important neurotransmitter systems for under-standing these functions, and potentially for understanding their disturbances in individuals with psychosis.

For many years, schizophrenia, the most important among the various psy-chotic disorders, was explained by the *dopamine hypothesis*, which proposed that the symptoms of this illness were due to a functional excess of dopamine. Because the efficacy of many of the neuroleptic drugs used to treat psychosis is highly correlated with their ability to block D_2 receptors (Figure 5–14), the dopamine

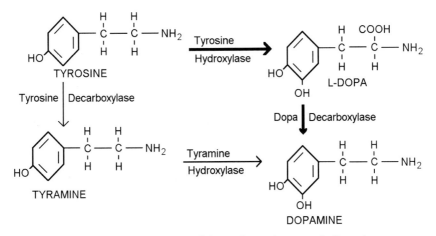

Figure 5–12.   Synthetic pathways of dopamine, primary and alternate.

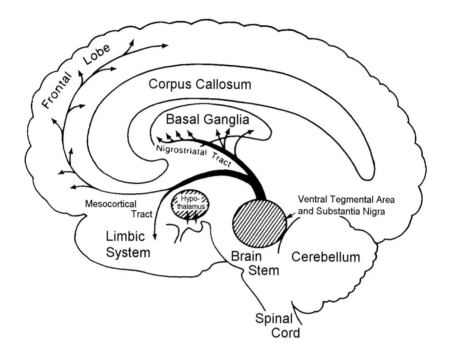

Figure 5–13.   The dopamine system. Reprinted with permission from Andreasen NC: The Broken Brain: The Biological Revolution in Psychiatry. New York, Harper & Row, 1984, p 134. Copyright 1984 Nancy C. Andreasen.

hypothesis also suggested that the abnormality in this illness might be specifically in D_2 receptors. There is a modest but much weaker correlation with their ability to block D_1 receptors (Figure 5–15). This hypothesis is currently being reappraised, however, in light of several new lines of evidence that have emerged. First, the distribution of D_1 and D_2 receptors has been more specifically mapped during recent years, and there appears to be a rather sparse density of D_2 receptors in critical brain regions that mediate cognition and emotion, such as the prefrontal cortex, the amygdala, and the hippocampus. These regions are, on the other hand, high in D_1 receptors. They are also high in serotonin type 2 (5-HT$_2$) receptors. This latter observation, coupled with the prominent effects on serotonin and D_1 of the new atypical neuroleptics, suggests that the traditional dopamine hypothesis must be revised.

Understanding the projections of the dopamine system, as well as the differential localization of D_1 and D_2 receptors, clarifies some of the other actions of neuroleptic drugs. Most of these drugs tend to have potent extrapyramidal effects as a consequence of blocking D_2 receptors in the nigrostriatal pathway. Drugs

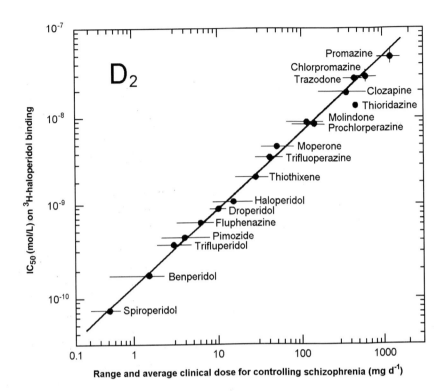

Figure 5–14. Correlation between drug potency and D_2 receptor blockade. Reprinted with permission from Seeman P: Dopamine receptors and the dopamine hypothesis of schizophrenia. Synapse 1:133–152, 1987.

that have a weak D_2 effect (of which clozapine and risperidone are recent examples) are more likely to have fewer extrapyramidal side effects as a consequence of their weak D_2 blockade. If only we understood more specifically the brain regions from which the symptoms of psychosis arise, it would be possible to design a rational psychopharmacology that might target drugs to specific regions on the basis of what we know about the chemical anatomy of the brain. Such a rational psychopharmacology could capitalize on knowledge about the neurotransmitters involved, the brain regions involved, and the chemical structure of the relevant receptors, as revealed through receptor cloning.

The Norepinephrine System

The norepinephrine system arises in the locus coeruleus and sends projections diffusely throughout the entire brain. These projections are summarized in Fig-

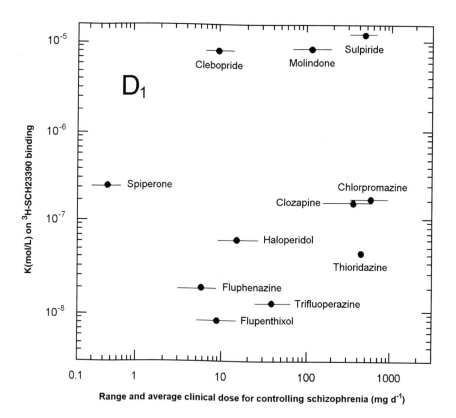

Figure 5–15.   Correlation between neuroleptic potency and D_1 receptor blockade. Reprinted with permission from Seeman P: Dopamine receptors and the dopamine hypothesis of schizophrenia. Synapse 1:133–152, 1987.

ure 5–16. As that figure illustrates, norepinephrine appears to exert effects on almost every region in the human brain, including the entire cortex, the hypothalamus, the cerebellum, and the brain stem. This distribution suggests that it may have a diffuse modulatory or regulatory effect within the CNS.

There is some evidence that norepinephrine may play a major role in mediating symptoms of major mental illnesses, especially mood disorders. Soon after they were developed, the tricyclic antidepressants were demonstrated to inhibit norepinephrine reuptake, thereby enhancing the amount of norepinephrine available for stimulating postsynaptic receptors. Likewise, the MAOIs also enhance noradrenergic transmission by inhibiting neurotransmitter breakdown. As is described below, however, it is also clear that many antidepressants have mixed noradrenergic and serotonergic activities or purely serotonergic effects (i.e., the serotonin reuptake inhibitors). Thus, the original catecholamine hypothesis of

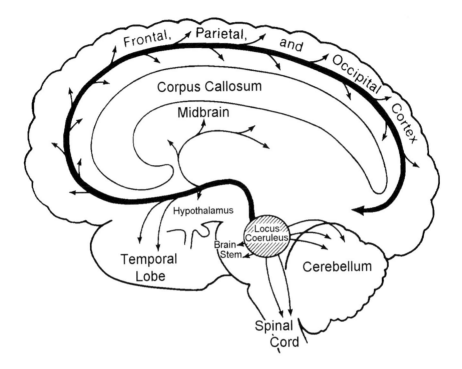

Figure 5–16. The norepinephrine system. Reprinted with permission from Andreasen NC: The Broken Brain: The Biological Revolution in Psychiatry. New York, Harper & Row, 1984, p 134. Copyright 1984 Nancy C. Andreasen.

affective illness, which suggested that depression was due to a functional deficit of norepinephrine at crucial nerve terminals and mania was due to a functional excess, is clearly an oversimplification.

The Serotonin System

Serotonergic neurons have a distribution strikingly similar to that of norepinephrine neurons (Figure 5–17). Serotonergic neurons arise in the raphe nuclei, localized around the aqueduct in the midbrain. They project to a similar wide range of CNS regions, including the entire neocortex, the basal ganglia, temporolimbic regions, the hypothalamus, the cerebellum, and the brain stem. As is the case with the norepinephrine system, the serotonin system appears to be a general modulator.

A serotonin hypothesis of depression has also been proposed, largely because some antidepressant medications (e.g., fluoxetine) also facilitate serotonergic

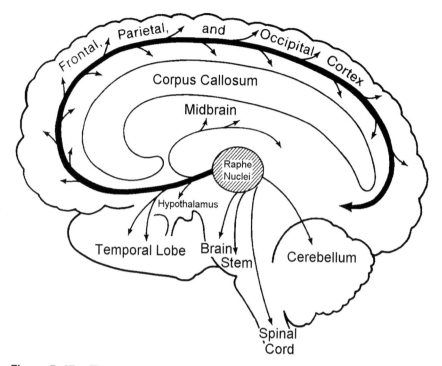

Figure 5–17.   The serotonin system. Reprinted with permission from Andreasen NC: The Broken Brain: The Biological Revolution in Psychiatry. New York, Harper & Row, 1984, p 135. Copyright 1984 Nancy C. Andreasen.

transmission by blocking reuptake. As discussed above, serotonin is probably also involved in schizophrenia and other psychotic disorders. Thus, there are probably no simple single neurotransmitter–single illness relationships.

The Cholinergic System

Like dopamine, acetylcholine has a relatively more specific localization in the human brain. This is shown schematically in Figure 5–18. The cell bodies of a major group of acetylcholine neurons are located in the nucleus basalis of Meynert, which lies in the ventral and medial regions of the globus pallidus. Neurons from the nucleus basalis of Meynert project throughout the cortex. The second group of acetylcholine neurons, originating in the diagonal band of Broca and the septal nucleus, project to the hippocampus and the cingulate gyrus. A third group of cholinergic neurons are local-circuit neurons that enter main structures within the basal ganglia.

The acetylcholine system plays a major role in the encoding of memory,

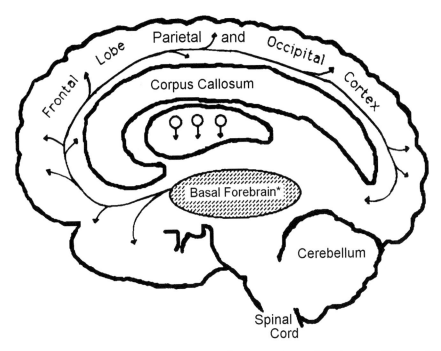

Figure 5–18. The acetylcholine system. *Includes the nucleus basilis of Meynert, the diagonal band of Broca, and the medial septal nucleus. Copyright 1989 Nancy C. Andreasen.

although the precise mechanisms are not understood. Patients with Alzheimer's disease show losses of acetylcholine projections both to the cortex and to the hippocampus, and blockade of muscarinic receptors produces impairment in memory. Dopamine and acetylcholine share heavy concentrations of activity within the basal ganglia, and the drugs used to block the extrapyramidal side effects of neuroleptics are cholinergic agonists, suggesting a possible reciprocal relationship between dopamine and acetylcholine in the modulation of motor activity and possibly of psychosis as well. These cholinergic agonists may also impair cognitive functions such as learning and memory in individuals for whom they are prescribed.

The GABA System

GABA is an amino acid neurotransmitter, as is glutamate. These two major amino acid neurotransmitters appear to serve complementary functions, with GABA playing an inhibitory role and glutamate playing an excitatory role.

GABAergic neurons are a mix of local-circuit and long-tract systems.

Within the cerebral cortex and the limbic system, GABAergic neurons are predominantly local circuit. The cell bodies of GABAergic neurons in the caudate and putamen project to the globus pallidus and the substantia nigra, making them relatively long tract, and long-tract GABA neurons also occur in the cerebellum.

The GABA system has substantial importance for the understanding of the neurochemistry of mental illness. Many of the anxiolytic drugs act as GABA agonists, thereby increasing the inhibitory tone within the CNS. Loss of the long-tract GABA neurons connecting the caudate to the globus pallidus releases the latter structure from inhibitory control, thereby permitting the globus pallidus to "run free" and produce the choreiform movements that characterize Huntington's disease.

The Glutamate System

Glutamate, an excitatory amino acid neurotransmitter, is produced by pyramidal cells throughout the cerebral cortex and hippocampus. It has already been noted, for example, that the projections from the prefrontal cortex to the basal ganglia are glutamatergic.

It has been observed for many years that glutamate, in addition to being a neurotransmitter, is also potentially a neurotoxin if present in amounts that produce excessive neuronal excitation. Recently this observation was coupled with observations about the psychological and biochemical effects of phencyclidine (PCP) to suggest a possible role for glutamate in either psychosis or neurodegenerative diseases such as Huntington's disease. PCP blocks the effects of activating one subgroup of glutamate receptors, the N-methyl-D-aspartate (NMDA) receptors, probably by blocking the cation channel that the NMDA receptor activates. PCP intoxication produces a psychosis characterized by withdrawal, stupor, disorganized thinking and speech, and hallucinations. The possible relationship between PCP, its characteristic psychosis, and its effects on the glutamate system suggest that glutamate may play some role in producing (or protecting against) the symptoms of psychosis. Such diseases could be produced by excessive glutamatergic activity, which might produce neuronal degeneration through excessive excitation.

The Genetics of Mental Illness

It has been recognized for many years that mental illnesses tend to run in families. Evidence that disorders are familial is sometimes said to imply that they are genetic as well, but this is not necessarily the case. Genetic disorders are precisely that: coded in segments of DNA. The history of research on the familial aggregation of mental illnesses has been one of an increasing ability to determine more specifically the degree to which mental illnesses are genetic in the literal sense. The era of molecular biology and molecular genetics has arrived. This era has been supported by a long history of research on the familial aggregation of mental illnesses, which has established that the study of familial transmission is relevant to understanding the mechanisms of mental illness. The newer molecular approaches offer substantial additional insights.

Studies of Familial Aggregation

Studies of familial aggregation have offered the first line of evidence for the familiality of major mental illnesses, as well as some indication that many mental illnesses may have a genetic component. The solid and increasingly methodologically rigorous studies of the prevalence of mental illnesses in families should not be minimized as we enter the era of molecular genetics; they have provided a major contribution. Such studies are usually divided into three broad groups: family studies, twin studies, and adoption studies. Each of these types of studies offers different perspectives on the genetics of disorders.

Family studies typically begin with the *proband method*. That is, individuals, or probands, are identified and used as the index cases because they have a particular disorder of interest, such as bipolar disorder or schizophrenia. Thereafter, all available first-degree relatives are typically evaluated. Early genetic studies used the *family history method*. This method involves interviewing the proband and one or two additional family members about whether other members of the family have any history of mental illness. This method is quick and simple, but less rigorous methodologically.

Gradually, the family history method has nearly been supplanted by the *family study method*, which involves directly interviewing all available first-degree relatives. The introduction of structured interviews and diagnostic criteria has presumably produced a steady increase in the accuracy of such family studies. In family studies, the prevalence of the specific disorder under investigation is also evaluated in some appropriately selected control group. For example, patients entering the hospital for hernia repair might represent the control group for the probands, and all the first-degree relatives of the hernia patients would serve as the control group for the first-degree relatives of the mentally ill probands. If an increased rate of the specific mental illness under study is observed in the first-degree relatives of the mentally ill probands, then investigators conclude that a disorder is familial and possibly genetic.

Such studies do not exclude the possibility that the disorder is purely familial, however, and not due to a specifically genetic cause. Disorders could run in families because of learned behavior, role modeling, or predisposing social environments. For example, depression tends to run in families, and this tendency could represent either genetic transmission or social learning; responding to stressful life events with a depressive coping style could easily be a learned adaptive mechanism passed on from parents to children through role modeling. Likewise, antisocial behavior also tends to run in families; although possibly genetic in origin, antisocial behavior could also be an adaptive response to social deprivation, nurtured by peer pressure from gangs, which tend to cluster in impoverished inner cities.

As discussed in more detail in the chapters on specific disorders (see Section II), many major mental illnesses have been shown through family studies to be highly familial. Alzheimer's disease, schizophrenia, bipolar and unipolar mood disorders, anxiety disorders, and antisocial personality all tend to have increased rates in first-degree relatives of probands with these various disorders. The test for the geneticist, however, is to determine whether they are also truly genetic.

Thus, investigators have turned to other methods in addition to family studies to identify a more purely genetic component. Before techniques were available to look directly at DNA, the best methods were *twin studies* and *adoption studies*.

Twin studies.   Twin studies typically begin with ascertainment of whether a proband twin (monozygotic or dizygotic) has the disorder of interest. The co-twin is then evaluated to determine whether he or she also has the illness (i.e., is concordant). The concordance rate in monozygotic twins can then be compared with that in dizygotic twins (using only same-gender twins among the dizygotic pairs to help control for random cultural and genetic "noise"). The higher the rate of concordance in monozygotic compared with dizygotic twins, the greater the degree of genetic influence.

The rationale behind twin studies is based on the fact that monozygotic twins have identical genetic material, whereas dizygotic twins theoretically share an average of 50% of their genetic material. (The percentage can actually run from 0% to 100%, but it should average to 50% across large numbers of twin pairs.) Thus, if a disorder was totally genetic and totally penetrant, the concordance rate in monozygotic twins would theoretically be 100%, whereas in dizygotic twins it would be 50%. In fact, the actual rates for both groups are lower for most major mental illnesses that have been studied using the twin method. Table 5–2 shows the concordance rates for schizophrenia in the various twin studies that have been conducted to date.

Table 5–2.   Pairwise rates of schizophrenia, schizoid disorder, other mental disorders, and normality among sets of monozygotic twins: a summary of study results

Study	Numbers of pairs	Schizophrenia[a] (%)	Schizoid[b] (%)	Other disorders[c] (%)	Normal (%)
Luxenburger 1928[d]	14	72	14	—	14
Rosanoff et al. 1934	41	61	—	7	32
Kallman 1946	174	69	21	5	5
Slater and Crowie 1971	37	64	—	14	22
Kringlen 1967	45	38	—	29	33
Fisher 1973	21	48	5	5	43
Gottesman and Shields 1982	22	50	9	9	23

[a]Includes both confirmed and presumptive diagnoses.
[b]So diagnosed by the investigators.
[c]Includes as examples alcoholic, psychopathic (Kallmann); psychopathic, suicide (Slater); alcoholic, character neurosis (Kringlen).
[d]Includes only co-twins of certain schizophrenic patients.

Although powerful, twin studies do not provide a perfect method for looking at the genetics of major mental illnesses. Because twins are reared together, role modeling could again be an influential factor, particularly for milder disorders, such as depression, that have a potentially prominent psychological component. This psychological component could theoretically be greater in monozygotic than in dizygotic twins, because monozygotic twins are often treated as identical by their parents and peers. The development of major mental illness in one's identical co-twin is clearly a serious psychological stressor that could be influential in the development of a disorder in the unaffected twin. If the unaffected twin is led to believe that he or she is indeed identical to his or her co-twin, the unaffected twin might develop a mental illness as part of a self-fulfilling prophecy. Alternatively, the unaffected twin might develop it out of sympathetic identification with a co-twin with whom he or she has been intimately nurtured for most of his or her life. Thus, environmental factors are not completely disentangled from genetic ones through the use of the twin method.

The twin method has been used less for the study of major mental illnesses, because it is methodologically quite difficult. Nevertheless, twin studies have been completed for some disorders, including schizophrenia, mood disorders, and alcoholism. In general, the twin method has tended to support the familiality, and potentially the genetic aspect, of most disorders to which it has been applied.

Adoption studies.   Adoption studies represent the most refined technique for disentangling environmental and genetic influences. In adoption studies, the population targeted for study is children who were born to parents with a major mental illness, then adopted at birth and reared by parents without the disorder. These children can be compared with a control group consisting of children born to psychiatrically normal mothers, similarly adopted at birth, and reared by psychiatrically normal parents. To whatever extent the rate of illness is higher in the adopted children of the mothers with the specific mental illness, that mental illness can be considered to be transmitted genetically rather than environmentally. In this model, learned behavior and role modeling of parents with mental illness are excluded, because the child is reared apart from the ill parent.

Like all paradigms, however, this one has inherent limitations and problems. Accurate diagnosis of the father is sometimes difficult, often relying on case registries and historical information rather than direct interview. Of more concern is the fact that information about the biological mother of the child may not be available, or the mother may not be able to identify the specific biological father because she has had multiple sex partners. An additional problem with adoption studies (and of family studies in general) is *assortative mating*. This term refers to the tendency of individuals with a specific mental illness to mate with, or marry, a person who has a similar illness. This may occur because of a "like attracts like" phenomenon, or it may occur as a consequence of simple social convenience, because the partners often meet each other in mental hospitals and sometimes have few friends who are not mentally ill because of the social handicaps produced by some mental illnesses. Whatever the mechanism, assortative mating produces problems for family and genetic studies, because it gives the offspring a double genetic loading.

Adoption studies are the most difficult to complete, largely because of problems in obtaining access to appropriate samples. Some major adoption studies have been done in Scandinavian countries, which have excellent epidemiological registries. Adoption data are available for schizophrenia, mood disorders, and antisocial personality disorder. In all cases, they add to the evidence for genetic factors in these disorders.

Genes Versus Environment in Major Mental Illnesses

As the above summary indicates, there is considerable evidence indicating that some mental illnesses are familial and that some may be genetic as well. Twin and family data provide particularly strong evidence in this regard, although family studies provide the weakest evidence for a purely genetic cause. Nevertheless, it seems unlikely that a familial propensity toward very serious illnesses such as Alzheimer's disease or schizophrenia could be explained purely on the basis of role modeling and learned behavior.

To understand the potentially complicated interactions between genes and environment, however, one must recognize that environmental factors are not necessarily psychological. Recent research with brain-imaging techniques has suggested that other types of environmental factors, such as perinatal injuries, may influence the development of severe mental disorders, particularly schizophrenia and affective disorders. Because these studies—using both computed tomography (CT) and MRI—have shown that male patients have a significant increase in ventricular size compared with both female patients and healthy control subjects, and because males are more vulnerable to perinatal injuries, these findings from neuroimaging suggest that physical environmental factors may also play a role in the development of major mental illnesses such as affective disorders or schizophrenia. These environmental factors could be perinatal, infectious, or traumatic, because male children appear to be more vulnerable to developing birth injuries, to having prenatal problems (e.g., a higher rate of spontaneous abortion), and possibly to developing infections. Because one common complication of difficult labor and delivery is periventricular hemorrhage, mechanisms of this type might explain the increased incidence of larger ventricular size in male patients with either schizophrenia or bipolar illness. The mechanism by which periventricular injury might predispose to the later development of schizophrenia or mood disorder is unclear; significant major subcortical structures such as the thalamus lie on the borders of the ventricles, and many major neurochemical tracts arising in the reticular core send white matter projections along the borders of the ventricles (e.g., the dopamine system arising in the ventral tegmental area, the norepinephrine system arising in the locus coeruleus).

Twin studies using neuroimaging have also been done in several cohorts of individuals with schizophrenia. The earliest twin study examined ventricular size in a group of monozygotic twins discordant for schizophrenia, compared with both dizygotic twins and psychiatrically normal monozygotic twins. In this study, conducted in Britain by the Reveleys, the ill monozygotic twins were found to have larger ventricular size than the well twins. (A summary of the Reveleys' data is shown in Table 5–3.) Further, the well monozygotic twins who had a schizophrenic co-twin also tended to have larger ventricular size than did the monozygotic twin pairs who were both well.

Thus, these results appear to suggest a combined genetic and environmental interaction. Both twins from the ill cohort tended to have bigger ventricles than the psychiatrically normal twins, suggesting a genetic contribution to ventricular size that might reflect an underlying predisposition to the illness. Because the ill twin had bigger ventricles than the well co-twin, however, these findings also

Table 5–3. Ventricle-to-brain ratio (VBR) in psychiatrically normal twins and in monozygotic twins discordant for schizophrenia

| Twin status | n | Age ± SE (y) | VBR | | |
			Overall	Mean intrapair difference	r	h^2 (%)
MZ normal	22	39 ± 3	4.2 ± 0.6	0.36	.98	98
DZ normal	16	38 ± 4	5.1 ± 0.6	1.90	.35	70
MZ schizophrenic	7	38 ± 3	8.6 ± 0.2	2.16	.87	87
MZ schizophrenic co-twins	7	38 ± 3	6.5 ± 0.2			

Note. MZ = monozygotic. DZ = dyzygotic.
Source. Adapted from Reveley AM, Reveley MA, Clifford CA, et al: Cerebral ventricular size in twins discordant for schizophrenia. Lancet 1:540–541, 1982.

suggest that some type of environmental factor was necessary to release an underlying genetic diathesis that both twins shared, and that this release—presumably something like a birth injury—is what caused the ill co-twin to develop schizophrenia. These findings were replicated in a similar study conducted at the National Institute of Mental Health in the United States. In this study, the ill twin in a discordant monozygotic twin pair was consistently identified on the basis of structural brain abnormalities seen with neuroimaging (in this instance, MRI).

Thus, a number of sources of information suggest that it may be difficult to find purely genetic models to explain some major mental illnesses. In general, patterns of transmission within families do not appear to follow simple Mendelian patterns. The neuroimaging data suggest the importance of environmental factors, in this case biological environmental factors. Psychological factors such as role modeling certainly cannot be excluded and may also be highly relevant. In some (perhaps many) cases, it may be necessary to use multifactorial models to explain the causes of major mental illnesses. One of the most widely discussed models is the *two-hit theory*. This theory proposes that two hits are required to produce an illness such as schizophrenia. The first hit is genetic and provides the individual with a diathesis to develop the illness. This diathesis is not sufficient, however, and requires a second hit in order to be released; the second hit is some type of environmental factor. Most of the existing twin, adoption, and high-risk data are consistent with a model of this type.

Molecular Genetics

Molecular genetics provides an alternative approach to the descriptive studies discussed above. The techniques of molecular biology provide methods for looking directly at the genetic material itself. Molecular genetics offers the hope of being able to identify the gene or genes that might produce an illness, either by working in isolation or by interacting with environmental factors. Initially, pursuing the principles of parsimony, investigators sought a single major locus. In all likelihood, however, most forms of major mental illness are too complex to be explained on the basis of a single gene. Consequently, investigators are turning to more complex models and more ingenious designs to apply the techniques of molecular biology to the study of mental illnesses.

Methods of molecular genetics.   The techniques of molecular genetics depend on the fact that many genetic loci are polymorphic; that is, genes are not simply a continuous series of base sequences that provide coding information in order to produce proteins. Instead, the information coded by the base pairs is divided by *spacers* in the DNA that vary in length. The spacers themselves have no known function, and they are edited out when messenger RNA is produced to initiate protein synthesis. They exist, however, in the genomic DNA.

Genetic variation and transmission can be studied through the use of these restriction fragment length polymorphisms (RFLPs). RFLPs are small pieces of DNA, typically measured in kilobases and consisting of somewhere between 1,000 and 10,000 base pairs. They can be seen after the DNA is digested or cut with an enzyme known as a restriction endonuclease—a bacterial enzyme that recognizes a specific base sequence and digests or cuts it out specifically. Differences in the lengths of these restriction fragments are inherited in classic Mendelian patterns. Therefore, if a single gene producing a disease is embedded within an RFLP or itself represents an RFLP, its transmission can be mapped within families and the genetic pattern of transmission thereby identified. Thus, the term *restriction fragment length polymorphism* refers to the variation in fragment length (polymorphism) produced by the spacers occurring between coding information. They are referred to as restriction fragment length polymorphisms because they are identified through the use of the restriction enzymes that cut the DNA and permit the identification of these variable fragment lengths. Typically, these measurements are made in the laboratory by Southern blotting techniques and a variety of other methods.

Two different strategies are available for studying the genetics of major mental illnesses such as bipolar disorder or schizophrenia—sometimes referred to as the *candidate gene approach* and the *reverse genetics approach.*

The candidate gene approach starts with the identification of some specific gene that might have pathophysiological relevance to the disorder of interest. During the past decade, molecular biologists have been actively engaged in cloning a large number of genes. The cloned genes obviously have applications beyond those involved in the study of genetics; for example, they can be used as an inexpensive method for synthetically manufacturing medically useful products such as hormones. As described above, they can be applied in psychiatry to the development of new drugs that have the appropriate chemical structure to "dock" in receptors whose amino acid sequences have been identified by receptor cloning.

The strength of the candidate gene approach is that it directly permits investigators to decide whether the particular protein has any relevance to the production of a major mental illness. When families of sufficient size are studied and it is determined that the particular gene sorts with the individuals who have the illness, then that particular protein has been identified as a causative mechanism. Likewise, if the study is negative, the protein has been excluded as a cause. Not all genes are polymorphic, but those that are can also be used to study genetic transmission. Examples of such polymorphic genes that have been or can be used in the candidate gene strategy include neuropeptide Y, beta nerve growth factor, dopamine, and monoamine oxidase (MAO). Candidate genes that might be relevant to mental illness include those involved in neurotransmission and hormonal regulation. To date, no positive candidate gene studies have been reported for major mental illnesses, but several negative studies have been completed (e.g., neuropeptide Y, beta nerve growth factor).

The majority of the work reported to date has involved the second strategy, linkage studies using RFLPs. This approach is referred to as reverse genetics because the investigator does not begin with a particular specific gene in mind. Here the unit of interest is the RFLP.

Linkage studies with RFLPs must begin with large, informative families that involve multiple generations in which a substantial number of individuals have the disorder of interest. Samples of their DNA can be collected through creating cell cultures of lymphocytes. Their genomes can then be scanned to determine whether a specific variation in restriction fragment length is linked to the presence of the specific disorder at some chromosomal location. Because of the size of the human genome, this process is relatively labor intensive. Nevertheless, it has had a highly successful application in Huntington's disease, where linkage was relatively quickly established on chromosome 4 through the study of a large Venezuelan pedigree. This led to the development of a premorbid test for the disease 2 years later. Nevertheless, illustrating the intransigent puzzles inherent in human biology, the gene itself has not yet been identified; we still do not know what abnormal structural or regulatory protein produces this illness. Thus, even with a clear, relatively simple, autosomal-dominant disease for which the chromosomal locus has been identified, the final answer we seek has not come easily.

Studying the genetics of major mental illnesses with RFLPs has presented much more complex problems, because in general these illnesses are not fully penetrant and are not clearly due to single loci. The pattern to date has been the reporting of positive findings, followed by nonreplications in other samples. Two types of studies of mood disorder have been reported. One suggested linkage between bipolar illness and chromosome 11, whereas another showed close linkage between bipolar illness and the X chromosome marker for color blindness. Both of these reports are controversial, however, and have not been replicated. A linkage for schizophrenia has been reported on chromosome 5, but many nonreplications were subsequently reported.

The results of these linkage studies illustrate some of the problems involved in applying molecular genetics to the study of mental illness, as well as the requirements for a good linkage study. One fundamental requirement, which is not easily obtained, is the availability of informative families. An informative family has large numbers of family members who are ill, and it also has the illness running through only one side of the family (i.e., only through the father or the mother of the proband). If the illness is contributed through both sides, it becomes much more difficult to determine linkage, because the illnesses diagnosed may be genetically heterogeneous. Theoretically, the disorder that runs within a single family and derives from one side is considered to be homogeneous in the literal sense (i.e., deriving from the same gene).

Heterogeneity is a serious problem in linkage studies. If a disorder is relatively common and affects large numbers of the population, and if it is caused by several different genes, then substantial noise is added to the system, because it becomes difficult or impossible to tell whether the clinical manifestations are linked to one gene or the other. Depression in particular is a very common disorder. Thus, for the study of mood disorder, a genetic isolate such as the Old Order Amish (used in the study of bipolar disorder and chromosome 11) is an ideal sample because there has been very little marriage in or out, and the disorder is more likely to be homogeneous within a family. Such genetic isolates are, of course, difficult to find. Further, isolates have their own inherent problems with respect to genetic research, because findings may not be generalizable. Nevertheless, if a gene is identified in an isolate and its metabolic pathway is studied and found to be informative, this might yield useful information concerning the pathophysiology of more common forms of the disorder. This hope has informed the study of Huntington's disease, for example.

The disorders within such informative families must be reliably and accurately diagnosed, and ideally, environmental phenocopies should be relatively rare. For this reason severe disorders such as bipolar disorder and schizophrenia present much easier cases than do depression and anxiety.

The application of molecular genetics to the study of mental illnesses to date has been somewhat frustrating and disappointing, apart from the case of Huntington's disease. Nevertheless, investigators continue to pursue this line of investigation because of its long-term promise. If an abnormal gene is found and its product identified, then the potential exists for either improved treatment or perhaps ultimately prevention. If a locus can be identified with linkage studies, it becomes possible to do genetic counseling and to identify unaffected individuals susceptible to developing the disease who may transmit it to their children. Measured against what was known and what could be done 30 years ago, recent achievements in genetics have been substantial. Measured against what remains to be done both scientifically and morally, however, these achievements seem quite modest.

Bibliography

Andreasen NC: Brain imaging: applications in psychiatry. Science 239:1381–1388, 1988

Andreasen NC (ed): Brain Imaging: Applications in Psychiatry. Washington, DC, American Psychiatric Press, 1989

Baron M, Risch N, Hamburger R, et al: Genetic linkage between X-chromosome markers and bipolar affective illness. Nature 326:289–292, 1987

Björklund A, Hökfelt T, Swanson LW: Handbook of Chemical Neuroanatomy, Vol 5: Integrated Systems of the CNS, Part I. Amsterdam, Elsevier, 1987

Botstein D, White RL, Skolnick MH, et al: Construction of a genetic linkage map in man, using restriction fragment length polymorphisms. Am J Hum Genet 32:314–331, 1980

Cooper JR, Bloom FE, Roth RH: The Biochemical Basis of Neuropharmacology, 6th Edition. New York, Oxford University Press, 1991

Coyle JT: Neuroscience and psychiatry, in The American Psychiatric Press Textbook of Psychiatry. Edited by Talbot JA, Hales RE, Yudofsky SC. Washington, DC, American Psychiatric Press, 1994, pp 3–32

Creese I, Burt DR, Snyder SH: Dopamine receptor binding predicts clinical and pharmacological potencies of anti-schizophrenic drugs. Science 192:481–483, 1972

Doane BK, Livingston KF: The Limbic System: Functional Organization and Clinical Disorders. New York, Raven, 1986

Egeland JA, Gerhard DS, Pauls DL, et al: Bipolar affective disorders linked to DNA markers on chromosome 11. Nature 323:646–650, 1987

Emson PC: Chemical Neuroanatomy. New York, Raven, 1983

Fischer M: Genetic and environmental factors in schizophrenia: a study of schizophrenic twins and their families. Acta Psychiatr Scand Suppl 238:9–142, 1973

Fuster JM: The Prefrontal Cortex: Anatomy, Physiology, and Neuropsychology of the Frontal Lobe, 2nd Edition. New York, Raven, 1989

Gottesman II, Schields J: Schizophrenia: The Epigenetic Puzzle. New York, Cambridge University Press, 1982

Gusella JF, Wexler NS, Conneally PM, et al: A polymorphic DNA marker genetically linked to Huntington's disease. Nature 306:234–238, 1983

Heaton R: Wisconsin Card Sorting Test. Odessa, TX, Psychological Assessment Resources, 1985

Heston LL: The genetics of schizophrenic and schizoid disease. Science 167:249–256, 1970

Isaacson RL: The Limbic System, 2nd Edition. New York, Plenum, 1982

Jones EG, Peters A: Cerebral Cortex, Vol 6: Further Aspect of Cortical Function, Including Hippocampus. New York, Plenum, 1987

Kallman FJ: The genetic theory of schizophrenia: an analysis of 691 schizophrenic twin index families. Am J Psychiatry 103:309–322, 1946

Kandel ER, Schwartz JH: Principles of Neural Science, 3rd Edition. New York, Elsevier, 1991

Kelsoe JR, Ginns EI, Egeland JA, et al: Re-evaluation of the linkage relationship between chromosome 11p loci and the gene for bipolar affective disorder in the Old Order Amish. Nature 342:238–243, 1989

Kety SS, Rosenthal D, Wender PH, et al: Mental illness in the biological and adoptive families of adopted schizophrenics. Am J Psychiatry 128:302–306, 1971

Kringlen E: Heredity and Environment in the Functional Psychoses: An Epidemiological-Clinical Twin Study. Oslo, Universitetsforlaget, 1967

Luxenburger H: Vorläufiger bericht über psychiatrische Serienuntersuchungen und Zwillinge. Zeitschrift fur die Gesamte Neurologie und Psychiatrie 116:1167–1171, 1928

Nauta WJH, Feirtag M: Fundamental Neuroanatomy. New York, WH Freeman, 1986

Rosanoff AJ, Handy LM, Plesset IR, et al: Etiology of so-called schizophrenic psychoses with special reference to their occurrence in twins. Am J Psychiatry 91:247–286, 1934

Rosvold HE, Mirsky AF, Sarason I, et al: A continuous performance test of brain damage. J Consult Clin Psychol 20:343–350, 1956

Seeman P, Lee T, Chau-Wong M, et al: Antipsychotic drug doses and neuroleptic-dopamine receptors. Nature 261:717–719, 1976

Shallice T: Specific impairments of planning. Philos Trans R Soc Lond Biol 298:199–209, 1982

Slater E, Crowie V: The Genetics of Mental Disorders. London, Oxford University Press, 1971

Stuss DT, Benson DF: The Frontal Lobes. New York, Raven, 1986

Suddath RL, Christison GW, Torrey EF et al: Anatomical abnormalities in the brains of monozygotic twins discordant for schizophrenia. N Engl J Med 322:789–794, 1990

Watson JD, Tooze J, Kurtz DT: Recombinant DNA: A Short Course. New York, WH Freeman, 1983

Yudofsky SC, Hales RE: The American Psychiatric Press Textbook of Neuropsychiatry. Washington, DC, American Psychiatric Press, 1992

Self-Assessment Questions

1. What is the standard anatomical definition of the prefrontal cortex? Describe the functions performed by the prefrontal cortex. Contrast the euphoric syndrome with the apathetic syndrome. List several neuropsychological tests used to assess prefrontal function.

2. Describe the limbic system, listing the structures included in it, and describe the functions of the amygdala and the hippocampus in relation to memory.

3. Discuss possible relationships between abnormalities in the frontal system, the memory system, and the language system in relation to the symptoms of psychosis.

4. Define a classic neurotransmitter and give five examples.

5. Describe the two receptor "superfamilies."

6. Discuss the ways that knowledge of receptor structure can influence the development of drugs used to treat mental illnesses.

7. Describe the location of cell bodies and projections for the dopamine system, the norepinephrine system, the serotonin system, and the acetylcholine system.

8. Describe the concept of atypical antipsychotics, their pharmacological profile, and the possible impact of this pharmacological profile on patient care.

9. Describe the mechanisms by which abnormalities in GABA neurons may produce Huntington's disease. Describe the functions of glutamate and its possible relationship to the symptoms of the psychosis, using PCP as a model.

10. Describe the relative strengths of family studies, twin studies, and adoption studies as methods for determining the familiality of mental illnesses and the degree to which purely genetic factors play a causal role.

11. Discuss the possible interaction between genes and environmental factors in producing mental illness, using neuroimaging studies of schizophrenia as an example.

12. Describe the candidate gene strategy versus the reverse genetics strategy for studying molecular mechanisms of mental illness. Describe the two different positive linkage studies for bipolar illness and their implications for the possible heterogeneity of major mental illnesses.

Section II

Psychiatric Disorders

Chapter 6

Delirium, Dementia, Amnesia, and Other Cognitive Disorders

When age has crushed the body with its might, the limbs
collapse with weakness and decay, the judgment limps, and
mind and speech give way.

Lucretius

What historically have been termed the *organic disorders* have now been divided into 1) cognitive disorders and 2) specific mental disorders that either are substance induced (e.g., amphetamine-induced psychosis) or result directly from a general medical condition (e.g., stroke-induced depression). The new classification used in DSM-IV recognizes the fact that all major psychiatric disorders are organic to some extent (i.e., a psychological or behavioral abnormality associated with transient or permanent central nervous system [CNS] dysfunction); for this reason, the term is considered outdated. The so-called functional disorders (e.g., schizophrenia, bipolar disorder) are also clearly associated with CNS dysfunction, ranging from structural brain abnormalities to disordered neurochemistry. Therefore, with growing evidence that all major psychiatric disorders involve CNS abnormalities, the organic/functional dichotomy is often arbitrary and is no longer thought to be valid.

Delirium, dementia, and amnestic disorder comprise the *cognitive disorders*, because disordered cognition (e.g., memory, abstract thinking, judgment) is the prominent feature in these conditions. *Specific mental disorders* that result directly from a general medical condition or are substance induced may be associated with cognitive disturbance; however, the prominent feature is a specific or isolated symptom, such as psychosis, dysphoric mood, or anxiety. In DSM-IV, specific mental disorders induced by medical illnesses or substances are included within the diagnostic category with which they share phenomenology; for instance, mania induced by psychostimulants is included with the *mood disorders.*

Mental disorders due to CNS dysfunction have been recognized for centuries. In the seventeenth century, Morgagni, the great Italian anatomist, made correlations between the clinical picture of mental patients and postmortem changes in their brains. Bayle, a Frenchman, published the first systematic study of paresis in 1822; he was able to correlate changes in brain parenchyma with progressive dementia. Another milestone was Korsakoff's investigation of extreme amnesia associated with brain stem lesions due to chronic alcoholism. However, it was not until the late nineteenth century that brain syndromes and their pathology were systematically investigated and described, mostly by the great neuropathologist-psychiatrists Alzheimer, Pick, Nissl, and Brodmann. Their pioneering work established conclusively that changes in brain structure and histology underlay the dementing illnesses. Even Freud, who was active at that time, understood the importance of neuroanatomical studies, and he observed that most mental disorders would eventually be found to have a structural basis.

In this chapter, we describe delirium, dementia, and amnestic disorder, which are the three major disorders associated with cognitive impairment. Next we describe mental disorders that are substance induced or due to general medical conditions and are characterized by specific, or isolated, symptoms, such as dysphoric mood, anxiety, psychosis, or personality change (see Tables 6–1 and 6–2).

Cognitive Disorders

Delirium

Delirium is a syndrome characterized by disturbance of consciousness, impaired attention, and change in cognition. Delirium develops quickly over hours or days and tends to fluctuate during the course of the day. (See Table 6–3 for the diagnostic criteria for delirium due to a general medical condition.) Because of its acuity, the development of a delirium creates a sense of clinical urgency.

Delirium is surprisingly common, especially among persons who are medically ill. Among medical patients at general hospitals, approximately 10%–15% develop a delirium during their hospitalization, and delirium is particularly com-

Table 6–1. Cognitive disorders

Deliriums
- Due to a general medical condition
- Substance induced
- Due to multiple etiologies
- Not otherwise specified

Dementias
- Of the Alzheimer type
     With early onset (age 65 years or below)
     With late onset (after age 65 years)
- Vascular
- Due to other general medical conditions
     Human immunodeficiency virus (HIV) disease
     Head trauma
     Parkinson's disease
     Huntington's disease
     Pick's disease
     Creutzfeld-Jakob disease
     Other (e.g., normal-pressure hydrocephalus, brain tumor, vitamin B_{12} deficiency)
- Substance-induced persisting dementia
- Due to multiple etiologies
- Not otherwise specified

Amnestic disorders
- Due to a general medical condition
- Substance-induced persisting amnestic disorder
- Not otherwise specified

Cognitive disorder not otherwise specified

mon among postsurgical and elderly patients (especially those over 80 years old); intensive-care–unit psychosis is an example of delirium occurring in the hospital. Other risk factors for delirium include an existing dementia, a fracture, a systemic infection, and use of narcotics or antipsychotics. Delirium is also associated with high mortality—an estimated 40%–50% of delirious patients will die within 1 year.

Clinical Findings

The hallmark of delirium is the relatively rapid development of global cognitive impairment combined with disorientation and confusion. Although the presentation of delirium may differ among patients, several features are characteristic, including disturbance of consciousness evidenced by a reduced awareness of the environment; difficulty focusing, sustaining, or shifting attention; impaired cognition; or development of perceptual disturbances of environmental stimuli

Table 6–2. Other specific mental disorders that are substance induced or due to a general medical condition

Psychotic disorder
- Substance induced
- Due to a general medical condition

Mood disorder
- Substance induced
- Due to a general medical condition

Anxiety disorder
- Substance induced
- Due to a general medical condition

Catatonic disorder due to a general medical condition
Personality change due to a general medical condition
Mental disorder not otherwise specified due to a general medical condition

Table 6–3. DSM-IV diagnostic criteria for delirium due to a general medical condition

A. Disturbance of consciousness (i.e., reduced clarity of awareness of the environment) with reduced ability to focus, sustain, or shift attention.

B. Change in cognition (e.g., memory deficit, disorientation, language disturbance) or the development of a perceptual disturbance that is not better accounted for by a preexisting, established, or evolving dementia.

C. The disturbance develops over a short period (usually hours to days) and tends to fluctuate during the course of the day.

D. There is evidence from the history, physical examination, or laboratory findings that the disturbance is caused by the direct physiological consequences of a general medical condition.

Coding note: If delirium is superimposed on a preexisting dementia of the Alzheimer type or vascular dementia, indicate the dementia by coding the appropriate subtype of the dementia; for example, dementia of the Alzheimer type, with late onset, with delirium.
Coding note: Include the name of the general medical condition on Axis I; for example, delirium due to hepatic encephalopathy. Also code the general medical condition on Axis III.

(e.g., illusions). The disturbance develops even over a short period and tends to fluctuate during the course of the day. At times the patient may appear normal, but later in the day may be disoriented and hallucinating. Other symptoms seen in delirium include sleep-wake cycle disturbances characterized by worsening at night (sundowning); disorientation to place, date, or person; incoherence; restlessness; and agitation or excessive somnolence.

The following case illustrates the disturbance of consciousness and cognition typical of delirium:

An 84-year-old retired police chief was brought to the emergency room by his family, who reported a 4- to 5-day history of lassitude, lower-extremity weakness, bladder incontinence, and intermittent confusion and memory impairment. They reported that the patient had fallen 4 weeks earlier and had sustained a scalp laceration requiring suturing. There was no history of alcohol use. When examined, the patient was cooperative, but drowsy and easily distracted. Although oriented to person, he was disoriented to date and situation. Memory for recent events was poor, and he was unable to recall three objects either immediately or at 3 minutes. He could not name the current president, but remembered President Franklin Roosevelt. Interestingly, the patient was an acquaintance of one of the author's deceased grandfathers and was able to speak at length of this remote relationship.

A presumptive diagnosis of delirium was made and a workup for a medical cause was begun. A computed tomography scan showed the presence of bilateral chronic subdural hematomas. The patient was transferred to the neurosurgery service, where burr-hole evaluation was performed. The delirium cleared, but the patient had a residual dementia and was eventually transferred to a long-term nursing facility.

Etiology

Delirium almost always occurs in persons who have serious medical, surgical, or neurological illness or who are in a state of drug intoxication or withdrawal. In fact, the development of a delirium may precede other manifestations of an underlying physical disorder, so that the presence of an unexplained delirium should lead to an immediate search for the factors that may have initiated the disturbance. Because delirium is a syndrome and not a disease, it is best seen as the final common pathway of many potential causes. Most causes of delirium lie outside the CNS and include metabolic disturbances, such as those caused by infection, febrile illness, hypoxia, hypoglycemia, drug withdrawal states, hepatic encephalopathy, or postoperative changes. Other causes lie within the CNS, such as brain abscesses, trauma, and postictal states. Although delirium may be influenced by the environment, the environment should never be considered the main cause of delirium, except in rare cases of total sensory deprivation.

Because the differential diagnosis of delirium is so broad, an evaluation needs to be thorough. The history and physical examination, however, will probably steer the clinician in a particular way. A medical workup must include a complete physical examination in which attention is paid to focal neurological signs, papilledema, and frontal lobe release signs (e.g., suck, snout, palmomental, rooting reflexes) characteristic of global deficit states. Laboratory tests should include routine blood and urine studies (e.g., complete blood count, urinalysis), chest X ray, computed tomography (CT) scan or magnetic resonance imaging (MRI), electrocardiogram, lumbar puncture (in selected patients), toxic screen, blood gases, and an electroencephalogram (EEG). Although laboratory results will vary depending on the underlying cause of the delirium, delirious patients are likely to have temperature elevations and abnormal EEGs that are diffusely slow.

The major problem in differential diagnosis is distinguishing delirium from a functional confusional state, which may occur in patients with schizophrenia or mania. Typically, the delirious patient has a more acute presentation and is globally confused, and the hallucinations (if present) tend to be fragmented, visual, and disorganized. The delirious patient is less likely to have a personal or family history of psychiatric illness. The clinician should be cautioned, however, that the presence of a preexisting psychiatric illness does not preclude the possibility of developing a delirium.

Clinical Management

First, it is essential that the underlying general medical condition be corrected, if possible. Until the condition is corrected, measures must be taken to maintain the patient's health and safety, including constant observation, consistent nursing care, frequent reassurance, and repeated simple explanations. Restraints may be necessary, but they may increase agitation in some patients. It is wise to minimize external stimulation. Experience has shown that delirious patients tend to do better in quiet, well-lighted rooms, because shadows or darkness may frighten them. Medication should be used with caution, because delirious patients are exquisitely sensitive to side effects. Unnecessary medication should be discontinued, including sedatives or hypnotics (e.g., benzodiazepines), which may have induced the delirium and can exacerbate sleep-wake cycle disturbances. For the highly agitated patient, low doses of a high-potency antipsychotic (e.g., haloperidol, thiothixene) may be helpful, but agents with significant anticholinergic properties (e.g., chlorpromazine, thioridazine) should be avoided, as these can worsen or prolong the delirium. In fact, in surgical patients, plasma anticholinergic levels have been found to correlate with delirium. If sedation is absolutely necessary, low doses of short-acting benzodiazepines (e.g., oxazepam, lorazepam) may be helpful. Treatment recommendations are summarized in the box.

Dementia

Dementia is a syndrome of impairment of cognition and memory, accompanied by a general decline in social and occupational functioning, which occurs without a disturbance in consciousness or level of alertness (i.e., sensorium). Cognitive impairment may include the 4 A's: aphasia (language disturbance), amnesia, apraxia (inability to carry out motor activities), and agnosia (failure to

---

Recommendations for management of delirium

1. In the hospital, a quiet, restful setting that is well lighted is best for the confused patient.
2. Consistency of personnel is less likely to upset the delirious patient.
3. Reminders of day, date, time, place, and situation should be prominently displayed in the patient's room.
4. Medication for behavioral management should be limited to those cases in which behavioral interventions have failed.
   - Only essential drugs should be prescribed, and polypharmacy should be avoided.
   - Avoid sedative-hypnotics and anxiolytics.
   - Unmanageable behavior may also require low-dose neuroleptics, or alternatively benzodiazepines with short half-lives (e.g., lorazepam 0.5 mg twice daily).

---

recognize or identify objects despite intact sensory function). Dementias are acquired, unlike mental retardation (which may be associated with these symptoms), which is congenital. The impairment created by dementia differentiates it from the mild memory change (benign senescent forgetfulness) that occurs during normal aging.

Although the causes of dementia are many, its clinical presentations are remarkably similar. Most dementias are irreversible, but many can be controlled by therapeutic interventions. Although a smaller number (up to 15%) are potentially reversible, only 3% fully resolve. A search for treatable causes is mandatory in the patient with dementia.

Dementia is relatively uncommon in persons under 65 years of age. About 5% of persons over 65 have severe dementia, whereas 10% have mild dementia. At age 80, 20% or more have severe dementia, and by age 90, the figure is 30%. Among elderly hospitalized patients and physically ill persons, the rates of dementia are higher still. Unfortunately, the prevalence of dementia will be an even greater problem in the future, because the growth in the population of those over age 65 is outstripping the growth in the general population.

Clinical Findings

Dementia usually develops insidiously, and its early signs may be overlooked or attributed to normal aging. In its earliest stages, the only symptoms may be subtle changes in personality, a decrease in range of interests or apathy, or the development of labile or shallow emotions. Gradually, intellectual skills will be lost, which may be noticed initially in work settings where high performance is required; the loss may be denied by the patient. Characteristics that help to separate delirium from dementia are highlighted in Table 6–4.

As the dementia advances, memory impairment becomes more pronounced, affecting immediate or recent memory preferentially; the changes in mood and personality become more exaggerated; social skills may be lost (whereas in earlier stages they may have helped to preserve the patient's image of health); psychotic symptoms may arise; judgment becomes impaired; and eventually language impairment—leading to perseveration, vagueness, or frank aphasia—may develop. In advanced cases, patients with dementia may be unable to perform basic tasks such as feeding themselves or caring for their personal hygiene. Patients may forget names of friends and be unable to recognize close relatives. Regression may include the development of infantile behavior, such as incontinence and extreme emotional lability. Finally, patients may become totally mute and unresponsive. At this stage, death usually occurs within months, although some patients may linger.

It is necessary to separate dementia from *pseudodementia*, an important condition that sometimes accompanies depressive illness. In this disturbance, the depressed patient appears to have dementia. He or she is unable to remember correctly, cannot calculate well, and complains, often bitterly, of lost cognitive abilities and skills. Features that are helpful in differentiating dementia from pseudodementia are presented in Table 6–5. The importance of this distinction is obvious; the patient with pseudodementia has a treatable illness and does not truly have dementia. The dementia is an artifact of the depression.

The noncognitive symptoms of dementia are often the most troublesome, especially from the family members' viewpoint (see Table 6–6). In some form of dementia, such as Alzheimer's disease, nearly two-thirds develop psychotic symptoms (e.g., hallucinations and delusions). As many as 20% develop major depression, although perhaps an equal number have milder depressive symptoms. Depression is even more common in patients with multi-infarct dementia. Because symptoms of dementia and depression overlap, the distinction between the two disorders may be difficult to determine. Clues to the diagnosis of depression

Table 6–4. Clinical features differentiating dementia from delirium

Dementia	Delirium
Chronic or insidious onset	Acute or rapid onset
Level of consciousness unimpaired early on	Level of consciousness clouded
Normal level of arousal	Agitation or stupor
Usually progressive and deteriorating	Often reversible
Common in nursing homes and psychiatric hospitals	Common on medical, surgical, and neurological wards

include recent weight loss (in the absence of cancer or apraxia in swallowing), worsening sleep, frequent crying spells, self-deprecating comments ("I can't do anything!"), and recent behavioral changes such as withdrawal, agitation, or negativism.

Diagnosis

The best diagnostic test for dementia is a careful history, physical examination, and mental status examination. The Mini-Mental State Examination, a quick, at-the-bedside test, can be used to get a rough index of cognitive impairment. (This test is included in the Appendix.) Assessing orientation, memory, constructional ability, and ability to read, write, and calculate, the test can be administered in 5 minutes. Thirty points are possible: a score of less than 25 is suggestive of impairment, and a score of less than 20 usually indicates definite impairment.

Laboratory testing is an important part of the evaluation. All patients with new onset of dementia should have a complete blood cell count, serum electrolytes, serum glucose, blood urea nitrogen, serum creatinine, liver and thyroid function tests, sedimentation rate, vitamin B_{12} and folate levels, serological tests for syphilis and human immunodeficiency virus (HIV), urinalysis, electrocardiogram, and chest X ray. Most of the readily reversible metabolic, endocrine, vitamin deficiency, and infectious states, whether causal or complicating, will be uncovered by these simple tests, when combined with the history and physical findings. Other tests are helpful in carefully chosen patients: a CT scan (or MRI)

Table 6–5. Clinical features differentiating pseudodementia from dementia

Pseudodementia	Dementia
Short duration	Long duration
Complaints of cognitive loss	Few complaints of cognitive loss
Complaints of cognitive dysfunction usually detailed	Complaints of cognitive dysfunction, usually imprecise
Communications of distress	Often appear unconcerned
Memory gaps for specific periods or events	Memory gaps for specific periods unusual
Attention and concentration usually well preserved	Attention and concentration faulty
"Don't know" answer typical	Near-miss answers frequent
Little effort to perform simple tasks	Patients struggle to perform tasks
Patients highlight failures	Patients delight in trivial accomplishments
Early loss of social skills	Social skills often retained
Mood change pervasive	Affect shallow and labile
History of prior psychiatric illness common	History of previous psychiatric illness uncommon

Table 6–6.   Behavior problems of 55 patients cited by family members

Behavior	Families reporting problems (%)
Memory disturbance	100
Temper outbursts	87
Demanding or critical behavior	71
Night awakening	69
Hiding things	69
Communication difficulties	68
Suspiciousness	63
Making accusations	60
Poor meal habits	60
Daytime wandering	59
Poor hygiene	53
Hallucinations	49
Delusions	47
Physical violence	47
Incontinence	40
Difficulty with cooking	33
Hitting or assaults	32
Problems driving	20
Problems smoking	11
Inappropriate sexual behavior	2

Source.   Adapted from Rabins PV, Mace NC, Lucas MJ: The impact of dementia on the family. JAMA 248:333–335, 1982.

of the brain is appropriate in the presence of a history suggestive of a mass, focal neurologic signs, or a dementia that is very brief in duration; EEGs are appropriate for patients with altered consciousness or suspected seizures. In some situations, other tests may be useful, including cerebral blood flow, lumbar puncture, and arterial blood gases. In particular, cerebral blood flow as measured by single photon emission computed tomography can be useful in the differential diagnosis of Alzheimer's dementia, because these patients have a relatively characteristic bilateral decrease in posterior temporoparietal blood flow. Undue weight should not be placed on isolated test results, however. The medical workup is summarized in Table 6–7.

Although the evaluation of most patients with dementia can be done on an outpatient basis, some patients will need hospitalization. In practice, most hospital admissions are for the evaluation and treatment of behavioral and psychological complications such as aggression, violence, wandering, psychosis, or depression. Other reasons for hospitalization include suicidal threats or behaviors, rapid weight loss or acute deterioration without apparent cause, or a social situation that precludes adequate observation.

Table 6–7.   Medical workup for dementia

1. Complete history
2. Thorough physical examination, including neurological examination
3. Mental status examination
4. Laboratory studies
   • Complete blood count, with differential
   • Serum electrolytes
   • Serum glucose
   • Blood urea nitrogen
   • Creatinine
   • Liver function tests
   • Serology for syphilis and HIV
   • Thyroid function tests
   • Serum vitamin B_{12}
   • Folate
   • Urinalysis and urine drug screen
   • Electrocardiogram
   • Chest X ray
   • Brain computed tomography or magnetic resonance imaging
5. Neuropsychological testing
6. Optional tests
   • Cerebral blood flow (i.e., single photon emission computed tomography)
   • Lumbar puncture

Neuropsychological testing can often be very useful in the evaluation of dementia. Testing may be done to obtain baseline data by which to measure change both before and after treatment. Testing can also be helpful in evaluating bright individuals suspected of developing an early dementia and when other test results (i.e., imaging studies) are ambiguous. Testing may also help distinguish delirium from dementia and depression.

Irreversible Causes of Dementia
Alzheimer's disease is the most common cause of the degenerative dementias and accounts for 50%–60% of all cases of dementia. It affects approximately 2.5 million Americans. In DSM-IV, Alzheimer's disease is divided into early (age 65 years and younger) and late (over 65 years) onset types; however, the natural history and pathology of cases arising before and after age 65 years are identical, so there is no clear basis for such a distinction. The diagnostic criteria for dementia of the Alzheimer type are presented in Table 6–8.

Alzheimer's disease usually begins insidiously in the 50s, 60s, or beyond and

Table 6–8.   DSM-IV criteria for dementia of the Alzheimer's type

A. The development of multiple cognitive deficits manifested by both:
1. Memory impairment (impaired ability to learn new information and to recall previously learned information)
2. One (or more) of the following cognitive disturbances:
    a. Aphasia (language disturbance)
    b. Apraxia (inability to carry out motor activities despite intact motor function)
    c. Agnosia (failure to recognize or identify objects despite intact sensory function)
    d. Disturbance in executive functioning (i.e., planning, organizing, sequencing, abstracting)

B. The cognitive deficits in A1 and A2 each cause significant impairment in social or occupational functioning and represent a significant decline from a previous level of functioning.

C. The course is characterized by gradual onset and continuing cognitive decline.

D. The cognitive deficits in A1 and A2 are not due to any of the following:
1. Other central nervous system conditions that cause progressive deficits in memory and cognition (e.g., cerebrovascular disease, Parkinson's disease, Huntington's disease, subdural hematoma, normal-pressure hydrocephalus, brain tumor)
2. Systemic conditions that are known to cause dementia (e.g., hypothyroidism, vitamin B_{12} or folic acid deficiency, niacin deficiency, hypercalcemia, neurosyphillis, HIV infection)
3. Substance-induced conditions

E. The deficits do not occur exclusively during the course of delirium.

F. The disturbance is not better accounted for by another Axis I disorder (e.g., major depressive disorder, schizophrenia).

Code based on type of onset and predominant features:
   With Early Onset: if onset is at age 65 years or below
      290.11 With Delirium: if delirium is superimposed on the dementia
      290.12 with Delusions: if delusions are the predominant feature
      290.13 With Depressed Mood: if depressed mood (including presentations that meet full symptom criteria for a major depressive episode) is the predominant feature. A separate diagnosis of mood disorder due to a general medical condition is not given.
      290.10 Uncomplicated: if none of the above predominates in the current clinical presentaiton

   With Late Onset: if onset is after age 65 years
      290.3 With Delirium: if delirium is superimposed on the dementia
      290.20 With Delusions: if delusions are the predominant feature
      290.21 With Depressed Mood: if depressed mood (including presentations that meet full symptom criteria for major depressive episode) is the predominant feature. A separate diagnosis of mood disorder due to a general medical condition is not given.
      290.0 Uncomplicated: if none of the above predominates in the current clinical presentation.

Specify if:
   With Behavioral Disturbance

Coding note: Also code 331.0 Alzheimer's disease on Axis III.

usually leads to death 8–10 years after onset. Estimates of the prevalence of Alzheimer's disease range from 5% at age 65 years to 20% by age 90 years. Symptoms begin gradually and progressively worsen over many years, resulting in near collapse of intellectual functioning. Physical findings are generally absent, or they are present only in later stages and may include hyperactive deep tendon reflexes, Babinski's sign, and frontal lobe release signs. Many patients develop illusions, hallucinations, and delusions, findings that have been associated with accelerated cognitive deterioration. Cortical atrophy and enlarged cerebral ventricles are seen on CT scan or MRI.

The case of composer Maurice Ravel illustrates the tragedy of Alzheimer-type dementia:

> Ravel, a leader of the French musical impressionist movement, excelled at piano composition and orchestration. At age 56, after completing his most famous work, the Concerto in G Minor, he began to complain of fatigue and lassitude, symptoms that were in keeping with his chronic insomnia and lifelong hypochondriasis. His symptoms did not improve and his creative energy waned.
>
> The following year, after a minor auto accident, his cognitive abilities began to noticeably erode. His capacity to remember names, to speak spontaneously, and to write became impaired, and this impairment progressed rapidly. An eminent French neurologist noted that Ravel's ability to understand verbal speech was superior to his ability to speak or to write. Unfortunately, Ravel also developed amusia, the inability to comprehend musical sounds. His last public performance occurred shortly thereafter. He was no longer capable of the coordination, cognition, and speech necessary to lead an orchestra.
>
> His friends made futile attempts to help him, trying to stimulate him intellectually any way they could. But gradually his speech and intellectual functions declined further. Within 4 years of the onset of dementia, Ravel was more or less mute and incapable of recognizing his own music.
>
> His death occurred at 62 years, after a neurosurgical procedure, the indications for which are far from clear. There was no autopsy, but his neurologist had suspected a cerebral degenerative disease. Syphilis, a common illness of the day, had been ruled out. (Dalessio 1984)

Although Alzheimer's disease is not diagnosable during life, characteristic brain pathology is found at autopsy, including senile plaques (degenerating neurons tangled around an amyloid core), neurofibrillary tangles (helical filaments tangled within neurons), neuronal granulovacuolar degeneration of nerve cell bodies, and Hirano bodies (elongated red structures often found in the hippocampus). Research has implicated primary degeneration of cholinergic neurons in the nucleus basalis of Meynert as a possible cause of Alzheimer's disease. Age-related memory disturbance in animals and humans may also be associated with a cholinergic dysfunction. In response to these findings, investigators have tried to increase choline levels in Alzheimer's patients with orally administered lecithin or tacrine hydrochloride, an acetylcholinesterase inhibitor. Although tacrine has been approved for the treatment of Alzheimer's disease, only mild improvement has been reported.

Risk factors for Alzheimer's disease include female gender, a history of head injury, Down's syndrome, low educational and occupational level, and having a first-degree relative with Alzheimer's disease. In fact, up to 50% of first-degree relatives are affected with the disorder by age 90 years. In the familial form of the disease, molecular genetic studies have found defects on chromosome 21 that may be responsible for the accumulation of amyloid in blood vessels and neurons and may explain the connection between Alzheimer's disease and Down's syndrome. This finding is important because recent research has focused on the protein amyloid, which may not be broken down properly in Alzheimer's patients.

Pick's disease accounts for about 5% of the irreversible dementias. It is clinically indistinguishable from Alzheimer's disease and can only be definitively diagnosed after death. At autopsy, the brain exhibits distinctive frontotemporal atrophy and ventricular dilatation. Microscopic examination discloses neuronal loss with gliosis and the presence of Pick's bodies in the neurons. Pick's bodies contain masses of cytoskeletal elements that bind polyclonal antibodies against neurotubules and a monoclonal antibody against neurofilaments. Pick's disease is more common in men and in first-degree relatives.

Huntington's disease is a neuropsychiatric disorder with autosomal-dominant inheritance. Its gene has been located on the short arm of chromosome 4. Psychiatric manifestations range from mild anxiety to hallucinations and delusions, which may precede the onset of choreiform movements. Dementia occurs in the terminal phase of the illness. The dementia is characterized by poor cognitive ability without a language disorder. These symptoms combined with pronounced apathy suggest that it is more subcortical than cortical.

Other degenerative illnesses associated with the dementia syndrome include diseases of the basal ganglia (Parkinson's disease), of the cerebellum (cerebellar, spinocerebellar, and olivopontocerebellar degeneration), and of the motor neuron (amyotrophic lateral sclerosis).

Other irreversible dementias include Parkinson-dementia complex of Guam, Creutzfeldt-Jakob disease, herpes simplex encephalitis, and the dementia of multiple sclerosis. Numerous hereditary metabolic diseases are associated with irreversible dementia, including Wilson's disease (hepatolenticular degeneration), metachromatic leukodystrophy, the adrenoleukodystrophies, and the neuronal storage diseases (e.g., Tay-Sachs disease).

Clinical Management

Other than tacrine, which has limited application, there are currently no drugs available that reverse the cognitive loss in Alzheimer's or other degenerative dementias. Tacrine may lead to modest improvements in cognition and ability to perform simple tasks, although not all patients benefit. Tacrine is started at 40 mg daily and gradually increased to between 120 and 160 mg in divided doses. Liver enzyme elevations, nausea and/or vomiting, diarrhea, and dyspepsia are the most common adverse effects; therefore, regular monitoring of hepatic transaminase levels is required.

Other medications may be used for the symptomatic treatment of associated anxiety, psychosis, or depression. In these cases, anxiolytics, antipsychotics, and antidepressants, respectively, can be helpful. The physician must find the lowest effective dose, a difficult task because these patients may not be able to tolerate side effects at relatively low doses.

Behavioral agitation consisting of irritability, hostility, aggression, uncooperativeness, and assaultiveness is the most difficult and vexing problem to manage. These disturbing and disruptive symptoms may make it difficult to keep the patient within his or her family or social situation and can lead to institutionalization. Antipsychotics are frequently prescribed to control behavioral problems in patients with dementia, as are the benzodiazepines. One recent study compared the efficacy of haloperidol, oxazepam, and diphenhydramine in controlling behavior. All agents were beneficial, with few differences among them.

Other medications may also be useful, including propranolol, lithium carbonate, or carbamazepine. Case reports suggest that trazodone and buspirone may also have a limited role in the management of disturbed behavior. Physostigmine has been reported to specifically ameliorate delusions in Alzheimer's patients.

In treating the depressed dementia patient, the clinician should avoid tertiary tricyclic antidepressants and use the better-tolerated secondary tricyclics (e.g., desipramine) or the newer serotonin-selective antidepressants (e.g., fluoxetine, paroxetine), which tend to be better tolerated in elderly persons. Whatever is used, dementia patients require lower doses than persons without dementia.

The behavioral goals of treatment should be the maintenance of the patient's socialization and provision of support for the family. Reality orientation may be worthwhile; reminiscence group therapy may be useful in maintaining socialization in selected patients. Even severely affected patients can react to familiar social activities and to music. Self-help groups for family members can provide educational and psychological support. Day care centers may provide needed relief for caregivers. A useful manual is *The 36-Hour Day* (Mace and Rabins 1981).

Recommendations for the management of dementia

---

1. Both at home and in care facilities, patients usually respond better to low-stimulus environments as opposed to high-stimulus situations.
   - Demented patients have difficulty interpreting sensory input and easily become overwhelmed.
2. Consistency and routine are important for reducing confusion and agitation.
3. Families are often overwhelmed by caring for a cognitively impaired relative.
   - Recommend that family members attend support groups available in most communities.
   - Provide appropriate reading material.
4. Families should be given psychological support if the dementia patient requires institutionalization, to lessen the guilt they almost inevitably feel.
5. Tacrine may help to slow the dementing process, but the benefits may not outweigh its adverse effects. Nonetheless, accompanying depression generally responds to antidepressants, and acute agitation or psychosis may respond to low-dose antipsychotics.
   - Avoid low-potency antipsychotics because of their anticholinergic side effects.
   - For long-term behavioral management, lithium carbonate, propranolol, carbamazepine, and other agents have been tried, but benefit is inconsistent.

Treatable Forms of Dementia

Vascular disorders.

Multi-infarct dementia is the second most common cause of dementia, accounting for about 10% of cases. Its differentiation from the degenerative dementias includes its history of rapid onset and a stepwise deterioration occurring in patients in their 50s or 60s. This deterioration may be accompanied by focal neurological impairment. The dementia is generally caused by multiple thromboembolic episodes occurring in persons with atherosclerotic disease of major vessels or heart valves. Patients with this disease commonly have high blood pressure or diabetes. There is generally a history of several strokes in the past, many of them silent. Atherosclerosis in major arteries may be surgically correctable, but because atherosclerosis occurs diffusely among smaller intracranial vessels, it is not amenable to any specific intervention. In most cases, however, hypertension can be controlled, and early treatment of asymptomatic patients can help prevent or arrest the development of a multi-infarct dementia. Patients who have had or are at risk for stroke may benefit from the administration of anticoagulants or aspirin, which may prevent thrombus formation.

Subdural hematoma may produce a dementia itself or may complicate other forms of dementia. Subdural hematomas are caused by a disruption of the veins that bridge the brain parenchyma and the meninges and are usually attributable to trauma. Risk factors for subdural hematoma include age over 60 years, alcoholism, epilepsy, and renal dialysis. The disorder is treated by evacuation of the hematoma through a burr hole in the skull.

Normal-pressure hydrocephalus. This disorder is caused by excessive accumulation of cerebrospinal fluid (CSF), which gradually dilates the ventricles of the brain in the presence of normal CSF pressure. The flow of CSF from the ventricles to its usual site of absorption becomes obstructed so that fluid collects within the ventricles, resulting in the characteristic syndrome of dementia, gait disturbance, and urinary incontinence. Normal-pressure hydrocephalus may result from brain trauma, but the cause is usually unknown. Some patients respond dramatically to shunting of the ventriculosubarachnoid reservoir.

Infections. Any infection that involves the brain is capable of producing a dementing illness. Many cases of dementia are prevented by the effective treatment of meningitis and encephalitis, whether caused by bacteria, fungi, protozoa, or viruses. Chronic infectious processes, for example, those caused by bacteria (e.g., Whipple's disease), fungi (e.g., cryptococcus), or other microorganisms (e.g., syphilis), may affect the brain in such a way that the process is reversible and arrestable, at least to some degree. The slow viruses responsible for conditions such as Creutzfeldt-Jakob disease and progressive multifocal leukoencephalopathy are resistant to any kind of treatment. A postinfectious encephalomyelitis occurring after a viral exanthem may produce enough brain damage to leave the patient with a dementia.

Dementia may also occur in patients with the acquired immunodeficiency syndrome (AIDS). The dementia may be caused by direct HIV infection of the nervous system, intracranial tumors, infections (e.g., toxoplasmosis, cryptococcus), or the indirect effects of systemic disease (e.g., septicemia, hypoxia, electrolyte imbalance). Because dementia may occur in the early stages of HIV infection, evaluation for HIV seropositivity is indicated for persons at high risk for infection (e.g., male homosexuals, drug addicts) who develop intellectual, mood, or behavioral changes. See Chapter 21 for a more complete discussion of the psychiatric aspects of HIV disease.

Metabolic disorders. Chronic diseases of the thyroid, parathyroid, adrenal, and pituitary glands can cause reversible dementias and are usually easily identified. Pulmonary diseases can produce dementia as a result of hypoxia or hypercapnia. Chronic or acute renal failure may cause a reversible dementia, as can liver failure (i.e., hepatic encephalopathy). Dementia is common in diabetic patients, particularly from either hypoglycemic or hyperosmolar coma.

Nutritional disorders.   Thiamine deficiency may lead to Wernicke-Korsakoff's syndrome and Korsakoff's psychosis, an amnestic disorder. Both disorders are discussed later in the chapter. There are different mechanisms by which pernicious anemia can produce dementia, not all of which are reversible. Folate deficiency is potentially reversible if recognized early. Pellagra (niacin deficiency), a major problem in underdeveloped countries, shows a dramatic response to niacin, even when mental changes have been present for a long time.

Treatable causes of dementia are summarized in Table 6–9.

Amnestic Disorder

The main feature of amnestic disorder is inability to learn new information or to recall previously learned information, leading to significant impairment in social and occupational functioning. The full criteria are shown in Table 6–10. Patients with this disorder may be oriented and alert, but cannot remember what happened a few hours earlier. This disorder may be caused by trauma, tumor, infection, infarction, seizures, or drugs, but the most common cause is alcohol abuse (Korsakoff's syndrome). Alcohol-induced amnesia is probably related to chronic thiamine deficiency; this syndrome may occur in association with

Table 6–9.   Treatable causes of dementia

Vascular	**Toxicity**
Multiple infarcts	Bromides
Subacute bacterial endocarditis	Mercury
Decreased cardiac output	Others
Myocardial infarction, heart failure	**Infections**
Collagen vascular diseases (e.g., lupus, polyarteritis)	General paresis
Metabolic and endocrine	Cryptococcal meningitis
Hypothyroidism	Encephalitis
Hyperparathyroidism	Sarcoid
Pituitary insufficiency	Postinfectious encephalomyelitis
Repeated hypoglycemia	HIV
Respiratory acidosis	**Mass effect**
Uremia	Lymphoma and leukemia (with or without pathologic change)
Hepatic encephalopathy	Intracranial tumor (e.g., subfrontal meningioma)
Porphyria	Subdural hematoma
Wilson's disease	**Subclinical seizures**
Nutrition	**Demyelinating disease**
Pernicious anemia	**Normal-pressure hydrocephalus**
Alcoholism and thiamine deficiency	
Pellagra	

Wernicke-Korsakoff's syndrome, characterized by the triad of gait ataxia, nystagmus, and mental confusion. This syndrome requires emergency treatment with thiamine, but once the condition is reversed, patients may have a residual amnestic disorder (i.e., Korsakoff's psychosis). Korsakoff's psychosis may not improve despite abstinence from alcohol and maintenance on thiamine, but it is reversible in up to 50% of patients. Autopsies of patients with this syndrome show hemorrhage and sclerosis of the hypothalamic mammillary bodies and nuclei of the thalamus, as well as more diffuse lesions in the brain stem, cerebellum, and the limbic system.

Specific Mental Disorders That Are Substance Induced or Due to a General Medical Condition

DSM-IV defines other specific syndromes that may be substance induced or due to a general medical condition: psychotic, mood, anxiety, and catatonic disorders and personality change (see Table 6–2). Cognitive or intellectual impairment is usually not prominent in these disorders, but it may be present. A residual category (mental disorder not otherwise specified due to a general medical condition) has been created for those patients whose disturbance does not meet criteria for a specific disorder, for example, a person with a dissociative disorder due to partial complex seizures.

Table 6–10. DSM-IV criteria for amnestic disorder due to a general medical condition

A. The development of memory impairment as manifested by impairment in the ability to learn new information **or** the inability to recall previously learned information.

B. The memory disturbance causes significant impairment in social or occupational functioning and represents a significant decline from a previous level of functioning.

C. The memory disturbance does not occur exclusively during the course of a delirium or a dementia.

D. There is evidence from the history, physical examination, or laboratory findings that the disturbance is the direct physiological consequence of a general medical condition (including physical trauma).

Specify if:

Transient (if memory impairment lasts for 1 month or less)

Chronic (if memory impairment lasts for more than 1 month)

Coding note: Include the name of general medical condition on Axis I, e.g., amnestic disorders due to head trauma; also code general medical condition on Axis III.

Psychotic Disorders

Psychotic disorders may occur and are often drug related. Ingestion of psychostimulants (e.g., cocaine, amphetamines) may cause a syndrome that can be indistinguishable from paranoid schizophrenia. It has been suggested that Hitler developed persecutory delusions and delusions of grandeur from psychostimulants, which he was known to abuse.

> Leonard and Renate Heston (1979) describe the personality change observed in Hitler, almost certainly due to the daily amphetamine injections that he was documented to have received from 1942 until his suicide in 1945. He was observed to become increasingly suspicious, rigid, distractible, and irritable. "He became unrestrained and reckless. He would lose his temper, flush deeply and in a rapid, loud voice breaking with excitement, denounce the incompetence and mendacious cowardice of the General Staff. After such an outburst he would have to pace the room furiously for a long time, wordlessly snapping his fingers until his agitation subsided somewhat." (p. 12) In addition to behavioral changes, he developed other signs of amphetamine toxicity, including a sleep disturbance, a tremor, and stereotypic behaviors, such as biting the skin around his fingernails.

Although an amphetamine psychosis is usually self-limited, delusions may persist for months or years after chronic abuse of psychostimulants. Psychotic disorders have also been associated with traumatic, metabolic, infectious, and other causes. The psychosis associated with temporal lobe epilepsy is often chronic and may not develop until 15 years or more have elapsed after the onset of psychomotor seizures.

Mood Disorders

The mood disturbance is characterized by either depressed mood or markedly diminished interest or pleasure, or by elevated, expansive, or irritable mood. Depression is a more common induced symptom than mania, although the latter has been attributed to causes such as head trauma, physical illness, or medication (e.g., zidovudine in patients with AIDS). In typical cases of induced mood disorder, patients tend to be older and less likely to have a family history of mood disturbance.

The following patient illustrates a relatively typical case of an induced mood disorder.

> Renee, a 29-year-old woman, was transferred for evaluation of depression and suicidal ideations. Although Renee had a long history of reclusiveness and undue social anxiety, she was otherwise psychiatrically well until 4 months before admission,

when she developed a depressive syndrome. One year earlier she had been diagnosed with multiple sclerosis on the basis of slurred speech, gait ataxia, and multiple sclerotic plaques visualized by MRI.

At admission, Renee admitted to low mood, appetite loss, poor energy, and low self-esteem, and she had psychomotor retardation. Before admission, Renee had written a suicide note and had been found in her room with insecticide sprays that she had been planning to kill herself with.

Renee's mood disorder was felt to be due to her multiple sclerosis. She was treated with eight bilateral electroconvulsive treatments after she had failed to respond to antidepressants. Her mood normalized, but she remained odd and reclusive.

As many as one-third of the patients who have a cerebrovascular stroke will experience depression in the 6- to 12-month period after the event. Interestingly, left-hemisphere strokes appear to result in more depression than right-hemisphere or brain stem strokes. Within the left hemisphere, the closer the lesion is to the frontal pole, the more likely it is to produce depression. These depressions are probably due to the direct structural and biochemical effects of the stroke, not the psychological reaction to a medical disorder. These patients tend to respond to tricyclic antidepressants (e.g., nortriptyline).

Anxiety Disorders

Anxiety disorders can result from general medical conditions or the direct effects of a substance, or from withdrawal from a substance. According to DSM-IV, prominent anxiety, panic attacks, or obsessions or compulsions may be seen. Examples commonly seen by clinicians include generalized anxiety or panic attacks caused by hyperthyroidism and the jitteriness caused by excessive caffeine intake. Withdrawal of a substance to which a person has become habituated (e.g., alcohol, benzodiazepines) may cause intense but transient anxiety.

Personality Change Due to a General Medical Condition

This category recognizes the fact that personality change can result from general medical conditions. Resulting changes in attitudes and behavior often represent an exaggeration of preexisting personality characteristics. By definition, the personality disturbance represents a change from the patient's previous personality pattern, and the change is not better accounted for by another mental disorder, such as major depression. See Table 6–11 for the criteria and subtypes.

A remarkable example of an induced personality change is that of Phineas Gage, whose case is discussed in Chapter 5. The case illustrates the frontal lobe syndrome, typically associated with impaired judgment, disinhibition, amotivation, and witzelsucht, or silly humor and punning, but no intellectual impair-

Table 6–11. DSM-IV criteria for personality change due to a general medical condition

A. A persistent personality disturbance that represents a change from the individual's previous characteristic personality pattern. (In children, the disturbance involvesa marked deviation from normal development or a significant change in the child's usual behavior patterns lasting at least 1 year.)

B. There is evidence from the history, physical examination, or laboratory findings that the disturbance is the direct physiological consequence of a general medical condition.

C. The disturbance is not better accounted for by another mental disorder (including other mental disorders due to a general medical condition).

D. The disturbance does not occur exclusively during delirium and does not meet criteria for dementia.

E. The disturbance causes clinically significant distress or impairment in social, occupational, or other important areas of functioning.

Specify type:

Labile type: if the predominant feature is affective lability

Disinhibited type: if the predominant feature is poor impulse control as evidenced by sexual indiscretions, etc.

Aggressive type: if the predominant feature is aggressive behavior

Apathetic type: if the predominant feature is marked apathy and indifference

Paranoid type: if the predominant feature is suspiciousness or paranoid ideation

Other type: if the predominant feature is not one of the above, e.g., personality change associated with a seizure disorder

Combined type: if more than one feature predominates in the clinical picture

Unspecified type

Coding note: Include the name of the general medical condition on Axis I, e.g., personality change due to temporal lobe epilepsy; also code general medical condition on Axis III.

ment. Before the injury that destroyed his frontal lobes, Gage was a sober, responsible family man, and afterward he became loud, obnoxious, and foul mouthed and was unable to keep a job.

The diagnosis is often used to describe the personality profile of some patients with temporal lobe epilepsy. These patients are described as *viscous*, a term that reflects their tendency to become fixated on philosophical concerns and talk endlessly, unaware that the listener may not share their enthusiasm. Patients may display hypergraphia, hyperreligiosity, and disturbed sexuality (e.g., hyper- or hyposexuality). Several historical figures appear to fit this description, including Dostoyevsky and Rasputin. Aggressive behavior may also occur as an interictal phenomenon, but it is rarely a manifestation of a seizure. Anticonvulsants such as carbamazepine have been used to treat these interictal changes in the belief that if the seizure disorder is better controlled, the personality changes will stabilize or reverse. Carbamazepine has also been used to reduce aggressive tendencies in these patients. Although case reports suggest benefit, controlled trials are still needed.

Catatonic Disorder Due to a General Medical Condition

This category, introduced in DSM-IV, is used when catatonic symptoms (e.g., motoric immobility, excessive motor activity, extreme negativism, mutism, peculiar voluntary movement, echolalia, or echopraxia) are judged to be related to a general medical condition. Conditions associated with catatonic features have included viral encephalitis, brain trauma, status epilepticus, Wernicke's encephalopathy, and tuberous sclerosis. Metabolic conditions have included diabetic ketoacidosis, acute intermittent porphyria, and hepatic encephalopathy.

Bibliography

Barnes R, Veith R, Okimoto J, et al: Efficacy of antipsychotic medications in behaviorally disturbed dementia patients. Am J Psychiatry 139:1170–1174, 1982

Black DW, Warrack G, Winokur G: The Iowa Record-linkage study, II: excess mortality in organic mental disorders. Arch Gen Psychiatry 42:78–81, 1985

Breitner JCS: Clinical genetics and genetic counseling in Alzheimer's disease. Ann Intern Med 115:601–606, 1991

Caine ED, Shoulson I: Psychiatric syndromes in Huntington's disease. Am J Psychiatry 140:728–733, 1983

Clarfield AM: The reversible dementias: do they reverse? Ann Intern Med 109:476–486, 1988

Coccaro EF, Kramer E, Zemishlany Z, et al: Pharmacologic treatment of non-cognitive behavioral disturbances of elderly demented patients. Am J Psychiatry 147:1640–1645, 1990

Consensus Conference: Differential diagnosis of dementing diseases. JAMA 258:3411–3416, 1987

Council on Scientific Affairs: Dementia. JAMA 256:2234–2238, 1986

Cummings JL, Gorman DG, Shapira J: Physostigmine ameliorates the delusions of Alzheimer's disease. Biol Psychiatry 33:536–541, 1993

Dalessio DJ: Maurice Ravel and Alzheimer's disease. JAMA 252:3412–3413, 1984

Davison K: Schizophrenia-like psychoses associated with organic cerebral disorders: a review. Psychiatric Developments 1:1–34, 1983

Drevets WC, Rubin EH: Psychotic symptoms and the longitudinal course of senile dementia of the Alzheimer type. Biol Psychiatry 25:35–48, 1989

Dubin WR, Weis KJ, Zeccardi JA: Organic brain syndrome—the psychiatric impostor. JAMA 249:60–62, 1983

Fallow M, Gracon SI, Hersey LA, et al: A controlled trial of tacrine in Alzheimer's disease. JAMA 268:2523–2529, 1992

Francis J, Martin, D, Kapoor WN: A prospective study of delirium in hospitalized elderly. JAMA 263:1097–1101, 1990

Golinger RC, Peet T, Tune LE: Association of elevated plasma anticholinergic activity with delirium in surgical patients. Am J Psychiatry 144:1218–1220, 1987

Greendyke RM, Kanter DR, Schuster DB, et al: Propranolol treatment of assaultive patients with organic brain disease—double-blind cross over, placebo controlled study. J Nerv Ment Dis 174:290–294, 1986

Heston L, Heston R: The Medical Casebook of Hitler. New York, Stein and Day, 1979

Heston LL, White JA, Mastri AR: Pick's disease—clinical genetics and natural history. Arch Gen Psychiatry 44:409–411, 1987

Knapp MJ, Knopman DS, Solomon PR, et al: A 30 week randomized controlled trial of high-dose tacrine in patients with Alzheimer's disease. JAMA 271:985–991, 1994

Levine AM: Case report: buspirone and agitation in head injury. Brain Injury 2:165–167, 1988

Lipsey JR, Robinson RG, Pearlson GD, et al: Nortriptyline treatment of poststroke depression: a double blind study. Lancet 1:297–300, 1984

Mace NL, Rabins PV: The 36-Hour Day. Baltimore, MD, Johns Hopkins University Press, 1981

Mayeux R, Stern Y, Williams JBW, et al: Clinical and biochemical features of depression in Parkinson's disease. Am J Psychiatry 143:756–759, 1986

McAllister TW: Overview: pseudodementia. Am J Psychiatry 140:528–533, 1983

Medalia A, Scheinberg IH: Psychopathology in patients with Wilson's disease. Am J Psychiatry 146:662–664, 1989

Pinner C, Rich CL: Effects of trazodone on aggressive behavior in seven patients with organic mental disorders. Am J Psychiatry 145:1295–1296, 1988

Rabins PV, Folstein MF: Delirium and dementia: diagnostic criteria and fatality rates. Br J Psychiatry 140:149–153, 1982

Robinson RG, Kubose KL, Star LB, et al: Mood changes in stroke patients: relationship to lesion location. Compr Psychiatry 24:555–566, 1983

Schor JD, Levkoff SE, Lipsitz LA, et al: Risk factors for delirium in hospitalized elderly. JAMA 267:827–831, 1992

Simpson DM, Foster D: Improvement in organically disturbed behavior with trazodone treatment. J Clin Psychiatry 74:191–193, 1986

Stern Y, Gurland B, Tatemichi TK, et al: Influence of education and occupation on the incidence of Alzheimer's disease. JAMA 271:1004–1010, 1994

Williams KH, Goldstein G: Cognitive and affective response to lithium in patients with organic brain syndrome. Am J Psychiatry 136:800–803, 1979

Self-Assessment Questions

1. What are the differences between delirium and dementia?
2. What does the medical workup for delirium and dementia consist of?
3. Describe Alzheimer's disease. What are its histopathological findings?
4. What is the pathognomic finding in Pick's disease?
5. What triad of symptoms cluster in normal-pressure hydrocephalus?
6. List the different causes of dementia.
7. What is pseudodementia? What are its typical signs?
8. How are dementia patients clinically managed?
9. What general medical conditions have been associated with catatonia?
10. Describe the frontal lobe syndrome.

Chapter 7

Schizophrenia

The psychopathology of schizophrenia is one of the most intriguing, since it permits a many-sided insight into the workings of the diseased as well as the healthy psyche.

Eugen Bleuler

Schizophrenia is probably the most devastating illness that psychiatrists treat. An estimated 1% of the population has schizophrenia, which claims its victims at a youthful age and prevents their full participation in society. Schizophrenia also creates an enormous economic burden, costing society over $104 billion annually in both direct and indirect costs. Despite its emotional and economic cost, schizophrenia has yet to receive sufficient recognition as a major health concern or the necessary research support to investigate its causes, treatments, and prevention.

This chapter is adapted with permission from Black DW, Andreasen NC: Schizophrenia, schizophreniform disorder, and delusional (paranoid) disorder, in The American Psychiatric Press Textbook of Psychiatry, 2nd Edition. Edited by Talbott JA, Hales RE, Yudofsky SC. Washington, DC, American Psychiatric Press, 1994, pp 411–463. Copyright 1994 American Psychiatric Press, Inc.

History

Schizophrenia has been recognized in almost all cultures and described throughout much of recorded time. Its modern history dates to Emil Kraepelin, who is credited with identifying schizophrenia. His original term for schizophrenia, *dementia praecox*, was based on his observations that these patients developed their illness at a relatively early age (praecox) and were likely to have a chronic and deteriorating course (dementia). Kraepelin was also instrumental in separating dementia praecox from manic-depressive illness, which had its onset distributed throughout life and had a more episodic course. Dementia praecox was eventually renamed *schizophrenia*, a term coined by Eugen Bleuler to emphasize the cognitive impairment that occurs, which he conceptualized as a splitting of cognitive processes. Bleuler believed that certain symptoms were fundamental to the illness, including affective blunting, disturbance of association (i.e., fragmented thinking), autism, and ambivalence (i.e., fragmented emotional responses). Other symptoms such as delusions and hallucinations were regarded by him to be accessory because they could occur in other disorders, including manic-depressive illness.

Bleuler's ideas earned acceptance throughout the United States, and generations of psychiatrists were taught the importance of Bleulerian fundamental symptoms (the four A's). Unlike hallucinations and delusions, these symptoms are on a continuum with normality and can be present in relatively mild forms even in psychiatrically healthy persons. Consequently, the conceptualization of schizophrenia in the United States became increasingly broad. Later, the ideas of a German psychiatrist, Kurt Schneider, who emphasized first-rank or specific psychotic symptoms, were introduced, helping to reshape the concept of schizophrenia into one of a relatively severe psychotic disorder, bringing it back to the original ideas of Kraepelin. DSM-IV (American Psychiatric Association 1994) represents a convergence of varying points of view with its Kraepelinian emphasis on course, the emphasis on specific delusions and hallucinations thought important by Schneider, and acknowledgment of the importance of Bleuler's fundamental symptoms.

Definition

According to DSM-IV, schizophrenia is defined by a group of characteristic positive or negative symptoms; deterioration in social, work, or interpersonal relationships; and continuous signs of the disturbance for at least 6 months. In addition, schizoaffective disorder and mood disorder with psychotic features have been ruled out, and the disturbance is not due to the direct physiological effects of a substance or a general medical condition. (See Table 7–1 for more detail on the DSM-IV criteria.) If an illness otherwise meets the criteria, but has a duration of less than 6 months, it is called a *schizophreniform disorder*. If the duration is less than 4 weeks and more than 1 day, the illness may be classified as either a *brief psychotic disorder* or a *psychotic disorder not otherwise specified*, which is a residual category for psychotic disturbances that cannot be better classified.

Clinical Findings

The clinical findings in schizophrenia are protean and can change over time. Because of their variety, it has been said that to know schizophrenia is to know psychiatry. Although some symptoms (e.g., hallucinations) are obvious, others (e.g., affective flattening) are relatively subtle and easily missed by the casual observer.

Many clinicians have found it useful to describe typical schizophrenic symptoms as either positive or negative. In practice, patients usually have a mixture of the two. *Positive symptoms*—such as hallucinations, delusions, marked positive formal thought disorder (manifested by marked incoherence, derailment, tangentiality, or illogicality), and bizarre or disorganized behavior—reflect aberrant mental activity. *Negative symptoms* reflect deficiency of a mental function that is normally present, for instance, alogia (e.g., marked poverty of speech or poverty of content of speech), affective flattening, anhedonia-asociality (e.g., inability to experience pleasure, few social contacts), avolition-apathy (e.g., anergia, lack of persistence at work or school), and attentional impairment. The classification resembles Bleuler's original distinction between fundamental and accessory symptoms. One of the authors (N. C. A.) developed the Scale to Assess Positive Symptoms and the Scale to Assess Negative Symptoms to evaluate these symptoms. These scales are included in the Appendix. The frequency of common positive and negative symptoms found in a series of 111 patients is shown in Table 7–2.

Hallucinations have sometimes been considered the hallmark of schizophrenia, although they may occur in a variety of other disorders, including mood disorders and brain disorders induced by medical illnesses or the effects of a substance. Hallucinations are perceptions experienced without an external stimulus to the sense organs and have a quality similar to a true perception. Schizophrenic patients commonly report auditory, visual, tactile, gustatory, or olfactory halluci-

Table 7–1.   DSM-IV criteria for schizophrenia

A. Characteristic symptoms: Two (or more) of the following, each present for a significant portion of time during a 1-month period (or less if successfully treated).
   1. Delusions
   2. Hallucinations
   3. Disorganized speech (e.g., frequent derailment or incoherence)
   4. Grossly disorganized or catatonic behavior
   5. Negative symptoms (i.e., affective flattening, alogia or avolition)

Note: Only one criterion A symptom is required if delusions are bizarre or hallucinations consist of a voice keeping up a running commentary on the person's behavior or thoughts, or two or more voices conversing with each other.

B. Social/occupational dysfunction: For a significant portion of the time since the onset of the disturbance, one or more major areas of functioning such as work, interpersonal relations, or self-care is markedly below the level achieved before the onset (or, when the onset is in childhood or adolescence, failure to achieve expected level of interpersonal, academic, or occupational achievement).

C. Duration: Continuous signs of the disturbance persist for at least 6 months. This 6-month period must include at least 1 month of symptoms that meet criterion A (i.e., active-phase symptoms) and may include periods of prodromal or residual symptoms. During these prodromal or residual periods, the signs of the disturbance may be manifested by only negative symptoms or two or more symptoms listed in criterion A present in an attenuated form (e.g., odd beliefs, unusual perceptual experiences).

D. Schizoaffective and mood disorder exclusion: Schizoaffective disorder and mood disorder with psychotic features have been ruled out because either 1) no major depressive, manic, or mixed episodes have occurred concurrently with the active-phase symptoms, or 2) if mood episodes have occurred during active-phase symptoms, their total duration has been brief relative to the duration of the active and residual periods.

E. Substance/general medical condition exclusion: The disturbance is not clearly due to the direct physiological effects of a substance (e.g. drugs of abuse, medication) or a general medical condition.

F. Relationship to a pervasive developmental disorder: If there is a history of autistic disorder or another pervasive developmental disorder, the additional diagnosis of schizophrenia is made only if prominent delusions or hallucinations are also present for at least a month (or less if successfully treated)

Classification of longitudinal course (can be applied only after at least 1 year has elapsed since the initial onset of active-phase symptoms):
   Episodic with interepisode residual symptoms (episodes are defined by the reemergence of prominent psychotic symptoms); *also specify if:*
   With prominent negative symptoms
   Episodic with no interepisode residual symptoms
   Continuous (prominent psychotic symptoms are present throughout the period of observation); *also specify if:* with prominent negative symptoms
   Single episode in partial remisiion; *also specify if:* with prominent negative symptoms
   Single episode in full remission
   Other or unspecified pattern

nations or a combination of these hallucinations, although auditory hallucinations are the most frequent. The hallucinations are most commonly experienced as voices. The voices may be mumbled or heard clearly, and they may speak

Table 7–2. Frequency of symptoms in 111 schizophrenic patients

Symptom	%	Symptom	%
NEGATIVE SYMPTOMS		**POSITIVE SYMPTOMS**	
• Affective flattening		**• Hallucinations**	
Unchanging facial expression	96	Auditory	75
Decreased spontaneous	66	Voices commenting	58
movements		Voices conversing	57
Paucity of expressive gestures	81	Somatic-tactile	20
Poor eye contact	71	Olfactory	6
Affective nonresponsivity	64	Visual	49
Inappropriate affect	63		
Lack of vocal inflections	73	**• Delusions**	
		Persecutory	81
• Alogia		Jealous	4
Poverty of speech	53	Guilt, sin	26
Poverty of content of speech	51	Grandiose	39
Blocking	23	Religious	31
Increased response latency	31	Somatic	28
		Delusions of reference	49
• Avolition-apathy		Delusions of being controlled	46
Impaired grooming and hygiene	87	Delusions of mind reading	48
Lack of persistence at work or	95	Thought broadcasting	23
school		Thought insertion	31
Physical anergia	82	Thought withdrawal	27
• Anhedonia-asociality		**• Bizarre behavior**	
Few recreational interests/	95	Clothing, appearance	20
activities		Social, sexual behavior	33
Little sexual interest/activity	69	Aggressive-agitated	27
Impaired intimacy/closeness	84	Repetitive-stereotyped	28
Few relationships with friends/	96		
peers		**• Positive formal thought disorder**	
		Derailment	45
• Attention		Tangentiality	50
Social inattentiveness	78	Incoherence	23
Inattentiveness during testing	64	Illogicality	23
		Circumstantiality	35
		Pressure of speech	24
		Distractible speech	23
		Clanging	3

Source. Adapted from Andreasen NC: The diagnosis of schizophrenia. Schizophr Bull 13:9–22, 1987.

words, phrases, or sentences. Visual hallucinations may be simple or complex and include flashes of light, persons, animals, or objects. Olfactory and gustatory hallucinations are often experienced together, especially as unpleasant tastes or odors. Tactile hallucinations may be experienced as sensations of being touched or pricked, electrical sensations, or the sensation of insects crawling under the skin, which is called *formication*.

Delusions involve disturbance in thought rather than perception; they are firmly held beliefs that are untrue as well as contrary to a person's educational and cultural background. Delusions occurring in schizophrenic patients may have somatic, grandiose, religious, nihilistic, or persecutory themes (Table 7–3). The type and frequency of the delusions tend to differ according to one's culture. For example, in the United States, a patient might worry about being spied on by the FBI or CIA; a Bantu or Zulu patient would more likely worry about persecution by demons and spirits. Certain types of hallucinations and delusions were considered "first rank" by Schneider; these hallucinations include clearly audible voices commenting on a person's actions, arguing with each other about a patient, or repeating aloud the patient's thoughts. The delusions include thought broadcasting, thought withdrawal, thought insertion, or being controlled (passivity) (Table 7–4). Although these symptoms commonly occur in schizophrenic patients, they may also occur in patients with mood disorders or brain disorders induced by medical illnesses or the effects of a substance.

Disorganized speech, known as *formal thought disorder*, is also common in schizophrenic patients, but it is not specific to the illness. Common types of thought disorder include incoherence and derailment (loose associations). Other

Table 7–3. Varied content in delusions

Delusions	Foci of preoccupation
Grandiose	Possessing wealth or great beauty, or having a special ability (e.g., extrasensory perception); having influential friends; being an important figure (e.g., Napoleon, Hitler)
Nihilistic	Believing that one is dead or dying; believing that one does not exist or that the world does not exist
Persecutory	Being persecuted by friends, neighbors, or spouses; being followed, monitored, or spied on by the government (e.g., FBI, CIA) or other important organizations (e.g., the Catholic church)
Somatic	Believing that one's organs have stopped functioning (e.g., that the heart is no longer beating) or are rotting away; belief that the nose or other body part is terribly misshapen or disfigured
Sexual	Belief that one's sexual behavior is commonly known; that one is a prostitute, pedophile, or rapist; that masturbation has led to illness or insanity; that one's sexual abilities are legendary
Religious	Belief that one has sinned against God; that one has a special relationship to God or some other deity; that one has a special religious mission; that one is the Devil or is condemned to burn in Hell

types of formal thought disorder have been identified and include tangentiality, illogicality, and neologisms. All are described in Chapter 3.

An example of speech from a patient with a prominent thought disorder, especially derailment, follows:

> Let's see, there was one I would have liked if it wasn't for the instructor, well I go along with his, he was always wanted me to do the worse in class, it seemed like, and I'd always get bad, the grade, in my grading, and he tried to make other people like they were good enough to be in Hollywood or something, you know I's be the last one down the ladder. That, that's the way they wanted the grading to be in the first place according to whose, theirs, they, they have all different reasons that I, I, I think that they use that they want one, won't come out. (Andreasen, *The Broken Brain*, p. 61)

Many schizophrenic patients display various types of disorganized behavior, including both motor and social behavior. Abnormal motor behaviors range from catatonic stupor to excitement. In a *catatonic stupor,* the patient may be immobile, mute, and unresponsive, yet fully conscious. In a state of *catatonic excitement,* the patient may exhibit uncontrolled and aimless motor activity. Patients may assume bizarre or uncomfortable postures, such as squatting, and maintain them for long periods. Patients may exhibit a *stereotypy,* which is a repeated but non–goal-directed movement, such as rocking. They may display *mannerisms* that are normal goal-directed activities, but are either odd in appearance or out of context, such as grimacing. Other common symptoms are *echopraxia,* or imitating the movements and gestures of another person; *automatic obedience,* or carrying

Table 7–4. Schneider's first-rank symptoms

Hallucination of one's thoughts being spoken aloud
Hallucination of voices in the form of a running commentary about the patient
Hallucination of voices conversing about the patient ("third person" hallucination) or arguing
Somatic hallucination attributed to outside forces (e.g., X rays, hypnosis)
Delusions of thoughts being withdrawn from or inserted into the patient's mind by an outside person or force
Delusions of thoughts being broadcast so that the patient's private thoughts are known to others
Delusional perceptions in which highly personal meanings are attributed to perceptions
Delusions of being influenced or forced to do things or want things the patient does not wish to do and does not want
Delusions of being made to feel emotions or sensations (often sexual) that are not the patient's own

out simple commands in a robotlike fashion; and *negativism*, or refusing to cooperate with simple requests for no apparent reason.

Antipsychotics are often blamed for causing motor abnormalities, and they clearly cause extrapyramidal side effects, as well as tardive dyskinesia in some patients (see Chapter 26). However, many patients were reported to display extrapyramidal signs, or spontaneous and bizarre movements, before antipsychotics became available. Interestingly, when tardive dyskinesia is present, schizophrenic patients are often unaware of it.

Deterioration of social behavior often occurs along with social withdrawal. Patients may neglect themselves, become messy or unkempt, and wear dirty or inappropriate clothing. Patients may ignore their surroundings so that they become cluttered and untidy. Patients may develop other odd behaviors that break social conventions, such as masturbating in public, foraging through garbage bins, or shouting obscenities. Many of today's street people are schizophrenic.

Schizophrenic patients often develop a *reduced intensity of emotional response* that leaves them indifferent, apathetic, and anhedonic (i.e., unable to experience pleasure). Expression of affect that is inappropriate, such as giggling over a relative's death, is especially common in patients with the disorganized subtype of schizophrenia. Significant depressive symptoms may develop in up to 60% of schizophrenic patients. Depression is often difficult to diagnose because the symptoms of schizophrenia and depression frequently overlap. Antipsychotics may also cause what may appear to be a depression but is actually a drug-induced akinesia. The depression may go away when the dose of antipsychotic is reduced or an anticholinergic medication is added. According to DSM-IV, if major depression develops in a patient with well-established schizophrenia, it is diagnosed as *depressive disorder not otherwise specified*.

Alcohol and drug abuse is especially common in patients with schizophrenia. Drug-using patients tend to be young, male, and poorly compliant with treatment; they also tend to have frequent hospitalizations. It is believed that many abuse drugs in an attempt to treat their depression or their medication side effects (e.g., akinesia) or to ameliorate their lack of motivation and pleasure.

The following case vignette illustrates many of the symptoms found in schizophrenia:

Jane, a 55-year-old woman, was admitted to the hospital for evaluation after her landlord became concerned by her agitation. A former schoolteacher, Jane had lived in a series of rooming houses and had held only temporary jobs in the past 10 years. She was socially isolated and interacted with others only at her church.

Jane was born with a cleft palate that was surgically corrected at 4 years. She was teased unmercifully as a child due to her appearance, despite good cosmetic results from the surgery. She was shy and socially awkward and had few friends, but she was an avid reader and model student. Jane had little interest in boys, never dated, and after graduating from high school, briefly joined a convent. She eventually obtained her teaching certificate after graduating from college and lived with her mother. She was briefly hospitalized at age 25 after developing the belief that her neighbors were harassing her. Over the next 20 years, her beliefs evolved into a complex delusional system. She believed that she was at the center of a government cabal to change her identity. The FBI, the judicial system, the Roman Catholic church, hospital personnel, and, it seems, most of her neighbors were involved in the plot. Neighbors, she believed, were recruited to spy on her, harass her, and generally make her life miserable. She would often overhear them plotting to assault or rape her.

As a result of her beliefs, Jane changed her residence about every 6 months. Unfortunately, she discovered that wherever she went, her new neighbors were also part of the plot to harass her. Still, she continued working, but she was gradually relegated to substitute teaching positions until these opportunities eventually dried up. A doctor had suggested that she obtain disability benefits from the government, but because she denied having any mental illness, she refused to apply. She would obtain any temporary position that she could, and at admission she had been working for several weeks in telemarketing schemes.

At age 49, Jane was briefly hospitalized after pounding on her ceiling and walls with a broom and yelling, in an attempt to stop her neighbors from harassing her. Reasons for her present hospitalization were similar. Although her landlord had complained of her yelling and screaming, Jane reported that she was simply responding to the discomfort her landlord and neighbors had caused by "zapping" her with electronic beams in an effort to harass her. She believed that electromagnetic waves were being used to control her actions and thoughts and described a bizarre sensation of electricity moving around her body when the landlord was near. At the hospital, Jane wore simple clothing, but she was always neatly groomed and dressed.

She cooperated well with her physicians, had no evidence of depressed mood, but was clearly upset about her hospitalization, which she felt was unnecessary and inappropriate. Her speech was markedly circumstantial, but she spoke in the clear, strong voice that one might expect after years of teaching. She cooperated with her treatment plans. After 1 month of antipsychotic therapy, she remained delusional but was no longer as concerned about her perceived harassment. Due to Jane's poor insight and history of medication noncompliance, she was placed on an intramuscular antipsychotic before discharge.

A common symptom in schizophrenia is *lack of insight*. A patient may not believe that he or she is ill or abnormal in any way. The hallucinations and delusions are real—not imagined—to the patient. Poor insight is one of the most difficult symptoms to treat, and it may persist even when other symptoms (e.g., hallucinations, delusions) respond to treatment. Orientation and memory are usually normal, unless they are impaired by the patient's psychotic symptoms, inattention, or distractibility. Some patients have difficulty giving their correct age (age disorientation).

Schizophrenic patients often develop *physical symptoms* as well. Neurological soft signs occur in a substantial proportion of patients and include abnormalities in stereognosis, graphesthesia, balance, and proprioception. A disorder of the visual tracking of smoothly moving targets (i.e., smooth pursuit eye movement) has been observed in both schizophrenic patients and their relatives. Other ocular abnormalities commonly include the absence and avoidance of eye contact and staring for long periods. Decreased or rapid blink rates and bouts of rapid blinking may occur. Some patients display disturbances of sleep, sexual interest, and other bodily functions. A variety of disrupted sleep measures have been reported, but decreased delta sleep with diminished stage 4 is the most consistent finding. Many schizophrenic patients have inactive sex drives and derive little or no pleasure from sexual activity. Many patients develop chronic constipation, and cases of megacolon have been described.

As a group, chronic schizophrenic patients have *odd personalities* before the onset of their illness, characterized by paranoid traits, eccentricities, and lack of feeling or lack of empathy. A study of 52 chronic schizophrenic patients found that 35% met criteria for a personality disorder premorbidly; 44% of these personality disorders were the schizoid type, and the rest were a mix of avoidant, paranoid, histrionic, compulsive, or other personality disorders. Kraepelin believed that most schizophrenic patients became more cognitively impaired with time. Schizophrenic patients tend to have lower premorbid IQs than siblings and peers of similar social class origins, but the IQ does not characteristically decline premorbidly or after the onset of schizophrenia. It is likely that observed changes in IQ are related to the severity of a patient's symptoms, which may affect test performance.

Subtypes of Schizophrenia

DSM-IV recognizes five subtypes of schizophrenia: paranoid, disorganized, catatonic, undifferentiated, and residual (Table 7–5). Their usefulness is primarily descriptive, because their reliability and validity are not established. As a practical matter, many patients seem to fit several of these subtypes during the course of their illness.

The *paranoid* subtype involves preoccupation with one or more delusions and frequently auditory hallucinations; disorganized speech and behavior, catatonic behavior, and flat or inappropriate affect are not prominent. Compared

Table 7–5. DSM-IV subtypes of schizophrenia

Subtype	Criteria	Associated features
Paranoid	A. Preoccupation with one or more delusions or frequent auditory hallucinations B. None of the following is prominent: disorganized speech, disorganized or catatonic behavior, or flat or inappropriate affect	Often associated with unfocused anger, anxiety, argumentativeness, or violence Stilted, formal quality or extreme intensity of interpersonal interactions may be seen
Catatonic	The clinical picture is dominated by at least two of the following: A. Motoric immobility as evidenced by catalepsy or stupor B. Excessive motor activity (that is apparently purposeless and not influenced by extreme stimuli) C. Extreme negativism (an apparently motiveless resistance to all instructions or maintenance of a rigid posture against attempts to be moved) or mutism D. Peculiarities of voluntary movements as evidenced by posturing, stereotyped movements, prominent mannerisms, or prominent grimacing E. Echolalia or echopraxia	Marked psychomotor disturbance present (stupor of agitation), and unusual motor disturbances may be present May need medical supervision due to malnutrition, exhaustion, hyperpyrexia, or self-injury Interviewing patient while he or she is under the influence of amobarbital sodium ("Amytal interview") may be helpful diagnostically
Disorganized	A. All of the following are prominent: 1. Disorganized speech 2. Disorganized behavior 3. Flat or inappropriate affect B. Does not meet criteria for catatonic type	Silly and childlike behavior is common Associated with extreme social impairment, poor premorbid functioning, and poor long-term functioning
Undifferentiated	Symptoms meeting criterion A[a] are present, but the criteria are not met for paranoid, catatonic, or disorganized types	Probably the most common presentation in clinical practice
Residual	A. Absence of prominent delusions, hallucinations, disorganized speech, and grossly disorganized or catatonic behavior B. There is continuing evidence of the disturbance as indicated by the presence of negative symptoms or two or more symptoms listed in criterion A for schizophrenia present in an attenuated form	Active-phase symptoms (i.e., psychotic symptoms) are not present, but patient still exhibits emotional blunting, eccentric behavior, illogical thinking, and mild loosening of associations

[a]For definition of criterion A, see Table 7–1.

with patients who have disorganized schizophrenia, paranoid patients tend to be an older age at onset and are more likely to be married, to have children, and to be employed; both their premorbid functioning and their outcome tend to be better.

Disorganized (hebephrenic) schizophrenic patients exhibit disorganized speech and behavior and flat or inappropriate affect; they do not meet criteria for catatonic schizophrenia. Delusions and hallucinations, if present, tend to be fragmentary, unlike the often well-systematized delusions of the paranoid schizophrenic patient. The onset of this subtype occurs at an early age with the development of nonparanoid symptoms such as avolition, flat affect, deterioration of habits, and cognitive impairment. These patients often seem silly and childlike and occasionally grimace, giggle inappropriately, and appear self-absorbed; mirror gazing is frequently described.

Catatonic schizophrenia is a subtype dominated by at least two of the following: motoric immobility (e.g., catalepsy, stupor), excessive motor activity, extreme negativism, peculiarities of voluntary movement (e.g., stereotypies, mannerisms, grimacing), and echolalia or echopraxia. This subtype of schizophrenia is reported to be less common than it was in the past, which may be a benefit of the modern treatment era.

The *undifferentiated* subtype is a residual category for patients meeting criteria for schizophrenia but not criteria for the paranoid, disorganized, or catatonic subtypes.

Residual schizophrenia, as described in DSM-IV, is a diagnosis for patients who no longer have prominent psychotic symptoms but who once met criteria for schizophrenia and have continuing evidence of illness such as blunted affect or eccentric behavior.

Epidemiology

The prevalence of schizophrenia has been estimated at between 0.5% and 1%. In the early 1980s, the Epidemiologic Catchment Area study in the United States, however, found the lifetime prevalence for schizophrenia to range from 1% to 1.9%. This study found a preponderance of schizophrenia in women and persons aged 18–44 years. If these recent data are correct, there are between 2.5 and 4.8 million persons in the United States who have schizophrenia. Prevalence rates are similar among different countries, but pockets of high prevalence have been reported in areas of Croatia, Sweden, and Ireland, among Canadian Catholics, and among the Tamils in southern India. Low prevalence rates have been reported among the American Old Order Amish, Aboriginal tribes in Taiwan, and natives in Ghana. African-Americans have traditionally had higher rates of schizophrenia, but this finding may be due to a systematic bias to overdiagnose schizophrenia in blacks.

Schizophrenia can develop at any age, but the mean age of the first psychotic episode is usually in the early 20s for men and the late 20s for women. Of persons with schizophrenia, 9 of 10 men—but only 2 of 3 women—develop the illness by age 30 years. Age at onset is probably under both genetic and environmental control, but it is unknown why women develop the illness later than men. Patients with schizophrenia tend not to marry, and they are less likely to have children than persons in the general population. These facts are probably due to the illness itself, which impairs motivation, creates social isolation, and is associated with low sex drive. Schizophrenic patients also tend to be concentrated in low social classes, a finding most likely due to the downward drift resulting from impaired social and occupational functioning.

Schizophrenic patients are at high risk for committing suicidal acts. About one-third will attempt suicide, and about 1 in 10 will complete suicide. Risk factors for suicide include male gender, age under 30 years, unemployment, chronic course, prior depression, past treatment for a depression, and recent hospital discharge. Risk of homicide and other violent crime is probably the same for schizophrenic patients as it is for the general population, despite unfortunate and frequently lurid depictions of mental illness in the popular media.

Etiology and Pathophysiology

Hypotheses about the etiology and pathophysiology of schizophrenia can be grouped into genetic, developmental, and neurobiologic causes.

Genetics

Evidence for a genetic contribution is based on family studies, twin studies, and studies of adoptees. Summaries of individual family studies have shown siblings of schizophrenic patients to have about a 10% chance of developing schizophrenia, whereas children who have one parent with schizophrenia have a 5%–6% chance. The risk of family members developing schizophrenia increases markedly when two or more family members have the illness. The risk of developing schizophrenia is 17% for persons with one sibling and one parent with schizophrenia and is 46% for the children of two schizophrenic parents. Twin studies have been remarkably consistent in demonstrating high concordance rates for monozygotic twins, averaging 46% compared with 14% concordance in dizygotic twins. Adoption studies show that the risk for schizophrenia is greater in the biological relatives of index adoptees who had schizophrenia than in the biological relatives of mentally healthy control adoptees.

Studies are now under way to find the schizophrenia gene (or genes) via molecular genetic techniques. (See Chapter 5 for a description of these techniques.) Although a preliminary report suggested that the gene may lie on chromosome 5, this finding has not been replicated. Many experts believe that because schizophrenia is heterogeneous, its etiology must be multifactorial, so that single-gene transmission would, at best, explain only a small fraction of the total cases. As is the case with mental retardation, multiple mechanisms may lead to a similar clinical picture (i.e., phenotype), so that no single cause for schizophrenia is likely to emerge. In fact, polygenic models of the inheritance of schizophrenia tend to appear more consistent with published family and twin data than single-gene models.

Developmental Influences

Clinicians working with families of schizophrenic patients became aware of frequent discord and social maladjustment within the family. Early theorists believed that bad parenting could lead to schizophrenia. Fromm-Reichmann wrote of the "schizophrenogenic mother," and Bateson warned of the "double-bind" situation, in which schizophrenic patients were thought to be subjected to ambiguous or confusing messages by their parents. Although these theories have been abandoned, they have led to more sophisticated family research on *expressed emotion*. In a family environment, frequent and intense expression of emotion by relatives may occur. Although expressed emotion does not cause schizophrenia, it can lead to worsening of symptoms (e.g., agitation, hallucinations).

Several lines of evidence have supported speculation that schizophrenia is a neurodevelopmental disorder, resulting from brain injury occurring early in life. For example, schizophrenic patients are more likely than nonschizophrenic control subjects to have a history of birth injury and perinatal complications, which could result in a subtle brain injury setting the stage for the development of schizophrenia. Birth seasonality in schizophrenic patients has also suggested to some a neurodevelopmental etiology. Throughout the temperate northern latitudes, more schizophrenic persons are born in the winter than in any other season. This suggests that as fetuses or neonates many schizophrenic persons may have sustained central nervous system damage due to a viral illness.

Neurobiology

Schizophrenia is widely believed to have a neurobiological basis. The most popular pathophysiological explanation for schizophrenia is the *dopamine hypothesis*, which suggests that schizophrenia symptoms are due primarily to hyperactivity in the dopamine system. Evidence supporting this hypothesis includes the effectiveness of the antipsychotic medications that block postsynaptic dopamine receptors and the exacerbation of the symptoms of schizophrenia by stimulant drugs (e.g., amphetamine), which enhance dopamine transmission. Direct support for this hypothesis is provided by postmortem brain studies showing an increase in dopamine 2 (D_2) receptors in the caudate nucleus and the nucleus accumbens. Other neurotransmitter systems may be involved in the neurochemistry of schizophrenia, including norepinephrine, serotonin, glutamate, and γ-aminobutyric acid (GABA), but these systems have been much less actively studied.

Neuroanatomic studies, some of which are reviewed in Chapter 5, have confirmed the presence of structural brain abnormalities in patients with schizophrenia, including ventricular enlargement, sulcal enlargement, and cerebellar atrophy. These abnormalities have not been explained on the basis of treatment with medication, length of illness, or treatment with electroconvulsive therapy, but they may be explained in part by gender, because these abnormalities may predominantly occur in males. Some studies suggest that ventricular enlargement correlates with poor premorbid functioning, poor response to treatment, and cognitive impairment. Single photon emission computed tomography studies, in which regional cerebral blood flow is measured, have suggested that schizophrenic patients have a relative hypofrontality, whereas positron-emission tomography studies have shown decreased glucose utilization in the frontal lobes. These studies suggest that schizophrenia may be caused by abnormalities in prefrontal circuitry and function.

Electrophysiological studies are often abnormal in schizophrenic patients. Electroencephalography tracings may show decreased alpha and increased beta activity. Evoked potentials often show a decreased amplitude. This research suggests that schizophrenic patients have deficits in attention and information processing and an inability to properly filter out irrelevant stimuli, leading to sensory overload.

Course and Outcome

Schizophrenia begins with a *prodromal phase* that precedes the active phase of the illness, sometimes by many years. This phase consists of the gradual development of social withdrawal, peculiar behavior, deterioration in personal hygiene and grooming, and strange ideation. The prodrome is followed by an *active phase* in which psychotic symptoms, such as hallucinations and delusions, predominate. This phase is florid, alarms friends and relatives, and may lead to medical intervention. A *residual phase* follows, which is similar to the prodromal phase, although affective flattening and role impairment may be worse. Psychotic symptoms may persist during this phase, but at a lower level of intensity, and they may not be as troublesome to the patient. The residual phase may be interrupted by repeated recurrences of the active phase or *acute exacerbations*. The frequency and timing of these exacerbations are unpredictable, although stressful situations may precede them. The patient and family members may initially notice changes in thought, feeling, and behavior before psychotic symptoms emerge. There is a tendency for the symptoms of schizophrenia to change over time. Patients may show a preponderance of positive symptoms early in their illness, but over time develop more negative or defect symptoms. These stages are summarized in Table 7–6.

Studies of outcome in schizophrenia are difficult to compare directly, but according to a review of six outcome studies, 13% of patients had a good outcome, 42% had an intermediate outcome, and 45% had a bad outcome. Good outcome was defined as no hospital readmission during follow-up, and bad outcome was defined as continuous hospitalization during follow-up or moderate to severe intellectual or social impairment. In one of the best-known outcome studies, the "Iowa 500," 200 schizophrenic patients hospitalized in the 1930s and 1940s were followed up in the 1970s. Twenty percent of patients were psychiatrically well at follow-up, but 45% remained incapacitated; 21% were married or widowed, but 67% had never married; 35% were economically productive, but 58% had never worked. In general, this and other studies demonstrate that

Table 7–6.   Typical stages of schizophrenia

Stage	Typical features
Prodromal	Insidious onset over months or years; subtle behavior changes including social withdrawal, work impairment, inappropriate affect, avolition, and strange ideation.
Active phase	Psychotic symptoms develop including hallucinations, delusions, or disorganized speech and behavior. These florid symptoms are alarming and lead to medical intervention. Acute-phase symptoms may reemerge during the residual phase ("acute exacerbation").
Residual phase	Active-phase symptoms are absent or no longer prominent. There is role impairment, negative symptoms, or attenuated positive symptoms.

schizophrenia is a devastating illness that affects every aspect of the patient's life. Fortunately, as many as one in four or five patients with schizophrenia will avoid the severe deterioration considered by some a hallmark of the disorder.

Although it is difficult to predict outcome in individual cases, many prognostic factors have been reported and are listed in Table 7–7. It appears that definitions of schizophrenia that exclude patients with mood symptoms or a duration of illness under 6 months (such as the definition in DSM-IV) predict a poor prognosis at least partly because they exclude patients with mood or schizophreniform disorders, who tend to have better outcomes.

Interestingly, there has been a slight improvement in outcome for schizophrenic patients over the past 100 years, either because the illness has changed or because antipsychotic medication and other treatments have altered the natural history of the illness. Another possibility is that our definitions of good outcome have changed. For example, a good outcome now may include patients living in care facilities or nursing homes who have minimal symptoms but who clearly are not well. For reasons that are not well understood, cross-cultural studies have shown that patients in less-developed countries tend to have better outcomes than those in more-developed countries. It may be that the schizophrenic patient is better accepted in less-developed societies, has fewer external demands, and is more likely to be taken care of by family members. In general, women tend to have a better outcome than men in their response to medication and in their long-term course.

Table 7–7.   Features associated with good and poor outcome in schizophrenia

Feature	Good outcome	Poor outcome
Onset	Acute	Insidious
Duration	Short	Chronic
Psychiatric history	Absent	Present
Mood symptoms	Present	Absent
Sensorium	Clouded	Clear
Obsessions/compulsions	Absent	Present
Assaultiveness	Absent	Present
Premorbid functioning	Good	Poor
Marital history	Married	Never married
Psychosexual functioning	Good	Poor
Neurological functioning	Normal	Soft signs present
Structural brain abnormalities	None	Present
Social class	High	Low
Family history of schizophrenia	Negative	Positive

Differential Diagnosis

Because psychotic symptoms are common and frequently accompany both functional and organic disorders, a careful diagnostic assessment is necessary. Schizophrenia has no pathognomonic signs or symptoms or predictable laboratory abnormalities. Like most psychiatric diagnoses, schizophrenia remains a clinical diagnosis that rests on historical information and a careful mental status examination. Schizophrenia should be thought of as a diagnosis of exclusion, because the consequences of the diagnosis are severe and limit therapeutic options. First, it is important that a thorough physical examination and medical history rule out medical causes for schizophrenic symptoms (see Table 7–8 for differential diagnosis). Atypical presentations, such as a relatively recent onset, clouding of the sensorium, or onset occurring after 30 years, should be carefully investigated.

Psychotic symptoms are found in patients with many other illnesses, including substance abuse (e.g., hallucinogens, phencyclidine, amphetamines, cocaine, alcohol), intoxication due to commonly prescribed medications (e.g., corticosteroids, anticholinergics, levodopa), infections, metabolic and endocrine disorders, tumors and mass lesions, and temporal lobe epilepsy of many years' duration.

Routine lab tests may be helpful in ruling out medical etiologies. Testing may include a complete blood count, urinalysis, liver enzymes, serum creatinine,

Table 7–8. Differential diagnosis of schizophrenia

Psychiatric illness	Medical illness
Bipolar disorder with psychotic features	Temporal lobe epilepsy
Major depression with psychotic features	Tumor, stroke, brain trauma
Schizoaffective disorder	Endocrine/metabolic disorders (e.g., porphyria)
Brief psychotic disorder	Vitamin deficiency (e.g., B_{12})
Schizophreniform disorder	Infectious (e.g., neurosyphilis)
Delusional disorder	Autoimmune (e.g., systemic lupus erythematosus)
Induced psychotic disorder	
Panic disorder	Toxic (e.g., heavy metal poisoning)
Depersonalization disorder	**Drugs**
Obsessive-compulsive disorder	Stimulants (e.g., amphetamine, cocaine)
Personality disorders (e.g., "eccentric cluster")	Hallucinogens (e.g., phencyclidine [PCP])
	Anticholinergics (e.g., belladonna alkaloids)
	Alcohol withdrawal
	Barbiturate withdrawal

blood urea nitrogen, thyroid function tests, and serological tests for evidence of an infection with syphilis or human immunodeficiency virus. Electroencephalography, computed tomography, or magnetic resonance imaging may be useful in selected cases to rule out alternate diagnoses, such as a brain tumor, or during the initial workup for new-onset cases.

The major differential diagnosis involves separating schizophrenia from schizoaffective disorder, mood disorder with psychotic features, delusional disorder, and personality disorders. To rule out schizoaffective disorder and psychotic mood disorders, major depressive or manic episodes should have been absent during the active phase, or the mood episode should have been brief relative to the total duration of the psychotic episode. Unlike delusional disorder, schizophrenia is characterized by bizarre delusions, and hallucinations are common. Patients with personality disorders, particularly those disorders within the eccentric cluster (e.g., schizoid, schizotypal, paranoid), may be characterized by indifference to social relationships and restricted affect, bizarre ideation, or odd speech, but they are not psychotic.

Other psychiatric disorders that need ruling out include schizophreniform disorder, brief psychotic disorder, factitious disorder with psychological symptoms, and malingering. If symptoms persist for more than 6 months, schizophreniform disorder will have been ruled out. The history of how the illness presents will help to rule out a brief psychotic disorder, because schizophrenia generally has an insidious onset and recovery is incomplete. Factitious disorder may be difficult to separate from schizophrenia, especially when the person is knowledgeable about the disorder, but careful observation should enable the clinician to make the distinction. Furthermore, the disorganized speech of schizophrenia is very difficult to simulate. A malingerer could attempt to feign schizophrenia, and as with factitious disorder, careful observation is essential. In the malingerer, there will be evidence of obvious secondary gain, such as avoiding military conscription, and the history will often suggest an antisocial personality disorder.

Clinical Management

Somatic Treatment

The mainstay of treatment is antipsychotic medication. All antipsychotics, with minor exceptions, have proven to be superior to placebo in the treatment of schizophrenia, reportedly because they block postsynaptic dopamine receptors. Except for clozapine and risperidone, none has been demonstrated to be superior to another, so that the choice of drug depends on the patient and his or her illness. There is little reason to prescribe more than a single antipsychotic agent at a time, and controlled studies do not support using a specific agent for a specific subtype of schizophrenia. Rather, selection should rest on predicted side effects, prior treatment response, and perhaps family history of drug response. Both clozapine and risperidone are reported to be effective in many patients refractory to other antipsychotics, and these agents have the advantage of causing few of the extrapyramidal side effects typical of most other antipsychotics. Therefore, patients who receive either of these drugs should be considered treatment refractory, or they should have had severe extrapyramidal side effects from other agents. Because clozapine has the potential to induce agranulocytosis, blood counts need to be obtained weekly.

The acutely psychotic or agitated patient requires rapid control of symptoms. A daily dose of between 10 and 20 mg of haloperidol (or 500–600 mg of chlorpromazine) will produce improvement in many patients within several days or weeks; higher doses may increase the likelihood of adverse effects, and lower doses may be ineffective. Although attempts to correlate plasma concentration of antipsychotics and their metabolites with therapeutic response have been generally unsuccessful, both haloperidol level (i.e., 5–15 ng/ml) and clozapine level (i.e., greater than 500 ng/ml) have been associated with improvement.

Highly agitated patients who are out of control should be given frequent, equally spaced doses of an antipsychotic. High-potency antipsychotics (e.g., haloperidol) should be given every 30–120 minutes intramuscularly or orally until agitation is under control. Rarely is more than 20–30 mg of haloperidol required in a 24-hour period. It is likely that its effectiveness in subduing patients results from sedation, not from a specific antipsychotic effect. If sedation is the desired effect, a more rational approach to managing these patients is short-term combination of an antipsychotic with a benzodiazepine (e.g., 5 mg of haloperidol and 2–4 mg of lorazepam every 30 minutes). Once the patient has calmed down, the benzodiazepine can gradually be withdrawn.

Patients benefiting from short-term treatment with antipsychotics are candidates for long-term prophylactic treatment, which has as its goal the sustained control of psychotic symptoms. Due to the potential of these medications to produce tardive dyskinesia, a potentially irreversible movement disorder, continuing benefit must be clearly established. Maintenance antipsychotics can reduce the risk of relapse by a factor of nearly fourfold within the first year. Maintenance for 1–2 years is appropriate after an initial psychotic episode, usually at doses in the range of one-third to one-half of the original dose and generally not falling below 100 mg of chlorpromazine (or its equivalent) per day. After two such episodes, patients will probably benefit from longer prophylaxis (up to 5 years). Although

30%–50% of patients on maintenance neuroleptics ultimately relapse, 70% of patients who do not receive maintenance medication relapse. Of course, many patients relapse due to their noncompliance with medication regimens.

Clinicians should periodically reassess whether the patient requires continued maintenance treatment. Because many patients develop increased negative and decreased positive symptoms over time, they may have less need for antipsychotic medication, which tends to work most effectively in controlling positive symptoms. Further information about antipsychotics and their rational use is found in Chapter 26.

Adjunctive psychotropic medications are occasionally useful in the schizophrenic patient, but their role has not been clearly defined. Many patients benefit from anxiolytics (e.g., benzodiazepines) if anxiety is prominent. These agents have also been used to relieve the akathisia associated with antipsychotic medication. Lithium carbonate may be useful to reduce impulsive and aggressive behaviors, hyperactivity, or excitation and to stabilize mood. Antidepressants have been used to treat depressed schizophrenic patients. Although early studies suggested that antidepressants were not helpful and could cause a worsening of thought disorder, more recent work shows they may have a legitimate role in treating depressed schizophrenic patients. Other medications, including propranolol, carbamazepine, and clonidine, have been used experimentally, but they have no current role in the treatment of schizophrenia.

Electroconvulsive therapy is rarely useful in treating schizophrenia, unless a catatonic syndrome is present or the patient has developed a severe depression. Psychosurgery has no role in the treatment of schizophrenia. Other physical treatments, including insulin coma therapy and hemodialysis, have been abandoned because of their ineffectiveness.

Psychosocial Interventions

Psychosocial interventions play an important role in the management of schizophrenic patients. Like somatic treatments, these interventions must be tailored to fit individual needs. The fit will depend on the patient, the phase of illness, and the living situation.

Supportive therapy that is reality oriented and pragmatic can be enormously helpful. The clinician should assist the patient in developing new coping strategies, testing reality, resolving concrete problems, and identifying both stressors and prodromal symptoms of relapse. A strong therapeutic alliance may also help to boost medication compliance. Insight-oriented approaches are generally not helpful and in some cases may worsen symptoms.

A vexing problem facing patients, their family members, and clinicians is deciding when to enter the hospital. Long-term institutionalization is now rare, and most hospitalized patients stay briefly in special psychiatric hospitals or in psychiatric units found in general hospitals. Stays tend to be short (i.e., weeks to months), and the patients are returned to the community. Reasons for hospitalization include patients being a danger to themselves or others, refusal of patients to properly care for themselves (e.g., not eating or taking fluids), or the need for special medical observation, tests, or treatments. The reasons are summarized in Table 7–9. In some cases, a court order will need to be obtained for hospitalization if the patient is a danger to himself or others and refuses hospitalization.

In the hospital, an active milieu characterized by high levels of support, a practical problem-solving approach, and broad delegation of responsibility with clear lines of authority tends to be superior to a custodial milieu for schizophrenic patients. The milieu must not be overly stimulating, however. Token economies in which patients are provided with a high degree of ward structure and are rewarded for desired behaviors seem to be effective in controlling behavior in the hospitals, but this improvement may not generalize to situations outside the hospital.

Group therapy may be threatening to some patients, and counterproductive in paranoid patients, but it can help to provide social skills training and a format to allow friendships to develop. Family therapy has proven to be important. Research has shown that a family environment characterized by harsh criticism and emotional overinvolvement tends to precede schizophrenic relapse. Families must be educated about the nature of schizophrenia and the need for long-term management based on realistic expectations. They should also be given instruction on how to reduce expressed emotion.

Self-help organizations for family members can be very beneficial. They can provide a forum for relatives to learn about schizophrenia, to gain encouragement from others, and to learn how to cope with its manifestations. The best-known

Table 7–9. Reasons to hospitalize the schizophrenic patient

1. When the illness is new, to rule out alternate diagnoses, and to stabilize the dose of antipsychotic medication.
2. For special medical procedures such as electroconvulsive therapy.
3. When aggressive or assaultive behavior presents a danger to the patient or others.
4. When the patient becomes suicidal.
5. When the patient is unable to properly care for himself or herself (e.g., refuses to eat or take fluids).
6. When medication side effects become disabling or potentially life threatening (e.g., severe pseudoparkinsonism, severe tardive dyskinesia, neuroleptic malignant syndrome).

group in the United States is the Alliance for the Mentally Ill (AMI), and local chapters can be found in many communities.

Some patients are unable to live at home or may be better off living apart from their families. Group residential treatment centers (halfway houses) may be appropriate for them. Many patients will be unable to work regularly, but a sheltered workshop may provide simple repetitive work that will allow the patient to maintain contact with the community, allow the development of interpersonal relationships, and provide additional income. Some patients may benefit from more intensive efforts at vocational training. For those patients who are unable to work, the clinician's role will be to assist them in obtaining disability benefits. Social skills are usually deficient in schizophrenic patients. There are many settings where patients can be encouraged to develop more appropriate social behaviors, including specific programs in social skills training.

Alcohol and drug abuse is a problem for many patients and can aggravate

---

Recommendations for management of the schizophrenic patient

1. Treat psychotic symptoms aggressively with medication.
   - Remember that all antipsychotics are equally effective (except clozapine and risperidone, which may be more effective), so choice of drug depends on patient tolerance and side effects.
   - Intramuscular medication is useful in uncooperative or poorly compliant patients.
2. Engage the patient in an empathic relationship.
   - This task may be particularly challenging, because many schizophrenic patients are unemotional, aloof, and withdrawn.
   - Be practical; help the patient with problems that matter to him or her, such as finding adequate housing.
3. Help the patient find a daily routine that he or she can manage to help improve socialization and reduce boredom.
   - Day hospital programs are available in many areas.
   - Sheltered workshops that provide simple, repetitive chores may be helpful.
4. Develop a close working relationship with local social services.
   - Patients tend to be poor and disabled; finding adequate housing and food takes the skills of a social worker.
   - Assist the patient in obtaining disability benefits.
5. Family therapy is important for the patient living at home or for one who still has close family ties.
   - As a result of the illness, many patients will have broken their family ties.
   - Families desperately need education about schizophrenia and need to learn how to reduce their "expressed emotion."
   - Help family members find a support group through referral to a local chapter of the Alliance for the Mentally Ill (AMI).

symptoms of schizophrenia, lead to medication noncompliance, and undermine other interventions. Abstinence should be encouraged in all patients, and some should be referred for drug detoxification and rehabilitation once an acute psychotic episode has resolved.

The treatment of schizophrenia must be comprehensive and include both somatic and psychosocial interventions. The physician should become aware of available social resources that can help to reinforce, maintain, and support the gains achieved by more formal programs, of which antipsychotics are an essential element.

Bibliography

American Psychiatric Association: Diagnostic and Statistical Manual of Mental Disorders, 4th Edition. Washington, DC, American Psychiatric Association, 1994

Andreasen NC: The Broken Brain: The Biologic Revolution in Psychiatry. New York, Harper and Row, 1984

Andreasen NC: The diagnosis of schizophrenia. Schizophr Bull 13:9–22, 1987

Andreasen NC, Ehrhardt JC, Swayze VW, et al: Magnetic resonance imaging of the brain in schizophrenia: the pathophysiological significance of structural abnormalities. Arch Gen Psychiatry 47:35–44, 1990

Andreasen NC, Flaum M, Swayze VW, et al: Positive and negative symptoms in schizophrenia: a critical reappraisal. Arch Gen Psychiatry 47:615–621, 1990

Andreasen NC, Rezai K, Alliger R, et al: Hypofrontality in neuroleptic-naive patients and in patients with chronic schizophrenia. Arch Gen Psychiatry 49:943–958, 1992

Baldessarini RJ, Cohen BM, Teicher MH: Significance of neuroleptic dose and plasma level in the pharmacologic treatment of psychosis. Arch Gen Psychiatry 45:79–91, 1988

Baron M: Genetics of schizophrenia. Biol Psychiatry 21:1051–1066, 1986

Black DW, Boffeli TJ: Simple schizophrenia: past, present, and future. Am J Psychiatry 146:1267–1273, 1989

Black DW, Fisher R: Mortality in DSM-III-R schizophrenia. Schizophr Res 7:109–116, 1992

Breier A, Astrachan BM: Characterization of schizophrenic patients who commit suicide. Am J Psychiatry 141:206–209, 1984

Buchsbaum MS, DeLisi LE, Holcomb HH, et al: Anteroposterior gradients in cerebral glucose use in schizophrenia and affective disorders. Arch Gen Psychiatry 41:1159–1166, 1984

Cutting J: Outcome in schizophrenia: overview, in Contemporary Issues in Schizophrenia. Edited by Kerr TA, Snaith RP. Washington, DC, American Psychiatric Press, 1986, pp 433–440

Davis KL, Kahn RS, Ko G, et al: Dopamine in schizophrenia: a review and reconceptualization. Am J Psychiatry 148:1474–1486, 1991

Dixon L, Haas G, Weiden PJ, et al: Drug abuse in schizophrenic patients—clinical correlates and reasons for use. Am J Psychiatry 148:224–230, 1991

Falloon IRH, Boyd JL, McGill CW: Family Care for Schizophrenia: A Problem-Solving Approach to Mental Illness. New York, Guilford, 1984

Farde L, Wiesel FA, Stone-Elander S, et al: D2 dopamine receptors in neuroleptic naive schizophrenic patients. Arch Gen Psychiatry 47:213–219, 1990

Fenton WS, McGlashan TH: Natural history of schizophrenia subtypes, I: longitudinal study of paranoid, hebephrenic and undifferentiated schizophrenia. Arch Gen Psychiatry 48:969–977, 1991

Fenton WS, McGlashan TH: Antecedents, symptom progression, and long-term outcome of the deficit syndrome in schizophrenia. Am J Psychiatry 151:351–356, 1994

Gur R, Mozley D, Shtasel DL: Clinical subtypes of schizophrenia: differences in brain and CSF volume. Am J Psychiatry 151:343–350, 1994

Kane J, Honigfeld G, Singer J, et al: Clozapine for the treatment-resistant schizophrenic. Arch Gen Psychiatry 45:789–796, 1988

Kendler KS, McGuire M, Gruenberg AM, et al: An epidemiologic, clinical, and family study of simple schizophrenia in county Roscommon, Ireland. Am J Psychiatry 151:27–34, 1994

Hogarty GE, Anderson CM, Reiss DJ, et al: Family psychoeducation, social skills training and maintenance chemotherapy in the aftercare treatment of schizophrenia. Arch Gen Psychiatry 48:340–347, 1991

Machon RA, Mednick SA, Schulsinger F: The interaction of seasonality, place of birth, genetic risk and subsequent schizophrenia in a high risk sample. Br J Psychiatry 143:383–388, 1983

McGlashan TH: The Chestnut Lodge follow-up study, II: long-term outcome in schizophrenia and the affective disorders. Arch Gen Psychiatry 41:586–601, 1984

Sherrington R, Brynjolfsson J, Petursson H, et al: Localisation of a susceptibility locus for schizophrenia on chromosome 5. Nature 336:164–166, 1988

Sirus SG, Cutler J, Owen K, et al: Adjunctive imipramine maintenance treatment in schizophrenic patients in the treatment of post-psychotic depression—a controlled trial. Arch Gen Psychiatry 4:533–539, 1987

Torrey EF: Surviving Schizophrenia: A Family Manual. New York, Harper & Row, 1983

Torrey EF, Bowler AE, Rawlings R, et al: Seasonality of schizophrenia and stillbirths. Schizophr Bull 19:557–562, 1993

Tsuang MT, Woolson RF, Fleming JA: Long-term outcome of major psychoses, I: schizophrenia and affective disorder compared with psychiatrically symptom-free surgical conditions. Arch Gen Psychiatry 36:1295–1306, 1979

Van Putten T, Marder S, Mintz J: A controlled dose comparison of haloperidol in newly admitted schizophrenic patients. Arch Gen Psychiatry 47:754–758, 1990

Weinberger DR: Implications of normal brain development for the pathogenesis of schizophrenia. Arch Gen Psychiatry 44:660–669, 1987

Wong DF, Wagner HN, Tune LE, et al: Positron emission tomography reveals elevated D2 dopamine receptors in drug-naive schizophrenics. Science 234:1528–1563, 1986

Self-Assessment Questions

1. What were Bleuler's "four A's"? What were his fundamental and accessory symptoms?
2. How is schizophrenia diagnosed? What is its differential diagnosis?
3. What are typical signs and symptoms of schizophrenia?
4. What are the subtypes of schizophrenia?
5. What is the prevalence and gender distribution of schizophrenia? What is the age at onset?
6. What recent developments have occurred in the study of the genetics of schizophrenia?
7. What evidence supports a neurobiological basis for schizophrenia?
8. What is the natural history of schizophrenia?
9. How is schizophrenia managed, both pharmacologically and psychosocially?
10. When should the schizophrenic patient be hospitalized?

Chapter 8

Delusional Disorder and Other Psychotic Disorders

In a sense, the paranoiac's behavior is justified; he perceives something that escapes the normal person; he sees clearer than one of normal intellectual capacity, but his knowledge becomes worthless when he imputes to others the state of affairs he thus recognizes.

Sigmund Freud

Although schizophrenia is clearly the most significant psychotic disorder, and mood disorder with psychotic features is the most common, several less well known psychotic disorders are seen by psychiatrists and are briefly reviewed here (Table 8–1). These disturbances include delusional disorder, schizoaffective disorder, schizophreniform disorder, brief psychotic disorder, shared psychotic disorder, and psychotic disorder not otherwise specified. Psychotic disorders thought to be due to the effects of a substance or a general medical condition are discussed in Chapter 6.

Delusional Disorder

Delusional disorders constitute a small, but important, group of disturbances. They are characterized by the presence of well-systematized, nonbizarre delusions accompanied by affect appropriate to the delusion and occurring in the presence of a relatively well preserved personality.

The former term, *paranoid disorder,* was discarded due to the ambiguity inherent in the term *paranoid,* which is usually construed to mean "persecutory." Further, delusional disorders may include grandiose, erotomanic (i.e., delusions of being loved), and somatic themes and are not restricted to themes involving persecution or jealousy.

Paranoid disorders have a long history; the term itself is from the Greek *para nous* meaning a "mind beside itself," and it was originally used as a description for insanity. German psychiatrists interested in disorders characterized by delusions of persecution and grandeur revived the term in the nineteenth century. Kraepelin separated paranoia from dementia praecox (schizophrenia) and used the term to describe persons with systematized delusions, an absence of hallucinations, and a prolonged course without recovery, but not leading to mental deterioration. Bleuler also believed that paranoia was separate from dementia praecox but that hallucinations could occur in some cases.

Delusional disorder has an estimated prevalence in the general population of between 24 and 30 per 100,000 persons and is rare in psychiatric hospitals. In one study, only 0.14% of hospitalized patients admitted over a 55-year period had a delusional disorder. It is generally considered to be a disorder of middle to late adult life, and it affects more women than men. Most patients seen in hospitals are married at the time of the first admission; many are from lower social classes, are educationally deprived, and are immigrants.

The cause of delusional disorder is unknown, although genetic, environmental, and psychodynamic explanations have been provided. Family studies have generally concluded that delusional disorder is probably not related to either schizophrenia or mood disorders, but delusional disorder is so uncommon that it is difficult to demonstrate that it runs in families. However, paranoid personality has been found in relatives of delusional disorder probands.

The possibility that psychosocial stressors may lead to delusional disorder in some persons is illustrated by certain rare conditions. *Migration psychosis,* for in-

Table 8–1. Other psychotic disorders

Delusional disorder	Schizoaffective disorder
• Erotomanic type	Schizophreniform disorder
• Grandiose type	Brief psychotic disorder
• Jealous type	Shared psychotic disorder
• Persecutory type	Psychotic disorder not otherwise specified
• Somatic type	
• Mixed type	
• Unspecified type	

stance, which is generally persecutory in nature, has been described in persons migrating from one country to another (although it is possible that persons in whom paranoia is prone to develop may be more likely to emigrate than others). Isolation in prison, especially solitary confinement, has been described as leading to paranoia (prison psychosis). *Querulent paranoia* is characterized by litigiousness and is believed by Scandinavian investigators to occur in persons with deviant personalities who have had unlucky personal experiences.

Most psychodynamic formulations of paranoia stem from Freud's analysis of the Schreber case. Schreber, a distinguished jurist, developed persecutory delusions in midlife, which Freud believed came from unconscious homosexual urges defended against by the ego defense mechanisms of denial and projection. Although Freud's analysis may help us to understand delusional disorder in some patients, its interest is primarily historical.

Delusional disorder tends to run a chronic, unremitting course. Unlike patients with schizophrenia, patients with delusional disorder are generally self-supporting and remain employed. The disorder is diagnostically stable, and it is unlikely that these patients will develop schizophrenia.

The diagnosis of delusional disorder is appropriate when nonbizarre delusions are present, have lasted at least 1 month, and involve situations that occur in real life (Table 8–2). The patient's behavior is generally not odd or bizarre apart from the delusion or its ramifications, and functioning is not markedly impaired. In addition, there is an absence of the bizarre delusions that may occur in schizophrenia (i.e., impossible delusions, such as being controlled by Martians), as well as an absence of disorganized speech or behavior, prominent hallucinations, and negative symptoms such as avolition. In addition, a mood disorder (if

---

Table 8–2.   DSM-IV diagnostic criteria for delusional disorder

A. Nonbizarre delusion(s) (i.e., involving situations that occur in real life, such as being followed, poisoned, infected, loved at a distance, having a disease, being deceived by one's spouse or lover) of at least 1 month's duration.

B. Criterion A for schizophrenia has never been met.[a]

Note: Tactile and olfactory hallucinations may be present in delusional disorder if they are related to the delusional theme.

C. Apart from the impact of the delusion(s) or its ramifications, functioning is not markedly impaired and behavior is not obviously odd or bizarre.

D. If mood episodes have occurred concurrently with delusions, their total duration has been brief relative to the duration of the delusional periods.

E. The disturbance is not due to the direct psychological effects of a substance (e.g., drugs of abuse, medication) or a general medical condition.

---

[a]For definition of criterion A, see Table 7–1.

present) is brief relative to the duration of the delusions, and the effects of a substance (e.g., amphetamines) or a general medical condition (e.g., the acquired immunodeficiency syndrome) have been ruled out.

The core feature, however, is a well-systematized, encapsulated, nonbizarre delusion. The term *systematized* is used to indicate that the delusion and its ramifications fit into a complex, all-encompassing scheme that makes logical sense to the patient. The term *encapsulated* indicates that, apart from the delusion or its ramifications, the patient generally behaves normally, or at least is not obviously odd or bizarre.

Sexual problems and depressive symptoms are common in patients with delusional disorder, and patients may show overtalkativeness or circumstantiality, especially when discussing their delusions. Episodes of major depression are frequent complications. Patients with delusional disorder are often socially isolated, seclusive, and suspicious. Some patients—particularly those with persecutory or jealous delusions—are angry, hostile, or (rarely) violent. Many patients become litigious and end up as lawyers' clients rather than as psychiatrists' patients. The frequency of common symptoms in a series of 29 patients in Iowa is shown in Table 8–3.

According to DSM-IV, the following subtypes are assigned based on the predominant delusional theme: *persecutory type*, in which there is a belief that one is being malevolently treated in some way; *erotomanic type* (De Clerambault's

Table 8–3. Common symptoms in 29 patients with delusional disorder

Symptoms	%
Delusions of persecution	83
Delusions of reference	76
Chronic suspiciousness	66
Sexual problems or dysfunction	55
Delusional jealousy	48
Manic symptoms	48
Depressive symptoms	45
Overtalkativeness/circumstantiality	30
Suicide attempts	14
Somatic delusions	10
Suicide threats	7
Delusions of grandeur	7
Significant drinking history	3

Source.   Adapted from Winokur G: Delusional disorder (paranoia). Compr Psychiatry 18:453–479, 1977.

syndrome), in which there is a belief that another person, usually of a higher status, is in love with the patient; *grandiose type,* in which there is a belief that one's worth, power, knowledge, or identity is inflated or that one has a special relationship to a deity or famous person; *jealous type,* in which the delusion is that one's sexual partner is unfaithful; and *somatic type,* in which the delusion is that a person has some physical defect or medical condition, such as cancer. There is a residual category (*unspecified type*) for patients who do not fit the previous categories (for example, those who have been ill less than 1 month) and a category (mixed type) for those with delusions characteristic of more than one subtype, but without any single theme predominating. The following case illustrates the erotomanic subtype.

Doug, a 33-year-old restaurant manager, was brought to the hospital under court order for evaluation and treatment. The accompanying papers alleged that he had harassed and threatened a young woman.

The patient had an uneventful childhood in a small midwestern town. Although quiet and bookish, he had many friends. He excelled in school and graduated from college with honors. He later returned to school for a master's degree.

After admission, the following story unfolded. Doug had had a 4½ year fantasy relationship with a comely young shop clerk who had recently married. Doug was convinced that the young woman was in love with him, although they had never met. He took as evidence of her affection glances and smiles that they had exchanged when they occasionally crossed paths in their small town. After becoming convinced of her love, he mailed a "sexual business letter" to her after learning her name and address. Love letters continued over the next few years, and Doug kept careful track of her whereabouts. There were no other formal communications, but the letters indicated his belief that she was infatuated with him and his desire that she act on it. In one letter he wrote: "What do you think I am? A can of vegetables that can just sit on your shelf to open or throw away whenever it suits you?"

The young woman complained about these letters to the police, who warned Doug not to call or write her. This warning had little effect. Interestingly, Doug himself complained to the police about his imagined harassment by her. The woman and her husband finally sought a court order for Doug's hospitalization when the letters to her had developed a more threatening tone and a restraining order had failed to keep him away from the shop where she worked. Doug had felt jilted by the woman's relationship and subsequent marriage, and he had suggested in recent letters that the three get together to "work things out."

In the hospital, Doug was noted to be neatly groomed, articulate, and indignant about his hospitalization. Although he was notably circumstantial in describing his fantasy relationship, there was no evidence of a mood disorder, hallucinations, or bizarre delusions. He reported a history of a similar relationship 10 years earlier, consisting mostly of letters, which had ended when the girl had moved out of town.

Although Doug was a loner with few friends and had never had a sexual relationship, he was highly functional in his position at work and was active in several community organizations. At his hearing, Doug denied that his behavior was inappropriate, but he agreed to undergo psychiatric treatment on an outpatient basis. The young woman eventually moved out of town.

Two unusual syndromes have been observed in some patients with delusional disorder: *Capgras syndrome*, in which a patient believes that a person closely related to him or her has been replaced by a double (this belief was the theme of the 1950s grade B horror movie, *Invasion of the Body Snatchers*), and the *Fregoli syndrome*, in which the patient identifies a familiar person in various other people he or she encounters. The patient may maintain that although there is no physical resemblance between the familiar person and others, they are nonetheless psychologically identical. (Some persons with these syndromes may have schizophrenia, however.)

A careful diagnostic evaluation is necessary to rule out other psychiatric or medical illnesses that could have caused the delusions. The workup must include a physical examination to rule out alcoholism, drug-induced states, dementia, and infectious, metabolic, and endocrine disorders. Routine laboratory tests may be indicated, depending on the results of the history and physical examination. Computed tomography or magnetic resonance imaging may be useful in selected cases, especially when mass lesions are suspected.

The major differential diagnosis involves separating delusional disorder from mood disorders with psychotic features, schizophrenia, and paranoid personality. The chief distinction from psychotic mood disorders is that in delusional disorder a depressive or manic syndrome is absent, develops after the psychotic symptoms, or is brief in duration in relation to the psychotic symptoms. Unlike schizophrenia, delusional disorders are characterized by nonbizarre delusions and generally either an absence of hallucinations or hallucinations that are not prominent or are very brief in duration. Furthermore, patients with delusional disorders do not develop other symptoms typically associated with schizophrenia, such as incoherence or grossly disorganized behavior, and personality is generally preserved. Persons with paranoid personality may be suspicious and hypervigilant, but they are not delusional.

Recommendations for treatment are based on clinical observation, not empirical evidence, because there are no systematic data comparing treatments in patients with delusional disorder. Nonetheless, a combination of psychosocial and physical measures seems sensible. Because most patients have little insight about their illness and refuse to acknowledge having a problem, the initial obstacle is getting the patient to the physician. Patients' reluctance to seek care may account for the low frequency of cases reported by physicians. After establishing a therapeutic relationship, the physician may gently challenge the patient's beliefs by showing how they interfere with the patient's life. Tact and skill are necessary to persuade a patient to accept treatment, and the physician must neither condemn nor collude in the beliefs. The patient must be assured of the confidential nature of the doctor-patient relationship. Because suspiciousness and hypersensitivity may lead the patient to make misinterpretations, insight-oriented psychotherapy and group therapy are not recommended.

Most persons with delusional disorder can be treated as outpatients. Hospitalization is indicated if there is a potential for danger. In some cases, involuntary hospitalization will be necessary, especially when the threat of self-harm or harm to others is present. Unfortunately, involuntary hospitalization may increase a patient's distrust of his physician; the resentment that may result can add fuel to a patient's persecutory delusions.

For reasons that are not understood, delusional disorder is reported to have a poor response to antipsychotic medication, although these drugs should be tried. They may help relieve the agitation and anxiety that often accompany delusions, while leaving the core delusion untouched. Any of the standard antipsychotics may be used, but the selection of medication and dose will depend on the patient's age and anticipated side effects. Depot forms may help to prevent noncompliance in suspicious patients. Other medications, including anxiolytics or antidepressants, may be indicated for accompanying anxiety or depressive syn-

---

Recommendations for the management of delusional disorder

1. Because the delusional disorder patient is so suspicious, it may be very difficult to establish a therapeutic relationship.
   - Building a relationship will take time and patience.
   - The therapist must neither condemn nor collude in the delusional beliefs of the patient.
   - The patient must be assured of complete confidentiality.
2. Once rapport is established, gently challenge the delusional beliefs, and point out how they are interfering with the patient's functioning.
   - Tact and skill will be needed to convince the patient to accept treatment.
3. A patient with delusional disorder may be more accepting of medication if it is explained as treatment for the anxiety, dysphoria, and stress that the patient invariably experiences as a result of his or her delusions.
   - Patients with the somatic subtype may preferentially respond to pimozide.
4. Treatment for the jealous subtype may include separation and divorce. Unfortunately, the delusional beliefs of infidelity may transfer to future lovers or spouses.

dromes, respectively; however, these agents have not been systematically evaluated in patients with delusional disorder. Electroconvulsive therapy has no role in the treatment of delusional disorders, unless it is used to treat a superimposed depression.

Some experts believe that the somatic subtype (*monohypochondriacal paranoia*) may preferentially respond to the antipsychotic pimozide, which is usually prescribed to treat Tourette's disorder. In cases of erotomania, forced separation from the love object may be needed, through hospitalization, restraining orders, or jailing if criminal offenses are committed. Several states have enacted stalking laws prompted by widely publicized cases in which a celebrity was harassed by an aggressive fan.

Schizoaffective Disorder

The term *schizoaffective* was first used in 1933 by Kasanin to describe a group of patients with concurrent schizophrenic and affective symptoms, a history of a precipitating stressor, acute onset, and a family history of mood disorder. Kasanin believed that these patients had a subtype of schizophrenia, even though they recovered from their symptoms. After his initial description, patients with this mixture of symptoms tended to receive a variety of diagnoses such as atypical schizophrenia, good-prognosis schizophrenia, cycloid psychosis, and reactive schizophrenia, because there was little agreement about definition or the relationship of these disorders to schizophrenia or mood disorders. In the past decade, the concept of schizoaffective disorder has been better defined and has been subjected to more intensive study. In all likelihood, patients with schizoaffective disorders probably constitute two groups: patients with mood disorders and patients with schizophrenia. Schizoaffective disorder probably does not represent an independent psychosis.

Because of its relatively imprecise definition, it is impossible to know the distribution of schizoaffective disorder in the community, although its prevalence is probably less than 1%. It is more frequently diagnosed in women. Schizoaffective disorder is a commonly used diagnosis in psychiatric hospitals and clinics, but it is primarily a diagnosis of exclusion. According to DSM-IV, schizoaffective disorder is a disturbance during which, at some time, there is either a major depressive or manic episode concurrent with symptoms characteristic of schizophrenia. During the period of illness, hallucinations or delusions must be present for 2 or more weeks in the absence of prominent mood symptoms, but mood symptoms must be present for a substantial portion of the total duration of the illness. Further, the effects of medical illness and drug-induced states have been excluded. The criteria specify two subtypes: the bipolar type, marked by a current or previous manic syndrome; and the depressive type, marked by the absence of any manic syndromes. The DSM-IV criteria are presented in Table 8–4.

The differential diagnosis for schizoaffective disorder consists primarily of schizophrenia, mood disorders, and disorders induced by medical illness or drugs. In schizophrenia, the duration of all episodes of mood syndrome is brief relative to the total duration of the illness, and by definition, schizophrenia leads to poor functioning in areas such as work, social relations, and self-care. Although psychotic symptoms may occur in persons with mood disorders, they are generally not present in the absence of a depression or mania, helping to set the boundary between schizoaffective disorder and psychotic mania and depression. Disorders due to medical illness or drugs may be associated with psychoses and mood syndromes, but it is usually clear from the history, physical examination, or laboratory tests that a substance or general medical condition has initiated and maintained the disturbance (e.g., treatment with corticosteroids).

Because it is likely that schizoaffective disorder affects a heterogeneous group of patients, it is difficult to talk about etiology. Family studies have shown an increased prevalence of both schizophrenia and mood disorders in relatives of schizoaffective patients, but because most of the studies use different diagnostic criteria, it is hard to know what to make of their conclusions. In general, schizoaffective patients have higher rates of schizophrenia and lower rates of mood disorders in their families than patients with mood disorder, but they have higher rates of mood disorder and lower rates of schizophrenia in their families than

Table 8–4.   DSM-IV diagnostic criteria for schizoaffective disorder

A. An uninterrupted period of illness during which, at some time, there is either a major depressive episode[a] or a manic episode concurrent with symptoms that meet criterion A for schizophrenia.[b]

B. During the same period of illness, there have been delusions or hallucinations for at least 2 weeks in the absence of prominent mood symptoms.

C. Symptoms meeting criteria for a mood episode are present for a substantial portion of the total duration of the active and residual periods of the illness.

D. The disturbance is not due to the direct psychological effects of a substance (e.g., a drug of abuse, medication) or a general medical condition.

Specify type:

Bipolar type: if the disturbance includes a manic or mixed episode (or a manic or mixed episode and major depressive episodes)
Depressive type: if the disturbance only includes major depressive episodes

---

[a]The major depressive episode must include criterion A1: depressed mood (see Table 9–1).
[b]For definition of criterion A, see Table 7–1.

patients with schizophrenia. Most other etiological indicators also suggest that schizoaffective disorder is a mixed bag, consisting of schizophrenic patients with severe mood symptoms and mood disorder patients with severe psychoses. In these cases, the disorders may be clinically indistinguishable and, of course, etiologically heterogeneous.

The signs and symptoms of schizoaffective disorder include those seen in schizophrenia and the mood disorders. The symptoms may present together or in an alternating fashion, and psychotic symptoms may be mood congruent or mood incongruent. The course and prognosis of schizoaffective disorder are variable and represent a middle ground between outcome in schizophrenia and outcome in mood disorder. Some studies, however, suggest that schizoaffective disorder, bipolar type, has an outcome similar to that of bipolar disorder, and that schizoaffective disorder, depressed type, has a prognosis similar to that of schizophrenia. Poor prognosis is indicated by poor premorbid adjustment, insidious onset, lack of a precipitating factor, predominance of psychotic symptoms, early onset, unremitting course, and a family history of schizophrenia.

The treatment of schizoaffective disorder depends on the symptom cluster that is manifested. The principles that apply for treatment of these patients apply to all psychiatric patients. If the patient is suicidal, is a danger to self or others, or is unable to properly care for himself or herself, hospitalization is necessary. Antimanic agents (e.g., lithium carbonate, carbamazepine, sodium valproate) are useful in treating a manic syndrome, and antipsychotics are useful in treating psychosis. Lithium has been shown to be useful in the long-term prophylaxis of schizoaffective disorders, particularly the bipolar type. The depressed schizoaffective patient may benefit from concurrent treatment with antidepressants and antipsychotics. The schizoaffective bipolar patient who does not respond to lithium should have a trial of carbamazepine or sodium valproate, or possibly a combination of two agents. Patients not responding to medication often respond to electroconvulsive therapy.

Schizophreniform Disorder

The term *schizophreniform* was first used in 1939 by Langfeldt to describe acute, reactive psychoses that occurred in persons with normal personalities. The definition of schizophreniform disorder requires 1) characteristic symptoms of schizophrenia, 2) that the symptoms are not due to a substance or general medical condition, 3) that schizoaffective disorder and mood disorder with psychotic features have been ruled out, and 4) that duration is at least 1 month but less than 6 months.

The diagnosis changes to schizophrenia once the symptoms have extended past 6 months, even if the only symptoms remaining are residual ones. The disorder can be further subdivided into cases with or without good prognostic features (e.g., acute onset). See Table 8–5 for the complete list of criteria. The diagnosis is to be considered provisional in patients who have not recovered, because many persons who meet criteria for schizophreniform disorder will eventually meet criteria for schizophrenia. In the past, patients with schizophreniform disorder would have received a diagnosis of *acute schizophrenia.*

This relatively new diagnosis has little empirical support, and the few relevant studies have yielded conflicting data. For example, one study found schizophreniform and schizophrenia patients to have similar structural brain abnormalities, but another investigator concluded that at least a portion of schizophreniform patients have a mood disorder, based on family history, treatment response, and neuroendocrine testing.

One long-term follow-up study indicates that patients with schizophreniform disorder have a heterogeneous outcome. Outcome measures used in the study (e.g., living situation, marital status, psychiatric symptoms) show that outcome in schizophreniform patients was more similar to that in schizophrenic patients than to that in mood disorder patients. This finding implies that some patients with schizophreniform disorder actually have a mood disorder, and that the others, probably the majority, later develop schizophrenia. The study also found that the morbidity risk for mood disorder among first-degree relatives of schizophreniform patients was no different from that observed among relatives of schizophrenic patients, but that it was significantly lower than that observed among relatives of mood disorder patients. Clearly, the proper boundaries of this

---

Table 8–5. DSM-IV diagnostic criteria for schizophreniform disorder

A. Criteria A, D, and E for schizophrenia are met.[a]

B. An episode of the disorder (including prodromal, active, and residual phases) lasts at least 1 month but less than 6 months. (When the diagnosis must be made without waiting for recovery, it should be qualified as "provisional.")

Specify if:

Without good prognostic features
With good prognostic features: as evidenced by two or more of the following:

1. Onset of prominent psychotic symptoms within 4 weeks of the first noticeable change in usual behavior or functioning
2. Confusion or perplexity at the height of the psychotic episode
3. Good premorbid social and occupational functioning
4. Absence of blunted or flat affect

---

[a]For definitions of criteria A, D, and E, see Table 7–1.

disorder remain in question. Its main use is to guard against premature diagnosis of schizophrenia.

Treatment of schizophreniform disorder has not been systematically evaluated, but the principles for its management are similar to those for an acute exacerbation of schizophrenia, which is described in Chapter 7.

Brief Psychotic Disorder

In a brief psychotic disorder, a patient develops psychotic symptoms that last at least 1 day but no more than 1 month, with the eventual return of normal premorbid functioning. Additionally, a mood disorder, schizophrenia, and the effects of a substance or general medical condition have been ruled out as causing the symptoms. Signs and symptoms are similar to those seen in schizophrenia, including hallucinations, delusions, or grossly disorganized behavior (see Table 8–6). The criteria specify three subtypes: 1) with marked stressor(s), if the symptoms appear to occur in response to a severe emotional stressor; 2) without marked stressor(s), if no stressor is apparent; and 3) with postpartum onset, if the disturbance occurs within 4 weeks of delivery. In the past, patients with marked stressors would have received a diagnosis of a reactive, hysterical, or psychogenic

Table 8–6.   DSM-IV diagnostic criteria for brief psychotic disorder

A. Presence of one (or more) of the following symptoms:
   1. Delusions
   2. Hallucinations
   3. Disorganized speech (e.g., frequent derailment or incoherence)
   4. Grossly disorganized or catatonic behavior

Note: do not include a symptom if it is a culturally sanctioned response pattern.

B. Duration of an episode of the disturbance is at least 1 day but less than 1 month, with eventual full return to premorbid level of functioning.

C. The disturbance is not better accounted for by a mood disorder with psychotic features, schizoaffective disorder, or schizophrenia and not due to the direct physiological effects of a substance (e.g., drugs of abuse, a medication) or a general medical condition.

Specify if:

   With marked stressor(s) (brief reactive psychosis): if symptoms occur shortly after and apparently in response to events that, singly or together, would be markedly stressful to almost anyone in similar circumstances in the person's culture.

   Without marked stressor(s): if psychotic symptoms do *not* occur shortly after, or are not apparently in response to, events that, singly or together, would be markedly stressful to almost anyone in similar circumstances in the person's culture.

   With postpartum onset: if onset within 4 weeks postpartum.

psychosis. Although the diagnosis does not imply a relationship with schizophrenia, the disorder is similar to what Scandinavian psychiatrists regard as *reactive psychoses*, which arise in persons with vulnerable constitutions who are subjected to stress.

Patients with postpartum onset generally develop symptoms within 1–2 weeks after delivery, which may include disorganized speech, misperceptions, labile mood, confusion, and hallucinations. *Postpartum psychosis,* as it is often called, tends to arise in persons with otherwise normal personalities and resolves within 2 to 3 months. Hospitalization is often required. This should be distinguished from postpartum blues, which occurs in up to 80% of mothers, lasts for only a few days after delivery, and is not considered pathological.

Because brief psychotic disorder has not been well studied, its prevalence and sex ratio are not known. The disorder is thought to occur more often in the lower social classes and among persons with personality disorders, especially borderline and schizotypal disorders.

The differential diagnosis of brief psychotic disorder includes schizophrenia, mood disorders, factitious disorder with psychological symptoms, malingering, and disorders induced by medical illness or drugs. In schizophrenia, onset is usually insidious, and there is no precipitating event. In mood disorders, a full mood syndrome is present, although psychotic symptoms and a precipitating event may be found. In factitious disorder with psychological symptoms, there is evidence of intentional production of the symptoms coupled with the need to assume a sick role that may bring secondary gain (e.g., more attention from family members). In malingering, the symptoms are voluntarily produced in response to an external motivation (e.g., escaping from military duties). In some cases, the differential between brief psychotic disorder, factitious disorder, and malingering will be very difficult, and prolonged observation will be needed to help clarify the diagnosis. In cases induced by medical illness or drugs, there will be evidence from history, laboratory tests, or physical examination of a substance or a general medical condition (e.g., drug intoxication) that initiated and maintained the disturbance.

As in any acute psychosis, hospitalization may be necessary for the safety of the patient or others. Because brief psychotic disorders are probably self-limiting, no specific treatment is indicated, and the hospital milieu itself may be sufficient to help the patient recover. If the patient is highly agitated or experiencing great emotional turmoil, antipsychotic or anxiolytic medications may be helpful. Once the patient is sufficiently recovered, the therapist can help the patient to explore the meaning of the psychotic reaction he or she has experienced and the meaning of the triggering stressor itself. Supportive psychotherapy should help to restore morale and self-esteem.

Shared Psychotic Disorder

The essence of this disorder is the transmission of delusional beliefs from one person to another. According to DSM-IV, this disorder occurs when the delusional system of a patient (usually persecutory) develops in the context of a close, often intimate, relationship with another person or persons who already have an established delusion. The delusion in the patient is similar to that in the person who already has a delusion. Further, other psychiatric illnesses, medical illnesses and drug-induced states have been ruled out as causing the disorder (Table 8–7).

The disorder had initially been termed *shared paranoid disorder* in DSM-III to highlight the possibility that several persons may share a similar delusion. In the past, this disorder was also called *folie à deux*, which is a French term meaning "double insanity." The disorder, first described in the late nineteenth century, is apparently rare, and information is limited to case reports. Persons of any social class can be affected.

Most cases of this disorder involve two members of the same family, most commonly siblings, a parent and child, or a husband and wife. Its development requires the presence of a dominant person with an established delusional system and a more submissive and suggestible but nonpsychotic person who then gains the acceptance of the more dominant individual by adopting his or her delusional beliefs. Because it is rare, its natural history is unknown; clinical lore suggests that separation may result in rapid improvement of the submissive person.

Psychotic Disorder Not Otherwise Specified

Psychotic disorder not otherwise specified is a residual category for persons with psychotic symptoms such as hallucinations, delusions, or grossly disorganized be-

---

Table 8–7. DSM-IV diagnostic criteria for shared psychotic disorder *(folie à deux)*

A. A delusion develops in an individual in the context of a close relationship with another person(s), who has an already established delusion.

B. The delusion is similar in content to that of the person who already has the established delusion.

C. The disturbance is not better accounted for by another psychotic disorder (e.g., schizophrenia) or a mood idsorder with psychotic features and is not due to the direct physiological effects of a substance (e.g., drugs of abuse, medication) or a general medical condition.

---

havior who do not clearly fit into any of the other better-defined categories. For example, a person with persistent auditory hallucinations who is otherwise well adjusted, employed, and socially competent would fit this category. The category should also be used to classify psychoses about which there is inadequate information to make a specific diagnosis, or when there is contradictory information.

Certain culture-bound syndromes may fit this category, including the interesting condition known as *koro*. Indigenous to China and other parts of the Far East, an individual develops the belief that his or her genitals are retracting into the body. Typically, a man believes that his penis is retracting, whereas a woman may believe that her breasts are retracting. There is usually no history of psychopathology, and the disorder remits spontaneously, although folk remedies may be used. These remedies include having the relatives pull on the person's genitals to prevent them from retracting. Epidemics of koro have been documented to occur in remote parts of China.

Bibliography

Clayton PJ: Schizoaffective disorders. J Nerv Ment Dis 170:646–650, 1982

Coryell WH, Tsuang MT: Outcome after 40 years in DSM-III schizophreniform disorder. Arch Gen Psychiatry 43:324–328, 1986

Fogelson DL, Cohen BM, Pope HG: A study of DSM-III schizophreniform disorder. Arch Gen Psychiatry 39:1281–1285, 1982

Harding JJ: Postpartum psychiatric disorders: a review. Compr Psychiatry 30:109–112, 1989

Kasanin J: The acute schizoaffective psychoses. Am J Psychiatry 90:97–126, 1933

Kendler KS: The nosologic validity of paranoia (simple delusional disorder: a review). Arch Gen Psychiatry 37:699–707, 1980

Kendler KS: Demography of paranoid psychoses (delusional disorder). Arch Gen Psychiatry 39:890–902, 1982

Kendler KS, Masterson C, Davis K: Psychiatric illness in first degree relatives of patients with paranoid psychosis, schizophrenia, and medical illness. Br J Psychiatry 147:524–531, 1985

Kendler KS, Spitzer RL, Williams JBW: Psychotic disorders in DSM-III-R. Am J Psychiatry 146:953–962, 1989

Levitt JJ, Tsuang MT: The heterogeneity of schizoaffective disorder: implications for treatment. Am J Psychiatry 145:926–936, 1988

Maj M: Lithium prophylaxis in schizoaffective disorder—a prospective study. J Affect Disord 14:129–135, 1988

Manschreck TO: Delusional disorders: clinical concepts and diagnostic strategies. Psychiatric Annals 22:241–251, 1992

Munoz RA, Amado H, Hyatt S: Brief reactive psychosis. J Clin Psychiatry 48:324–327, 1987

Opjordsmoen S: Long-term course and outcome in delusional disorder. Acta Psychiatr Scand 78:556–586, 1988

Pope HG, Lipinski JF, Cohen BM: Schizoaffective disorder: an invalid diagnosis? A comparison of schizoaffective disorder, schizophrenia, and affective disorder. Am J Psychiatry 137:921–927, 1980

Sacks MH: Folie à deux. Compr Psychiatry 29:270–277, 1988

Segal JH: Erotomania revisited: from Kraepelin to DSM-III-R. Am J Psychiatry 141:1261–1266, 1989

Strakowski SM: Diagnostic validity of schizophreniform disorder. Am J Psychiatry 151:815–824, 1994

Targum SD: Neuroendocrine dysfunction in schizophreniform disorder—correlation with six month clinical outcome. Am J Psychiatry 140:309–313, 1983

Tseng WS, Kan-Ming M, Hsu J, et al.: A sociocultural study of koro epidemics in Guangdong, China. Am J Psychiatry 145:1538–1543, 1988

Tsuang D, Coryell WH: An eight-year follow-up of DSM-III-R psychotic depression, schizoaffective disorder and schizophrenia. Am J Psychiatry 150:1182–1188, 1993

Weinberger DL, DeLisi LE, Perman GP, et al: Computed tomography in schizophreniform disorder and other acute psychiatric disorder. Arch Gen Psychiatry 39:778–783, 1982

Winokur G: Delusional disorder (paranoia). Compr Psychiatry 18:453–479, 1977

Winokur G: Familial psychopathology and delusional disorder. Compr Psychiatry 26:241–248, 1985

Self-Assessment Questions

1. How does delusional disorder differ from schizophrenia?
2. What are systematized and encapsulated delusions?
3. What are the subtypes of delusional disorder?
4. How does schizoaffective disorder differ diagnostically from both schizophrenia and psychotic mood disorders?
5. Why is schizoaffective disorder a controversial diagnosis?
6. What evidence is there to link schizophreniform disorder to either schizophrenia or the mood disorders?
7. What is the differential diagnosis of a brief psychotic disorder?
8. How is a brief psychotic disorder managed?

9. What is the commonly accepted treatment in shared psychotic disorder for the patient who develops a delusion in the context of a close relationship with another person?
10. Give an example of a situation in which the diagnosis psychotic disorder not otherwise specified is used.
11. What is koro?

Chapter 9

Mood Disorders

I see the lost are like this, and their curse
To be, as I am mine, their sweating selves. But worse.

Gerard Manley Hopkins

The mood disorders are characterized primarily by a disturbance in emotions and feelings. The disturbance may manifest itself as either elation or unhappiness, and the two clinical syndromes associated with these extremes are referred to as mania and depression. Most people who have mood disorders have some type of depression, but a few experience mood swings between these two poles of mood disorder and are therefore referred to as bipolar. Mood disorders are very common, and they usually respond well to treatment. Learning to diagnose and treat these disorders is as basic and fundamental a skill in medicine as the diagnosis and management of myocardial infarction or streptococcal pharyngitis.

History

The recognition that some human beings have a recognizably abnormal syndrome characterized by a disorder in mood has been present for many millennia. Perhaps the oldest medical document available to us is from ancient Egypt, the Eber papyrus, and it describes a medical condition characterized by severe despondency that is equivalent to modern concepts of depression. In the Old Testament, the case of Saul is described in the book of Samuel during the eighth century B.C. Saul, King of Israel, develops periods of severe depression, guilt, and incapacity. Several different treatments are attempted, including placing a young woman in his bed and having the young shepherd David play soothing music for him. He responds to the music of David for a time and even accepts David as a member of the royal household. Later, however, he relapses again, becomes severely psychotic, and even attempts to kill David and his own son Jonathan.

The original name for this disorder, *melancholy*, appears in Hippocratic writings of the fourth century; the term *melancholy* literally means black bile, and it reflects the belief that this disorder was due to a chemical imbalance of the humors of the body. Clear and explicit references to disorders of mood continue from classical times up to the present. St. Augustine, St. John of the Cross, Shakespeare's Hamlet, John Keats, William James, and Leo Tolstoy are only a few of the many notable figures who have described their personal struggles with periods of depression or despondency.

Mood disorders are thus historically among the oldest psychiatric syndromes that have been recognized. They are also extremely common and psychologically understandable. We have all experienced mild periods of despondency after some personal loss or failure, and it is therefore very easy to identify with people who have the more severe forms of the illness. As later portions of this chapter indicate, effective treatments for these illnesses have become available during the past few decades, making these among the most treatment-responsive disorders in psychiatry and in medicine generally. As a result, working with patients with mood disorders tends to be very gratifying.

An additional aspect of mood disorders that makes them intriguing is their association with giftedness or creativity. As early as the fourth century B.C., Aristotle commented that "those who have become eminent in philosophy, politics, poetry, and the arts have all had tendencies toward melancholia." People with mood disorders may, as a group, be somewhat more creative or gifted than the general population. For example, in a group of successful creative writers selected from the rotating faculty at The University of Iowa Writers' Workshop, the rate of mood disorder was nearly three times greater than that of a socioeconomically and educationally equivalent control group. This finding, first reported in the 1970s, has been repeatedly replicated in subsequent studies by several different investigators. The list of notable writers who clearly have had a mood disorder is long, including Robert Lowell, Ernest Hemingway, Sylvia Plath, John Berryman, William Styron, and Anne Sexton.

Many eminent philosophers, scientists, and politicians have had mood disorder as well. Aristotle cites both Plato and Alexander the Great as examples. Oliver Cromwell, Martin Luther, and Abraham Lincoln are probably examples as well. It is a sad commentary on the stigma attached to mental illness in our society that American presidential candidates are screened for a history of psychiatric illness, and even the untrue attribution of such a history is considered to be an effective form of mudslinging. Many of our great leaders of the past would have been prevented from accomplishing their missions had a history of mood disorder been considered grounds for disqualification.

These disorders are variously referred to as either mood or affective disorders. DSM-IV uses the term *mood disorders*, but DSM-III and much of the older clinical and research literature use the alternate term. Although more traditional and more widely used, the concept of an abnormality of affect as a unifying principle for these disorders is somewhat problematic on several grounds. The term *affect* is sometimes used to refer to the external expression of an internal state (i.e., mood); the distinction between mood and affect also sometimes turns on transient versus sustained states, with affect being more transient and mood being more sustained (affect is to weather as mood is to climate). According to this distinction, the abnormality in affective or mood disorders is more often one of mood, because the change in emotion lends a constant and pervasive coloring to the individual's perception of reality during the period of illness. Further, patients with schizophrenia often have pronounced abnormalities in affect that are fundamental to the illness; therefore, schizophrenia is in some respects an affective disorder. Thus, although the terms *affective disorder* and *mood disorder* tend to be used interchangeably to refer to either depression or mania, mood disorder is probably the preferable term. Linguistic conventions are hard to wipe out, however, and so the term *affective disorder* is likely to be used in clinical and research literature as well.

Clinical Findings and Diagnostic Criteria

The mood disorders fall into two broad syndromes: depression and mania.

Major Depressive Episode

Because feelings of sadness and despondency are very much part of normal human experience, having diagnostic criteria to demarcate pathological sadness from normal responses to stress and injury is particularly important. The DSM-IV criteria for an episode of major depression appear in Table 9–1. These criteria specify that the patient must have at least five symptoms of depression (and one of them must be depressed mood or loss of interest or pleasure). These five symptoms are drawn from a list of nine in criterion A. These characteristic symptoms

Table 9–1. DSM-IV diagnostic criteria for major depressive episode

A. Five (or more) of the following symptoms have been present during the same 2-week period and represent a change from previous functioning; at least one of the symptoms is either 1) depressed mood, or 2) loss of interest or pleasure.

Note: Do not include symptoms that are clearly due to a general medical condition, or mood-incongruent delusions or hallucinations.

  1. Depressed mood most of the day, nearly every day, as indicated either by subjective account (e.g., feels sad or empty) or observation by others (e.g., appears tearful) **Note:** In children and adolescents, can be irritable mood.

  2. Markedly diminished interest or pleasure in all, or almost all, activities most of the day, nearly every day (as indicated by either subjective account or observation made by others)

  3. Significant weight loss when not dieting or weight gain (e.g., a change of more than 5% of body weight in a month), or decrease or increase in appetite nearly every day **Note:** In children, consider failure to make expected weight gains.

  4. Insomnia or hypersomnia nearly every day

  5. Psychomotor agitation or retardation nearly every day (observable by others, not merely subjective feelings of restlessness or being slowed down)

  6. Fatigue or loss of energy nearly every day

  7. Feelings of worthlessness or excessive or inappropriate guilt (which may be delusional) nearly every day (not merely self-reproach or guilt about being sick)

  8. Diminished ability to think or concentrate, or indecisiveness, nearly every day (either by subjective account or as observed by others)

  9. Recurrent thoughts of death (not just fear of dying), recurrent suicidal ideation without specific plan, or a suicide attempt or a specific plan for committing suicide

B. The symptoms do not meet criteria for a mixed episode.

C. The symptoms cause clinically significant distress or impairment in social, occupational, or other important areas of functioning.

D. The symptoms are not due to the direct physiological effects of a substance (e.g., a drug of abuse, a medication) or a general medical condition (e.g., hyperthyroidism).

E. The symptoms are not better accounted for by bereavement, i.e., after the loss of a loved one, the symptoms persist for longer than 2 months or are characterized by marked functional impairment, morbid preoccupation with worthlessness, suicidal ideation, psychotic symptoms, or psychomotor retardation.

define major depression, and they must be present for at least 2 weeks to rule out transient fluctuations in mood. Criteria B, D, and E serve to rule out other conditions, such as a bipolar disorder (e.g., presence of a mixed episode), abnormalities in mood due to abuse of a substance (e.g., amphetamines) or to a general medical condition (e.g., myxedema), or a disturbance in mood due to bereavement. To differentiate a *disorder* from normal fluctuations in mood, criterion C specifies that the symptoms must cause distress or impairment.

Because major depression is perhaps the most common psychiatric illness that clinicians in any branch of medicine are likely to encounter, it is worthwhile to commit the nine characteristic symptoms to memory. In interviewing patients to determine whether they are depressed, the clinician will repeatedly find himself or herself mentally running through this list of symptoms. Consequently, it is convenient to have it stored in an accessible memory bank so that the evaluation can be done fluently and smoothly. This can be facilitated through the use of a simple mnemonic: Depression Is Worth Studiously Memorizing Extremely Grueling Criteria. Sorry (DIWS MEGCS). The initials stand for: Depressed mood, Interest, Weight, Sleep, Motor activity, Energy, Guilt, Concentration, Suicide.

As the DSM-IV criteria imply, the basic abnormality in depression is an alteration in mood: a person who is depressed feels sad, despondent, down in the dumps, or full of despair. Although the dysphoric mood is most frequently expressed as a complaint of feeling sad, occasionally patients will complain of feeling tense or irritable, with only a small component of sadness, or of having lost their ability to feel pleasure or to experience interest in things they normally enjoy.

The depressive syndrome is frequently accompanied by a group of vegetative symptoms, such as decreased appetite or insomnia. The decreased appetite often leads to some weight loss, although occasionally people who are depressed will force themselves to eat in spite of decreased appetite, or they may be urged to eat by a parent or spouse so that the weight loss is minimal. Less frequently, depression expresses itself as a desire to eat excessively and is accompanied by weight gain.

Insomnia may be initial, middle, or terminal. *Initial insomnia* means that the patient has difficulty in falling asleep, often tossing or turning for several hours before dozing off. *Middle insomnia* refers to awakening in the middle of the night, remaining awake for an hour or two, and finally falling asleep again. *Terminal insomnia* refers to awakening early in the morning and being unable to return to sleep. Patients with insomnia will often worry and ruminate during the time when they are lying awake. Patients who have terminal insomnia may have more severe depressive syndromes. Depressed patients may also complain of restless sleep, indicating that they have awakened so frequently throughout the night that they scarcely got any sleep at all. These various types of sleep disturbance have been well documented by electroencephalography (EEG) research in sleep laboratories. Occasionally, the sleep difficulty may involve a need to sleep excessively: the patient may complain of feeling chronically tired and needing to spend 10–14 hours each day in bed.

Motor activity is often altered in depression. Patients may subjectively complain of feeling either slowed down or agitated, but objective evidence is required as well to ensure that the symptom is truly present. Patients with *psychomotor retardation* may sit quietly in a chair for hours without speaking to anyone, simply staring into space. When these patients get up and move about, they walk at a snail's pace, their speech is slow, and their replies are brief and laconic. If asked about their thinking, they may complain that it is markedly slowed down. On the other hand, patients with *psychomotor agitation* are restless and seem extremely nervous. Agitated patients may complain more of irritability or tenseness than of depression. They are unable to sit in a chair and frequently pace about. They may wring their hands or perform some other stereotyped and repetitive nervous gesture such as drumming their fingers on a table, pulling on their hair or clothing, or playing with objects in their hands. Their speech is usually somewhat rapid, and they may complain in a high-pitched and staccato whine about the various miseries from which they are suffering.

Depressed patients also complain frequently of tiring too easily or having a marked decrease in their energy level. In a general medical setting, this may be one of the most common presenting complaints of depression, and the clinician will need to probe to determine whether the easy fatigability is due to a depressive syndrome.

Feelings of worthlessness and guilt are also very common in depression. Depressed persons may lose confidence in themselves so that they are fearful of going to work, taking examinations, or assuming responsibility for household tasks. They may avoid answering the phone or returning phone calls to avoid responsibilities or social relationships that they feel unable to handle. They may become completely hopeless and full of despair, believing that their situation can never be improved, or even that they do not deserve to feel better. Depressed persons may feel quite guilty over actual or fantasized misdeeds that they committed in the past. Usually the misdeed is seen as more terrible than it actually was, so that depressed persons believe that they should be social pariahs because of a lie told as a child, or sent to prison for a long term because of a questionable deduction taken on an income tax return.

Complaints of difficulty in concentrating or thinking clearly are also common in depression. Depressed persons feel that they function less well at work, are unable to study, or (in severe cases) are even unable to perform simple cognitive tasks such as watching a football game on television or reading escape fiction.

Depressed patients may think a great deal about death or suicide. Death may be seen either as an escape from their suffering or a deserved punishment for their various misdeeds. The suicidal patient often expresses the notion that "everyone would be better off without me." Suicide risk is high in depressed patients and should always be assessed carefully. (See Chapter 20 for more detail on evaluation and management of the suicidal patient.)

In addition to the nine core symptoms summarized in the diagnostic criteria, other symptoms may also occur in patients with depression. *Diurnal variation*, another vegetative symptom, is a fluctuation in mood during the course of a 24-hour day; it may reflect some type of neuroendocrine abnormality in depression. Most typically, patients state that their mood is worse in the morning, but that it improves as the day progresses, so that they feel best in the evening. Less frequently, this problem is reversed, with the patient stating that he or she feels best in the morning.

Sex drive may decrease markedly, so that the patient has no interest in sex or even begins to experience impotence or anorgasmia. The depressed patient may also complain of other physical symptoms such as constipation or dry mouth. The frequency of some of the common symptoms of depression is summarized in Table 9–2.

Occasionally patients experience *masked depression*. This term means that the full depressive syndrome is not immediately obvious, because the patient does not report a depressed mood. With the introduction of diagnostic criteria, however, the diagnosis has been unmasked, because a thorough and systematic interview that runs through the various criteria will reveal the presence of decreased interest and a substantial clustering of symptoms. Masked depression may be especially important in a primary care setting. For example, an older person may

Table 9–2. Frequency of typical symptoms in depressed patients

Symptom	%
Insomnia	100
Sadness of mood	100
Tearfulness	94
Poor concentration	91
Suicidal thoughts	82
Fatigue	76
Irritability	76
Psychomotor retardation	76
Anorexia	66
Diurnal variation	64
Hopelessness	51
Poor memory	35
Delusions	33
Suicide attempts	15
Auditory hallucinations	6

Source. Adapted from Winokur G, Clayton P, Reich T: Manic Depressive Illness. St. Louis, MO, CV Mosby, 1969.

come in complaining primarily of many physical symptoms that are so troubling that he or she is unable to concentrate, unable to work, and unable to sleep. This patient will deny being in a despondent or irritable mood, stating that he or she is indeed upset but would feel fine if only the physical symptoms were corrected. These symptoms are often pain or gastrointestinal problems, such as piercing headache, burning pains in the rectum, or persistent heartburn. Although a careful medical workup reveals no physical abnormalities, the patient usually continues to insist on the troubling nature of the various somatic and depressive symptoms. When the masked depression clears with appropriate treatment, however, the physical complaints tend to disappear, making it clear that they were secondary to a depressive syndrome.

Patients who are severely depressed may experience psychotic symptoms such as delusions or hallucinations. These are usually consistent with the depressed mood; for example, people who are depressed may hear the voice of the Devil telling them that they have fallen so far from God's ways that their souls are forever lost and that they will be tormented in hell throughout eternity. They may begin to believe that the world is coming to an end and that they have seen various signs as indicators of its impending demise. They may develop the delusion that the FBI or police are following them and bugging their house or office to catch them in the various misdeeds that their excessive guilt makes them believe they have committed. They may think that a fatal disease is consuming their bodies and rotting away their internal organs. Less frequently, the delusions will not be consistent with depressed mood. For example, patients may report that they are being spied on because they are on the verge of developing some great invention that others are attempting to steal—a persecutory delusion that is not directly related to depressed mood.

The following history is relatively typical of a major depressive episode:

Wilma was brought to the hospital at the request of her family, and of her husband in particular. She described herself as being despondent and demoralized because her husband was having an affair with a woman who had previously been his secretary, but her husband adamantly denied this and indicated that this belief was a delusion due to his wife's depressed condition.

Wilma admitted to a depressed mood plus a full constellation of depressive symptoms, including feelings of worthlessness, suicidal thoughts, hypersomnia, increased appetite and weight gain, decreased interest in and enjoyment of activities she normally found pleasurable (such as following the many activities of her four teenage children), and decreased energy.

When interviewed alone, she indicated that she was absolutely convinced that her husband, a successful local insurance agent, was secretly involved with another woman. She attributed most of her depressive symptoms to this situation, which she believed had been going on for at least 6 months (as had her depression). She had no specific evidence to support the occurrence of the affair, but she indicated that her husband had been away more in the evenings, had a marked decrease in sexual interests, and had talked frequently about Lydia's secretarial skills until Wilma became jealous and angry. Due to pressure from Wilma, her husband eventually urged Lydia to seek another position, but Wilma believed that her husband was continuing to see Lydia secretly. Both in the presence of his wife and when interviewed alone, Bill adamantly denied the affair. He indicated that he was a devout Catholic (as was Wilma) and that such behavior was strongly discordant with his religious beliefs, as well as risky to his community position. Bill indicated that his sexual interest had decreased because Wilma had become increasingly overweight and less attractive. Wilma had had one prior episode of depression that had been successfully treated with antidepressants approximately 5 years earlier.

A diagnosis of depression was therefore made again, and Wilma was placed on imipramine, with the dose gradually increased to 150 mg/day. She showed some improvement on this medication, and both Bill and Wilma were also seen for marital counseling. Their relationship improved somewhat, but Wilma continued to be suspicious.

Wilma remained on antidepressants for the next 3 months and continued to see a psychotherapist at weekly intervals to learn techniques to decrease her chronic negative mind set, her suspicious attitude toward her husband, and her tendency to use food as a way of raising her spirits.

After 3 months of psychotherapy, she came in one day with a new firmness of step and her eyes flashing with anger. While cleaning out of the pockets of one of her husband's suits in preparation for sending it to the cleaners, she found a love letter from Lydia. She did not confront Bill immediately, but instead followed him the next night when he indicated that he was going back to the office to get caught up on some dictation. Ten minutes after his departure, Wilma left, drove past Lydia's house, and found Bill's car parked in her garage. Thereafter, she confronted him, and he finally confessed to an affair that had been going on for nearly 2 years.

The direction of marital counseling changed sharply, and Bill was urged to seek individual psychotherapy himself. Wilma continued to require antidepressant medication for another 6 months, as she gradually came to terms with the fact of her husband's infidelity (which was actually more painful than having her suspicions discounted by both her husband and the medical community). Eventually, however, the couple was able to work through this situation, to remain married, and eventually to establish a reasonably good relationship with one another.

Manic Episode

The DSM-IV criteria for a manic episode require the presence of an abnormally elevated, expansive, or irritable mood lasting at least 1 week, plus three from a list of seven characteristic symptoms. The criteria are similar to those used to define depression, in that the mood disturbance must be sufficiently severe to cause marked impairment or to require hospitalization. As in the case of depression, the symptoms cannot be due to the physiological consequences of drugs of abuse, medications, or a general medical condition. The criteria for a manic episode appear in Table 9–3.

The manic patient's mood is typically cheerful, enthusiastic, and expansive. The cheerfulness often has an infectious quality, making interviewing an enjoyable and sometimes amusing experience. Sometimes, however, the patient's mood is simply irritable, particularly when he or she is thwarted, and such irritable manic patients can be quite difficult to manage. Because of their euphoria, manic patients usually have very little insight into their problems. In fact, they may deny that anything is wrong with them and instead blame friends or family for attributing an abnormality to them that is in fact not present. Because manic disorder is characterized by other symptoms that are clearly pathological, such as

Table 9–3. DSM-IV diagnostic criteria for manic episode

A. A distinct period of abnormally and persistent elevated, expansive, or irritable mood, lasting at least 1 week (or any duration if hospitalization is necessary)

B. During the period of mood disturbance, three (or more) of the following symptoms have persisted (four if the mood is only irritable) and have been present to a significant degree:

  1. Inflated self-esteem or grandiosity

  2. Decreased need for sleep (e.g., feels rested after only 3 hours of sleep)

  3. More talkative than usual or pressure to keep talking

  4. Flight of ideas or subjective experience that thoughts are racing

  5. Distractibility (i.e., attention too easily drawn to unimportant or irrelevant external stimuli)

  6. Increase in goal-directed activity (either socially, at work or school, or sexually) or psychomotor agitation

  7. Excessive involvement in pleasurable activities that have a high potential for painful consequences (e.g., engaging in unrestrained buying sprees, sexual indiscretions, or foolish business investments)

C. The symptoms do not meet criteria for a mixed episode.

D. The mood disturbance is sufficiently severe to cause marked impairment in occupational functioning or in usual social activities or relationships with others, or to necessitate hospitalization to prevent harm to self or others, or there are psychotic features.

E. The symptoms are not due to the direct physiological effects of a substance (e.g., a drug of abuse, a medication, or other treatment) or a general medical condition (e.g., hyperthyroidism).

Note: Manic episodes that are clearly caused by somatic antidepressant treatment (e.g., medication, electroconvulsive therapy, light therapy) should not count toward a diagnosis of bipolar I disorder.

poor judgment and extreme grandiosity, it is usually not difficult for the clinician to differentiate manic euphoria from a normal good mood.

Manic patients typically have inflated self-esteem and grandiosity, which may reach delusional proportions. Manic patients may believe that they have special abilities or powers, which clearly are outside the normal range for their educational background or intellectual achievement. They may develop plans to write books, cut records, lead religious movements, or undertake expansive business ventures. When the grandiosity reaches delusional proportions, patients may report that they are rock stars, famous athletes or politicians, or even religious figures such as the Messiah.

The euphoria and grandiosity are typically accompanied by increased energy, activity levels, and cognitive speed. Patients with mania usually require less sleep than usual, often getting by on only 2 or 3 hours per night. Unlike the patient with depression, the manic patient does not feel tired and does not complain about his or her inability to sleep.

Manic patients tend to talk excessively and to manifest pressured speech. Thus, they answer questions at great length, continue to talk even when interrupted, and sometimes talk when no one is listening. Their speech is usually rapid, loud, and emphatic. Underlying the pressured speech, there is probably a rapid flow of thought, sometimes referred to as *flight of ideas*. This increased speed in cognitive functioning is inferred by listening to the patient's speech, which manifests derailment, incoherence, and distractibility. Manic patients tend to skip from one topic to another as they describe their experiences, ideas, or symptoms. Thus, positive formal thought disorder is quite common in mania. Distractibility is observed both in their speech and in their social behavior. While speaking, they may shift their topic in response to some stimulus in the environment, and they manifest the same pattern of distractibility when trying to perform tasks or complete activities. Unfortunately, the increased energy and cognitive productivity are usually not sufficiently well organized to produce the magnificent goals that are projected in the patients' grandiose plans.

People with mania are often more physically active than usual as well. Patients may become more social and gregarious, going to bars, planning parties, or calling friends at all hours of the night. Interest in sex is often increased, leading the manic patient to exhaust his or her partner or to make inappropriate overtures to casual acquaintances or strangers. Patients with mania are usually physically restless and unable to sit still. The increased level of activity is often accompanied by poor judgment. Patients with mania tend to overextend themselves in ways that lead them into serious trouble after the manic episode is over. They spend money excessively, commit themselves to projects that they are unable to complete, become involved in extramarital affairs, or engage in quarrels with business associates or family members who disagree with them or try to slow them down.

As in the case of depression, manic patients may manifest symptoms of psychosis. Indeed, psychotic symptoms are almost more the norm than the exception in mania. Approximately 50% of manic patients have psychotic symptoms, compared to only about 20% of patients with depression. Psychotic symptoms may include either delusions or hallucinations and typically express themes consistent with the mood, such as delusions about special abilities or powers. Less commonly the delusions may be mood incongruent and express themes that are not related to the euphoric and grandiose mood. Table 9–4 summarizes the frequency of some common symptoms of mania.

The following case history illustrates a relatively typical manic episode.

Charles was brought to the psychiatric emergency room by the local police, after he had jumped from his seat in the middle of a performance of *Les Miserables*, run onto

Table 9–4.   Frequency of typical symptoms in patients with mania

Symptom	%
Distractibility	100
Pressured speech	99
Euphoria	98
Lability	95
Flight of ideas	93
Insomnia	90
Grandiosity	86
Irritability	85
Hostility	83
Extravagance	69
Depression	68
Diurnal variation	67
Depression after mania	52
Delusions of any type	48
Increased alcohol consumption	42
Increased intercourse	32
Auditory hallucinations	21
Increased sexual contacts (noncoital)	12
Promiscuity	11
Suicidal thoughts	7

Source.   Adapted from Winokur G, Clayton P, Reich T: Manic Depressive Illness. St. Louis, MO, CV Mosby, 1969.

the stage, and begun yelling that the injustices of the Reagan Administration were as extensive and profound as those portrayed in the performance. He had begun conversing with Jean Valjean, urging him to leave the performance, to join the Democratic party, and to assist in the effort to place a Democrat in the American presidency. This speech was accompanied by an extensive speech on the injustice of packing the Supreme Court with a group of extreme conservatives.

In the emergency room he indicated that he did not reside in Iowa City but had come from Des Moines (100 miles away) to attend the performance and to consult with friends and colleagues at the law school. He described himself as a prominent lawyer, a graduate of Harvard Law School who had edited the *Law Review*, a close friend of the Kennedy family and other prominent Democrats, and a dedicated crusader against social injustice. He described the Reagan Administration as a rerun of the industrial-totalitarian axis that had been created in Nazi Germany, complained about a conspiracy that he believed was under way to destroy the Democratic party either by persecution or assassination of key figures, and indicated that one of the purposes of his trip to Iowa City was to warn his colleagues at the law school about these dangerous circumstances. He was organizing a campaign to assist a little-known Arkansas politician in his effort to run for president in the next election, believing that this person would be a reincarnation of John Kennedy.

His appearance was somewhat unkempt and disheveled, not consistent with his description of his prominent status. Although he was attired in an expensive-appearing pinstripe suit, his hair was uncombed, his eyes were red, and he was unshaven. He talked excitedly in a rapid manner, and his voice rose to a shout at times. His speech was disjointed and difficult to follow, as his topic changed from his own special importance and abilities to the various conspiracies that he thought were under way in the Reagan government. He described a complex internal structure in the Reagan Administration that he believed would "lead to another Watergate," and he marshaled evidence to support this position by referring to special implications in programs that had recently run on television such as *Dynasty* and *David Letterman*. When admission to the hospital was proposed, he became physically agitated and tried to run away. He became physically combative at attempts to restrain him, asserting in a threatening manner that he was a former state wrestling champion who was also a finalist for the Olympic team in his weight class.

Because of his agitation, a decision was made to obtain an emergency holding order. His claims of special importance and abilities were discounted and attributed to his manic state. Later, as more history was obtained, it became evident that he was indeed a prominent attorney with many important national connections and also had been a star wrestler. The conspiracy against the Democratic Party, although potentially bearing some credence, contained enough implausible elaborations to qualify as delusional thinking. (The beliefs about the Arkansas politician were also thought to be delusional!) Interviews with his family members revealed that he had had one prior hospitalization for mania and had been treated for depression as an outpatient. He had been taking maintenance lithium, but he had decided to discontinue it abruptly approximately 3 days before coming to Iowa City to attend the performance of *Les Miserables*. Within a day after discontinuing the lithium, he became increasingly euphoric, irritable, and grandiose. His wife had been reluctant to let him go alone, but he had insisted that he would be fine and left against her wishes.

He was placed on a therapeutic dose of lithium, and his symptoms cleared rapidly over the course of 4–5 days. He was able to leave the hospital and to return to work within 1 week. His second episode of mania helped him appreciate the importance of maintenance lithium, because his insight about his illness increased, and he has been able to prevent subsequent relapses and to function effectively.

Mixed and Hypomanic Episodes

A small number of patients present with a mixture of both manic and depressive symptoms within a single episode of illness. When this occurs, it is referred to as a *mixed* episode. The clinical presentation of mixed episodes can be quite confusing because the patient's mood and symptom picture tend to alternate rapidly. At one moment, the patient will be talkative, energetic, and expansive, and yet minutes later he or she may burst into tears and complain of feeling hopeless and suicidal. DSM requires that full criteria for both a manic episode and a depressive episode be met within a 1-week period to diagnose the presence of a mixed episode. Patients with a mixed episode are difficult to treat, because medications must target both poles of mood disorder simultaneously.

Hypomania is another less common but important form of mood disorder. The syndrome is similar to mania, but is milder, briefer, and less florid. During a hypomanic episode, the patient experiences the elevated mood and other classic symptoms that define mania, but they are not accompanied by delusional beliefs or hallucinations, and their severity is not great enough to require hospitalization or to markedly impair social and occupational functioning. The criteria for a hypomanic episode appear in Table 9–5. Most patients with hypomania also are depressed, so it can sometimes be difficult to determine whether they are back to their usual selves or are just feeling good for a change. Obtaining information from family and friends is usually helpful in determining whether the presence of a good mood is indeed pathological rather than a patch of normal happiness in the midst of feeling chronically blue. Examining the level and quality of social and occupational functioning can provide a clue as to whether the episode is hypomania; the hypomanic person is clearly mildly impaired and suboptimal in these functions, in spite of subjectively feeling good or even great. Subtle clues, such as tactlessness in a usually sensitive person or flirtatious behavior in a typically discreet person, indicate that the hypomanic episode reflects a real and pathological change from the normal baseline level of functioning.

DSM-IV also recognizes two forms of mood disorder that are somewhat

Table 9–5. DSM-IV diagnostic criteria for hypomanic episode

A. A distinct period of persistently elevated, expansive, or irritable mood lasting throughout at least 4 days, that is clearly different from the usual nondepressed mood

B. During the period of mood disturbance, three (or more) of the following symptoms have persisted (four if the mood is only irritable) and have been present to a significant degree:
   1. Inflated self-esteem or grandiosity
   2. Decreased need for sleep (e.g., feels rested after only 3 hours of sleep)
   3. More talkative than usual or pressure to keep talking
   4. Flight of ideas or subjective experience that thoughts are racing
   5. Distractibility (i.e., attention too easily drawn to unimportant or irrelevant external stimuli)
   6. Increase in goal-directed activity (either socially, at work or school, or sexually) or psychomotor agitation
   7. Excessive involvement in pleasurable activities that have a high potential for painful consequences (e.g., the person engages in unrestrained buying sprees, sexual indiscretions, or foolish business investments)

C. The episode is associated with an unequivocal change in functioning that is uncharacteristic of the person when not symptomatic.

D. The disturbance in mood and the change in functioning are observable by others

E. The episode is not severe enough to cause marked impairment in social or occupational functioning, or to necessitate hospitalization, and there are no psychotic features.

F. The symptoms are not due to the direct physiological effects of a substance (e.g., a drug of abuse, a medication, or other treatment) or a general medical condition (e.g., hyperthyroidism)

Note: Hypomanic-like episodes that are clearly caused by somatic antidepressant treatment (e.g., medication, electroconvulsive therapy, light therapy) should not count toward a diagnosis of bipolar II disorder.

milder than those discussed: *dysthymic disorder* and *cyclothymic disorder.*

Dysthymic disorder (sometimes referred to as *depressive neurosis*) is a chronic and persistent disturbance in mood that has been present for at least 2 years and is characterized by relatively typical depressive symptoms, such as anorexia, insomnia, decreased energy, low self-esteem, difficulty concentrating, and feelings of hopelessness. Because dysthymic disorder is a mild chronic disorder, only two of these symptoms are necessary, but they must have persisted more or less continuously for at least a 2-year period. Criteria for dysthymic disorder appear in Table 9–6.

Patients with dysthymic disorder are chronically unhappy and miserable. Some of them also develop the relatively more severe major depressive syndrome; when the major depressive episode clears, these patients subsequently return to their chronic state of dysthymia. The coexistence of these mild and severe forms of depression is sometimes referred to as *double depression.*

Table 9–6.   DSM-IV diagnostic criteria for dysthymic disorder

A. Depressed mood for most of the day, for more days than not, as indicated either by subjective account or observation by others, for at least 2 years.

Note: In children and adolescents, mood can be irritable and duration must be at least 1 year.

B. Presence, while depressed, of two (or more) of the following:
   1. Poor appetite or overeating
   2. Insomnia or hypersomnia
   3. Low energy or fatigue
   4. Low self-esteem
   5. Poor concentration or difficulty making decisions
   6. Feelings of hopelessness

C. During a 2-year period (1 year for children and adolescents) of the disturbance, the person has never been without the symptoms in criteria A and B for more than 2 months at a time.

D. No major depressive disorder during the first 2 years of the disturbance (1 year for children and adolescents); i.e., the disturbance is not better accounted for by chronic major depressive disorder or major depressive disorder, in partial remission.

Note: There may have been a previous major depressive episode provided there was a full remission (no significant signs or symptoms for 2 months) before development of the dysthymic disorder. In addition, after the initial 2 years (1 year in children and adolescents) of dysthymic disorder, there may be superimposed episodes of major depressive disorder, in which case both diagnoses may be given when the criteria are met for a major depressive episode.

E. There has never been a manic episode, a mixed episode, or a hypomanic episode, and criteria have never been met for cyclothymic disorder.

F. The disturbance does not occur exclusively during the course of a chronic psychotic disorder, such as schizophrenia or delusional disorder.

G. The symptoms are not due to the direct physiological effects of a substance (e.g., a drug of abuse, a medication) or a general medical condition (e.g., hyperthyroidism).

Specify if:
    Early onset: if onset is before age 21 years
    Late onset: if onset is age 21 years or older

Specify (for most recent 2 years of dysthymic disorder):
    With atypical features

A second mild affective syndrome is *cyclothymic disorder*, a condition in which the patient has mild swings between the two poles of depression and hypomania. While in the manic phase, the person appears to be high, but not so high as to be socially or professionally incapacitated. During the depressed phase, the person has some symptoms of depression, but these are not severe enough to meet criteria for a full major depressive episode (i.e., five symptoms persisting for 2 weeks). Thus, the individual with cyclothymic disorder tends to swing from high to low with a chronic mild instability of mood. The criteria for cyclothymic disorder appear in Table 9–7.

Table 9–7. DSM-IV diagnostic criteria for cyclothymic disorder

A. For at least 2 years, the presence of numerous periods with hypomanic symptoms and numerous periods with depressive symptoms that do not meet criteria for a major depressive episode.

Note: In children and adolescents, the duration must be at least 1 year.

B. During the above 2-year period (1 year in children and adolescents) the person has not been without the symptoms in criterion A for more than 2 months at a time.

C. No major depressive episode, manic episode, or mixed episode has been present during the first 2 years of the disturbance.

Note: After the initial 2 years (1 year in children and adolescents) of cyclothymic disorder, there may be superimposed manic or mixed episodes (in which case both bipolar I disorder and cyclothymic disorder may be diagnosed) or major depressive episodes (in which case both bipolar II disorder and cyclothymic disorder may be diagnosed).

D. The symptoms in criterion A are not better accounted for by schizoaffective disorder and are not superimposed on schizophrenia, schizophreniform disorder, delusional disorder, or psychotic disorder not otherwise specified.

E. The symptoms are not due to the direct physiological effects of a substance (e.g., a drug of abuse, a medication) or a general medical condition (e.g., hyperthyroidism).

F. The symptoms cause clinically significant distress or impairment in social, occupational, or other important areas of functioning.

Classification and Subtypes

Controversy exists about the best way to define and classify the various disorders of mood. This controversy arises because the major mood syndromes exist on a continuum of severity with normality and even with one another. Very mild periods of depression are probably normal, because most people experience them. Once an arbitrary dividing line is set to distinguish mild normal blues from pathological blues, then it is not clear whether the remainder of the depressive syndromes are a single disorder on a continuum of severity or whether they represent discrete disorders. If discrete, are there subtypes, and what are they? The transition from mania to hypomania to normal creative highs presents similar problems. Further, there is even controversy about whether bipolar disorder is simply a more severe form of depression or whether it represents a different and discrete disorder. This controversy arises largely because of patterns of familiality and heredity, which are often helpful in delineating syndromes and disorders in medicine: family studies indicate that many relatives of bipolar patients have only depression, suggesting that bipolar and purely depressive mood syndromes may simply be more and less severe forms of the same underlying disorder.

The DSM-IV classification of mood disorders is summarized in Table 9–8. It represents the best compromise that can be achieved concerning subtypes of

Table 9–8. DSM-IV classification of mood disorders

Bipolar disorders	Depressive disorders
Bipolar disorder, manic	Major depression, single episode
Bipolar disorder, depressed	Major depression, recurrent
Bipolar disorder, mixed	Dysthymic disorder
Cyclothymic disorder	Depressive disorder not otherwise
Bipolar disorder not otherwise specified	specified

mood disorders based on existing evidence. The mood disorders may be subdivided into two main groups: those that are characterized by depression only (i.e., with a major depressive episode or some milder mood disturbance) and those that are bipolar; the latter are characterized by mania (i.e., with a manic episode or a hypomanic episode), either alone or in combination with depression. Thus, this classification initially defines the types of mood disorders as *bipolar* and *unipolar*.

The term *unipolar* is not included in DSM-IV, but it is widely used by clinicians to refer to patients who have depression only. Thus, patients are subdivided in the DSM-IV on a syndromal basis: those who have had an episode of mania are referred to as having bipolar disorder (even if they have not yet had a depression), whereas those who have had depression only are classified as having a depressive disorder. This subdivision is based on its predictive power. These two subforms of mood disorder typically have different familial patterns, require different treatments, and perhaps have a different pathophysiology and etiology.

The depressive disorders include major depressive disorder and dysthymic disorder, as well as a residual category (depressive disorder not otherwise specified). Major depressive disorder is defined by the presence of at least one episode of major depression. The disorder can be further characterized by a variety of specifiers, as described below. Dysthymic disorder is defined on the basis of the criteria enumerated above. The residual category is used for the occasional odd case that does not fit any of the criteria, but seems to fit the overall syndrome.

The bipolar disorders include bipolar I disorder, bipolar II disorder, cyclothymic disorder, and bipolar disorder not otherwise specified.

Bipolar I disorder is defined by the occurrence of at least one manic or mixed episode. Typically, bipolar I disorder is characterized by recurrent episodes of both mania and depression, which may be separated by intervals of months to years. Although the episodes may lead to psychosocial morbidity because of the impact of a severe recurrent illness on interpersonal relationships or work functioning, interepisode functioning may be good or even excellent. When well, individuals with bipolar disorder can be high achievers. As described below, both the most recent episode and the longitudinal course can be characterized by a variety of specifiers.

Bipolar II disorder is characterized by periods of hypomania that typically occur either before or after periods of depression but also may occur independently. These mild manic episodes are not sufficiently severe to require hospitalization, although they may lead to personal, social, or work difficulties. During the mild bipolar phase, the patient is upbeat, shows signs of poor judgment, and has other indices of mania such as increased energy or insomnia, but the illness does not meet full criteria for a manic episode. Bipolar II disorder appears to breed true within families, in that relatives of bipolar II patients themselves have higher rates of bipolar II disorder than either bipolar I (i.e., criteria are met for a full manic episode) or unipolar major depression. Bipolar II patients also tend to have a high rate of comorbidity with other disorders, such as substance abuse.

As defined above, *cyclothymic disorder* is the mildest form of bipolar disorder, whereas *bipolar disorder not otherwise specified* is a residual category.

The nature of the mood disorder is further characterized in a variety of ways. Because mood disorders tend to be recurrent, the various additional specifiers give the clinician a way of characterizing the most recent episode (for which the patient is currently in treatment) and the overall lifetime course of the disorder.

It is very useful to characterize the most recent manic or depressive episode in terms of its severity. This way of subdividing depression is summarized in Table 9–9. The subdivision for mania or for mixed episodes is similar. The episode is classified as mild, moderate, severe, or in partial or full remission. This classification recognizes the continuum of severity within the mood disorders and permits the clinician to indicate where a particular patient falls on that continuum. The

---

Table 9–9. Types of major depressive episode

Mild: Few, if any, symptoms in excess of those required to make the diagnosis, **and** symptoms result in only minor impairment in occupational functioning or in usual social activities or relationships with others.

Moderate: Symptoms or functional impairment between "mild" and "severe."

Severe, Without Psychotic Features: Several symptoms in excess of those required to make the diagnosis, **and** symptoms markedly interfere with occupational functioning or with usual social activities or relationships with others.

Severe, With Psychotic Features: Delusions or hallucinations. If possible, specify whether the psychotic features are mood congruent or mood incongruent.

    Mood-congruent psychotic features: Delusions or hallucinations whose content is entirely consistent with the typical depressive themes of personal inadequacy, guilt, disease, nihilism, or deserved punishment.

    Mood-incongruent psychotic features: Delusions or hallucinations whose content does not involve typical depressive themes of personal inadequacy, guilt, disease, death, nihilism, or deserved punishment. Included are symptoms such as persecutory delusions (not directly related to depressive themes), thought insertion, thought broadcasting, and delusions of control.

most severe form is psychotic mania or depression, which is characterized by florid psychotic symptoms such as delusions or hallucinations. Sometimes the psychotic symptoms are consistent with the patient's mood. For example, a depressed patient who feels guilty and despondent may have elaborate religious delusions of sin and guilt, or may hear voices condemning him or her. A manic patient may develop grandiose delusions that he or she is a deity, a rock star, or an important political figure. Such delusions are characterized as *mood congruent*, and the subtype of mania or the subtype of manic or depressive episode is therefore classified as manic/psychotic/mood congruent or depressed/psychotic/mood congruent. A very disturbed patient with mania or depression may display psychotic features that are not congruent with his or her mood; for example, a manic patient may believe that he or she is being tormented by demons. *Mood incongruent* delusions or hallucinations are a relatively worse prognostic feature, and so this form of psychotic mood disorder is delineated as a separate category.

Several additional descriptors of the depressive episode are also used: chronic, with catatonic features, with melancholic features, with atypical features, and with postpartum onset.

Melancholia

Among these various specifiers, "melancholic features" is perhaps the most important. The criteria for melancholic features appear in Table 9–10. The concept of *melancholia* is thought to identify a relatively severe form of depression that is more likely to respond to somatic therapy. The concept is based on an older historic distinction between endogenous versus reactive depression, a distinction that was based both on presumed etiology and a characteristic clustering of symptoms. In the original definition of *endogenous depression*, it had no

Table 9–10.   DSM-IV diagnostic criteria for melancholia

A. Either of the following, occurring during the most severe period of the current episode:
 1. Loss of interest or pleasure in all, or almost all, activities
 2. Lack of reactivity to usually pleasurable stimuli (does not feel much better, even temporarily, when something good happens)
B. Three (or more) of the following:
 1. Distinct quality of depressed mood (i.e., the depressed mood is experienced as distinctly different from the kind of feeling experienced after the death of a loved one)
 2. Depression regularly worse in the morning
 3. Early morning awakening (at least 2 hours before usual time of awakening)
 4. Marked psychomotor retardation or agitation
 5. Significant anorexia or weight loss
 6. Excessive or inappropriate guilt

precipitating factors (endo-genous = grows from within), whereas a *reactive depression* occurred in reaction to some stressful life event such as a divorce or loss of a job. The term *endogenous* has been abandoned, because increasing evidence has suggested that severe depressions may also be triggered by a variety of physiological or psychological stressors.

As traditionally defined, endogenous depression has a characteristic set of symptoms, most of which are used to specify the presence of melancholic features in DSM-IV. Two specific characteristic features are required: pervasive loss of interest or pleasure and inability to respond to pleasurable stimuli. Three from a list of six additional features are also required: distinct quality to the mood, diurnal variation, terminal insomnia, severe psychomotor retardation or agitation, anorexia or weight loss, and excessive guilt. Many of these symptoms are predominantly somatic or vegetative, and sometimes this form of depression is referred to as vegetative. A substantial body of research has suggested that this clustering of symptoms predicts a good response to antidepressant medication or electroconvulsive therapy (ECT). Frequently, patients with this clustering of symptoms have a past history of somatic therapy with good response.

Atypical Features

Other specifiers highlight other aspects of the most recent episode that may also be clinically useful and guide decisions about management. The *atypical features specifier* identifies a group of patients who are diametrically opposed to those with endogenous features; they do not present with the classic vegetative symptoms such as insomnia, weight loss, or anorexia, but instead have weight gain and hypersomnia. In addition, instead of having a nonreactive mood, they are quite responsive to their life situation, and they are particularly sensitive to slights or rejections. This rejection sensitivity often leads to difficulties in interpersonal relationship, with a stormy love life characterized by being easily hurt, having many partners, and experiencing frequent breakups. Subjectively, these patients often express their somatic state by complaining of "leaden paralysis," the feeling that their arms and legs weigh them down and make activities difficult for them. Patients with atypical features are difficult to treat and may require a mixture of psychotherapy and medications. Monoamine oxidase (MAO) inhibitor antidepressants have proved especially useful with this group of patients (see Chapter 26). The criteria for atypical features appear in Table 9–11.

Chronic, Postpartum, and Catatonic Specifiers

The other specifiers identify other aspects of the recent episode that may also be clinically important. The *chronic specifier* simply indicates that the full criteria for a major depressive episode have been present for 2 years; patients in this group are treatment refractory and clinically challenging. The *postpartum-onset specifier* identifies those patients who experience a depressive, manic, or mixed episode within the first 4 weeks postpartum. Although feeling a bit depressed after delivery is common (referred to as the postpartum blues), some women develop a full mood syndrome that requires medical attention with either somatic therapy or psychotherapy or both. At its most severe, the mood episode may become psychotic and/or life-threatening to the mother or child; such severe abnormalities have been estimated to occur in 1 of 500 to 1 of 1,000 deliveries; the risk of recurrence in subsequent deliveries is great—between 30% and 50% of cases. The *catatonic features specifier* identifies a subgroup of patients who display catatonic features similar to those that historically have been observed primarily in schizophrenia (e.g., posturing, waxy flexibility, catalepsy, negativism, and mutism). The presence of this specifier serves to remind the clinician that such symptoms may also occur in other disorders and that they are not pathognomonic of schizophrenia. These types of symptoms tend to occur primarily in the mood disorders at the severe and psychotic end of the continuum.

Longitudinal Course Descriptors

DSM-IV also provides a system for specifying the longitudinal course of the disorder, as well as the clinical characteristics of the most recent episode. The clinician is usually asked to specify whether the disorder involves only a single episode (usually the first episode, for which the patient is currently being treated) or whether the condition is recurrent. If recurrent, the clinician is re-

---

Table 9–11.   DSM-IV diagnostic criteria for atypical features

Specify if:

With atypical features (can be applied when these features predominate during the most recent 2 weeks of a major depressive episode in major depressive disorder or in bipolar I or bipolar II disorder when the major depressive episode is the most recent type of mood episode, or when these features predominate during the most recent 2 years of dysthymic disorder)

A. Mood reactivity (i.e., mood brightens in response to actual or potential positive events)

B. Two (or more) of the following features:
1. Significant weight gain or increase in appetite
2. Hypersomnia
3. Leaden paralysis (i.e., heavy, leaden feelings in arms or legs)
4. Long-standing pattern of interpersonal rejection sensitivity (not limited to episodes of mood disturbance) that results in significant social or occupational impairment

C. Criteria are not met for "with melancholic features" or "with catatonic features" during the same episode.

minded that closer follow-up is needed and that the prognosis may be more guarded. The need for prophylactic long-term medications to prevent relapse is also substantially increased. Because the various specifiers permit description of many different permutations and combinations of features, the classification of mood disorders may appear quite complicated. A summary of the various combinations appears in Table 9–12. An example of some typical patterns of longitudinal course is shown in Figure 9–1, which displays the various combinations of major depression and dysthymia that may occur. Similar variations in pattern are also seen in the bipolar disorders.

The various longitudinal descriptors also permit identification of two other facets of long-term course: *with seasonal pattern* and *with rapid cycling*. The criteria for the seasonal pattern specifier are summarized in Table 9–13. Clinicians have recognized for many decades that some individuals have a characteristic onset of mood symptoms in relation to changes of season, with depression typically oc-

Table 9–12. DSM-IV episode specifiers that apply to mood disorders

	Severity/ psychotic/ remission	Chronic	With catatonic features	With melancholic features	With atypical features	With postpartum onset
Major depressive disorder, single episode	X	X	X	X	X	X
Major depressive disorder, recurrent	X	X	X	X	X	X
Dysthymic disorder					X	
Bipolar I disorder, single manic episode	X		X			X
Bipolar I disorder, most recent episode hypomanic						
Bipolar I disorder, most recent episode manic	X		X			X
Bipolar I disorder, most recent episode mixed	X		X			X
Bipolar I disorder, most recent episode depressed	X	X	X	X	X	X
Bipolar I disorder, most recent episode unspecified						
Bipolar II disorder, hypomanic						
Bipolar II disorder, depressed	X	X	X	X	X	X
Cyclothymic disorder						

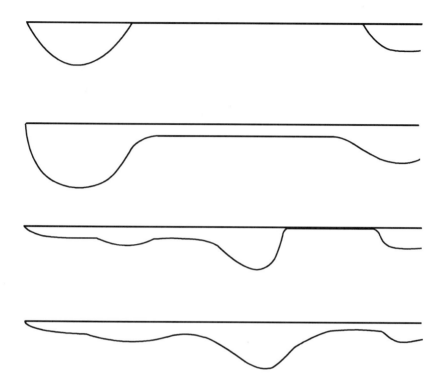

Figure 9–1. DSM-IV patterns of longitudinal course of mood disorders. *Top,* recurrent, with full interepisode recovery, with no dysthymic disorder. *Second,* recurrent, without full interepisode recovery, with no dysthymic disorder. *Third,* recurrent, with full interepisode recovery, superimposed on dysthymic disorder (also code 300.4). *Bottom,* recurrent, without full interepisode recovery, superimposed on dysthymic disorder (also code 300.4).

Table 9–13. DSM-IV diagnostic criteria for seasonal pattern

A. There has been a regular temporal relationship between the onset of major depressive episodes in bipolar I or bipolar II disorder or major depressive disorder, recurrent, and a particular time of the year (e.g., regular appearance of depression in the fall or winter).

Note: Do not include cases in which there is an obvious effect of seasonal-related psychosocial stressors (e.g., regularly being unemployed every winter).

B. Full remissions (or a change from depression to mania or hypomania) also occur at a characteristic time of the year (e.g., depression disappears in the spring).

C. In the last 2 years, two major depressive episodes have occurred that demonstrate the temporal seasonal relationship defined in criteria A and B, and no nonseasonal major depressive episodes have occurred during that same period.

D. Seasonal major depressive episodes (as described above) substantially outnumber the nonseasonal major depressive episodes that may have occurred over the individual's lifetime.

curring more frequently during the winter months and remissions or changes from depression to mania during the spring. This seasonal pattern also has important implications for prevention and treatment, in that medications can be adjusted appropriately once the pattern is recognized. The rapid cycling descriptor identifies those patients who have had at least four episodes of major depression, mania, hypomania, or a mixed episode during the past 12 months. This specifier also warns the clinician of the need for close follow-up and careful medication management. Rapid cyclers are clearly at high risk for relapse and also have a high suicide risk.

Other Approaches to Subtyping Mood Disorders

There are other important ways of classifying or describing the mood disorders that do not appear in DSM-IV. They are sufficiently widely discussed that the clinician should have at least some familiarity with them.

Patients with depression are sometimes subdivided into *primary* and *secondary* subtypes. Primary depression is depression occurring in a person who has never had any other psychiatric illness. Secondary depression is depression occurring in a person who previously has had another psychiatric diagnosis, the most common being alcoholism, other substance abuse, panic disorder and other anxiety disorders, and antisocial personality. This subclassification was originally introduced to facilitate research, because investigators seeking genetic patterns of transmission or neurochemical indicators of depression wanted to study relatively pure examples of depression. Patients with secondary depression were thought to have a disorder more closely related to their antecedent diagnosis (e.g., alcoholism) than to the depressive disorders. Secondary depression is, however, clinically important in its own right. Studies have indicated rather consistently that patients with secondary depression tend to be more difficult to manage, in that they have more suicidal thoughts and suicide attempts, are less compliant with treatment, tend to improve less with treatment, and have a higher relapse rate. No doubt some of this increased morbidity in secondary depression is related to the fact that the patient has two illnesses, depression and some other disorder such as alcoholism, both of which have their own inherent morbidity.

A distinction between *neurotic depression* and *psychotic depression* is also sometimes made. This subdivision was originally developed as a way of identifying the two extremes of severity that are seen in the mood disorders. Neurotic depression is usually defined as a mild mood disorder that tends to be chronic and to be accompanied by personality problems such as a tendency toward obsessional worrying; many patients classified as dysthymic in DSM-IV would be considered to have a neurotic depression. The use of the term *neurotic* highlights the possibility that the patient is likely to require treatment with some form of psychotherapy, either as an adjunct to somatic therapy or in lieu of it. Psychotic depression is usually defined as a severe depression that is extremely incapacitating; although the depression is called psychotic, this term does not necessarily require that the patient have delusions or hallucinations. When the neurotic versus psychotic distinction is used, the term *psychotic* typically means that the patient is severely impaired in psychosocial function, is more likely to need inpatient treatment, and will definitely require medication or ECT.

Epidemiology

Because epidemiological surveys of the prevalence or incidence of mood disorder have not used identical criteria to define mood disorders, the incidence and prevalence are uncertain. One study done in New Haven, Connecticut, which used diagnostic criteria closely equivalent to those in the DSM-IV, indicated that approximately 4.3% of the population has depression at any given time. A lifetime prevalence for major depression of about 6% was found in the Epidemiologic Catchment Area (ECA) study, and about 18% was found in the more recent National Comorbidity Study. Estimates of lifetime prevalence vary, but it seems likely that somewhere between 8% and 20% of the population will experience a significant depression at some time, depending on how narrowly or broadly *significant depression* is defined. Depression is more common in women than in men (currently, the ratio in the United States is approximately 2:1). The age at onset of major depression appears to be getting steadily lower, a phenomenon referred to as the *cohort effect*. That is, a proportionately larger number of individuals in the baby boom generation have had episodes of major depression compared with older individuals. In the baby boomers, the age at onset is reported to be earlier than it is in older individuals.

Bipolar disorder is much less common than unipolar major depression. The lifetime prevalence for bipolar disorder is between 0.5% and 1%. Bipolar disorder is also more common in women than men, with a ratio of approximately 3:2.

Data from the ECA study show that dysthymic disorder has a lifetime prevalence of approximately 3%, and it is more common in women under age 65, unmarried persons, and persons with low income. A recent study indicates that dysthymic disorder may also be quite common in elderly persons. There are no comparable figures for cyclothymic disorder.

Etiology and Pathophysiology

Many different ideas have been proposed to explain the pathophysiology and etiology of mood disorders. These explanations encompass the domains of genetics, social and environmental factors, and neurobiological factors.

Genetics

It has been recognized for many years that mood disorders tend to run in families. As discussed in Chapter 5, however, familiality does not necessarily indicate genetic transmission, because role modeling, learned behavior, social environmental factors such as economic deprivation, and physical environmental factors such as prenatal and perinatal birth complications may all provide nongenetic contributions to the development of a disorder, and these contributions could themselves be familial. (For example, before the advent of antibiotics, tuberculosis tended to run in families for environmental rather than genetic reasons.)

Studies of familial aggregation in mood disorders have provided empirical evidence that these disorders run in families. Data from family studies are summarized in Figures 9–2 and 9–3. Figure 9–2 summarizes data based on studies that used bipolar patients as the index case. Figure 9–3 shows the rates of bipolar illness in the first-degree relatives of unipolar patients. Nearly all studies show significantly increased rates of mood disorder (especially bipolar disorder) in the

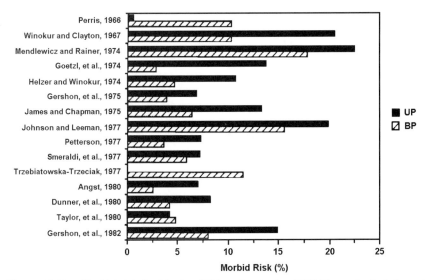

Figure 9–2. Morbid risk for bipolar (BP) and unipolar (UP) illness in first-degree relatives of bipolar probands.

first-degree relatives of bipolar patients compared with psychiatrically normal control subjects. Unipolar patients tend to have much less bipolar illness among their first-degree relatives, but a high rate of unipolar illness. Control rates vary from study to study, but they are typically around 1% in the psychiatrically normal population for bipolar disorder and between 5% and 15% for unipolar disorder; rates vary depending on the methods of definition. As these figures indicate, the first-degree relatives of bipolar patients tend to have a higher rate of bipolar illness than unipolar illness, although unipolar illness is also quite common in the first-degree relatives of bipolar patients. The opposite effect is seen in the first-degree relatives of unipolar patients. Thus, not only are these disorders familial, but they also tend to breed true. The fact that they do not breed *perfectly* true (i.e., bipolar illness *only* in the relatives of bipolar patients and unipolar illness *only* in the relatives of unipolar patients) also suggests that these two forms of mood disorder may not be totally distinct from each other.

Twin and adoption studies have complemented these family studies and provided evidence to suggest that mood disorders are genetic in addition to familial. The twin studies are summarized in Table 9–14. The total number of available twin pairs is under 500; the overall monozygotic to dizygotic ratio in this entire sample is approximately 4:1 (65:14). Within individual studies the monozygotic-to-dizygotic ratio ranges from 75:0 to 57:23. These data are certainly sufficient to indicate that affective illness must have a strong genetic component. Adoption studies also support this conclusion.

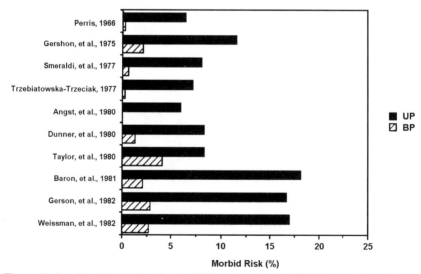

Figure 9–3. Morbid risk for bipolar (BP) and unipolar (UP) illness in first-degree relatives of unipolar probands.

Mood disorders were the first among the major mental illnesses to be studied with the techniques of molecular biology using the linkage method. Two types of linkage have been reported. In a study of the Old Order Amish, linkage to the short arm of chromosome 11 was reported for bipolar disorder, a finding not supported by a subsequent reanalysis. In several other studies, X linkage has been reported for bipolar disorder. It is quite possible that several different genetic mechanisms could produce different forms of bipolar illness, so that a finding of linkage to different chromosomes is not unlikely.

It seems virtually certain that if a single gene exists for mood disorder, its penetrance is incomplete and is likely to be variable. The fact that monozygotic twins are not 100% concordant is just one piece of evidence that indicates a lack of full penetrance. Operationally, this means that individuals are carrying the gene but not expressing it clinically, a fact that makes it difficult to identify a case and reduces the strength of the statistical analyses on which linkage studies depend. Many other problems are likely to continue to plague the search for a bipolar gene or a depression gene, including environmental phenocopies (especially a problem for depression), lack of clarity about the boundaries between unipolar and bipolar forms of mood disorder, clinical heterogeneity of the disorders, and probable genetic heterogeneity as well.

Social and Environmental Factors

Early empirical research focused extensively on the question of whether stressful life events might be considered to cause mood disorders, particularly depression. The questions pursued in this research are supported by intuition and common sense, which suggest that misfortune is likely to produce sadness, particularly if

Table 9–14. Concordance rates for affective illness in monozygotic and dizygotic twins

Study	Monozygotic twins		Dizygotic twins	
	Concordant pairs/ total pairs	Concordance %	Concordant pairs/ total pairs	Concordance %
Luxenberger 1930	3/4	75.0	0/13	0.0
Rosanoff et al. 1935	16/23	69.6	11/67	16.4
Slater 1953	4/7	57.1	4/17	23.5
Kallmann 1954	25/27	92.6	13/55	23.6
Harvald and Hauge 1965	10/15	66.7	2/40	5.0
Allen et al. 1974	5/15	33.3	0/34	0.0
Bertelsen 1979	32/55	58.2	9/52	17.3
Totals	95/146	65.1	39/278	14.0

the misfortunes are severe, multiple, or persistent and if the individual experiencing them is vulnerable or predisposed either because of a genetic vulnerability or because of a variety of early life experiences producing greater sensitivity to stress, such as the loss of a parent early in life.

The results of this research are conflicting, with some studies suggesting that life events may indeed influence the development of mood disorders, whereas others have found no relationship. These conflicting results are difficult to interpret because many of the studies (both positive and negative) have methodological problems, due largely to the inherent difficulty of the topic being studied. Some of the early explanations of this question approached it from an either/or perspective: that is, some studies conceived of psychosocial stressors as the *only* cause of depression and did not explore the role of familial predisposition, and other studies tended to assume that depression could only be caused by biological factors and did not adequately examine the effects of psychosocial stressors.

A major confounder in many of these studies is the effect of depression itself on life events. Once an individual has developed an episode of depression or mania, the occurrence of the illness may produce many changes in psychosocial status, such as divorce, loss of job, or poor academic performance. The prior experience of a depressive episode may color future perceptions as well, making individuals who have had depression perceive relatively neutral life events in a more grim or pathological way. Thus, the only truly rigorous approach to examining the effects of the life events on depression is to assess their frequency *before* the onset of a first episode of depression. Because this approach would require large epidemiological samples, it has not been applied.

Perhaps the best approach to the psychosocial and life-event literature is to return to the intuitive and common sense perspective with which this research endeavor began. That is, individuals who experience losses are likely to feel sad or despondent, and a sufficient accumulation of losses may produce demoralization and depression. Indeed, the neuroendocrinological research described below provides some support for this point of view. It seems distinctly possible that a series of stressful life events could induce a biological reaction (e.g., an outpouring of cortisol) that, once initiated, is difficult to stop and could trigger or exacerbate a depressive syndrome that is based on both social-psychological and biological factors. One genetic factor that could be transmitted within families might be a tendency to be neurobiologically oversensitive to the effects of psychosocial stress.

The cohort effect for mood disorders, described above, also provides some evidence to suggest that psychosocial factors may have some influence on the development of mood disorders. This cohort effect was observed in a very large collaborative study of more than 1,000 patients with mood disorder, their first-degree relatives, and a sample of psychiatrically normal control subjects. When the subjects in this study were divided into cohorts based on their current age, and the age at onset of major depression was plotted, it became clear that people in the younger age ranges had a steadily earlier age at onset and an increased rate of mood disorder.

Various possible explanations for this cohort effect have been explored. It does not appear to be a consequence of better memory in younger individuals, involving a more recent approximation to the actual age at onset in these younger people. Because most of the people with an early onset of mood disorder are in the baby boom generation, it may reflect the impingement of a variety of economic and social stresses on this cohort. The baby boomers have experienced more intensive competition in a variety of spheres than any generation in recent history. Because of the large number of individuals in this cohort, they have had to compete with one another for college admission and jobs in an economy that has declined substantially from that of their parents, due to pressures of recession and inflation. They have been through the Age of Aquarius and its subsequent abandonment, seen a variety of cultural heros assassinated, and participated in the tragedy of the Vietnam War. It is not clear how these various economic and social stresses would produce a high rate of depression in this cohort, but the cohort effect is not consistent with any purely genetic explanation of depression, and it is one piece of evidence suggesting the continuing importance of social and environmental factors in the development of mood disorders.

Psychodynamic and other purely psychological explanations for mood disorders have also been proposed. Depression may be usefully conceptualized as anger turned inward. Individuals vulnerable to depression may find it socially or ethically unacceptable to overtly express anger that they feel about unfairnesses or misfortunes that they have experienced; instead of ventilating and eliminating their anger, they instead turn it in against themselves, criticize and castigate themselves, and become depressed. Mania is sometimes conceptualized as a defense against an underlying depression. According to this view, a person experiencing mania has in fact an underlying depression, but fights against it psychologically by artificially elevating both mood and activity level. Nevertheless, periods of depression tend to break through from time to time. This interpretation of mania is consistent with some well-observed clinical phenomena, such as the occurrence of mixed episodes and rapid cycling.

Neurobiology

Neurobiological studies of mood disorders have pursued four major areas of investigation: abnormalities in neurotransmission, neuroimaging of brain structure and blood flow, abnormalities in neurophysiological function (especially sleep), and abnormalities in neuroendocrine function.

Abnormalities in Neurotransmission

Studies of neurotransmitter function in depression originally emphasized the *catecholamine hypothesis*. This hypothesis postulates that depression is caused by a deficit of norepinephrine at crucial nerve terminals throughout the brain. As for the neurotransmitter theories of other illnesses, much of the support has come from studies of the mechanism of action of medications used to treat depression. Many antidepressants (e.g., imipramine) have been shown to increase the amount of norepinephrine functionally available at nerve terminals by inhibiting reuptake. The monoamine oxidase inhibitors (MAOIs), which are effective in treating depression, also increase the amounts of norepinephrine available to receptors by inhibiting breakdown of norepinephrine through monoamine oxidase. Reserpine, known to deplete monoamines, tends to worsen depression. Finally, some studies (but not all) have demonstrated that patients with depression may have a decrease in 3-methoxy-4-hydroxyphenylglycol (MHPG), a major metabolite of brain norepinephrine. There is some suggestion that the finding of decreased MHPG is more prominent in bipolar patients with depression than in unipolar and especially nonmelancholic patients.

However, other neurotransmitters may also play a role in depression, as evidenced by the action of other types of medication. Some antidepressants, particularly the newer ones such as fluoxetine, have potent and relatively specific effects on the serotonin system. These medications are selective serotonin reuptake inhibitors (SRIs) and appear to exert their therapeutic effect chiefly by increasing the amount of serotonin functionally available at the terminal, suggesting that a functional deficit of serotonin may contribute to the development of depression. Patients with severe depression have also been noted to have a decrease in the major serotonin metabolite, 5-hydroxyindoleacetic acid (5-HIAA), in their cerebrospinal fluid, and decreased numbers of serotonin type 2 (5-HT_2) receptors have been observed in postmortem brains of individuals who have committed suicide.

Dysregulation in the acetylcholine system has also been proposed as another possible neurochemical mechanism for the symptoms of depression. Acetylcholine appears to have an interactive relationship with the monoamine neurotransmitters: increased tone in the monoamine system leads to a decrease in cholinergic tone; conversely, increased cholinergic tone leads to a decrease in monoamine activity. Administration of cholinergic agonists tends to produce a variety of symptoms characteristic of depression, such as psychomotor slowing or the subjective experience of dysphoria.

Neuroimaging Studies

Both structural and functional imaging techniques have been applied to study the mechanisms of mood disorders. Computed tomography studies of stroke patients have applied the lesion method to determine the possible anatomic substrates of mood abnormalities; these studies suggest that anterior left-hemisphere strokes are likely to induce dysphoria, perhaps by disconnecting noradrenergic circuits projecting to the left prefrontal cortex; right-hemisphere strokes are more likely to induce euphoria. Positron-emission tomography (PET) studies provide some additional support for these findings, in that induction of dysphoria in psychiatrically normal individuals appears to activate left frontal regions, and areas of decreased metabolic activity or perfusion have also been noted in these regions in individuals with depression. The most consistently noted abnormality to date with magnetic resonance imaging has been an increased number of focal signal hyperintensities in white matter; the functional significance of this abnormality is unclear, but it has been noted in both bipolar and unipolar mood disorders.

Abnormalities in Neurophysiology

Neurophysiological abnormalities have also been extensively studied in mood disorders. The largest and most consistent body of data involves the use of sleep EEG. (The sleep EEG, or polysomnography, is further discussed in Chapter 23.) Studies have consistently demonstrated that patients with depression have a variety of EEG abnormalities during sleep, including decreased slow-wave sleep (i.e., deep sleep), a shortened time before the onset of rapid eye movement (REM) sleep (the period when dreams and nightmares occur), and longer periods of REM sleep than do psychiatrically normal subjects. These three types of abnormality are referred to as decreased delta sleep, decreased REM latency, and increased REM density. All these abnormalities in sleep EEG are consistent with the subjective complaints of insomnia that depressed patients express. Depressed patients typically state that they do not sleep very deeply or very long; their decreased delta sleep indicates that their sleep is indeed not as deep as normal sleep, and the abnormalities in REM sleep are consistent with their complaints of light, fitful sleep.

Abnormalities in Neuroendocrine Function

Neuroendocrine abnormalities have also been extensively explored in patients with depression. Early research in this area suggested that depressed patients had larger quantities of cortisol metabolites in their urine than did psychiatrically normal subjects, as well as higher blood levels of cortisol and abnormal diurnal variation in cortisol production. The dexamethasone suppression test (DST) has been used extensively to explore the possibility of neuroendocrine dysregulation in depression and to attempt to determine the place on the hypothalamic-pituitary-adrenal axis where this abnormality might occur.

The accumulated evidence suggests that somewhere between 30% and 70% of patients with severe depression do not show normal suppression of cortisol secretion after the administration of dexamethasone. For a time, an abnormal DST was thought to provide a potential tool in the differential diagnosis of depression, but it has become clear that the test is quite nonspecific; there are also relatively high rates of DST nonsuppression in other psychiatric conditions such as anorexia nervosa, dementia, and substance abuse. (The DST is further discussed in Chapter 4.)

Other aspects of the neuroendocrine system have been explored in addition to the hypothalamic-pituitary-adrenal axis. Depressed patients have been shown to have a blunting of growth hormone output in response to insulin challenge, as well as blunted production of thyroid-stimulating hormone in response to thyrotropin-releasing hormone. The abnormalities across a variety of neuroendocrine target organs (e.g., adrenals, pancreas, thyroid) indicate that the abnormality does not lie in these organs, and the patterns of abnormal response to challenge also suggest that the abnormality is not in the pituitary. More likely, the abnormality is at the level of the hypothalamus, a brain region regulated largely through monoamine neurotransmitters. The neuroendocrine data are consistent with a hypothesis of neurochemical dysregulation in the brain, perhaps reflecting a dysregulation within the catecholamine system.

Course and Outcome

Depressive Episode

A depressive episode may begin either suddenly or gradually. The duration of an untreated episode may range from a few weeks to months or even years, although it is suspected that most depressive episodes clear spontaneously within about 6 months. Although the prognosis for any single depressive episode is quite good, particularly in view of the efficacy of the various antidepressant medications, most patients experience a recurrence of depression at some time. About 20% of patients become chronically depressed. Thus, for most people who become depressed, depression is either chronic or recurrent.

Suicide is the most serious complication. About 15% of all hospitalized patients with depression die by suicide. Several factors suggest an increase in risk: being divorced or living alone, history of alcohol or drug abuse, age over 40, history of a prior attempt, and an expression of suicidal ideation (particularly when detailed plans have been formulated). Suicidal risks should always be carefully evaluated in any patient with depression, beginning with a direct inquiry whether the patient has considered taking his or her life. A patient considered at risk for suicide usually should be treated as an inpatient rather than an outpatient to minimize the risk. Suicide is discussed in more detail in Chapter 20.

Although suicide is the most important serious complication of depression, other social and personal complications may also occur. Decreased energy, poor concentration, and lack of interest may cause poor performance at school or work. Apathy and decreased sexual interest may lead to marital discord. Patients may attempt to treat depressive symptoms themselves with sedatives, alcohol, or stimulants, thereby initiating problems with drug and alcohol abuse.

Manic Episode

The onset of mania is frequently abrupt, although it may begin gradually over the course of a few weeks. The episodes usually last from a few days to months. They tend to be briefer and to have a more abrupt termination than depressive episodes. Although the prognosis for any particular episode is reasonably good, especially with the availability of effective treatments such as lithium and antipsychotics, the risk for recurrence is significant. Not uncommonly, an episode of mania is followed by an episode of depression. Some patients with bipolar disorder recover relatively fully, but a substantial subset continue to have chronic mild instability of mood, particularly recurrent episodes of mild depression.

The complications of mania are primarily social: marital discord, divorce, business difficulties, financial extravagance, and sexual indiscretions. Drug or alcohol abuse may occur during a manic episode. When mania is severe, the patient may be almost completely incapacitated and require protection from the consequences of poor judgment or hyperactivity. In the past, mania sometimes resulted in death from physical exhaustion. Excessive activity level continues to be a significant risk in patients with cardiac problems. A manic syndrome can switch rapidly to depression, and the risk of suicide is heightened when the patient becomes remorsefully aware of inappropriate behavior that occurred during the manic episode. Patients rarely commit suicide while manic.

Differential Diagnosis

When evaluating a patient with a mood disorder, the physician should always consider the possibility that the illness may result from some specific extrinsic factor that can induce a manic or depressive syndrome, such as drugs of abuse, sedatives, tranquilizers, antihypertensives, oral contraceptives, and glucocorticoids. General medical conditions such as myxedema or systemic lupus erythematosus may also present with prominent depressive symptoms. If the episode of mood disorder is judged to be the result of a specific drug or medical illness, the disorder is diagnosed as secondary to it. Treatment usually involves withdrawing or reducing the drug or treating the underlying general medical illness.

A depressive episode in elderly persons may be difficult to distinguish from the various dementias, because both may be characterized by apathy, difficulty concentrating, and complaints of poor memory. If the features suggesting a depressive episode are at least as prominent as those suggesting a dementia, it is usually best to treat such patients for depressive symptoms, because a successful treatment will result in the disappearance of symptoms suggesting a possible dementia. Neuroimaging techniques such as single photon emission computed tomography and neuropsychological testing may also assist in the differential diagnosis. (See Chapter 4 for more details on laboratory assessment and Chapter 6 for a discussion of pseudodementia.)

Dysphoric mood is a common symptom in schizophrenia. A depressive disorder can usually be distinguished from schizophrenia through use of several different clues. The dysphoric mood in schizophrenia is more typically apathetic or empty, whereas the person with depression usually experiences his or her mood as intensely painful. The onset of schizophrenia is usually more gradual, but patients with schizophrenia also typically have a more severe deterioration in function than do patients with depression. Patients with schizophrenia and patients with major depression may both have psychotic symptoms; thus, severe psychotic depression is often very difficult to distinguish from schizophrenia with acute onset. In this relatively difficult case, it is often best to treat the patient for depression and to observe the course of illness over time. If psychotic symptoms tend to persist after mood symptoms remit, then the diagnosis of schizophrenia or schizoaffective disorder is more likely.

The differential diagnosis between mania and schizophrenia is also quite important. Several features are useful in making this distinction. Personality and general functioning are usually satisfactory before and after an episode of manic disorder, even though mild disturbances in mood may occur. Although manic episodes may present with disorganized speech that is indistinguishable from the speech sometimes observed in schizophrenia, speech abnormalities in mania are always accompanied by a disturbance in mood and usually by overactivity and physical agitation. Although manic patients may experience delusions or hallucinations, these typically reflect the underlying disturbance in mood. (Of course, mood-incongruent psychotic symptoms occur occasionally, making the differential diagnosis more difficult.) It may be particularly difficult to distinguish an irritable and angry manic patient from an excited patient with paranoid schizophrenia, based on a simple cross-sectional evaluation. As in the case of a difficult differential diagnosis of depression, it is usually best to defer definitive diagnosis and to treat the patient for mania, because mania carries a better prognosis. Additional guidelines that make the diagnosis of manic episode more likely include a family history of affective disorder, good premorbid adjustment, and a previous episode of affective disorder from which there was complete or substantial recovery. On the other hand, if psychotic symptoms persist in the absence of an abnormality in mood, the diagnosis of schizophrenia or schizoaffective disorder is more likely.

People experiencing bereavement may have many depressive symptoms and experience them for a sufficient duration to meet criteria for a depressive episode. Nevertheless, such patients are not diagnosed as having depressive disorder because the presence of the symptoms is considered to be a normal reaction. Further, the symptoms are usually self-limiting, clear spontaneously over time, have a cause and prognosis different from those of major depression, and usually do not respond to antidepressant medication. Consequently, such individuals are referred to as having *uncomplicated bereavement*.

Clinical Management

Good psychopharmacological management is fundamental to the treatment of mood disorders. Both depression and mania usually respond remarkably well to the wide array of medications that are available. A more detailed discussion of antidepressant and antimanic medications, as well as ECT, appears in Chapter 26.

Treatment of Depression

In the management of depression, the clinician's first decision must be whether the patient has an adjustment disorder or chronic personality problem (e.g., borderline personality) that either mimics or is accompanied by a major depressive episode (indicating that psychotherapy would be more effective), or whether the patient has a syndrome that is likely to respond to medications. The DSM-IV criteria are helpful in this regard, but not all patients who meet criteria for major depression or dysthymic disorder will require medication. Likewise, some patients with adjustment or personality disorders may benefit from medication. Some features suggestive of a good response to antidepressant medications include the presence of vegetative symptoms such as insomnia or weight loss, meeting criteria for melancholia, history of prior episodes of depression (particularly if they have responded well to antidepressants), relatively acute onset of symptoms, and a family history of mood disorder.

Various medications are available to treat depression: tricyclic antidepressants, MAOIs, and newer antidepressants, including the SRIs. In addition, ECT may be used for severe depressions, particularly if the patient is suicidal. Lithium is often used as a maintenance medication to prevent relapse in patients with a history of recurrent depression.

The available antidepressant medications vary in both their side effects and their pharmacological mechanisms of action. They may be thought of as existing on a continuum, ranging from those that are more sedating (e.g., amitriptyline, doxepin, nortriptyline) to those that are less sedating and may even have psychostimulant effects (e.g., desipramine, fluoxetine). In general, the more sedating antidepressants tend to be anticholinergic, and the less sedating ones tend to be less anticholinergic.

Although the neuropharmacology of antidepressants is increasingly understood, and may eventually lead to rational approaches to treating depression as

---

Recommendations for management of the depressed patient

1. Establish a hopeful, optimistic tone at the initial interview.
   - Assess the severity of the depressive syndrome, remembering that there may be individual and cultural differences in the way depression is experienced and expressed.
   - Do not attempt extensive psychological probing when the patient is deeply depressed.
   - Determine suicidal risk initially and reassess frequently.

2. Treat severe to moderate depression aggressively with somatic therapy.
   - Severely depressed or suicidal patients may require hospitalization.
   - Severely depressed outpatients may need frequent (e.g., twice-weekly) brief (e.g., 10- to 15-minute) contacts for support and medication management until their depression lifts.
   - Most patients will require at least 16–20 weeks of maintenance medication after an initial episode, and thereafter should be given a trial of decreasing or discontinuing the medication. If symptoms reemerge, medication should be reinstituted.

3. Determine whether psychosocial stressors are present that are contributing to the depressed mood, and counsel the patient on ways to cope with them.

4. Depressed patients tend to "get down" on themselves because they have been depressed; help the patient learn to abandon negative or self-deprecating attitudes toward his or her depression through cognitive therapy or other psychotherapeutic techniques.

our knowledge of specific neurochemical mechanisms in individual patients increases, at present the choice of an antidepressant medication is largely empirical. Thus, clinicians typically select an antidepressant based primarily on the patient's presenting complaints. Patients with insomnia or anorexia may do better with more sedating medications, perhaps largely because they will begin to sleep better almost immediately, whereas patients with lethargy and lower levels of tension and anxiety may prefer the less-sedating medications such as imipramine or fluoxetine. Fluoxetine, in particular, has a specific tendency to produce insomnia and weight loss, making it a useful drug for those patients with atypical depressions characterized by hypersomnia and weight gain.

Most antidepressant medications have a relatively long half-life, as well as a relatively long latency for clinical response. The long half-life permits physicians to prescribe antidepressants in a single daily dose, which is usually taken at bedtime for the more sedating antidepressants but may be taken in the morning for the less sedating. Patients should be warned about the various side effects of antidepressants, which some patients often find particularly discomforting. It is helpful to explain to patients that they may feel worse before they feel better, and that they should not expect to see any clear response for 2–4 weeks—although patients sometimes do feel a slight improvement of some symptoms shortly after beginning their medication regimen. This message offers some hope, but it also encourages patients to stick with the medication even if they find the side effects unpleasant. It is also helpful to convey the fact that most patients who present with depression do respond eventually to some type of antidepressant medication and obtain relief from their symptoms.

The specific dose of antidepressant varies depending on the antidepressant, the patient's body size and ability to tolerate side effects, and the severity of the depression. For most patients, it is best to begin with a moderate dose (e.g., 50 mg of imipramine at bedtime for the first few days) and then to titrate the dose up after the patient's ability to tolerate side effects has been assessed. This approach is particularly important in the management of outpatients, who may find it difficult to remain alert at work or while studying if the medications are extremely sedating. Treatment can be more aggressive with inpatients, because they are not attempting to maintain a work schedule and because potentially dangerous side effects on the cardiovascular system can be monitored closely. Because some antidepressants (e.g., nortriptyline) appear to have a therapeutic window, blood levels may be useful in monitoring dosages. A more detailed description of this issue and of the pharmacology of antidepressants is provided in Chapter 26.

If patients do not respond to a specific antidepressant within 6–8 weeks, a clinical trial of another antidepressant or recourse to ECT may be appropriate.

This decision will be guided by the clinical picture of the patient. If the syndrome is severe and worsening, then ECT may be chosen. If the patient shows more characterological or atypical features, a MAOI may be tried. Most often, however, the clinician will choose to try at least one other antidepressant, often with a different pharmacological profile (i.e., a different balance of effects on norepinephrine, serotonin, and acetylcholine) from that of the drug to which the patient has not responded. A patient thought to be at risk for impulsive suicide attempts should be given an SRI, because overdoses are rarely lethal, unlike overdoses of tricyclics or MAOIs.

Patients who respond to a given antidepressant should usually be maintained on it for at least 16–20 weeks. Thereafter, the clinician may choose to attempt to discontinue the medication while monitoring the patient closely. Because some antidepressants produce undesirable side effects such as weight gain, and because conservative prescription of medications is always a good clinical guideline, discontinuance should almost always be attempted in patients who do not have a history of recurrent depression. The medication should be discontinued gradually because many patients experience some mild withdrawal effects if tricyclics or shorter-acting SRIs are discontinued abruptly. In particular, insomnia is a problem. Patients sometimes subjectively experience these withdrawal symptoms as a recurrence or relapse. Other symptoms that occur on abrupt withdrawal of antidepressants include increased tension and nervousness, nightmares, and gastrointestinal symptoms such as nausea or even vomiting.

Patients with recurrent depressions will often need long-term maintenance. Some patients benefit from lithium augmentation of antidepressants to enhance therapeutic response. Lithium prophylaxis to prevent depressive relapse may be particularly useful for those patients who have had three or four previous episodes of depression. Maintenance lithium doses may range from 600 to 1,200 mg/day, and blood levels are usually maintained in the 0.6–0.8 mEq/L range.

MAOIs may be used to treat those patients who do not respond to the first-line antidepressants (i.e., tricyclics, SRIs) or who are unable to tolerate their side effects. MAOIs should be used with caution because they have potentially more dangerous side effects and interactions than do the other antidepressants. Nevertheless, for a subset of patients, MAOIs may be useful. These patients tend to be those characterized by *atypical depression*, with symptoms such as hypersomnia, increased appetite, and personality difficulties such as rejection sensitivity.

ECT is the treatment of choice for some patients with severe depression. Methods for administering and monitoring ECT, as well as its side effects, are described in more detail in Chapter 26. In general, indications for ECT include very severe depression, psychotic depression, high potential for suicide, cardiovascular disease (which may preclude use of antidepressants), and pregnancy.

ECT is highly effective in producing a rapid remission of depressive symptoms. Response occurs relatively consistently in approximately 80% of patients. Patients will need maintenance antidepressant treatment after the course of ECT is completed.

Treatment of Mania

Lithium carbonate is the first-line treatment for manic disorder. Mania usually is a severe syndrome that requires hospitalization; consequently, aggressive treatment can be initiated in the closely supervised hospital environment. Patients are typically placed on a dose of 1,200–2,400 mg/day, with a goal of achieving serum blood levels between 0.9 and 1.4 mEq/L. Blood levels are usually monitored at least twice weekly at first. If the patient is severely agitated and psychotic, antipsychotics should be added to lithium to provide adequate behavioral control. Antipsychotic doses are typically in the range of 5–20 mg per day of haloperidol; a combination of a benzodiazepine and an antipsychotic may work even better to subdue the patient. As the psychotic symptoms or agitation clear, the antipsychotics and/or benzodiazepines can be gradually discontinued. Manic patients will almost always require maintenance lithium.

Patients who do not respond to lithium or antipsychotics may be given a

---

Recommendations for management of the manic patient

1. Use somatic therapies aggressively to treat manic symptoms as rapidly as possible.

2. Follow the patient closely as the mania "breaks" to determine whether a subsequent depression is emerging; if this occurs, treat it with antidepressants as needed.

3. After an episode of mania, patients should be placed on maintenance lithium; typically they will continue to take lithium for a number of years, and perhaps for the remainder of their life, to prevent subsequent relapses.

4. Even when they are stable, patients should be followed regularly to ensure continued compliance with lithium prophylaxis and to monitor blood levels.

5. Manic episodes can have devastating personal, social, and economic consequences; patients will usually require (at a minimum) supportive psychotherapy to help them cope with these consequences and maintain their self-esteem.

6. Family members should be provided with both psychological support, as needed, and educational materials to help them understand the disorder, its symptoms, and its need for continued treatment.

7. Patients with bipolar illness are often appreciative of being told about the "good side" of their illness: its association with creativity and high achievement.

variety of alternate treatments. ECT is also highly effective for mania, and it is indicated as a treatment of choice in the subset of patients who cannot be given lithium or antipsychotics (e.g., patients who are pregnant or who have severe cardiovascular disease). The most effective alternate medications used to treat mania are carbamazepine and sodium valproate. They have consistently proved effective in a subset of lithium nonresponders. Treatment of mania is more fully explored in Chapter 26.

Other Treatments

Experiencing an episode of mood disorder is often a major blow to the patient's confidence and self-esteem. Consequently, most patients will require some supportive psychotherapy in addition to whatever medications are prescribed. During the acute episode, the clinician will typically let the depressive wound begin to heal, but as the patient recovers, the clinician may begin to review with him or her the various social and psychological factors that may be causing distress or that may have worsened as a consequence of depression. Work, school performance, and interpersonal relationships may all be impaired because of a mood disorder. It is important to help patients assess these problems, recognize that their illness is responsible rather than they themselves are responsible, and instill confidence that they can now begin to restore and repair whatever injuries have occurred as a consequence of their episode of mood disorder.

Some patients will respond well to this type of brief supportive psychotherapy used as an adjunct to medications. Others may require more intensive psychotherapy depending on their personality structure, social situation, disability induced by the mood disorder, and environmental supports. These psychotherapies may include psychodynamic psychotherapy, cognitive therapy, or behavior therapy. These various psychotherapies are described in more detail in Chapter 25.

Some patients may respond to psychotherapy alone. In particular, a patient with a brief, situation-based depression may respond well to crisis intervention. A person presenting with depressive symptoms who is attempting to cope with a stressful life event, such as separation or divorce, may have a relatively painful and persistent mood disorder for weeks to months, yet not require the use of medications. These patients may also benefit substantially from supportive and psychodynamic therapy. Patients with chronic mild depression (e.g., dysthymic disorder) may also be more likely to benefit from a treatment regimen that emphasizes psychotherapy as its primary tool. In particular, these patients are likely to benefit from cognitive therapy, interpersonal therapy, behavior therapy, or long-term psychodynamic therapy.

Bibliography

Allen MG, Cohen S, Pollin W, et al: Affective illness in veteran twins: a diagnostic review. Am J Psychiatry 131:1234–1239, 1974

Andreasen NC, Rice J, Endicott J, et al: Familial rates of affective disorder: a report from the National Institute of Mental Health Collaborative Study. Arch Gen Psychiatry 44:461–469, 1987

Angst J, Frey R, Lohmeyer B, et al: Bipolar manic-depressive psychoses: results of a genetic investigation. Hum Genet 55:237–254, 1980

Asberg M, Thoren P, Traskman L, et al: "Serotonin depression"—a biochemical subgroup within the affective disorders? Science 191:478–480, 1976

Baron M, Risch N, Hamburger R, et al: Genetic linkage between X-chromosome markers and bipolar affective illness. Nature 326:289–292, 1987

Baxter LR, Schwartz JM, Phelps ME, et al: Reduction of prefrontal cortex glucose metabolism common to three types of depression. Arch Gen Psychiatry 46:243–250, 1989

Bertelsen A: A Danish twin study of manic-depressive disorders, in Origin, Prevention and Treatment of Affective Disorders. Edited by Schou M, Stromgren E. London, Academic Press, 1979, pp 227–239

Black DW, Nasrallah A: Hallucinations and delusions in 1,715 patients with unipolar and bipolar affective disorders. Psychopathology 22:28–34, 1989

Black DW, Winokur G, Nasrallah A: Treatment and outcome in secondary depression: a naturalistic study of 1,087 patients. J Clin Psychiatry 48:438–411, 1987

Blazer DG, Kessler RC, McGonagle KA, et al: The prevalence and distribution of major depression in a national community sample: the National Comorbidity Survey. Am J Psychiatry 151:979–986, 1994

Cadoret RJ: Evidence of genetic inheritance of primary affective disorder in adoptees. Am J Psychiatry 135:463–466, 1978

Carney MWP, Roth M, Garside RF: The diagnosis of depressive syndromes and the prediction of ECT response. Br J Psychiatry 111:659–674, 1966

Carroll BJ: The dexamethasone suppression test for melancholia. Br J Psychiatry 140:292–304, 1982

Coppen AJ, Doogan DP: Serotonin and its place in the pathogenesis of depression. J Clin Psychiatry 49 (suppl 8):4–11, 1988

Davis JM, Koslow SH, Gibbons RD, et al: Cerebrospinal fluid and urinary biogenic amines in depressed patients and healthy controls. Arch Gen Psychiatry 45:705–717, 1988

Drevets WC, Videen TO, Price JL, et al: A functional anatomical study of unipolar depression. J Neurosci 12:3628–3641, 1992

Gershon ES, Bunney WE, Leckman JF, et al: The inheritance of affective disorders: a review of data and hypotheses. Behav Genet 6:227–261, 1976

Gillin JC, Byerley WA: Sleep: a neurobiological window on affective disorders. Trends Neurosci 8:537–542, 1985

Glassman AH: Indoleamines and affective disorders. Psychosom Med 31:107–114, 1969

Gold PW, Goodwin FK, Chrousos GP: Clinical and biochemical manifestation of depression: relation to the neurobiology of stress (parts 1 and 2). N Engl J Med 319:348–353, 1988

Goodwin FK, Jamison KR: Manic-Depressive Illness. New York, Oxford University Press, 1990

Harvald B, Hauge M: Genetics and the epidemiology of chronic diseases (PHS Publ No 1163). Edited by Neal JV, Shaw W, Shull WJ. Washington, DC, Department of Health, Education and Welfare, 1965, pp 61–76

Huston PE, Locher LM: Manic-depressive psychosis: course when treated and untreated with electric shock. Arch Neurol Psychiatry 50:37–48, 1948

Kallmann FJ: Genetic principles in manic-depressive psychosis, in Depression: Proceedings of the American Psychopathologic Association. Edited by Zubin J, Hock P. New York, Grune & Stratton, 1954, pp 1–24

Kendell RE: The Classification of Depressive Illnesses. London, Oxford University Press, 1968

Klein DF: Endogenomorphic depression: a conceptual and terminological revision. Arch Gen Psychiatry 34:447–454, 1974

Klerman GL, Lavori PW, Rice J, et al: Birth cohort trends in rates of major depressive disorder among relatives of patients with affective disorder. Arch Gen Psychiatry 42:689–693, 1985

Kraepelin E: Manic-Depressive Insanity and Paranoia. Edinburgh, E and S Livingstone, 1921

Krishnan KRR, Manepalli AN, Ritchie JC, et al: Growth hormone-releasing factor stimulation test in depression. Am J Psychiatry 145:90–92, 1988

Luxenberger H: Psychiatrisch-neurologische Zwillings-pathologie. Zentralblatt fur Diagesamte Neurologie und Psychiatrie 14:56–57, 145–180, 1930

Meltzer HY: Lithium mechanisms in bipolar illness and altered intracellular calcium functions. Biol Psychiatry 21:492–510, 1986

Meltzer HY, Lowy MT: The serotonin hypothesis of depression, in Psychopharmacology: The Third Generation of Progress. Edited by Meltzer HY. New York, Raven, 1987, pp 513–526

Mendlewicz J, Rainer JD: Adoption study supporting genetic transmission in manic-depressive illness. Nature 268:327–329, 1977

Nemeroff CB: The role of corticotropin-releasing factor in the pathogenesis of major depression. Pharmacopsychiatry 21:76–82, 1988

Paykel ES (ed): Handbook of Affective Disorders, 2nd Edition. New York, Guilford, 1992

Post RM, Ballenger JC: Neurobiology of Mood Disorders. Baltimore, MD, Williams & Wilkins, 1984

Robinson RG, Szetela B. Mood change following left hemisphere brain injury. Ann Neurol 9:447–453, 1981

Rosanoff AJ, Handy L, Plesset IR: The etiology of manic-depressive symptoms with special reference to their occurrence in twins. Am J Psychiatry 91:725–762, 1935

Schildkraut JJ: The catecholamine hypothesis of affective disorder: a review of supporting evidence. Am J Psychiatry 122:509–522, 1965

Schildkraut JJ, Orsulak PJ, Schatzburg AF, et al: Toward a biochemical classification of depressive disorders, I: differences in urinary excretion of MHPG and other catecholamine metabolites in clinically defined subtypes of depression. Arch Gen Psychiatry 35:1427–1433, 1978

Slater E: Psychotic and neurotic illness in twins (Medical Research Council Special Report Series No 278). London, Her Majesty's Stationery Office, 1953

Stahl SM: Regulation of neurotransmitter receptors by desipramine and other antidepressant drugs: the neurotransmitter receptor hypothesis of antidepressant action. J Clin Psychiatry 45:37–44, 1984

Starkstein SE, Robinson RG (eds). Depression in Neurological Disease. Baltimore, MD, Johns Hopkins University Press, 1993

Swayze VW, Andreasen NC, Alliger RJ, et al: Structural brain abnormalities in bipolar affective disorder: ventricular enlargement and focal signal hyperintensities. Arch Gen Psychiatry 47:1054–1059, 1990

Weissman MM, Kidd KK, Prusoff BA: Variability in rates of affective disorders in relatives of depressed and normal probands. Arch Gen Psychiatry 39:1397–1403, 1982

Weissman MM, Leaf PJ, Bruce ML, et al: The epidemiology of dysthymia in five communities: rates, risks, comorbidity, and treatment. Am J Psychiatry 145:815–819, 1988

Whybrow PC, Akiskal HS, McKinney WT Jr: Mood Disorders: Toward a New Psychobiology. New York, Plenum, 1984

Winokur G, Black DW, Nasrallah A: Depressions secondary to other psychiatric disorders and medical illnesses. Am J Psychiatry 154:233–237, 1988

Winokur G, Clayton P, Reich T: Manic Depressive Illness. St. Louis, MO, CV Mosby, 1969

Self-Assessment Questions

1. What are the nine symptoms used to define a major depressive episode in DSM-IV?

2. What is the difference between mood-congruent and mood-incongruent delusions?

3. What are some symptoms that typically predict a good response to antidepressants?

4. What is the lifetime prevalence for bipolar disorder and for (unipolar) major depressive disorder?

5. Why have variable rates been reported for depression?

6. What is the cohort effect?

7. Review the evidence that suggests that mood disorders are familial and may be genetic.

8. Which neurotransmitter systems have been proposed to be dysfunctional in mood disorders?

9. Which brain region has been found to be abnormal in both lesion and positron-emission tomography (PET) studies?

10. What is the evidence indicating that neuroendocrine abnormalities occur in patients with mood disorders?

11. What is the difference between bereavement and a depressive episode?

12. Describe the first-line treatments for depression, as well as the various alternative treatments and their indications.

13. Describe the appropriate program of treatment for a manic episode. What alternative treatments are available?

Chapter 10

Anxiety Disorders

I stood stunned, my hair rose, the voice stuck in my throat.

Virgil

Unlike depression, a syndrome recognized for centuries, the syndrome of anxiety has been recognized only in relatively recent times. DaCosta was first credited with describing anxiety as a disorder that he called *irritable heart* in the *American Journal of Medical Sciences* in 1871. Because chest pain, palpitations, and dizziness were the main symptoms of this syndrome, DaCosta thought the disorder was due to a functional cardiac disturbance characterized by hypersensitivity and sympathetic overreactivity. Physicians frequently diagnosed this syndrome in patients undergoing significant stress, such as warfare. In fact, DaCosta first described this syndrome in a soldier who developed the disorder during the Civil War. Shortly thereafter, the condition was identified in many other settings, and it was variously referred to as *soldier's heart*, the *effort syndrome*, or *neurocirculatory asthenia*.

While internists were emphasizing cardiovascular aspects of the anxiety syndrome, psychiatrists and neurologists became more concerned with its psychological aspects. Freud was responsible for recognizing anxiety as the core symptom in the syndrome and for introducing the term *anxiety neurosis*. Freud's conceptualization brought the patient's inner subjective feelings to the forefront, emphasizing the sense of fearfulness, terror, panic, and impending doom.

The relative relationship between the physical and psychological symptoms of anxiety has remained a matter of debate. Early in the twentieth century, psychologist William James postulated that the psychological experience of anxiety is nothing more than an awareness of the physical symptoms of anxiety, thus implying that the physical experience is primary. Freud, on the other hand, believed that the psychological symptoms of anxiety were primary and led to the development of physical symptoms. Whichever is primary, the relationship is probably interactive once the symptoms have begun.

Because nervousness and fear are common human emotions that nearly everyone has experienced at one time or another, defining the boundaries of anxiety disorder is a matter of some debate. It is important that physicians recognize the difference between pathological anxiety and anxiety as a normal or adaptive response. Feeling anxiety when being attacked by a grizzly bear is a normal and natural response and prepares the individual for the classic flight or fight response. Feeling anxiety before taking an examination or giving a talk is also normal and adaptive as long as the alertness or tension does not become excessive or handicapping. Even classic phobias, such as fear of heights, may reflect some primitive adaptive response. The potentially adaptive mechanism of anxiety or arousal, so useful in human beings in coping with the stresses and threats of life, becomes a disorder only when the anxiety becomes crippling or disabling.

Until 1980, panic disorder and generalized anxiety were classified together as *anxiety neurosis*. In DSM-III, anxiety neurosis was divided, because it had been discovered that panic disorder and generalized anxiety disorder were each associated with a different natural history, familial aggregation, and response to treatment. At the same time, a new diagnosis, posttraumatic stress disorder (PTSD), was introduced. In this chapter we review panic disorders, agoraphobia, specific and social phobias, generalized anxiety, and both PTSD and acute stress disorder. A residual category, anxiety disorder not otherwise specified, may be used to diagnose conditions that do not meet criteria for a specific disorder, such as mixed symptoms of anxiety and depression. Anxiety disorders thought to be due to the effects of a substance or a general medical condition are discussed in Chapter 6. Although obsessive-compulsive disorder (OCD) is classified as an anxiety disorder, there is considerable uncertainty about its true relationship to the other anxiety disorders. OCD is discussed in Chapter 11. The anxiety disorders listed in DSM-IV are presented in Table 10–1.

Panic Disorder and Agoraphobia

Panic disorder consists of recurrent unexpected panic (or anxiety) attacks accompanied by at least 1 month or more of persistent concern about having an-

Table 10–1. Anxiety disorders

Panic disorder	Generalized anxiety disorder
With agoraphobia	Posttraumatic stress disorder
Without agoraphobia	Acute stress disorder
Agoraphobia	Anxiety disorder due to a general medical condition (see Chapter 6)
Social phobia	
Specific phobia	Substance-induced anxiety disorder (see Chapter 6)
Obsessive-compulsive disorder (see Chapter 11)	Anxiety disorder not otherwise specified

other attack, worry about the implications of having an attack, or significant behavioral change related to the attack. The requirement for unexpected attacks is to help rule out those triggered by specific situations that might cause anxiety in normal persons, such as being robbed at gunpoint. As a practical matter, patients with unexpected attacks generally have situational attacks as well. Additionally, during the attacks at least 4 of 13 characteristic symptoms occur, such as shortness of breath, dizziness, palpitations, and trembling or shaking. Finally, the clinician should determine that the attacks are not due to the direct physiological effects of a substance or to a general medical condition and that the anxiety is not better accounted for by another mental disorder, such as OCD. Panic disorder is further classified as occurring with or without agoraphobia, a condition explained below. Diagnostic criteria for panic attacks are presented in Table 10–2, and the criteria for panic disorder without agoraphobia are presented in Table 10–3.

Agoraphobia is a disabling complication of panic disorder characterized by phobic avoidance; its criteria are listed in Table 10–4. Although originally conceptualized as separate disorders, a variety of evidence suggests that panic disorder and agoraphobia represent a single illness. The term *agoraphobia* derives from Greek, meaning "fear of the marketplace," and although many patients with agoraphobia are uncomfortable in shops and markets, their true fear is to be separated from their source of security. Agoraphobic patients may fear having a panic attack in a public place and embarrassing themselves, or having a panic attack and not being near their physicians or medical clinics. These patients tend to avoid crowded places, such as shops, restaurants, theaters, and church. Many have difficulty driving long distances (i.e., being away from help should a panic attack occur), crossing bridges, and driving through tunnels. Many agoraphobic patients insist on being accompanied to places they might otherwise avoid. Severe agoraphobia leads many patients to become housebound. Many of the common situations that either provoke or relieve anxiety in people with agoraphobia are shown in Table 10–5.

Table 10–2.   DSM-IV criteria for a panic attack

A discrete period of intense fear or discomfort, in which four (or more) of the following symptoms developed abruptly and reached a peak within 10 minutes:

1. Palpitations, pounding heart, or accelerated heart rate
2. Sweating
3. Trembling or shaking
4. Sensations of shortness of breath or smothering
5. Feeling of choking
6. Chest pain or discomfort
7. Nausea or abdominal distress
8. Feeling dizzy, unsteady, light-headed, or faint
9. Derealization (feelings of unreality) or depersonalization (being detached from oneself)
10. Fear of losing control or going crazy
11. Fear of dying
12. Paresthesias (numbness or tingling sensations)
13. Chills or hot flushes

Table 10–3.   DSM-IV criteria for panic disorder without agoraphobia

A. Both 1 and 2:
　　1. Recurrent unexpected panic attacks
　　2. At least one of the attacks has been followed by at least 1 month (or more) of one (or more) of the following: a) persistent concern about having additional attacks, b) worry about the implications of the attack or its consequences (e.g., losing control, having a heart attack, "going crazy"), or c) a significant change in behavior related to the attacks

B. Absence of agoraphobia.

C. The panic attacks are not due to the direct physiological effects of a substance (e.g., a drug of abuse, medication) or a general medical condition (e.g. hyperthyroidism).

D. The panic attacks are not better accounted for by another mental disorder, such as social phobia (e.g., occurring on exposure to feared social situations), specific phobia (e.g., on exposure to a specific phobic situation), obsessive-compulsive disorder (e.g., on exposure to dirt in someone with an obsession about contamination), posttraumatic stress disorder (e.g., in response to stimuli associated with a severe stressor), or separation anxiety disorder (e.g., in response to being away from home or close relatives).

The following case example illustrates how these common disorders affected one of our patients.

Susan, a 32-year-old housewife, presented to the outpatient clinic for evaluation of anxiety. She reported the onset of panic attacks at age 13, which she remembered as

Table 10–4. DSM-IV criteria for agoraphobia

A. Anxiety about being in places or situations from which escape might be difficult (or embarrassing) or in which help may not be available in the event of having an unexpected or situationally predisposed panic attack or panic-like symptoms. Agoraphobic fears typically involve characteristic clusters of situations that include being outside the home alone; being in a crowd or standing in a line; being on a bridge; and traveling in a bus, train, or automobile.

Note: Consider the diagnosis of specific phobia if the avoidance is limited to one or only a few specific situations, or social phobia if the avoidance is limited to social situations.

B. The situations are avoided (e.g., travel is restricted), or else endured with marked distress or with anxiety about having a panic attack or panic-like symptoms, or require the presence of a companion.

C. The anxiety or phobic avoidance is not better accounted for by another mental disorder, such as social phobia (e.g., avoidance limited to social situations because of fear of embarrassment), specific phobia (e.g., avoidance limited to a single situation like elevators), obsessive-compulsive disorder (e.g., avoidance of dirt in someone with an obsession about contamination), posttraumatic stress disorder (e.g., avoidance of stimuli associated with a severe stressor), or separation anxiety disorder (e.g., avoidance of leaving home or relatives).

Table 10–5. Common situations that either provoke or relieve anxiety in 100 agoraphobic patients

Situations that provoke anxiety		Situations that relieve anxiety	
Situation	**%**	**Situation**	**%**
Standing in line at a store	96	Being accompanied by spouse	85
An appointment	91	Sitting near the door in church, etc.	76
Feeling trapped at hairdresser, etc.	89	Focusing thoughts on something else	63
Increasing distance from home	87	Taking the dog, baby carriage, etc., along	62
Particular places in neighborhood	66	Being accompanied by friend	60
Cloudy, depressing weather	56	Reassuring self	52
		Wearing sunglasses	36

Source. Adapted from Burns LE, Thorpe GL: The epidemiology of fears and phobias (with particular reference to the National Survey of Agoraphobics). J Int Med Res 5 (suppl 5):1–7, 1977.

terrifying. She could still remember her very first attack, which occurred during a history class. "I was just sitting in class when my heart began to beat wildly, my skin began to tingle, and I began feeling shaky. There was no need for me to feel nervous," she observed. For the next 19 years, attacks had been chronic and unrelenting, occurring up to 6–10 times daily. To Susan, the panic was devastating: "I grew up all those years feeling that I wasn't quite normal."

Soon after the onset of panic attacks, Susan developed phobic avoidance of crowded places, particularly shopping centers, grocery stores, movie theaters, and restaurants. A religious person, she attended church, but would sit in a pew near an exit. Her agoraphobia waxed and waned over the years, and although she had never been housebound, at times she would insist on having her husband or a friend accompany her when she went shopping.

Susan had never sought treatment before and thought that no one could help her. She had gone to emergency rooms for evaluation, but she had never received a diagnosis of panic disorder. As Susan got older, she tried to ignore her feelings, believing that to admit them was a sign of weakness. She never told her husband of 15 years about her panic.

Susan was treated with a then-experimental medication (fluvoxamine), and within 1 month she was free of panic attacks; within 3 months she was no longer agoraphobic. At a 6-month follow-up, she remained free of all anxiety-related symptoms. Susan reported feeling like a new person and felt much better about herself. Six years later, Susan continued to be well, although in the interim she had switched to fluoxetine.

Epidemiology and Clinical Findings

According to the Epidemiologic Catchment Area study, 2%–3% of women and 0.5%–1.5% of men have panic disorder. The prevalence of agoraphobia is slightly higher. Panic disorder and agoraphobia each typically have an onset in the middle 20s, although age at onset may vary; 79% of patients with panic disorder develop the disorder before age 30 years.

There are usually no precipitating stressors before the onset of either panic disorder or agoraphobia. Many patients, however, will report that panic attacks came on after an illness, accident, or the breakup of a relationship; developed postpartum; or occurred after taking mind-altering drugs such as LSD or marijuana.

The initial panic attack is generally alarming to people and may provoke a visit to a nearby emergency room, where results of routine laboratory tests such as an electrocardiogram are inevitably found to be normal. The person is usually told that the symptoms are due to "nerves."

If the panic attacks recur, the patient may be referred for an extensive medical workup. When no obvious physical cause for the anxiety is found, a psychiatrist is generally consulted. Typically, the psychiatrist's consultation is preceded by six or seven other evaluations, especially by cardiologists, neurologists, or gastroenterologists, depending on the target symptoms that the patient develops (see Table 10–6).

Attacks generally have a sudden onset, peak within minutes, and last 5–30 minutes. Although many patients claim that their attacks may last hours or even all day, it is likely that their continuing symptoms represent either a recurrence of panic or mild symptoms that persist after an attack. Common symptoms in panic disorder are presented in Table 10–7.

Etiology and Pathophysiology

Neurobiological models are currently the most popular explanations for the etiology of panic disorder. Possible biological disturbances underlying panic may include increased catecholamine levels in the central nervous system, an abnormality in the locus coeruleus (an area of the brain stem regulating alertness), carbon dioxide hypersensitivity, disturbances in lactate metabolism, and abnormalities of the γ-aminobutyric acid (GABA) neurotransmitter system. Experi-

Table 10–6. Specialists consulted depending on target symptoms of panic disorder

Specialist	Target symptoms
Pulmonologist	Shortness of breath, hyperventilation, smothering sensations
Dermatologist	Sweating, cold, clammy hands
Cardiologist	Palpitations, chest pain or discomfort
Neurologist	Tingling and numbness, imbalance, dizziness, derealization or depersonalization, tremulousness or jitteriness, light-headedness
Otolaryngologist	Choking sensation, dry mouth
Gynecologist	Hot flashes, sweating
Gastroenterologist	Nausea, diarrhea, abdominal pain or discomfort (i.e., "butterflies")
Urologist	Frequent urination

Table 10–7. Common symptoms reported by patients with panic disorder and agoraphobia

Symptoms	%	Symptoms	%
Fearfulness or worry	96	Restlessness	80
Nervousness	95	Trouble breathing	80
Palpitations	93	Easy fatigability	76
Muscle aching or tension	89	Trouble concentrating	76
Trembling or shaking	89	Irritability	74
Apprehension	83	Trouble sleeping	74
Dizziness or imbalance	82	Chest pain or discomfort	69
Fear of dying or going crazy	81	Numbness or tingling	65
Faintness/light-headedness	80	Tendency to startle	57
Hot or cold sensations	80	Choking or smothering sensation	54

Source. Adapted from Noyes R, Clancy J, Garvey MJ et al: Is agoraphobia a variant of panic disorder or a separate illness? J Affect Disord 1:3–13, 1987.

mental data support each of these disturbances to some extent, but none explains all of the manifestations of panic disorder. Many of the competing theories are based on the ability of different substances to induce panic attacks, such as isoproterenol (a β antagonist), yohimbine (an α_2-receptor blocker), carbon dioxide, and sodium lactate. Recent theories highlight the role of GABA, an inhibitory neurotransmitter.

Family and twin studies suggest that panic disorder may be hereditary. If the results of family studies are pooled, the morbidity risk for panic disorder is about 18% among relatives of patients with panic disorder compared to only 2% among relatives of control subjects. Early twin studies showed a higher concordance rate for anxiety disorder among monozygotic twins than dizygotic twins, roughly 45% compared to 15%, a finding that indicates that genetic influences predominate over environmental influences. However, these early studies were flawed by including a mixed group of anxiety patients. Another study, however, found that anxiety disorders accompanied by panic attacks were five times more frequent in monozygotic twins than in dizygotic twins. There have been no adoption studies specifically of panic disorder.

Psychodynamic formulations of panic have stressed the importance of *repression*, a common defense mechanism. Freud believed that repression was the mental mechanism that holds out of conscious reach all unacceptable sexual thoughts, impulses, or desires. When the psychic energy attached to these unacceptable elements becomes too strong to be held back by repression, they are brought into consciousness in a distorted way and are manifested by anxiety.

Meanwhile, learning theorists argue that anxiety is conditioned by the fear of certain environmental stimuli. Anxiety attacks, for example, are believed to be a conditioned response to a fearful situation; a car accident might be paired with the experience of heart palpitations and anxiety. Long after the accident, palpitations alone, whether during vigorous exercise or minor emotional upset, become capable in themselves of provoking the *conditioned response* of an anxiety attack.

Course and Outcome

Different studies of panic disorder tend to describe different outcomes, due in part to the varied criteria used. In an early study, 173 patients were followed over 20 years. On follow-up, nearly 12% of the patients were well; 73% had symptoms, but no or mild disability; and 15% had moderate to severe symptoms. A 5-year follow-up of patients seen on a psychiatric consultation service found that 16% were well and 51% were mildly impaired. These studies suggest that over a long period, it is not unreasonable to expect that 50%–70% of patients with panic disorder will show some amount of improvement, although total remission is uncommon. There is some increased risk for peptic ulcer and hypertension in panic disorder patients and higher mortality rates, higher suicide rates, and a larger number of deaths due to circulatory disease than expected.

The course of agoraphobia tends to parallel that of panic disorder, as the two are usually related. It tends to be chronic, but it may wax and wane. If panic disorder is treated, the agoraphobia usually improves as well, as is illustrated in the case of Susan.

The most common complications of panic disorder are depression and alcohol abuse. Depression occurs in up to 50% of patients with panic disorder or agoraphobia, but it usually tends to be mild and reactive to situational circumstances. Alcohol abuse complicates panic disorder in about 20% of cases and may start in an attempt at self-medication. This complication is important to keep in mind when evaluating patients with substance abuse, because it is possible that their illness began with spontaneous panic attacks or chronic anxiety.

Differential Diagnosis

In the evaluation of panic disorder, it is essential to rule out other physical and psychiatric disorders that may mimic panic (see Table 10–8). The physical manifestations of panic disorder are compatible with many physical disorders, for example, hyperthyroidism, hyperparathyroidism, pheochromocytoma, diseases of the vestibular nerve, hypoglycemia, and supraventricular tachycardia.

A relationship between mitral valve prolapse and panic disorder has been

Table 10–8. Differential diagnosis of anxiety

Medical illness	Personality disorders
Angina	Adjustment disorder with anxious mood
Cardiac arrhythmias	**Drugs**
Congestive heart failure	Caffeine
Hypoglycemia	Aminophylline and related compounds
Hypoxia	Sympathomimetic agents (e.g.,
Pulmonary embolism	decongestants and diet pills)
Severe pain	Monosodium glutamate
Thyrotoxicosis	Psychostimulants and hallucinogens
Carcinoid	Alcohol withdrawal
Pheochromocytoma	Withdrawal from benzodiazepines and
Menière's disease	other sedative-hypnotics
Psychiatric illness	Thyroid hormones
Schizophrenia	Antipsychotic medication
Mood disorders	

proposed. Mitral valve prolapse is usually a benign condition that occurs more frequently in panic disorder patients than in psychiatrically normal persons, leading many clinicians to regard panic symptoms as a manifestation of mitral valve prolapse. However, studies have shown that panic disorder patients with or without mitral valve prolapse have a similar natural history, course of illness, and response to treatment. The presence of mitral valve prolapse does not preclude a diagnosis of panic disorder.

Other psychiatric disorders must also be ruled out, particularly depression. Patients with primary depression often have panic attacks and anxiety. Panic attacks may also occur in patients with generalized anxiety disorder, schizophrenia, depersonalization disorder, somatoform disorder, and personality disorders.

Clinical Management

Panic disorder has traditionally been treated with a combination of individual psychotherapy and medication. Cognitive-behavior psychotherapy, which was recently applied to panic disorder, appears to have promise in treating the condition. This approach usually combines distraction and breathing exercises, along with education to help the patient in making more appropriate attributions for distressing somatic symptoms. For example, the patient learns that panic-induced chest pain will not lead to a heart attack. Supportive psychotherapy is helpful in boosting the generally low morale of patients and improving their self-esteem. In addition, the therapist can help the patient to problem-solve and can recommend books and other reading materials about panic and agoraphobia.

Patients with agoraphobia, with or without panic attacks, should receive behavioral therapy. Exposure in vivo is the most effective intervention and in its most basic form may consist of gentle encouragement for patients to enter feared situations, such as shopping in a grocery store. Some patients may require supervision by the therapist to expose themselves to different situations.

Antidepressant medication—including tricyclic antidepressants, monoamine oxidase inhibitors (MAOIs), and serotonin reuptake inhibitors (SRIs)—are effective in the treatment of panic and agoraphobia. MAOIs are generally reserved for patients who do not respond to the other agents. These medications will generally block panic attacks in up to 80% of patients. The benzodiazepine alprazolam is also effective in blocking panic attacks, but it has a tendency to become habit forming. These medications are discussed in more detail in Chapter 26. β-adrenergic–blocking drugs such as propranolol are often prescribed to patients with anxiety disorders, but they are much less effective than antidepressants or alprazolam.

Although these medications are effective and most patients do improve, there are few predictors of response. In general, patients who respond well tend to have milder anxiety symptoms, have fewer panic attacks, and have a normal personality. Depressed mood is not a requirement for antidepressant medications to be effective in blocking panic attacks.

Doses of antidepressants will depend on the specific medication, but are usually similar to doses used to treat depression. For example, imipramine is prescribed in a range of 150–300 mg/day, whereas fluoxetine may be effective at 20 mg. Doses of alprazolam typically range from 2 to 6 mg/day. Once panic attacks have remitted, the patient should remain on medication for 6 months to 1 year to prevent early relapse. After this period, it is advisable to taper the dose of medication. Although panic disorder tends to recur, up to two-thirds of patients will not relapse immediately after cessation of medication. Some patients, however, will need to take medication chronically.

Panic disorder patients should be advised to eliminate caffeine from their diets, because its anxiogenic effects tend to exacerbate the disorder. Patients often fail to realize how much caffeine they are taking in with coffee (50–150 mg), tea (20–50 mg), some sodas (30–60 mg), and even milk chocolate (1–15 mg).

Generalized Anxiety Disorder

Generalized anxiety disorder (GAD) is a relatively new disorder, having been first included in DSM-III in 1980. It is characterized by excessive anxiety and worry that is difficult to control, without the specific symptoms that characterize phobic disorders, panic disorder, or OCD (i.e., phobias, panic attacks, obsessions, and compulsions). Patients with GAD usually worry excessively about life circumstances, such as health, finances, social acceptance, job performance, and marital adjustment.

The diagnostic criteria require that GAD should not be diagnosed when the symptoms occur exclusively during the course of another illness such as major depression or schizophrenia, or when the generalized anxiety occurs in the context of a panic disorder, social phobia, or OCD. The anxiety or worry in GAD should not relate purely to having a panic attack, being embarrassed in public, being contaminated, or gaining weight as in anorexia nervosa. The criteria also require that the individual have at least three of six symptoms, including restlessness or feeling keyed up or on edge, being easily fatigued, having difficulty concentrating or feeling that one's mind is going blank, irritability, muscle tension, and sleep disturbance. Additionally, the symptoms must cause significant distress or impairment in social, occupational, or other important domains of functioning. Finally, the direct effects of a substance (e.g., caffeinism) or a general medical condition (e.g., hyperthyroidism) must be ruled out as a cause of the symptoms. The condition must exist for 6 months or longer. The complete DSM-IV criteria for GAD are listed in Table 10–9. If the disturbance occurs in a child, it is usually referred to as an *overanxious disorder.*

Epidemiology

Community surveys have shown that generalized anxiety disorder is common and has a lifetime prevalence between 4.1% and 6.6% of the general population. Rates are higher in women, African-Americans, and persons under age 30 years. The disorder tends to start in the early 20s, although persons of any age may develop the disorder. Few patients with the disorder seek treatment, and many see cardiologists or pulmonary specialists for specific symptoms. The disorder ap-

Table 10–9.   DSM-IV criteria for generalized anxiety disorder (includes overanxious disorder of childhood)

A. Excessive anxiety and worry (apprehensive expectation), occurring more days than not for at least 6 months, about a number of events or activities (such as work or school performance).

B. The person finds it difficult to control the worry.

C. The anxiety and worry are associated with three (or more) of the following six symptoms (with at least some symptoms present for more days than not for the past 6 months).

Note: Only one item is required in children.

   1. Restlessness or feeling keyed up or on edge
   2. Being easily fatigued
   3. Difficulty concentrating or mind going blank
   4. Irritability
   5. Muscle tension
   6. Sleep disturbance (difficulty falling or staying asleep, or restless unsatisfying sleep)

D. The focus of the anxiety and worry is not confined to features of an Axis I disorder, e.g., the anxiety or worry is not about having a panic attack (as in panic disorder), being embarrassed in public (as in social phobia), being contaminated (as in obsessive-compulsive disorder), being away from home or close relatives (as in separation anxiety disorder), gaining weight (as in anorexia nervosa), having multiple physical complaints (as in somatization disorder), or having a serious illness (as in hypochondriasis) and the anxiety and worry do not occur exclusively during posttraumatic stress disorder.

E. The anxiety, worry, or physical symptoms cause clinically significant distress or impairment in social, occupational, or other important areas of functioning.

F. The disturbance is not due to the direct physiological effects of a substance (e.g., a drug of abuse, medication) or a general medical condition (e.g., hyperthyroidism), and does not occur exclusively during a mood disorder, a psychotic disorder, or a pervasive developmental disorder.

pears to have a prolonged course, with symptoms that fluctuate in severity over time. One study showed that over 25% of these patients develop panic disorder on follow-up. Compared with panic disorder and depression, GAD is a relatively mild disorder; about 10% of the anxious patients seen by psychiatrists have GAD.

The most common complications are depression or substance abuse. Many patients experience one or more episodes of major depression over the course of the illness, and many will meet criteria for social phobia or a specific phobia. Some patients use alcohol or drugs to control their symptoms, which can lead to substance abuse.

Etiology

The etiology of GAD is unknown, although a preliminary family study showed that approximately 25% of first-degree relatives are affected, females more often than males; male relatives were likely to have alcoholism. The same study showed that life events were also important in the development of GAD. One twin study failed to find a difference in the concordance rate among monozygotic twins compared with dizygotic twins. Several different neurotransmitter systems have been implicated in the disorder, including the noradrenergic, GABA, and serotonergic systems in the frontal lobe and limbic system, but at present the cause of GAD is unknown.

The hyperarousal of patients with GAD is evident in electroencephalographic and sleep recordings (e.g., reduced alpha activity, increased beta activity, and reduced stage I and rapid eye movement sleep). The increased arousal appears to be associated with inhibition of the autonomic system.

Differential Diagnosis

The differential diagnosis of GAD is the same as for panic disorder and agoraphobia. It is particularly important to rule out drug-induced conditions such as caffeine intoxication, stimulant abuse, alcohol withdrawal, and sedative-hypnotic withdrawal. The mental status examination and history should explore the diagnostic possibilities of panic disorder, simple phobias, specific phobias, OCD, schizophrenia, and major depression.

Clinical Management

Behavioral therapy (e.g., relaxation training) may help the patient recognize and control anxiety symptoms, especially if the condition is mild. The patient should be educated about the chronic nature of the disorder and the tendency of

symptoms to wax and wane, often together with external stressors that the patient may be having. The following case presents a typical patient at our clinic
who benefited from these techniques.

> Kelly, a 19-year-old college student, presented for evaluation of "nerves." He was
> mildly tremulous and swallowed frequently, and sweat beaded up on his brow. He said
> that he had been anxious for as long as he could remember, but he denied that he
> was sad or blue. The problem had been worse since he had finished high school and
> moved away from home to attend college.
>
> Kelly seemed to worry about everything. He worried about his physical appear-
> ance, his grades in school, whether he had the right kind of friends, the health of his
> parents, his finances, and even his lack of sexual experience.
>
> He acknowledged, when asked, that he was usually tense and unable to relax. He
> had recently been evaluated for stress headaches. He often had dry mouth (he
> chewed gum to counter it), clammy hands, and a feeling of a lump in his throat.
>
> Although there was no apparent precipitant to his problems, added stress made
> his condition worse. He requested tranquilizers but agreed to try progressive muscle
> relaxation and guided imagery as an initial treatment. Although he remained anx-
> ious after learning and using these techniques, he said he no longer thought he
> needed tranquilizers.

Minor tranquilizers are the medications of choice for GAD. Benzodiazepines
should be prescribed in a maintenance dose (e.g., diazepam 5 mg three times
daily, or 5–10 mg at bedtime) for short periods (e.g., weeks or months) when the
anxiety is particularly severe. β-adrenergic blockers such as propranolol (e.g.,
40–160 mg/day) may be effective, but these agents are not as well studied in
GAD. Treatment with benzodiazepines should be time limited to prevent the
complications of tolerance and dependence.

An alternative is buspirone, a nonbenzodiazepine anxiolytic. Its onset of
action is relatively slow (i.e., weeks), but it has the advantage over benzodiazepines of having little abuse potential. Tricyclic antidepressants may also be useful, particularly sedating ones such as doxepin or amitriptyline, often in low doses
(e.g., 25–100 mg at bedtime). The antipsychotic trifluoperazine has been effective, but it should not be used due to its potential to cause tardive dyskinesia. In
general, antipsychotics should be used only in psychotic patients.

Phobic Disorders

A phobia is an irrational fear of specific objects, places, situations, or activities.
Although fear itself is to some degree adaptive, particularly for animals and

primitive humans, the fear in phobias is irrational, excessive, and disproportionate to any actual danger. Three categories of phobia are described in DSM-IV: *agoraphobia*, which has already been described; *social phobias*, in which there is fear of humiliation or embarrassment in public places; and *specific phobias*, a category that includes isolated phobias such as the irrational and intense fear of snakes.

Persons with social phobia tend to have multiple fears of situations where they may be observed by other people, which is why the disturbance is also referred to as *social anxiety disorder*. Patients with social phobia also commonly fear speaking in public, eating in public restaurants, writing in front of other persons, or using public rest rooms. Sometimes the fear becomes generalized, so that the phobic person avoids almost all social situations. Specific phobias are usually isolated and involve objects that conceivably may cause harm such as snakes, heights, flying, or blood, but the person's reaction to them is excessive.

Diagnostic criteria for social and specific phobias are presented in Tables 10–10 and 10–11, respectively. Examples of common specific phobias are presented in Table 10–12.

Epidemiology

Phobias are quite common in the general population. Social phobias reportedly affect 3%–5% of the population, but specific phobias may affect up to 25% of the population at some point during their lives. Specific phobias are more prevalent among women, but social phobias affect men and women equally. Specific phobias tend to have their onset in childhood, most starting before age 12 years. Social phobias begin during adolescence, the majority having their onset before age 25 years. Among specific phobias, the most commonly feared objects or situations include animals, storms, heights, illness, injury, and death.

Despite the frequency of phobias in the general population, few phobic persons receive treatment; most people are likely to perceive their phobias as trivial and are rarely limited by them. Fear of snakes, for example, will hardly keep a person from succeeding socially or occupationally, unless the person is employed as a zookeeper. Consequently, patients with phobias comprise only 2%–3% of psychiatric outpatients.

Etiology

Phobic disorders tend to run in families, although there are few studies that deal specifically with social or specific phobias. Most studies lump all phobias together, including agoraphobia. A recent study of specific phobias showed that

Table 10–10. DSM-IV criteria for social phobia (social anxiety disorder)

A. A marked and persistent fear of one or more social or performance situations in which the person is exposed to unfamiliar people or to possible scrutiny by others. The individual fears that he or she will act in a way (or show anxiety symptoms) that will be humiliating or embarrassing. **Note:** In children, there must be evidence of the capacity for age-appropriate social relationships with familiar people and the anxiety must occur in peer settings, not just in interactions with adults.

B. Exposure to the feared social situation almost invariably provokes anxiety, which may take the form of a situationally bound or situationally predisposed panic attack. **Note:** In children, the anxiety may be expressed by crying, tantrums, freezing, or shrinking from social situations with unfamilar people.

C. The person recognizes that the fear is excessive or unreasonable. **Note:** In children, this feature may be absent.

D. The feared social or performance situations are avoided or else are endured with intense anxiety or distress.

E. The avoidance, anxious anticipation, or distress in the feared social or performance situation(s) interferes significantly with the person's normal routine, occupational (academic) functioning, or with social activities or relationships with others, or there is marked distress about having the phobia.

F. In individuals under age 18 years, the duration is at least 6 months.

G. The fear or avoidance is not due to the direct physiological effects of a substance (e.g., a drug of abuse, medication) or a general medical condition, and is not better accounted for by another mental disorder (e.g., panic disorder with or without agoraphobia, separation anxiety disorder, body dysmorphic disorder, a pervasive developmental disorder, or schizoid personality disorder).

H. If a general medical condition or other mental disorder is present, the fear in criterion A is unrelated to it, e.g., the fear is not of stuttering, trembling in Parkinson's disease, or exhibiting abnormal eating behavior in anorexia nervosa or bulimia nervosa.

Specify if:

Generalized: If the fears include most social situations (e.g., initiating or maintaining conversations, participating in small groups, dating, speaking to authority figures, attending parties). Note: Also consider the additional diagnosis of avoidant personality disorder.

---

relatives of subjects with a phobia were more than three times as likely to have phobias as were relatives of nonphobic control subjects. Further, twin studies have generally shown a higher rate of concordance for anxiety and phobic disorders in monozygotic twins than in dizygotic twins.

Learning may play an important role in the etiology of phobias. Behaviorists have pointed out that many phobias tend to arise in association with traumatic events, such as developing a fear of heights after sustaining a fall. Learning theory appears to explain many, but not all, cases of phobia, so that other explanations are likely. Psychoanalysts have long held that phobias result from unresolved conflicts in childhood and attribute phobias to the use of *displacement* and *avoidance* as defense mechanisms against castration anxiety.

Table 10–11. DSM-IV criteria for specific phobia (simple phobia)

A. Marked and persistent fear that is excessive or unreasonable, cued by the presence or anticipation of a specific object or situation (e.g., flying, heights, animals, receiving an injection, seeing blood).

B. Exposure to the phobic stimulus almost invariably provokes an immediate anxiety response, which may take the form of a situationally bound or situationally predisposed panic attack. **Note:** In children, the anxiety may be expressed by crying, tantrums, freezing, or clinging.

C. The person recognizes that the fear is excessive or unreasonable. **Note:** in children, this feature may be absent.

D. The phobic situation(s) is avoided or else is endured with intense anxiety or distress.

E. The avoidance, anxious anticipation, or distress in the feared situations significantly interferes with the person's normal routine, occupational (academic) functioning, or with social activities or relationships with others, or there is marked distress about having the phobia.

F. In individuals under age 18 years, the duration is at least 6 months.

G. The anxiety, panic attacks, or phobic avoidance associated with the specific object or situation is not better accounted for by another mental disorder, such as obsessive-compulsive disorder (e.g., fear of dirt in someone with an obsession about contamination), posttraumatic stress disorder (e.g., avoidance of stimuli associated with a severe stressor), separation anxiety disorder (e.g., avoidance of school), social phobia (e.g., avoidance of social situations because of fear of embarrassment), panic disorder with agoraphobia, or agoraphobia without history of panic disorder.

Specify type:

Animal type
Natural environment type (e.g., heights, storms, water)
Blood, injection, injury type
Situational type (e.g., planes, elevators, enclosed places)
Other type (e.g., phobic avoidance of situations that may lead to choking, vomiting, or contracting an illness; or in children, avoidance of loud sounds or costumed characters)

Clinical Findings

People with social and specific phobias experience fear when exposed to specific phobic objects or situations, manifest autonomic arousal, and develop avoidance. Initially, exposure leads to an unpleasant subjective state of anxiety. This state, in turn, leads to typical physiological manifestations of anxiety, such as rapid heartbeat, shortness of breath, and jitteriness. In the dreaded situation, socially phobic people develop overwhelming anxiety and fear that others will recognize this anxiety. They soon learn to avoid these unpleasant situations, and they may eventually learn to avoid public speaking engagements, eating in public, riding in public, or using public toilets. Socially phobic persons may gradually learn to avoid social gatherings, meeting with superiors, and eventually almost any social encounter.

Table 10–12.   Common specific phobias by type

Phobia	Focus of fear	Phobia	Focus of Fear
Animal type		**Blood, injection, injury type**	
Ailurophobia	Cats	Hemophobia	Blood
Arachnophobia	Spiders	Odynephobia	Pain
Cynophobia	Dogs	Poinephobia	Punishment
Entomophobia	Insects		
Ophidiophobia	Snakes	**Situation type**	
		Apeirophobia	Infinity
Natural environment type		Claustrophobia	Closed spaces
Acrophobia	Heights	Topophobia	Stage fright
Amathophobia	Dust		
Frigophobia	Cold weather	**Other**	
Keraunophobia	Thunder	Gynephobia	Women
Nyctophobia	Night	Homophobia	Homosexuals
Phonophobia	Loud noises	Kakorrhaphiophobia	Failure
Photophobia	Light	Logophobia	Words
Pyrophobia	Fire	Theophobia	God
		Triskaidekaphobia	Number 13

For the person with a specific phobia, the degree of distress varies with the prevalence of the avoided situation. For example, a hospital employee who fears blood may be in constant distress because of the availability of blood at hospitals. Apart from contact with the feared stimulus, the phobic person is usually free of symptoms. A case example of a boy with a specific phobia follows:

John, a 13-year-old boy, was brought to the clinic by his mother. His mother reported that John would not wear shirts that had buttons on them and was worried that this peculiarity would cause problems for John when he was older. Already, his mother pointed out, not being able to wear regular collared shirts had kept John out of scouting troops and the school orchestra because of the uniforms he would have to wear. Doctors had told John's mother in the past that he would outgrow this fear. John clearly was uncomfortable and appeared embarrassed by his mother's recitation of the story but admitted that it was all true. John said that at about age 4 he had developed a fear of buttons, but was not sure why. Since then, he had worn only T-necked shirts or sweaters and had refused to wear collared shirts. In fact, John said, just thinking about such shirts bothered him, and he even avoided touching his brother's shirts that hung in the closet that they shared.

Ten years later, John had finished college and had enrolled in graduate school. He had overcome the phobia by himself at age 16, and he was able to wear regular collared shirts, but he still reported that he avoided wearing these shirts when possible.

Course and Outcome

Social phobias tend to develop slowly, have no obvious precipitating stressors, and are chronic but fluctuating. Variable degrees of disability may occur depending on the nature and extent of the feared situation. Degree of disability also depends on the occupation and position of the phobic person. For example, a business executive whose job requires meeting with the public would face much greater disability from a social phobia than would a lighthouse keeper.

Specific phobias tend to remit spontaneously with age, as illustrated in the case of John. When specific phobias persist into adulthood, they often become chronic, but they rarely cause disability.

Complications of phobic disorders include depression or substance abuse. Many persons with social phobia become dependent on alcohol or sedative drugs and use them to reduce their anxiety in feared situations. Phobic symptoms may precede the onset of pathological drinking, suggesting that these disorders have a role in the development of alcohol dependence in some patients.

Differential Diagnosis

The differential diagnosis of phobic disorders includes other anxiety disorders such as panic disorder or GAD, mood disorders, schizophrenia, OCD, and avoidant personality disorder. Phobias may occur in the context of these disorders but tend to appear after the onset of the primary disorder. The irrational fear that characterizes phobias must be separated from a schizophrenic delusion. The differentiation of a simple phobia from OCD is often difficult, but in the obsessive-compulsive person the phobia tends to be just one of many obsessional concerns. The differentiation between avoidant personality disorder and social phobia may be difficult, and in fact, there is great overlap between the two disorders. In general, the avoidant person has no specific fears of objects or situations but has a general discomfort in social situations and requires continual reassurance.

Phobic symptoms are common in depression. Ones that arise in the context of a depressive episode are generally mood congruent (e.g., fear of failure) and usually disappear when the depression has been successfully treated.

Clinical Management

Mild cases of social phobia may respond to behavioral therapy alone, but many patients will need medication. Patients with social phobia have been treated with some success with MAOIs, alprazolam, and the newer SRIs. Tricyclic anti-depressants appear to be somewhat less effective, and persons with social phobia tend to be sensitive to their side effects and may develop jitteriness, irritability, and insomnia on relatively low doses. Patients tend to relapse when the drugs are discontinued.

Behavioral therapy is useful in the treatment of both social phobias and specific phobias. *Systematic desensitization* and *flooding* are the most widely used forms of exposure. In the former, patients learn to gradually reduce their anxiety associated with feared situations. In flooding, patients are instructed to enter situations or do things that are generally associated with anxiety until the anxiety associated with the exposure (e.g., eating in restaurants) subsides. It is unlikely that patients will improve unless they are persuaded to confront feared situations. Behavioral techniques are discussed further in Chapter 25.

Supportive psychotherapy is also helpful, especially when combined with behavioral therapy or medication to help restore morale and self-confidence. Cognitive techniques can be used to help modify dysfunctional thoughts about fear of failure, humiliation, or embarrassment. For example, socially phobic persons tend to overestimate the extent of others' scrutiny of them. Marriage or family counseling may be indicated when disturbed marital or family situations are contributing to the symptoms.

Posttraumatic Stress Disorder

PTSD develops in persons who have experienced a traumatic event that has involved experiencing, witnessing, or being confronted with actual or threatened death, serious physical injury, or a threat to one's physical integrity. Examples include combat, physical assault, rape, and disasters such as home fires. The three major elements of PTSD include reexperiencing the trauma through dreams or recurrent and intrusive thoughts, emotional numbing such as feeling detached from others, and symptoms of autonomic arousal such as irritability and exaggerated startle response. Two subtypes are specified: acute if the duration of the symptoms is less than 3 months and chronic if the symptoms last 3 months or longer. If onset is delayed more than 6 months after the stressor, that delay is specified. The diagnostic criteria for PTSD are listed in Table 10–13.

The term *posttraumatic stress disorder* was introduced in 1980 in DSM-III, although the concept of this disturbance has a long history. In the past, this syndrome was recognized in wartime as shell shock or war neurosis, because it was seen most commonly in wartime situations. Many of its typical symptoms, however, such as intrusive thoughts and autonomic arousal, were also recognized in

Table 10–13. DSM-IV criteria for posttraumatic stress disorder

A. The person has been exposed to a traumatic event in which both of the following were present:
   1. The person experienced, witnessed, or was confronted with an event or events that involve actual or threatened death or serious injury, or a threat to the physical integrity of self or others
   2. The person's response involved intense fear, helplessness, or horror.
      Note: In children, it may be expressed instead by disorganized or agitated behavior.

B. The traumatic event is persistently reexperienced in one (or more) of the following ways:
   1. Recurrent and intrusive distressing recollections of the event, including images, thoughts, or perceptions. **Note:** In young children, repetitive play may occur in which themes or aspects of the trauma are expressed.
   2. Recurrent distressing dreams of the event. **Note:** In children, there may be frightening dreams without recognizable content.
   3. Acting or feeling as if the traumatic event were recurring (includes a sense of reliving the experience, illusions, hallucinations, and dissociative flashback episodes, including those that occur on awakening or when intoxicated). **Note:** In young children, trauma-specific reenactment may occur.
   4. Intense psychological distress at exposure to internal or external cues that symbolize or resemble an aspect of the traumatic event.
   5. Physiological reactivity on exposure to internal or external cues that symbolize or resemble an aspect of the traumatic event

C. Persistent avoidance of stimuli associated with the trauma and numbing of general responsiveness (not present before the trauma), as indicated by three (or more) of the following:
   1. Efforts to avoid thoughts, feelings, or conversations associated with the trauma
   2. Efforts to avoid activities, places, or people that arouse recollections of the trauma
   3. Inability to recall an important aspect of the trauma
   4. Markedly diminished interest or participation in significant activities
   5. Feeling of detachment or estrangement from others
   6. Restricted range of affect (e.g., unable to have loving feelings)
   7. Sense of a foreshortened future (e.g., does not expect to have a career, marriage, or children, or a normal life span)

D. Persistent symptoms of increased arousal (not present before the trauma), as indicated by two (or more) of the following:
   1. Difficulty falling or staying asleep
   2. Irritability or outbursts of anger
   3. Difficulty concentrating
   4. Hypervigilance
   5. Exaggerated startle response

E. Duration of the disturbance (symptoms in criteria B, C, and D) is more than 1 month.

F. The disturbance causes clinically significant distress or impairment in social, occupational, or other important areas of functioning.

Specify if:
   Acute: if duration of symptoms is less than 3 months
   Chronic: if duration of symptoms is 3 months or more

Specify if:
   With delayed onset: If onset of symptoms is at least 6 months after the stressor

victims of other traumatic events, such as natural disasters. In DSM-I, the disorder was diagnosed as *gross stress reaction*, a diagnosis dropped from DSM-II.

Epidemiology and Clinical Findings

The prevalence of PTSD in the general population has been estimated to be 0.5% among men and 1.2% among women. Most men with the disorder have experienced combat. For women, the most frequent precipitating stressor is a physical assault or rape. The disorder can occur at any age, and children have been reported to develop the disorder, such as after the Chowchilla school bus kidnapping incident in 1976. The prevalence of PTSD among survivors of catastrophes varies, but in one well-studied tragedy, the Coconut Grove nightclub fire in the 1940s, 57% of patients followed up 1 year later experienced an acute posttraumatic syndrome.

PTSD may begin within hours or days of the stressor, but it may be delayed for months or years. The disorder can be chronic and has been reported to last in some cases for 30 or 40 years. Symptoms tend to fluctuate and worsen during periods of stress. Predictors of good outcome include rapid onset of symptoms, adequate premorbid functioning, strong social supports, and an absence of psychiatric or medical comorbidity.

We recently saw a woman who had developed PTSD after a sexual assault:

> Doris, a 21-year-old college student, presented to our clinic for evaluation of depression and flashbacks. Three months earlier, at a fraternity party, Doris had become intoxicated and begun to neck with one of the men. The kissing continued, and the man suggested that they go elsewhere to have sexual intercourse. Doris objected, but the man persisted; he forcibly took her to another room, tore off her clothing, and raped her. After sobering up, and feeling embarrassed and humiliated, Doris said nothing to her friends, nor did she seek a medical evaluation. She thought that what happened would be considered date rape and be ignored by the authorities.
>
> Although she never missed a class or her part-time clerical job, she began to have inexplicable episodes of anger and irritability; began to ruminate about the rape, remembering every unpleasant detail; and began to withdraw from her friends and refuse social invitations. Her symptoms of depression and anxiety, as well as the concern of her friends, led her to seek help.
>
> The diagnosis of PTSD was made and explained to the patient; she was referred for group therapy at a local rape crisis advocacy center.

Etiology

The major etiological event leading to PTSD is the stressor. Because not all persons who experience a major stressor develop the disorder, other variables such as underlying personality and biological vulnerability are undoubtedly important. Stressors of all types may contribute to the development of PTSD, but they must be severe enough to be outside the range of normal human experience. Business losses, marital conflicts, or the death of a loved one, for example, are not considered stressors that lead to PTSD. At least for war, certain experiences are highly linked to the development of PTSD: witnessing a friend being killed in action, witnessing wartime atrocities, and especially, participating in atrocities.

Individual differences that can predispose to the development of PTSD include age, history of emotional disturbance, social support, and proximity to the stressor. Eighty percent of young children who sustain a burn injury, for example, show symptoms of posttraumatic stress 1–2 years after the initial injury, but only 30% of adults who sustain this injury have symptoms after 1 year. Persons with prior history of psychiatric treatment have a greater likelihood of developing the syndrome, presumably because the previous illness reflects a greater sensitivity to stress; and persons with adequate social support are less likely to develop the disorder than persons with poor support. Certain biological abnormalities have been found in persons with PTSD, such as decreased rapid eye movement latency in stage IV sleep, and these abnormalities may play a role in its development.

Complications

Complications of PTSD may include violence and aggression, alcohol and drug abuse, and poor impulse control. Although many war veterans have claimed that PTSD has led them to commit criminal offenses, one study found that felonious behavior in combat veterans occurred only in those who had had similar behavior before their military service.

Differential Diagnosis

The differential diagnosis for PTSD includes major depression, adjustment disorder, panic disorder, GAD, acute stress disorder, OCD, depersonalization disorder, factitious disorder, or malingering. Occasionally, a physical injury may have occurred during the stressor so that a mental disorder secondary to brain injury must be considered as well. Many patients with PTSD meet criteria for another Axis I disorder (e.g., major depression, panic disorder), in which case both disorders should be diagnosed.

Clinical Management

There are few controlled studies of the pharmacological and psychotherapeutic strategies for the treatment of PTSD. However, research indicates that tricyclic antidepressants, MAOIs, and alprazolam are all helpful clinically. Medication helps to decrease depression, to reduce intrusive symptoms such as nightmares and flashbacks, and to normalize sleep. Other medications have been the subject of case reports, including carbamazepine, lithium carbonate, antipsychotics, and SRI antidepressants. More study is needed before specific recommendations can be made. Medications are probably best reserved for patients with specific psychiatric syndromes in addition to PTSD, for example, antidepressants to treat major depression or antipsychotics to treat psychotic symptoms.

Psychotherapy can be enormously helpful. Behavioral techniques involving direct therapeutic exposure (i.e., flooding), are particularly helpful in reducing the intrusive symptoms of PTSD. Cognitive therapies may also help to reduce anxiety by providing patients with the skills to control anxiety. More psychody-

Table 10–14. DSM-IV criteria for acute stress disorder

A. The person has been exposed to a traumatic event in which both of the following were present:
   1. The person has experienced, witnessed, or been confronted with an event or events that involve actual or threatened death or serious injury, or a threat to the physical integrity of self or others
   2. The person's response involved fear, helplessness, or horror

B. Either while experiencing or after experiencing the distressing event, the individual has three (or more) of the following dissociative symptoms:
   1. A subjective sense of numbing, detachment, or absence of emotional responsiveness
   2. A reduction in awareness of one's surroundings (e.g. "being in a daze")
   3. Derealization
   4. Depersonalization
   5. Dissociative amnesia (i.e., inability to recall an important aspect of the trauma)

C. The traumatic event is persistently reexperienced in at least one of the following ways: recurrent images, thoughts, dreams, illusions, flashback episodes, or a sense of reliving the experience; or distress on exposure to reminders of the traumatic event.

D. Marked avoidance of stimuli that arouse recollections of the trauma (e.g., thoughts, feelings, conversations, activities, places, people).

E. Marked symptoms of anxiety or increased arousal (e.g., difficulty sleeping, irritability, poor concentration, hypervigilance, exaggerated startle response, motor restlessness).

F. The disturbance causes clinically significant distress or impairment in social, occupational, or other important areas of functioning, or impairs the individual's ability to pursue some necessary task, such as obtaining necessary assistance or mobilizing personal resources by telling family members about the traumatic experience.

G. The symptoms last for a minimum of 2 days and a maximum of 4 weeks and occur within 4 weeks of the traumatic event.

H. The disturbance is not due to the direct physiological effects of a substance (e.g., a drug of abuse, medication) or a general medical condition, is not better accounted for by brief psychotic disorder, and is not merely an exacerbation of a preexisting Axis I or Axis II disorder.

namic approaches may help persons to integrate the traumatic event into their understanding of the meaning of life and their self-concept. Hypnosis and intravenous amobarbital sodium (i.e., "Amytal interview") have been used to facilitate this approach. Group and family therapy have been advocated, particularly in association with Vietnam veterans. The Veterans Administration has organized groups for distressed veterans across the country.

Acute Stress Disorder

Acute stress disorder is a newly defined condition. According to DSM-IV, the disorder occurs in response to a traumatic event and is accompanied by typical dissociative symptoms, such as emotional numbing, derealization, amnesia, and depersonalization (see Table 10–14).

Because the disorder was recently defined, there is little information about its prevalence, gender distribution, or risk factors. By definition, the disorder lasts at least 2 days and at most 1 month. The differential diagnosis is between PTSD, brief psychotic disorder, a dissociative disorder, or an adjustment disorder. PTSD lasts more than 1 month, and although dissociative symptoms may be present,

---

Recommendations for treatment of anxiety disorders

1. Mild cases of panic may respond to behavioral interventions, but many patients will need medication (e.g., tricyclic antidepressants [TCAs], monoamine oxidase inhibitors [MAOIs], alprazolam).

2. The agoraphobic patient should be gently encouraged to get out and explore the world.
   - Progress will not occur unless the phobic patient confronts the feared places or situations.

3. Behavioral techniques (i.e., exposure, flooding, desensitization) will help most persons with specific and social phobias.
   - Some people with social phobias respond well to medication (e.g., TCAs, MAOIs, serotonin reuptake inhibitors, alprazolam).

4. Generalized anxiety may respond to simple behavioral techniques (e.g., relaxation training), but many patients will need medication (e.g., benzodiazepines).
   - Be sure that the benzodiazepine is prescribed for a limited time only (e.g., weeks or months).

5. Posttraumatic stress disorder tends to be chronic, but many patients will benefit from the support available in group therapy.
   - Group therapy has become especially popular with Vietnam veterans, and most veteran organizations can offer help in finding a group.

they are usually not prominent. Although brief psychotic disorder lasts less than 1 month, it is characterized by hallucinations, delusions, or bizarre behavior. A dissociative disorder does not necessarily occur in response to a traumatic situation or involve emotional numbing, reexperiencing of the trauma, or autonomic arousal. An adjustment disorder occurs in response to stressful situations (e.g., personal bankruptcy), but not necessarily a traumatic event involving serious personal threats; adjustment disorders may last up to 6 months, and the diagnosis is mainly used when criteria for other Axis I disorders are not met. In this case, a diagnosis of acute stress reaction would preempt a diagnosis of adjustment disorder.

Bibliography

Andreasen NJC, Norris AS, Hartford CE: Incidence of long-term psychiatric complications in severely burned adults. Ann Surg 174:785–793, 1971

Barlow DH: Anxiety and Its Disorders—The Nature and Treatment of Anxiety and Panic. New York, Guilford, 1988

Ballenger JC, Burrows GD, DuPont RL, et al: Alprazolam in panic disorder and agoraphobia: results from a multicenter trial, I: efficacy in short-term treatment. Arch Gen Psychiatry 45:413–422, 1988

Black DW, Wesner R, Bowers W, et al: A comparison of fluvoxamine, cognitive therapy, and placebo in the treatment of panic disorder. Arch Gen Psychiatry 50:44–50, 1993

Brawman-Mintzer O, Lydiard B, Emmanuel N, et al: Psychiatric comorbidity in patients with generalized anxiety disorder. Am J Psychiatry 150:1216–1218, 1993

Breslau N, Davis GC: Post-traumatic stress disorder: the etiologic specificity of war time stressors. Am J Psychiatry 144:578–583, 1987

Brown TA, Barlow DH, Liebowitz MR: The empirical basis of generalized anxiety disorder. Am J Psychiatry 151:1281–1288, 1994

Friedman MJ: Toward rational pharmacotherapy for post-traumatic stress disorder: an interim report. Am J Psychiatry 145:281–285, 1988

Fyer AJ, Mannuzza S, Gallops MS, et al: Familial transmission of simple phobias and fears—a preliminary report. Arch Gen Psychiatry 47:252–256, 1990

Gorman JM, Liebowitz MR, Fyer A, et al: A neuroanatomical hypothesis for panic disorder. Am J Psychiatry 146:148–161, 1989

Greist JH, Jefferson JW, Marks IM: Anxiety and Its Treatment—Help Is Available. Washington, DC, American Psychiatric Press, 1986

Heimberg RG, Barlow DH: Psychosocial treatments for social phobias. Psychosomatics 29:27–37, 1988

Helzer JE, Robins LE, McEvoy L: Post-traumatic stress disorder in the general population: findings of the epidemiologic catchment area survey. N Engl J Med 317:1630–1634, 1987

Katon WJ, Van Korff M, Lin E: Panic disorder: relationship to high medical utilization. Am J Med 92 (suppl 1A):7S–11S, 1992

Lee MA, Flegel P, Greden JF, et al: Anxiogenic effects of caffeine in panic and depressed patients. Am J Psychiatry 145:632–635, 1988

Liebowitz MR, Fyer J, Gorman JM: Social phobia: review of a neglected anxiety disorder. Arch Gen Psychiatry 42:729–736, 1985

Marks IM: Fears, Phobias, and Rituals: Panic, Anxieties, and Their Disorders. New York, Oxford University Press, 1987

Meibach RC, Dunner D, Wilson LG, et al: Comparative efficacy of propranolol, chlordiazepoxide, and placebo in the treatment of anxiety. J Clin Psychiatry 48:355–358, 1987

Noyes R: Suicide and panic disorder: a review. J Affect Disord 22:1–11, 1991

Noyes R, Clancy J, Garvey MJ, et al: Is agoraphobia a variant of panic disorder or a separate illness? Journal of Anxiety Disorders 1:3–13, 1987

Noyes R, Clarkson C, Crowe R, et al: A family study of generalized anxiety disorder. Am J Psychiatry 144:119–124, 1987

Pittman RK, Orr SP, Forgue D: Psychophysiologic assessment of post-traumatic stress disorder imagery in Vietnam combat veterans. Arch Gen Psychiatry 44:970–975, 1987

Reich J, Yates W: A pilot study of treatment of social phobia with alprazolam. Am J Psychiatry 145:590–594, 1988

Ross RJ, Ball WA, Sullivan KA, et al: Sleep disturbance as the hallmark of post-traumatic stress disorder. Am J Psychiatry 146:697–707, 1989

Roy-Byrne P (ed): Anxiety: New Findings for the Clinician. Washington, DC, American Psychiatric Press, 1989

Schneier FR, Heckelman LR, Garfinkel R, et al: Functional impairment in social phobia. J Clin Psychiatry 55:322–331, 1994

Shaw DM, Churchill CM, Noyes R, et al: Criminal behavior and posttraumatic stress disorder in Vietnam veterans. Compr Psychiatry 28:403–411, 1987

Smith EM, North CS, McCool RE, et al: Acute post-disaster psychiatric disorders: identification of persons at risk. Am J Psychiatry 147:202–206, 1990

Solomon SD, Gerrity ET, Muff AM: Efficacy of treatments for post-traumatic stress disorder—an empirical review. JAMA 268:633–638, 1992

Terr LC: Chowchilla revisited: the effects of psychic trauma four years after a school bus kidnapping. Am J Psychiatry 140:1543–1550, 1983

Thyer BA, Parrish RT, Curtis GC, et al: Ages of onset of DSM-III anxiety disorder. Compr Psychiatry 26:113–122, 1985

Torgerson S: Genetic factors in anxiety disorders. Arch Gen Psychiatry 40:1085–1089, 1983

Van Amerigen M, Mancini C, Streiner DC: Fluoxetine efficacy in social phobia. J Clin Psychiatry 54:27–32, 1993

Self-Assessment Questions

1. What is the relationship between panic disorder and agoraphobia?
2. What is the irritable heart syndrome?
3. What are the findings in genetic studies of panic disorder?
4. What is the differential diagnosis of panic disorder?
5. What is the pharmacological treatment of panic disorder? Generalized anxiety disorder? Social phobia?
6. What are social and specific phobias? How do they differ?
7. What is the natural history of the different anxiety disorders?
8. When does posttraumatic disorder develop? What factors predispose to its development?
9. What behavioral treatments are useful in the different anxiety disorders?
10. When is anxiety normal and when is it abnormal?

Chapter 11

Obsessive-Compulsive Disorder

He had another peculiarity—This was his anxious care to
go out or in at a door or passage by a certain number of
steps from a certain point. . . .

Boswell's Life of Johnson

Johnson, whose ritualistic behavior was so carefully observed by Boswell, probably had obsessive-compulsive disorder (OCD). Shakespeare, in describing the
guilt-laden hand-washing rituals of Lady Macbeth, appears to have had some
familiarity with the symptoms of the disorder. More recently, industrialist Howard Hughes developed crippling contamination obsessions in late adulthood that
resulted in a fanatic preoccupation with germs and a bizarre life of filth and neglect. Like most mental illnesses, OCD had been recognized for centuries, but it
was first described in 1838 by Esquirol, a French psychiatrist. Earlier, rituals were
probably regarded as personal quirks or, worse, as evidence of possession by the
Devil. One wonders how many luckless victims of OCD were burned at the
stake!

By the end of the nineteenth century, obsessions and compulsions were generally believed to be manifestations of depressive illness. Later, in part due to the
influence of Freud, these symptoms were recognized as a syndrome, *obsessional
neurosis*, believed to result from intrapsychic conflicts. This view remained prominent until recently, when biologically oriented research supported the disease
model of OCD, and behaviorally oriented clinicians began to reconceptualize
OCD in terms of learning theory. In 1980, obsessional neurosis was renamed

321

obsessive-compulsive disorder, reflecting these new etiological concepts. Although the cause of OCD is still unknown, its study has been reinvigorated by new research methods, as well as by the development of effective treatments that have altered its formerly poor prognosis.

Definition

The essential features of OCD are obsessions or compulsions, or more commonly both. According to DSM-IV (see Table 11–1), obsessions are recurrent or persistent ideas, thoughts, impulses, or images that are experienced as intrusive and inappropriate and that cause marked anxiety and distress. Common obsessions include fears of harming other persons or sinning against God. For example, a person may have an obsessional thought to kill a loved one, or a religious person may have blasphemous thoughts. The content of typical obsessions is explained in Table 11–2.

Compulsions, on the other hand, are repetitive, purposeful, and intentional behaviors or mental acts performed in response to obsessions or according to rules that must be rigidly applied. Common examples of compulsions include repetitive hand washing or checking rituals. Compulsive rituals are meant to neutralize or reduce discomfort or to prevent a dreaded event or situation. The rituals are not connected in a realistic way to the event or situation, or they are clearly excessive. For example, a person might think that if he failed to reread the directions on a box of detergent, harm would come to his child. In short, obsessions cause anxiety, which is relieved by compulsive rituals. The frequency of common obsessions and compulsions in a series of 250 patients is presented in Table 11–3.

To receive a diagnosis of OCD, a person must have either obsessions or compulsions that cause marked distress, are time consuming (more than 1 hour daily), or significantly interfere with the person's normal routine, occupational functioning, or usual social activities and relationships. In addition, at some point the patient must recognize that the obsessions and compulsions are unreasonable, and the clinician will have determined that the symptoms are not due to another Axis I disorder, such as major depression, and that they are not due to the direct physiological effects of a substance or a general medical condition.

Many psychiatrically normal persons, especially children, have occasional obsessional thoughts or repetitive behaviors, but they tend not to cause distress or interfere with living. In fact, in many ways rituals add structure to our lives. Most of us have daily routines that have probably changed little in years (e.g., drinking coffee in the morning, having lunch at noon, having dinner at 6 P.M.,

Table 11–1. DSM-IV criteria for obsessive-compulsive disorder

A. Either obsessions or compulsions:

Obsessions as defined by 1, 2, 3, and 4:

1. Recurrent and persistent thoughts, impulses, or images that are experienced at some time during the disturbance as intrusive and inappropriate, and that cause marked anxiety or distress

2. The thoughts, impulses, or images are not simply excessive worries about real-life problems

3. The person attempts to ignore or suppress such thoughts, impulses, or images or to neutralize them with some other thought or action

4. The person recognizes that the obsessional thoughts, impulses, or images are a product of his or her own mind (not imposed from without as in thought insertion)

Compulsions as defined by 1 and 2:

1. Repetitive behaviors (e.g., hand washing, ordering, checking) or mental acts (e.g., praying, counting, repeating words silently) that the person feels driven to perform in response to an obsession, or according to rules that must be applied rigidly

2. The behaviors or mental acts are aimed at preventing or reducing distress or preventing some dreaded event or situation; however, these behaviors or mental acts either are not connected in a realistic way with what they are designed to neutralize or prevent or are clearly excessive

B. At some point during the course of the disorder, the person has recognized that the obsessions or compulsions are excessive or unreasonable. **Note:** This does not apply to children.

C. The obsessions or compulsions cause marked distress; are time consuming (take more than an hour a day); or significantly interfere with the person's normal routine, occupational (or academic) functioning, or usual social activities or relationships.

D. If another Axis I disorder is present, the content of the obsessions or compulsions is not restricted to it (e.g., preoccupation with food in the presence of an eating disorder; hair pulling in the presence of trichotillomania; concern with appearance in the presence of body dysmorphic disorder; preoccupation with drugs in the presence of a substance use disorder; preoccupation with having serious illness in the presence of hypochondriasis; preoccupation with sexual urges or fantasies in the presence of a paraphilia; or guilty ruminations in the presence of major depressive disorder).

E. The disturbance is not due to the direct physiological effects of a substance (e.g., a drug of abuse, medication) or a general medical condition.

Specify if:

Poor insight type: if, for most of the time during the current episode, the person does not recognize that the obsessions and compulsions are excessive or unreasonable.

and retiring at 11 P.M.). Many of us double-check locks, avoid stepping on cracks, and say prayers before meals. Rituals also enhance the spiritual life of many (e.g., religious catechism). These daily rituals are accepted, desirable, and easily adapted to changing circumstances. To the obsessive-compulsive patient, however, rituals are a distressing and unavoidable way of life.

The following is a case history of a patient treated in our clinic who suffered the crippling effects of OCD:

Table 11–2.   Varied content in obsessions

Obsession	Foci of preoccupation
Aggression	Physical or verbal assault on self or others (includes suicidal and homicidal thoughts); accidents; mishaps; wars and natural disasters; death
Contamination	Excreta, human or otherwise; dirt, dust; semen; menstrual blood; other bodily excretions; germs; illness, especially venereal diseases; acquired immunodeficiency syndrome (AIDS)
Symmetry	Orderliness in arrangements of any kind (e.g., books on the shelf, shirts in the dresser)
Sexual	Sexual advances toward self or others; incestuous impulses; genitalia of either sex; homosexuality; masturbation; competence in sexual performance
Hoarding	Collecting items of any kind (e.g., string, shopping bags); inability to throw things out
Religious	Existence of God; validity of religious stories, practices, or holidays; committing sinful acts
Somatic	Preoccupation with body parts (e.g., nose); concern with appearance; belief in having disease or illness (e.g., cancer)

Source.   Adapted from Akhtar S, Wig NN, Varma VK, et al: A phenomenological analysis of symptoms in obsessive-compulsive neurosis. Br J Psychiatry 127:342–348, 1975.

Todd, a 24-year-old male, was accompanied to the psychiatric outpatient clinic by his mother for evaluation of obsessions and compulsive rituals. According to Todd, the rituals began in childhood and included touching objects a certain number of times and rereading prayers in church, but these symptoms were not disabling. After graduating from college, he moved to a large midwestern city to work as an accountant for a major firm. Soon after moving there, he began to check the locks on his doors frequently and to check his automobile for signs of intruders. Eventually, he began to check other things around his apartment such as appliances, water faucets, and electrical switches, fearing that they might be unsafe. Fearing contamination, he also developed extensive grooming and bathing rituals. Because of his time-consuming rituals, he was often late for work. In fact, his work load became too much for him, and he was forced to quit his job. As an accountant, he would find himself adding columns of numbers over and over to make sure that he had "done it right."

In addition to extensive rituals, Todd also developed substantial obsessional thinking, such as having thoughts of losing control and assaulting someone, yelling embarrassing words in public, becoming contaminated, and possibly contracting acquired immunodeficiency syndrome. He also worried about the arrangement and symmetry of objects. Much of the time his rituals consisted of debating whether he needed to actually conduct a ritual and, in fact, mentally rehearsing rituals. Todd admitted that his rituals were irrational and excessive, but he felt powerless to control

Table 11–3.   The frequency of common obsessions and compulsions in 250 patients with obsessive-compulsive disorder

Obsessions	%	Compulsions	%
Contamination	45	Checking	63
Pathological doubt	42	Washing	50
Somatic	36	Counting	36
Need for symmetry	31	Need to ask or confess	31
Aggressive impulse	28	Symmetry and precision	28
Sexual impulse	26	Hoarding	18
Multiple obsessions	60	Multiple compulsions	48
Other	13		

Source.   Adapted from Rasmussen SA, Eisen JL: Epidemiology and clinical features of obsessive-compulsive disorder, in Obsessive-Compulsive Disorders: Theory and Management, 2nd Edition. Edited by Jenike MA, Baer L, Minichiello WE. Littleton, MA, Year Book Medical Publishers, 1990, pp. 10–27.

them. Efforts to resist them merely increased his anxiety, ultimately making the rituals worse.

Todd moved back into his parents' home, but his rituals became more extensive and eventually took up nearly his entire day, literally from sunrise to when he retired at night. By this time, the rituals mostly involved bathing (he showered for half an hour and had to wash his body in a specific fashion), dressing in a certain way, and repeating rituals, such as walking in and out of the door a certain number of times.

Todd presented as a slender, unkempt young man with a scraggly beard, long hair, and unclipped fingernails. His shoes were untied, and he wore several layers of clothing. Because his rituals had became so time consuming, Todd found it easier not to shave or wash at all. He wore the same clothes every day for the same reason.

Todd began treatment with fluoxetine 80 mg daily and quickly improved. Within 2 months his rituals were reduced to less than 1 hour per day, and his grooming had improved. After 6 months Todd still had minor rituals, but reported that he felt like his old self. He had obtained a job and was coaching track at a nearby high school.

At follow-up 6 years later, Todd remained well. Attempts to stop the medication had always led to an increase in symptoms. In the interim, Todd had completed law school and had entered practice.

Epidemiology

OCD typically begins in the late teens or early 20s; about one-third of OCD patients will have developed the illness by age 15 and nearly three quarters by age 30. Onset of the illness is generally gradual, but may be sudden, occurring over a period of 1 month, generally in the absence of any obvious stressor or precipitant. In the past, it was calculated that about 7½ years passed between onset of obsessions and compulsions and the initiation of treatment. The delay may now be less because of the availability of effective treatments and the growing public awareness of OCD.

The prevalence of OCD was once thought to be as low as 0.05% in the community and between 1% and 4% in a psychiatric clinic population. However, data from the Epidemiologic Catchment Area study suggest that as many as 2%–3% of the general population meet criteria for OCD at some point during their lives.

Men and women appear to be affected equally by OCD, although there may be a slight female preponderance. One interesting study showed that 75% of childhood-onset patients were male, which suggests that there may be more than one form of OCD. Patients with OCD have a normal range of intelligence, despite early reports (drawn from samples of persons seeking treatment) that they possess above-average intellect.

Most patients with OCD have relatively normal social and occupational functioning. However, those with a more severe, full-time illness have a high frequency of marital maladjustment and job disability.

Etiology and Pathophysiology

Over the years, OCD has been explained in genetic, psychodynamic, behavioral, and neurobiological terms. No explanation accounts for all of the richness of OCD, and it is likely that a combination of these explanations will be found to account for the disturbance.

Some family studies have shown that up to 20% of first-degree relatives of OCD patients have obsessive-compulsive symptoms, whereas others have shown an increased prevalence of anxiety and mood disorders in relatives. Family studies have linked OCD and Tourette's disorder. Twin studies have generally found a higher concordance of OCD among monozygotic twins than among dizygotic twins, suggesting that there may be an inherited predisposition to OCD. More careful studies on this subject are needed before definite conclusions about the genetics of OCD can be made.

Dynamically oriented clinicians have long explained OCD as stemming from a fixation at the genital stage of development and regression to the earlier anal stage, which involves a preoccupation with anger, dirt, magical thinking, and ambivalence. This leads to an overdeveloped superego and a variety of neurotic defense mechanisms—such as isolation, undoing, reaction formation, and displacement—to control these patients' internal anxious state. (These defense mechanisms are explained in Chapter 25.) Although obsessions and ritualistic behaviors often appear laden with symbolic meaning, psychodynamic approaches have not been helpful in treating this disorder and are primarily of historical interest.

Behaviorists have explained the development of OCD in terms of learning theory. They believe that anxiety, at least initially, becomes paired with specific environmental events (i.e., classical conditioning), for example, becoming dirty or contaminated. The person then engages in compulsive rituals designed to decrease the anxiety (e.g., hand washing). When the rituals successfully reduce the anxiety, the compulsive behavior is believed more likely to occur in the future (i.e., operant conditioning). Although behavioral models of OCD have had little empirical support, behavioral techniques have become a mainstay in treating the disorder.

The neurobiological model of OCD has received wide support in the past decade. Evidence supporting this model includes the fact that OCD occurs with increased frequency in a number of neurological disorders, including cases of head injury, epilepsy, Sydenham's chorea, and Huntington's chorea. Further, many who had encephalitis during an epidemic after World War I subsequently developed OCD. OCD has also been linked to birth injury, abnormal electroencephalograms, abnormal auditory evoked potentials, growth delay, and abnormalities in neuropsychological test results. Additional support for a biological origin comes from animal studies in which bilateral hippocampal lesions or chronic amphetamine administration leads to stereotypic behaviors that resemble compulsive rituals.

New imaging techniques have provided evidence of basal ganglia abnormalities in patients with OCD. Using positron-emission tomography scanning, two groups of investigators showed increased glucose metabolism in the caudate nuclei and the orbital cortex of the frontal lobes; these abnormalities partially normalized following successful treatment. Computed tomography scanning has shown a mild decrease in the volume of the caudate nuclei, whereas magnetic resonance imaging studies have revealed abnormalities of the white matter of the frontal lobes. It has been hypothesized that basal ganglia dysfunction may lead to the complex motor programs involved in OCD, whereas the prefrontal hyperactivity may be related to the tendency to ruminate and plan excessively or to think in an overly abstract way. As discussed in Chapter 5, the prefrontal cortex has important connections with the basal ganglia.

The most widely studied biochemical model has focused primarily on the neurotransmitter serotonin, which has been implicated as mediating a variety of behaviors including impulsivity, suicidality, aggression, and obsessive-compulsive symptoms. The antiobsessional effect of clomipramine and other agents (i.e., fluoxetine, fluvoxamine, paroxetine, sertraline) that potently block serotonin reuptake supports a role for serotonin in OCD. A reduction in obsessive-compulsive symptoms has been correlated with a reduction of platelet serotonin and cerebrospinal fluid 5-hydroxyindoleacetic acid (5-HIAA) during clomipramine treatment. However, data on other serotonin measures, such as platelet tritiated imipramine binding, have been inconclusive. Clearly, more research is needed, and it is unlikely that serotonin will account for all of the manifestations of OCD.

The Relationship Between OCD And Obsessive-Compulsive Personality

Although obsessive-compulsive personality disorder and OCD share a similar name, the two should not be confused. Obsessive-compulsive personality—which is characterized by perfectionism, obstinacy, and orderliness—was once thought by psychoanalysts to lead to OCD, although research has shown that this rarely happens. In fact, most persons with OCD do not have obsessive-compulsive personality traits and are more likely to have dependent and passive-aggressive character traits.

In some cases of obsessive-compulsive personality disorder, compulsive behaviors such as hoarding may develop. We recently evaluated a 45-year-old man brought in by his wife. She was "sick and tired" of putting up with his tendency to collect books, which she described as "taking over their house." He saw nothing wrong with his hobby; in fact, he enjoyed it and saw no reason to give it up. In this case, the obsessive-compulsive traits were ego-syntonic and were not resisted. Based on his history of a rigid and aloof demeanor, miserliness, and perfectionism, in addition to the collecting, he received a diagnosis of obsessive-compulsive personality disorder. A further discussion of this personality disorder is found in Chapter 16.

Course and Outcome

In a study of 250 patients, 85% were reported to have a continuous course, 10% a progressive or deteriorating course, and 2% an episodic course with periods of remission. Because effective treatments are a relatively recent development, future outcome studies may yield more favorable results. A recent follow-up study of children and adolescents with OCD who had received clomipramine seems to bear this trend out. Although most were still symptomatic, symptoms were less severe, and 6% had achieved full remission.

A good outcome appears to be related to having mild or typical symptoms and a well-adjusted premorbid personality. An early onset and severe personality disorders—especially the schizotypal, borderline, and avoidant types—have been associated with poor prognosis. Obsessive-compulsive symptoms are usually worsened by depressed mood and stressful events. In fact, it is frequently depression that leads the OCD patient to seek help, not the obsessions or compulsions. Recurrent episodes of major depression occur in up to 80% of patients with OCD. Although suicidal thoughts often figure prominently in obsessional thinking, the rate of suicide among persons with OCD is not increased.

Differential Diagnosis

The diagnosis of OCD rests on the patient's history and the mental status examination, not laboratory or psychological tests. The disorder overlaps with many other psychiatric syndromes (see Table 11–4), which need to be ruled out. Schizophrenia is the most important disorder to rule out, and several features are common to both conditions. OCD and schizophrenia both tend to be chronic and (at least in the past) to respond poorly to treatment. Severe obsessional thoughts can resemble delusional thinking. This was illustrated for us by Earl, a 38-year-old disabled truck driver who had extensive cleaning and checking rituals and felt compelled to describe the rituals in a loud voice as he was performing them—so loudly, in fact, that neighbors complained. Earl firmly believed that harm would come to his family if he did not announce his rituals in this fashion. Although we tried, we were unable to reassure him that his belief was unreasonable. The distinction between obsessions and delusions is usually clear, because obsessions are unwanted, resisted, and recognized by the patient as having an internal origin, whereas delusions are typically not resisted and are looked on as being of external origin. Obsessive-compulsive patients may occasionally develop hallucinations or delusions, particularly in the context of a severe depression, but follow-up studies show that these patients are not at increased risk for developing schizophrenia.

Cases of OCD in which depression develops (i.e., secondary depression) need to be distinguished from cases of primary depression in which obsessional thinking develops, usually in the form of morbid preoccupations and guilty ruminations (e.g., "I'm a terrible person and have sinned!"). In these situations, the

Table 11–4.   Differential diagnosis of obsessive-compulsive disorder

Disorder	Similarities and differences
Anorexia nervosa	Both involve rituals and tend to be chronic; with anorexia, symptoms are generally not resisted or thought unreasonable; anorexia mainly affects women
Autistic disorder	Stereotypies in autism resemble rituals, but they are not resisted; autism mainly affects males, and many are mentally retarded
Hypochondriasis	Both may involve recurrent thoughts about physical illness, but this is the main symptom in hypochondriasis; hypochondriacal symptoms are rarely resisted or thought unreasonable
Major depression	Depressed patients may develop transient obsessions or compulsions, but the disorder is episodic and mainly affects women; depressive ruminations often resemble obsessions, but are generally considered appropriate
Posttraumatic stress disorder	Both involve intrusive, unwanted thoughts, which cause physiological arousal and anxiety; precipitating stressors are rare in OCD, and many symptoms in posttraumatic stress disorder, such as emotional numbing and depersonalization, tend to be uncommon in OCD
Schizophrenia	Both tend to be chronic and develop in the late teens or early 20s; schizophrenia tends to be severely disabling and is associated with psychotic symptoms
Specific phobia	Both involve fears and avoidance, but the fear is well circumscribed in phobias; phobias tend to come on in childhood and are rarely resisted
Tourette's disorder	Both tend to be chronic, and many Tourette's patients have rituals; Tourette's disorder mostly affects males, and usually has a childhood onset
Trichotillomania	Both involve excessive, unreasonable behaviors, and may respond to similar treatments; trichotillomania mainly affects women and has a childhood onset; obsessional thoughts are uncommon

ruminations are viewed as not unreasonable, although perhaps exaggerated, and are seldom resisted. Whereas the depressed patient tends to focus on past events, the obsessional patient focuses on the prevention of future events. In general, obsessive-compulsive symptoms arising in the context of a depression will resolve completely when the depression is treated.

There is also a close association between OCD and phobias or other anxiety disorders. Both OCD and anxiety disorder patients have avoidant behavior, show intense subjective and autonomic responses to certain objects or situations, and respond to behavioral interventions. Many persons with OCD do in fact have simple phobias such as a fear of snakes, which may be unrelated to the content of their obsessions. Social phobia is also common in some patients with OCD who worry about public scrutiny and embarrassment.

Other disorders need to be ruled out as well. Tourette's disorder, characterized by vocal and motor tics, may coexist with OCD. Autistic disorder, a childhood disorder characterized by repetitive or stereotyped behaviors, may resemble OCD. Posttraumatic stress disorder is characterized by recurrent, intrusive, unwanted thoughts that may suggest obsessional thinking. Trichotillomania, or compulsive hair pulling, is classified as an impulse control disorder, but it has many features in common with OCD, such as an irresistible urge to pull, which is usually unsuccessfully resisted. Anorexia nervosa may also resemble OCD, because both disorders involve ritualistic behavior; however, in the anorexic patient the behavior is viewed as desirable and is rarely resisted. Some patients with anorexia nervosa will meet criteria for OCD, but in addition to rituals involving eating and food will have symptoms typical of OCD, such as frequent hand washing and checking.

Clinical Management

The treatment of OCD has traditionally been viewed as difficult and unsatisfactory. Recent developments in the treatment of OCD have changed this picture dramatically and have instilled a greater sense of optimism. The mainstays of treatment are pharmacotherapy and behavioral therapy (see box). Behavioral therapies, which tend to be more successful for ritualizers, emphasize exposure paired with response prevention. As an example, a patient might be exposed to a dreaded situation, event, or stimulus by means of a number of techniques (e.g., imaginal exposure, systematic desensitization, flooding) and then prevented from carrying out the compulsive behavior that usually results. For example, a compulsive washer may be asked to handle "contaminated" objects (e.g., a dirty tissue) and then be prevented from washing his hands. Thought-stopping techniques may be used to interrupt obsessional thoughts (e.g., the therapist may announce in a loud voice "Stop!" to interrupt the cycle of thinking). Proponents of behavioral therapies state that 60%–70% of patients who stick with the treatment have marked improvement. Unfortunately, many patients will refuse to participate in the therapy, fearing the increase in anxiety, or will drop out. (See Chapter 25 for a more detailed description of behavioral therapy.)

Pharmacotherapy has been growing in importance, primarily due to studies showing that certain antidepressant medications have clear antiobsessional properties. The first agent studied, clomipramine, a tricyclic antidepressant, is administered in doses ranging from 150 to 300 mg daily. Nearly 60% of patients receiving clomipramine experience marked or moderate improvement, although side effects may limit its usefulness. Many patients develop sedation, orthostatic hypertension, and anticholinergic side effects such as dry mouth, constipation, visual blurring, and urinary hesitancy. (See Chapter 26 for a more complete discussion of tricyclic antidepressants.) Clomipramine works well for both obsessions and compulsions, irrespective of the presence of depressive symptoms, and a range of improvement is seen. Treatment may need to be long term, because

---

Recommendations for management of obsessive-compulsive disorder

1. Educate the patient about his or her illness.
   - To reduce the patient's feelings of isolation, fear, and confusion.
   - To reassure the worried patient that people with OCD rarely act on their frightening or violent obsessions.
   - By pointing out the "up" side of OCD—that people with this disorder are usually conscientious, dependable, and likable.
   - By recommending lay literature and suggesting that they join the OCD foundation (Milford, CT).

2. Establish an empathic relationship.
   - Do not tell patients to stop their rituals. They can't. That's why they are seeing you.
   - Explain that talking about the obsessions and compulsions will not make them worse.

3. Set limited goals with behavior therapy—don't tackle all rituals at once.
   - Find out what makes the rituals worse and what alleviates them.
   - Work on rituals one at a time and start with simple goals (e.g., reducing the amount of time spent in the shower from 40 to 35 minutes).
   - It may be best to refer the patient to an experienced behavior therapist, particularly when compulsive rituals are prominent.

4. Use medication in moderate and severe cases.
   - Use clomipramine or a serotonin reuptake inhibitor (e.g., fluoxetine, paroxetine) and be patient. A full response may take months.
   - Have realistic expectations for the treatment. Understand that most patients will still have substantial symptoms after successful treatment.

5. Patient support groups, family therapy, and marital counseling may be helpful adjuncts.
   - Family therapy can be helpful in educating the family about OCD, as well as addressing other problems such as anger, guilt, and hostility. Similarly, marital therapy can be helpful when OCD has disrupted the spousal relationship.
   - Support groups can provide patients with a supportive atmosphere, where they can meet others with the disorder.

patients tend to relapse (often within weeks) when the drug is discontinued.

The serotonin reuptake inhibitors (SRIs), a relatively new group of antidepressants including fluoxetine, sertraline, paroxetine, and fluvoxamine, are antiobsessional as well. Although it is unclear what doses produce the best results, patients with OCD may need higher doses than do depressed patients (e.g., fluoxetine 60–80 mg/day, sertraline 150–200 mg/day, paroxetine 40–60 mg/day, fluvoxamine 200–300 mg/day) and may take several months to respond. Other psychoactive medications have been the subject of case reports, but it is not clear that they have any role in the treatment of OCD. There is little evidence that augmenting strategies are helpful, such as combining fluoxetine with buspirone or lithium. An exception is the addition of an antipsychotic when the patient has a schizotypal personality or a tic disorder.

In treating OCD, the clinician should be patient, because obsessive-compulsive symptoms tend to resolve slowly. Typically, patients will first notice improved mood and a reduction in their level of anxiety. Eventually, the amount of time spent obsessing or ritualizing decreases, and the patient's ability to resist these symptoms increases. Patients responding to medication can expect a 50%–70% reduction in symptoms. A medication trial should last 3 to 4 months; most improvement will have occurred by the end of the third month.

In the past, psychosurgery was reported to benefit up to 80% of patients receiving the surgery; more recent research shows that 25%–30% of treatment-refractory patients benefit from stereotactic cingulotomy, the most commonly used surgical procedure. Patients should not be referred for psychosurgery unless they fail to respond to other proven therapies. Some patients may need to have the surgery repeated, and weeks or months are typically required for optimal improvement.

Supportive psychotherapy is an important adjunct to both behavioral and pharmacological treatments. It is particularly useful in guiding rehabilitative efforts by helping to restore morale, helping with problem solving, and encouraging treatment compliance. Patients must also be encouraged to take risks, such as exposing themselves to dreaded situations.

Family therapy can also be helpful. Family members are often woefully ignorant about OCD and may be unwittingly drawn into their relative's rituals or obsessional thoughts. A mother, for example, may be asked by her son to check the house before bedtime to make sure it is safe. In the setting of family therapy, relatives can learn to accept the illness, learn to cope with its manifestations, and learn how not to perpetuate or encourage obsessive-compulsive behavior. Patient support groups are now available in many parts of the country. They are helpful in providing education about the illness, assistance in solving day-to-day problems, and an atmosphere of mutual support.

Bibliography

Baer L, Jenike MA, Black DW, et al: Effect of Axis II diagnoses on treatment outcome in 55 patients with obsessive-compulsive disorder. Arch Gen Psychiatry 49:862–866, 1992

Baxter LR, Phelps ME, Mazziotta JC, et al: Local cerebral glucose metabolism rates in obsessive-compulsive disorder. Arch Gen Psychiatry 44:211–218, 1987

Baxter LR, Schwartz JM, Bergman KS, et al: Caudate glucose metabloic rate changes with both drug and behavior therapy for obsessive-compulsive disorder. Arch Gen Psychiatry 49:681–689, 1992

Black DW, Blum NS: Obsessive-compulsive support groups: The Iowa Model. Compr Psychiatry 33:65–71, 1992

Black DW, Noyes R, Goldstein RB, Blum W: A family study of obsessive-compulsive disorder. Arch Gen Psychiatry 49:362–368, 1992

Black DW, Noyes R, Pfohl B, et al: Personality disorder in obsessive-compulsive volunteers, well comparison subjects and their first-degree relatives. Am J Psychiatry 150:1226–1232, 1993

Clomipramine Collaborative Study Group: Clomipramine in the treatment of patients with obsessive-compulsive disorder. Arch Gen Psychiatry 48:730–738, 1991

Foa EB, Wilson R: Stop Obsessing! How to Overcome Your Obsessions and Compulsions. New York, Bantam Books, 1991

Insel TR: Toward a neuroanatomy of obsessive-compulsive disorder. Arch Gen Psychiatry 49:739–744, 1992

Jenike MA, Buttolph L, Baer L, et al: Open trial of fluoxetine in obsessive-compulsive disorder. Am J Psychiatry 146:909–911, 1989

Jenike MA, Baer L, Minichiello WE: Obsessive-Compulsive Disorders, 2nd Edition. Littleton, MA, Year Book Medical Publishers, 1990

Jenike MA, Baer L, Ballantine T, et al: Cingulotomy for refractory obsessive-compulsive disorder. Arch Gen Psychiatry 48:548–555, 1991

Karno M, Golding JM, Sorenson SB, et al: The epidemiology of obsessive-compulsive disorder in five U.S. communities. Arch Gen Psychiatry 45:1094–1099, 1988

Leonard HL, Swedo SE, Lenane MC, et al: A 2- to 7-year follow-up study of 54 obsessive-compulsive children and adolescents. Arch Gen Psychiatry 50:427–439, 1993

Luxenberg JS, Swedo SE, Flament MF, et al: Neurochemical abnormalities in obsessive-compulsive disorder detected with quantitative x-ray computed tomography. Am J Psychiatry 145:1089–1093, 1988

Pato MT, Zohar-Kadouch R, Zohar T, et al: Return of symptoms after discontinuation of clomipramine in patients with obsessive-compulsive disorder. Am J Psychiatry 145:1521–1525, 1988

Perse TL, Greist JH, Jefferson JW, et al: Fluvoxamine treatment of obsessive-compulsive disorder. Am J Psychiatry 144:1543–1548, 1987

Rappoport JL: The neurobiology of obsessive-compulsive disorder. JAMA 260:2888–2890, 1988

Rappoport JL: The Boy Who Couldn't Stop Washing. New York, EP Dutton, 1989

Swedo SE, Pietrini P, Leonard HL, et al: Cerebral glucose metabolism in childhood-onset obsessive-compulsive disorder: revisualization during pharmacotherapy. Arch Gen Psychiatry 49:690–694, 1992

Tollefson GD, Rampey AH Jr, Potvin JH, et al: A multicenter investigation of fixed-dose fluoxetine in the treatment of obsessive-compulsive disorder. Arch Gen Psychiatry 51:559–567, 1994

Zohar J, Insel TR, Zohar-Kadouch RC, et al: Serotonergic responsivity in obsessive-compulsive disorder. Arch Gen Psychiatry 45:167–172, 1988

Self-Assessment Questions

1. How is OCD diagnosed?
2. What is the prevalence and gender distribution of OCD?
3. What defense mechanisms are thought to operate in OCD?
4. What evidence supports a neurobiological model?
5. What is the prognosis in OCD? What may change the prognosis of OCD in the future?
6. What is the differential diagnosis of OCD?
7. How are obsessions distinguished from delusions?
8. What are some of the behavioral techniques used to treat OCD?
9. What is the purported mechanism of action of antiobsessional medications?
10. What type of psychosurgery is occasionally performed in patients with OCD?

Chapter 12

Somatoform and Related Disorders

So it is that a patient can confront his doctor with his
symptoms, and put on him the whole onus of their cure.

Mayer-Gross, Slater, and Roth, Clinical Psychiatry

Somatoform disorders are characterized by physical complaints that occur in the absence of identifiable physical pathology. These conditions have been noted throughout recorded time and continue to baffle patients and practitioners alike. Typically, these disorders are seen by primary care physicians and other specialists, such as neurologists and cardiologists, rather than by psychiatrists. Patients with these disorders take up an extraordinary amount of the clinician's time and energy. In several studies of primary care patients, the proportion with somatic complaints for which no physical cause was detected has ranged from 10% to 30%; in specialty clinics this proportion is even higher.

There are seven somatoform disorders, which are listed in Table 12–1. These disorders share the common feature of excessive concern with bodily symptoms that is not explainable on the basis of physical or laboratory evidence.

Portions of this chapter are adapted with permission from Black DW: Somatoform disorders. Prim Care 4:711–724, 1987. Copyright 1987 W. B. Saunders Company.

Table 12–1.   DSM-IV somatoform disorders

Somatization disorder
Conversion disorder
Hypochondriasis
Pain disorder
  With psychological factors
  With both psychological factors and a general medical condition
Undifferentiated somatoform disorder
Somatoform disorder not otherwise specified

History

Although we now recognize several discrete somatoform disorders, their history has been intertwined. Somatization disorder, formerly known as *hysteria,* was recognized in the ancient world, when Greek physicians thought it resulted from a displaced uterus. Their treatment was to attract the "wandering uterus" back to its proper place by putting aromatic substances in the region of the vagina. Although Galen rejected this idea, the theory of uterine pathology persisted until Willis suggested that hysteria was caused by a disorder of the brain.

Hypochondriasis, meanwhile, is a term that derives from the Greek, having the literal meaning of "below the cartilage," referring to the area under the ribs housing various organs. The term has been used since the seventeenth century to associate changes in mental state with changes in the organs of the hypochondria, which, it was believed, led to a preoccupation with bodily symptoms. In the seventeenth century, Sydenham suggested a close relationship between hysteria and hypochondriasis, and over the next two centuries, clinicians viewed hypochondriasis as the masculine version of hysteria, which occurred mostly in females.

In the nineteenth century, Charcot, a French neurologist working at the Salpêtrière, became interested in the bizarre and baffling manifestations of hysteria. He believed that strange emotions could produce hysterical symptoms in vulnerable people. Hysteria later became Freud's main interest in the early years of psychoanalysis, his interest having developed while working in Paris with Charcot, who was treating hysteria with hypnosis. Psychoanalysts became very interested in hysteria, which they viewed as an illness designed to work out unconscious conflicts.

In their seminal book on hysteria, Freud and his associate Breuer argued that hysterical patients have emotionally charged memories stored out of reach in the unconscious mind. *Conversion* was believed to be the ego-defense mechanism responsible for converting psychic energy into bodily symptoms, thereby leading to hysteria, and was thought to give rise to both *primary gain* (i.e., the anxiety arising from a psychological conflict is kept from the patient's conscious mind) and *secondary gain* (i.e., support and sympathy from family and friends).

Over the years, the term *hysterical* was used to describe any demanding patient whose symptoms were unexplained. So many different meanings had developed that by the 1960s, a neutral term, *Briquet's syndrome,* was proposed. The term derived from the work of Paul Briquet, a French physician, who in 1859 had described hysteria as a polysymptomatic disorder. His concepts were used to develop diagnostic criteria (i.e., Briquet's checklist, developed in 1962), which were later modified for inclusion in DSM-III, DSM-III-R, and DSM-IV as somatization disorder.

Although hysteria and hypochondriasis had been thought to be similar, use of the term *hypochondriasis* became restricted to less clearly delineated complaints of pain and discomfort. It was believed that the hypochondriac was morbidly preoccupied with bodily function, unlike the hysteric, who exhibited *la belle indifférence* (i.e., a strange lack of concern with the symptoms). Freud furthered the distinction between the two disorders by classifying hypochondriasis as a true neurosis, which implied that common everyday disturbances (e.g., sexual frustration) played a role in its etiology, whereas hysteria was conceptualized as a psychoneurosis (e.g., determined by early life experiences).

The acceptance of hypochondriasis as a distinct disorder continued to wax and wane. In the early twentieth century, it was argued that hypochondriasis was a valid disorder. This view was later challenged, because patients with hypochondriacal symptoms were often felt to have other primary disorders, such as depression. Although the term has been little used and was, in fact, excluded from DSM-I, the term was restored in DSM-II and subsequent editions. Its validity as a primary disorder has still not been adequately determined.

Somatization Disorder

Somatization disorder is a malady beginning early in life, affecting mostly women. It is characterized by recurrent and multiple somatic symptoms involving most of the organ systems. The physical complaints, often dramatically described, are unexplained and typically include pain, anxiety and mood-related symptoms, gastrointestinal disturbance, and psychosexual symptoms. To fulfill the criteria for the diagnosis of somatization disorder, patients must have at least eight unexplained symptoms including four pain, two gastrointestinal, one sexual, and one pseudoneurological symptom (see Table 12–2). For symptoms to

Table 12–2.   DSM-IV criteria for somatization disorder

A. A history of many physical complaints beginning before age 30 years that occur over a period of several years and result in treatment being sought or significant impairment in social, occupational, or other important areas of functioning.

B. Each of the following criteria must have been met, with individual symptoms occurring at any time during the course of the disturbance:

   1. *Four pain symptoms:* A history of pain related to at least four different sites or functions (e.g., head, abdomen, back, joints, extremities, chest, rectum, during menstruation, during sexual intercourse, or during urination)

   2. *Two gastrointestinal symptoms:* A history of at least two gastrointestinal symptoms other than pain (e.g., nausea, diarrhea, bloating, vomiting other than during pregnancy, or intolerance of several different foods)

   3. *One sexual symptom:* A history of at least one sexual or reproductive symptom other than pain (e.g., sexual indifference, erectile or ejaculatory dysfunction, irregular menses, excessive menstrual bleeding, vomiting throughout pregnancy)

   4. *One pseudoneurological symptom:* A history of at least one symptom or deficit suggesting a neurological disorder not limited to pain (conversion symptoms such as impaired coordination or balance, paralysis or localized weakness, difficulty swallowing or lump in the throat, aphonia, urinary retention, hallucinations, loss of touch or pain sensation, double vision, blindness, deafness, seizures; dissociative symptoms such as amnesia; or loss of consciousness other than fainting)

C. Either (1) or (2):

   1. After appropriate investigation, each of the symptoms in criterion B cannot be fully explained by a known general medical condition or the direct effects of a substance (e.g., a drug of abuse, a medication)

   2. When there is a related general medical condition, the physical complaints or resulting social or occupational impairment are in excess of what would be expected from the history, physical examination, or laboratory findings

D. The symptoms are not intentionally produced or feigned (as in factitious disorder or malingering).

meet the criteria, they must not be fully explained by a general medical condition, and the complaints or impairment must be greater than would be expected from the history, physical examination, or laboratory findings. In making the diagnosis, it is useful to have old medical charts available and to interview the patient on more than one occasion. Because of their many symptoms, patients may not recall old ones and may not have sufficient time to report new symptoms in one sitting. The frequency of common symptoms in somatization disorder is summarized in Table 12–3, and complaints from a typical patient are presented in Table 12–4.

Although a simple count of symptoms appears arbitrary, several studies have shown that this approach identifies a homogeneous group of patients who have a predictable course and outcome. The diagnosis is highly reliable and stable over time. The following case example illustrates the variety and stability of symptoms found in somatization disorder:

Table 12–3. Common symptoms in somatization disorder

Symptom	%	Symptom	%
Nervousness	92	Sexual indifference	44
Back pain	88	Dysuria	44
Weakness	84	Aphonia	44
Joint pain	84	Other bodily pains	36
Dizziness	84	Vomiting	32
Extremity pain	84	Anesthesia	32
Fatigue	84	Thoughts of suicide	28
Abdominal pain	80	Burning pains in rectum, vagina,	
Nausea	80	mouth	28
Headache	80	Lump in throat	28
Dyspnea	72	Felt life was hopeless	28
Trouble doing anything because	72	Weight loss	28
of feeling bad		Anorgasmia	24
Chest pain	72	Diarrhea	20
Abdominal bloating	68	Vomiting all 9 months of pregnancy	20
Constipation	64	Blindness	20
Anxiety attacks	64	Fits of convulsions	20
Depressed feeling	64	Fluctuations in weight	16
Visual blurring	64	Unconsciousness	16
Anorexia	60	Paralysis	12
Palpitations	60	Visual hallucinations	12
Fainting	56	Attempted suicide	12
Dyspareunia	52	Amnesia	8
Menstrual irregularity	48	Urinary retention	8
Food intolerances	48	Dysmenorrhea (prepregnancy only)	8
Excessive menstrual bleeding	48	Dysmenorrhea (premarital only)	4
Dysmenorrhea (other)	48	Deafness	4
Phobias	48		

Source. Adapted from Perley MJ, Guze SB: Hysteria—the stability and usefulness of clinical criteria. N Engl J Med 266:421–426, 1962.

A 26-year-old housewife first presented for medical evaluation with a chief complaint of weakness and malaise of 1 year's duration. Other symptoms were soon unraveled: burning pain in her eyes, muscular aches and pains in her lower back, headaches, a stiff neck, abdominal pain "on both sides and below the navel," and vomiting "glassy white stuff—as if I were poisoned." Nine months earlier she had been hospitalized for evaluation of the abdominal pain and had a barium enema examination and upper gastrointestinal X-ray series, both negative.

Table 12–4. Complaints from a typical somatization disorder patient

Organ system	Complaint
Neuropsychiatric	"The two hemispheres of my brain aren't working properly." "I couldn't name familiar objects around the house when asked." "I was hospitalized with tingling and numbness all over and the doctors didn't know why."
Cardiopulmonary	"I had extreme dizziness after climbing stairs." "It hurts to breathe." "My heart was racing and pounding and thumping. . . . I thought I was going to die."
Gastrointestinal	"For 10 years I was treated for nervous stomach, spastic colon, and gall bladder and nothing the doctor did seemed to help." "I got a violent cramp after eating an apple and felt terrible the next day." "The gas was awful—I thought I was going to explode."
Genitourinary	"I'm not interested in sex, but I pretend to be to satisfy my husband's needs." "I've had red patches on my labia and I was told to use boric acid." "I had difficulty with bladder control and was examined for a tipped bladder, but nothing was found." "I had nerves cut going into my uterus because of severe cramps."
Musculoskeletal	"I have learned to live with weakness and tiredness all the time." "I thought I pulled a back muscle, but my chiropractor says it's a disk problem."
Sensory	"My vision is blurry. It's like seeing through a fog, but the doctor said glasses wouldn't help." "I suddenly lost my hearing. It came back, but now I have whistling noises, like an echo."
Metabolic/ endocrine	"I began teaching half days because I couldn't tolerate the cold." "I was losing hair faster than my husband."

Six months before her clinic visit she had developed blurry vision and a sharp shooting pain in her rectum with walking, and she had noted passing blood and mucus in her stools. Sigmoidoscopic examinations were unremarkable, but she was nevertheless diagnosed as having mild ulcerative colitis and was treated with azulfidine. Another barium enema examination was negative. Five months before her clinic visit she noted "wasting" of her hands and reported needing a larger glove size for the right hand, where she had noticed a pulsating vessel and whitish nodules for the first time.

Other medical complaints developed, including joint pains, malaise, blotching and red spots on her skin in response to sun exposure, and swelling of her right ankle, both knees, elbows, wrists, and shoulders. She began to notice multiple bruises that were slow to heal. Three months before her clinic visit a physician diagnosed rheumatoid arthritis despite a normal sedimentation rate and administered injections of cortisone and corticotropin, which did not help. At her clinic visit she identified other symptoms, including a burning pain in her pelvis, hands, and feet; heavy vaginal bleeding passing "clots as large as a fist"; abdominal bloating; malodorous stools with "bits of sudsy mucus"; urinary urgency; cough incontinence; tingling and burning in hands and feet; and a belief that her bowel movements "just don't look right." She also disclosed a 10-year history of recurrent tonsillitis and quinsy during her childhood.

She was next seen at the same clinic 21 years later, after referral by her primary care physician for evaluation of multiple somatic complaints. Her symptoms were remarkably similar to those reported earlier, and it soon became clear that she had never been free of them. Her main complaint was a right-sided tremor that caused her to spill food. She also reported migratory aches and pains, feeling cold in her extremities, and heavy menstrual flow: "I used 48 sanitary pads in a single day." In addition, she noted feeling sick, abdominal bloating, flatulence, frequent nausea and vomiting, constipation, her skin becoming darker, and her scalp hair falling out.

A protracted medical workup followed, including thyroid function studies, a thyroid uptake scan, rheumatoid factor, antinuclear antibody titer, electromyography, and consultations from neurology, ophthalmology, and gynecology. She reported to the neurologist a history of convulsions 10 years earlier, which she believed left her with a residual tremor. Several years later she had experienced episodes of weakness, headache, and nausea and vomiting that would wax and wane over the following 2 years. She reported having been concerned with her face sagging, which had alerted a previous neurologist to consider the diagnosis of myasthenia gravis. The ophthalmologist obtained a history of double vision and discovered that she had had six changes in her eyeglass prescription during the past year because of deteriorating vision. She confirmed a history of heavy and painful bleeding to the gynecologist and also a history of five dilation and curettage procedures during the previous 10 years. She also complained of a yellowish discharge during the last 4 days of her cycle that had an "odor of semen."

Six years later she was admitted to a psychiatric hospital. She had had a total hysterectomy and oophorectomy in the interim, but apart from menstrually related symptoms, she continued to have the same unrelenting physical complaints. Again, a protracted medical workup was negative.

This woman's remarkable history of illness spanning 27 years leaves little doubt that she had an unrecognized somatization disorder. Her complaints were consistent over the years and had resulted in multiple evaluations and procedures. Despite the multiplicity of complaints, many quite alarming, the patient remained fit and physically healthy.

In the Epidemiologic Catchment Area study, somatization disorder was shown to have a lifetime prevalence of about 0.4% in the general population. The disorder is more common in rural areas and among the educationally deprived; many female patients report a history of sexual molestation as children. Few patients experience significant improvement or complete remission of symptoms.

Unfortunately, somatization disorder often leads to repeated surgeries, drug abuse, marital instability, depression, and suicide attempts. Most patients with somatization disorder also have personality disorders; between one-half and two-thirds meet criteria for histrionic personality.

Somatization disorder is probably hereditary and is found in about 20% of the first-degree female relatives of patients with somatization disorder. Family studies also show a link between somatization disorder and antisocial personality. First-degree male relatives of patients with somatization disorder have high rates of both antisocial personality and alcoholism. These findings have led to the observation that depending on the gender of the individual, underlying genetic or environmental factors may lead to different, but overlapping, clinical manifestations.

The differential diagnosis includes other psychiatric syndromes such as panic disorder, major depression, and schizophrenia. The panic patient typically has many physical symptoms, but they occur almost exclusively during panic attacks. The depressed patient may have physical complaints, but they are usually overshadowed by dysphoria and prominent vegetative symptoms of depression (e.g., appetite loss, lack of energy, insomnia). Schizophrenic patients often have physical complaints, but they are typically delusional (e.g., "my spine is a set of twirling plates"). Although somatic complaints are common to these disorders, the syndromes are sufficiently distinctive that diagnosis should not be difficult.

Conversion Disorder

According to DSM-IV, conversion disorder involves symptoms or deficits affecting motor or sensory functions that suggest a neurological or general medical condition; pain is not included in the definition. Further, the physician has determined that the symptom is not under voluntary control and cannot, after appropriate investigation, be explained by a known neurological or general medical condition. Psychological factors are judged to be associated with the symptom, as suggested by its initiation or exacerbation after stressful situations. Further, the symptom must not be intentionally produced or feigned, and it is not a culturally sanctioned behavior or experience. The complete criteria are listed in Table 12–5.

Typical conversion symptoms include paralysis, abnormal movements, inability to speak (aphonia), blindness, and deafness. Conversion symptoms usually conform to the patient's concept of disease rather than to typical physiological patterns. For example, anesthesia may follow a stocking-and-glove pattern, not a dermatomal distribution. Symptoms may occur in isolation, but generally

Table 12–5. DSM-IV criteria for conversion disorder

A. One or more symptoms or deficits affecting voluntary motor or sensory function that suggest a neurological or general medical condition.

B. Psychological factors are judged to be associated with the symptom or deficit because the initiation or exacerbation of the symptom or deficit is preceded by conflicts or other stressors.

C. The symptom or deficit is not intentionally produced or feigned (as in factitious disorder or malingering).

D. The symptom or deficit cannot, after appropriate investigation, be fully explained by a neurological or general medical condition, or by the direct effects of a substance, or as a culturally sanctioned behavior or experience.

E. The symptom or deficit causes clinically significant distress or impairment in social, occupational, or other important areas of functioning or warrants medical evaluation.

F. The symptom or deficit is not limited to pain or sexual dysfunction, does not occur exclusively during the course of somatization disorder, and is not better accounted for by another mental disorder.

Specify type of symptom or deficit:

With motor symptom or deficit
With sensory symptom or deficit
With seizures or convulsions
With mixed presentation

occur within the context of a primary illness (e.g., major depression, somatization disorder, schizophrenia). When a conversion disorder occurs along with another disorder, both diagnoses are made.

An estimated 20%–25% of patients admitted to general medical services have had conversion symptoms at some time during their lives. In a survey of consecutive psychiatric consultations in a general hospital, 5% of patients were found to have conversion symptoms. Conversion symptoms are more common in women than men, in patients from rural areas, and in persons having low socioeconomic status.

Psychodynamic, biological, cultural, and behavioral mechanisms have been invoked to explain conversion symptoms. According to psychodynamic interpretations, patients with certain developmental predispositions respond to particular types of stress with conversion symptoms. The stress causes anxiety by awakening unconscious conflicts, usually over issues involving sexuality, aggression, or dependency. The high frequency of conversion symptoms in patients with a history of brain injury, however, argues for a biological etiology. The predisposition of various ethnic and social (generally non-European) groups to respond to emotional stress with conversion of symptoms illustrates the sociocultural contributions to etiology. Behaviorists have explained conversion symptoms as a learned excess or deficit that follows a particular event or psychological state and is reinforced by a particular event or set of conditions.

The diagnosis of conversion disorder is established by ruling out medical or neurological illness as a cause of the symptoms, as well as demonstrating the presence of psychological factors involved in the initiation or exacerbation of the symptom. It is usually not difficult to rule out medical illness when a patient's physical symptoms are inconsistent with physical findings and the psychological stress is unmistakable. The diagnosis needs to be made with caution, however, because up to 30% of patients diagnosed with conversion disorder are later found to have a medical or neurological illness that in retrospect accounts for the symptom. Further, many patients who receive a diagnosis of conversion disorder also have a history of a brain injury or illness. A study of psychiatric patients in Australia and Great Britain who had received a diagnosis of conversion hysteria found that 63.5% of patients, but only 5.5% of control subjects, had coexisting or antecedent brain disorders such as epilepsy, tumor, or stroke.

There are many useful clues that the clinician can use to help establish a diagnosis of conversion. Studies of patients with conversion symptoms indicate a high prevalence of comorbidity with major depression, somatization disorder, schizophrenia, and various personality disorders. Thus, an unexplained symptom in a patient with a serious psychiatric disorder or a prior history of conversion symptoms is likely to represent a new conversion symptom. Patients sometimes model symptoms based on their experience with a prior illness or model them on the symptoms of an illness experienced by an important figure in their life (e.g., a figure from childhood).

Several psychological factors that were once thought to be helpful in distinguishing conversion symptoms from genuine medical or neurological illness have not been confirmed by research. These include emotional stress before the onset of symptoms, a history of disturbed sexuality, sibling position, the presence of primary gain, the presence of secondary gain, the presence of histrionic personality, and *la belle indifférence*. Most patients with conversion symptoms do not have any specific personality type. Further, most patients with conversion symptoms do not show *la belle indifférence*. Instead, they are deeply interested in their symptoms.

Favorable prognosis is generally associated with acute onset, definite precipitation by a stressful event, good premorbid health, and the absence of medical or neurological comorbidity or a major psychiatric disorder. Among favorable prognostic studies, one found that 83% of inpatients and outpatients were well or improved at a 4- to 6-year follow-up; in another, 100% of outpatients with conversion symptoms had an immediate favorable response to treatment, with only 20% experiencing a relapse at the end of a 1-year follow-up. Other studies have had less optimistic findings. One study from Britain noted that of 85 patients, 4 committed suicide, and of 60 patients still alive, 82% had a brain disorder, schizophrenia, a mood disorder, or severely disabling conversion symptoms. Because conversion disorder rarely occurs as an isolated event and usually occurs in the context of another disorder, it is likely that the outcome reflects the natural history of the primary disorder, such as major depression, somatization disorder, or schizophrenia.

Hypochondriasis

Hypochondriasis is defined as a preoccupation with fears of having a serious disease, based on a person's misinterpretation of bodily symptoms. This preoccupation persists after an appropriate medical evaluation has ruled out the presence of a physical disorder that could account for the symptoms; further, other mental disorders such as schizophrenia, major depression, or somatization disorder have been ruled out as a cause of the disturbance. Hypochondriasis has a duration of 6 months or more. See Table 12–6 for the complete set of criteria.

Hypochondriacal patients display an abnormal concern with their health and tend to amplify normal physiological sensations and misinterpret them as indicators of disease. These patients often fear a particular disease such as cancer or the acquired immunodeficiency syndrome (AIDS) and cannot be reassured despite careful and repeated examinations. The following description illustrates a typical case of hypochondriasis seen in our hospital:

Table 12–6. DSM-IV criteria for hypochondriasis

A. Preoccupation with fears of having, or the idea that one has, a serious disease based on the person's misinterpretation of bodily symptoms.

B. The preoccupation persists despite appropriate medical evaluation and reassurance.

C. The belief in criterion A is not of delusional intensity (as in delusional disorder, somatic type) and is not restricted to a circumscribed concern about appearance (as in body dysmorphic disorder).

D. The preoccupation causes clinically significant distress or impairment in social, occupational, or other important areas of functioning.

E. The duration of the disturbance is at least 6 months.

F. The preoccupation does not occur exclusively during the course of generalized anxiety disorder, obsessive-compulsive disorder, panic disorder, a major depressive episode, separation anxiety, or another somatoform disorder.

Specify if:

With poor insight: if, for most of the time during the current episode, the person does not recognize that the concern about having a serious illness is excessive or unreasonable.

Mabel, an 80-year-old retired school teacher, was admitted for evaluation of an 8-month preoccupation with having colon cancer. The patient had a history of single vessel coronary artery disease and diabetes mellitus controlled by oral hypoglycemic agents, but was otherwise well. There was no history of mental illness. On admission, Mabel reported her concern about having colon cancer like her two brothers. As evidence of possible cancer, she reported having mild diffuse abdominal pain and cited an abnormal barium enema examination that she had had a year earlier. (The examination revealed diverticulosis.) Because of her concern about having cancer, Mabel had seen 11 physicians, but each in turn had been unable to reassure her that she did not have cancer.

Despite her complaint, Mabel denied depressed mood, displayed a full affect, and appeared to enjoy life. She reported sleeping less than usual, but she attributed this to her abdominal discomfort.

At the hospital, Mabel was pleasant and cooperative, but she chose not to socialize with other patients, whom she characterized as "crazy." She continued to be preoccupied with the possibility that she had cancer despite our reassurance. A benzodiazepine was prescribed for her sleep disturbance, but she refused any other type of psychiatric treatment.

Despite the popularity of the term *hypochondriasis* and the frequency with which physicians see patients with unexplained physical symptoms, not much is known about the disorder. Unlike somatization disorder, which starts early in life and affects mostly women, hypochondriasis may begin at any age (but peaks in the middle years) and may be equally common in males and females. There usually is no precipitating stressor. The prevalence of hypochondriasis in the general population is unknown, but between 60% and 80% of healthy individuals have unexplained somatic symptoms in any given week; intermittent worry about illness occurs in about 10%–20% of psychiatrically normal persons and in about 45% of psychiatric outpatients. Although most patients can be reassured by physicians that their symptoms are benign, many will doubt the physician's reassurance.

Like patients with somatization disorder, hypochondriacal patients may have complaints involving most organ systems, doctor-shop, receive many evaluations and unnecessary surgery, and become addicted to drugs as a result of their ongoing physical complaints. The distinction between hypochondriasis and somatization disorder rests on age at onset and the number of symptoms that a patient reports.

Like conversion symptoms, hypochondriacal symptoms may occur in the course of psychotic, mood, or anxiety disorder, all of which need to be ruled out. When they occur in the course of another illness, such as panic disorder, treatment of the primary disorder will often lead to a reduction of hypochondriacal symptoms. When hypochondriasis is the primary disorder, remission appears un-likely, and a waxing and waning course is typical.

One particular form of hypochondriasis, *illness phobia*, may respond to anti-depressant medication. Patients with illness phobia have an unreasonable fear that they have a specific or serious illness. A study of 14 patients showed that imipramine was an effective treatment.

Pain Disorder

Pain in one or more anatomic sites is the major symptom in pain disorder, and psychological factors are believed to have an important role in its etiology (see Table 12–7 for the criteria). Two subtypes are specified: pain associated with psychological factors and pain associated with psychological factors and a gen-eral medical condition. The disorder is termed *acute* if the duration is less than 6 months and *chronic* if the duration is 6 months or more. Some researchers be-lieve that pain disorder is a conversion symptom. Among pain patients, pain is

Table 12–7.   DSM-IV criteria for pain disorder

A. Pain in one or more anatomical sites is the predominant focus of the clinical presentation and is of sufficient severity to warrant clinical attention.

B. The pain causes clinically significant distress or impairment in social, occupational, or other important areas of functioning.

C. Psychological factors are judged to have an important role in the onset, severity, exacerbation, or maintenance of the pain.

D. The symptom or deficit is not intentionally produced or feigned (as in factitious disorder or malingering).

E. The pain is not better accounted for by a mood, anxiety, or psychotic disorder and does not meet criteria for dyspareunia.

Code as follows:

Pain disorder associated with psychological factors: psychological factors are judged to have a major role in the onset, severity, exacerbation, or maintenance of the pain. (If a general medical condition is present, it does not have a major role in the onset, severity, exacerbation, or maintenance of the pain.) This type of pain disorder is not diagnosed if criteria are also met for somatization disorder.

Pain disorder associated with both psychological factors and a general medical condition: both psychological factors and a general medical condition are judged to have important roles in the onset, severity, exacerbation, or maintenance of the pain. The associated general medical condition or anatomical site of the pain (see below) is coded on Axis III.

Specify if:

Acute: duration of less than 6 months
Chronic: duration of 6 months or more

often related to environmental stress, such as the breakup of a relationship, and it generally occurs in the absence of identifiable medical or neurological illness or is grossly out of proportion to that expected from the physical pathology. A patient seen in our clinic illustrates this disorder.

> Nancy, a 34-year-old school teacher, developed disabling lower back pain coincidental to a work-related lawsuit in which she alleged unfair treatment by her coworkers. She attributed the back pain to a trivial fall 6 months earlier in which she had twisted her ankle; extensive neurological and orthopedic workups had failed to document any physiological abnormality. She became preoccupied by her back pain, had to quit working, and joined a support group for persons who have chronic pain.

Patients with these disorders are more commonly seen by internists and general practitioners because their complaints are physical, and psychiatric symptoms, such as depressed mood, are often denied.

Pain disorders have been explained by psychoanalysts as a defect in ego functioning underlying the experience and expression of feelings. They believe that psychologically stressful events are converted into somatic symptoms rather than allowing the individual to develop and elaborate appropriate emotions. The inability to express emotion is called *alexithymia* and is thought to underlie other neurotic symptoms such as somatization, anxiety, dissociation, and conversion.

Unexplained pain often occurs in the course of other psychiatric disorders, such as schizophrenia, somatization disorder, and major depression. In one report, 60% of depressed patients had subjective complaints of pain when asked. On the other hand, depression frequently accompanies chronic pain, although most pain patients do not have fulminant vegetative symptoms of depression. Therefore, the clinician must take care to determine whether a major depression is also present in the patient with a pain disorder. If present, the depression may respond well to antidepressants, and the subjective experience of pain may also be reduced.

Other Somatoform Disorders

There are three residual categories in DSM-IV for patients who do not clearly manifest the characteristics of the four major somatoform disorders; these categories are body dysmorphic disorder, undifferentiated somatoform disorder, and somatoform disorder not otherwise specified.

A patient with *body dysmorphic disorder* is usually preoccupied with an imagined defect in appearance rather than having diffuse complaints involving multiple organ systems; this condition is often called *dysmorphophobia*. Patients believe that they have a serious disease on the basis of a minor local lesion such as a freckle on a nose. Patients who focus on perceived defects in their facial appearance may seek plastic surgery. This condition needs to be differentiated from *monohypochondriacal paranoia* (delusional disorder, somatic type), in which a patient has the delusional belief that a body part, such as the nose, is grossly deformed or distorted. In body dysmorphic disorder, the patient is not delusional and is willing to acknowledge the possibility that the perceived defect is trivial. In some cases, body dysmorphic disorder has been shown to respond to serotonin reuptake inhibitors (SRIs) such as fluoxetine.

The following case example is of a patient seen in our clinic.

Arthur first began to think of his face as a problem when he was a senior in high school. He noticed that when his face was in repose, his brows would droop over his eyes and give him a "devious look." He also noticed that his jawline seemed weak and receding. He tried to camouflage these "defects" by keeping his lower jaw jutted forward and his eyebrows raised. His attempts at camouflage became almost habitual, but he consulted a surgeon to obtain a jaw augmentation and have his eyebrows raised because he felt that the camouflaging made him self-conscious and decreased his spontaneity. He did not feel the cosmetic surgery would materially affect his work or social life.

Arthur was a very good student in high school, participated in a few activities, and dated occasionally. He had not had a close relationship with a girl and had not had sexual intercourse. He described a brief "bad period" in high school during which he rebelled against family standards, quit studying, and smoked marijuana. After several months of this behavior, he began to feel depressed, apathetic, guilt ridden, and paranoid. He did not have a full set of depressive symptoms, nor did he have any delusions or hallucinations, and the episode passed when he stopped rebelling and smoking marijuana. He returned readily to his usual life-style. He completed 1 year of college but then dropped out to work to obtain money for cosmetic surgery. After the surgery was completed, he planned to return to college and perhaps go to medical school and pursue a career in psychiatry.

The patient was actually a rather handsome young man with heavy, dark eyebrows, but a perfectly normal, perhaps even prominent, jawline. He related his motivation for seeking surgery to his general pattern of pursuing perfection in all aspects of life. He considered himself well adjusted and normal, in fact, superior to most people. He saw no need for psychiatric treatment and refused a recommendation for a trial of SRIs.

The diagnosis of *undifferentiated somatoform disorder* is reserved for patients who have one or more physical complaints that are not explained by a known general medical condition or pathophysiological mechanism and that last at least 6 months, but who do not meet criteria for another somatoform disorder. The category *somatoform disorder not otherwise specified* is reserved for somatoform symptoms that do not meet criteria for a more specific disorder. Because these three residual categories are relatively new, information about their frequency and course is not available.

Clinical Management of the Somatoform Disorders

The development of effective treatments has caused a minor revolution in contemporary psychiatric practice, particularly for patients with psychotic, mood, or anxiety disorders. The same cannot be said of patients with somatoform disorders. The fundamental management of patients with these disorders has not changed substantially in the past 25 years. However, physicians are now more aware of these disorders and recognize that simple measures can have a profound impact on the care and treatment of patients who have these disorders.

Recommendations for the treatment of somatization disorder, hypochondriasis, and somatoform pain disorder are similar. There is general agreement on treatment approaches among experienced clinicians. These recommended approaches are not based on controlled clinical trials, but on everyday experience. First, it is essential the physician follow the Hippocratic oath and "do no harm."

Recommendations for management of somatoform disorders

1. Schedule the patient for brief but frequent visits.
   - As the patient improves, the time between visits can be extended.
2. Establish an empathic relationship to reduce the patient's tendency to doctor-shop.
   - Try to be the patient's only physician.
3. Focus on psychosocial problems, not the physical symptoms.
   - Don't try to talk patients out of their symptoms or tell them it is "all in their head."
   - To the patient, the symptom is real and distressing.
4. Minimize the use of psychotropic drugs.
   - No medication has proven value in somatoform disorders.
   - These patients may tend to become dependent on drugs easily, particularly sedative-hypnotics.
5. Minimize medical evaluations to reduce expense as well as iatrogenic complications.
   - Simple (i.e., conservative) management is proven to reduce costs.

Somatoform disorders often lead to repeated evaluations, surgeries, and medication that may have little or no relevance to the underlying disorder. Because symptoms may be exaggerated or misidentified (e.g., minor spotting during the menses may be reported as "gushing"), physicians may overreact and pursue the diagnostic equivalent of a wild goose chase. Therefore, it is essential that physicians who encounter patients with multiple unexplained symptoms make a proper diagnosis. The nonpsychiatric physician may find a psychiatric consultation to be extremely helpful in pinpointing the diagnosis and in helping to formulate treatment plans. A proper diagnosis and treatment plan will help to place the patient's symptoms in context so that unnecessary evaluations and surgeries will be avoided.

Second, it is important to see patients at regular intervals so that they will not need to acquire new symptoms to see a physician. The purpose of the visit is to listen attentively and respond to historical data without inquiring in detail about the physical symptoms reported. By avoiding placing the focus on symptoms, the physician is able to convey the message that physical complaints are not the most important or interesting thing about the patient. It is advisable to set specific appointments at brief intervals.

Third, it is important to minimize the use of psychotropic agents and prescription analgesics. Somatoform patients often request medications, but there is usually little indication for them. Whether medication is ever justified, particularly as these patients are at risk for substance abuse, is debatable. There are almost no data to show that medication is beneficial in treating either somatization disorder or hypochondriasis; therefore, medication is not indicated unless another psychiatric syndrome develops that may be amenable to treatment (e.g., major depression).

Depression is common in these patients, but there are few empirical data about the effectiveness of antidepressants in somatoform disorders. In general, depressions that occur secondary to other psychiatric disorders do not respond well to antidepressant medication; therefore, physicians should not have unrealistically high expectations for the treatment. There is some evidence that pain disorders may be relieved by antidepressant medication, but more careful research is needed. Occasionally, somatoform patients will develop an anxiety syndrome such as generalized anxiety disorder and benefit from the short-term use of a benzodiazepine (e.g., diazepam, alprazolam). Because of the potential for abuse of benzodiazepines, their use should be sharply limited and closely monitored. Ground rules need to be established from the outset so that the patient is aware that the anxiolytic therapy is considered temporary.

Finally, it is important to realize that the lives of patients with these disorders revolve around their symptoms and that patients are highly resistant to referral for psychiatric treatment. Thus, the most important therapeutic approach available to the primary physician is a sound long-term doctor-patient relationship. Ideally, he or she should become the patient's primary and only physician. These patients have a tendency to doctor-shop, which only leads to more evaluations, greater expense, and the possibility of iatrogenic complications.

These simple measures (see box) have been demonstrated to lower health care costs in patients with somatization disorder. A group of patients receiving a psychiatric consultation with recommendations for conservative care (i.e., essentially these five measures) experienced a 53% drop in health care costs, mostly due to fewer hospitalizations. There was no change in the patients' health status or satisfaction with their health care. Health care costs of control subjects did not change.

Systematic treatment of conversion symptoms has not been well established, but reassurance and suggestion are usually appropriate, along with efforts to resolve any stressful situation that may have provoked the reaction. The spontaneous remission rate for individual conversion symptoms is high, so that even without intervention most patients will improve and not have any serious complications. A treatment using behavioral modification has been described in which the patient is placed at complete bed rest with the use of a bedpan and is informed that use of ward facilities will parallel his or her improvement. As the patient improves, the time out of bed is gradually increased until full privileges are restored. Nearly all patients (84%) who had conversion symptoms ranging from blindness to bilateral wrist drop experienced full remission. By allowing the patient to save face, this method may have the advantage of keeping secondary gain (e.g., escaping from noxious activities, obtaining desired attention from family, friends, and others) to a minimum and reducing the opportunity for acting out.

In treating the conversion disorder patient, hospital staff should remain supportive and demonstrate concern while encouraging self-help. It may be explained to the patient that the disorder is caused by psychological factors. It is rarely helpful to confront patients about their symptoms or make them feel ashamed or embarrassed. To them, their pain, weakness, or whatever is experienced is quite real, and it may be helpful for the physician to communicate awareness of this as he or she explains that the treatment will be conservative and will stress rehabilitation rather than medication.

Some experts believe that hypnosis or intravenous amobarbital sodium (e.g., the "Amytal interview") may help the patient to relive the events that provoked the conversion symptoms and to abreact (or express) accompanying emotions. Psychodynamically oriented clinicians have recommended insight-oriented psychotherapy, focusing on childhood sexual behavior and other problems that they believe central to the etiology of conversion. These techniques, however, have not proven to be any more effective than conservative approaches.

The patient with hypochondriasis may additionally benefit from individual psychotherapy that involves education about illness and selective perception of symptoms. Cognitive techniques that help to correct misinterpretations of internal stimuli are reported to be helpful. Some experts have noted the similarity between hypochondriasis and obsessive-compulsive disorder (i.e., the hypochondriacal person is obsessed with fearful thoughts of having a dreaded disease and may feel compelled to check with friends and physicians to confirm its presence or absence). On the basis of these observations, cases have been reported in which SRI antidepressants that are effective in treating obsessive-compulsive disorder were also effective in treating hypochondriasis. Additional study is now warranted based on these reports.

Related Disorders

There are several conditions related to the somatoform disorders in which physical illnesses are mimicked. In DSM-IV, factitious disorders and malingering are categorized separately from somatoform disorders. Another common clinical syndrome, *compensation neurosis*, does not appear in DSM-IV, but it is discussed briefly because of its clinical importance.

Factitious Disorders

Factitious disorders result in the intentional production or feigning of physical or psychological symptoms. Patients with these disturbances presumably have a psychological need to assume the sick role, as evidenced by the lack of external incentives for the behavior, such as economic gain, better care, or improved physical well-being. Thus, patients with factitious disorders knowingly fake physical or emotional illnesses for reasons that are presumably unconscious. The criteria are listed in Table 12–8.

Many persons with the disorder appear to make hospitalization a way of life and have been called "hospital hobos" or "peregrinating problem patients." The term *Munchausen syndrome* has also been applied to this condition to describe the disorder of the patient who moves from hospital to hospital simulating a variety of illnesses. The name Munchausen comes from the fictitious peregrinations of the nineteenth-century Baron Von Munchausen, who was known for his tall tales and fanciful exaggeration. Cases of Munchausen syndrome by proxy have even been noted: a parent repeatedly induces illness or simulates illness in his or

Table 12–8.   DSM-IV criteria for factitious disorders

A. Intentional production or feigning of physical or psychological signs or symptoms.

B. The motivation for the behavior is to assume the sick role.

C. External incentives for the behavior (such as economic gain, avoiding legal responsibility, or improving physical well-being, as in malingering) are absent.

Code based on type:

With predominantly psychological signs and symptoms: if psychological signs and symptoms predominate in the clinical presentation.

With predominantly physical signs and symptoms: if physical signs and symptoms predominate in the clinical presentation.

With combined psychological and physical signs and symptoms: if both psychological and physical signs and symptoms are present but neither predominates in the clinical presentation.

---

her child so that the child is repeatedly hospitalized.

The incidence of factitious disorder is unknown because many cases probably go undetected. However, in one study involving fever of unknown origin, up to 10% of the fevers were diagnosed as factitious. Factitious symptoms can occur in almost any organ system, and the variety of symptoms produced is limited only by the imagination of the patient. Patients with factitious disorders will generally use one of three strategies: 1) report symptoms suggesting an illness, without having them; 2) present false evidence of an illness (e.g., a factitious fever produced by applying friction to a thermometer to raise the temperature); or 3) intentionally produce symptoms of illness (e.g., by injecting feces into a knee joint or taking warfarin orally to induce a bleeding disorder). Common methods for producing a factitious disorder are presented in Table 12–9.

Although most cases of factitious disorder involve the simulation of physical illness, patients sometimes feign mental illness. This form of factitious disorder is apparently less common, and its diagnosis can be extremely difficult, due in part to the lack of objective physical or laboratory abnormalities in psychiatric illness. Patients may report depression, delusions, or auditory hallucinations, or they may behave in a bizarre manner—all in an attempt to simulate mental illness. In a follow-up of nine patients with factitious psychosis, patients remained emotionally disturbed and had poor social functioning. All patients had severe personality disorders.

Studies suggest that factitious disorder is a chronic condition that starts early in adulthood in persons who may have had prior experience with hospitalization or severe illness, either involving themselves or someone close to them, such as a parent. The disorder causes severe impairment of social and occupational functioning, because these patients spend a great deal of time in the hospital. Facti-

Table 12–9. Methods used to produce factitious disorders in 41 patients

Method	%
Injection or insertion of contaminated substance	29
Surreptitious use of medications	24
Exacerbation of wounds	17
Thermometer manipulation	10
Urinary tract manipulation	7
Falsification of medical history	7
Self-induced bruises or deformities	2
Phlebotomy	2

Source. Adapted from Reich P, Gottfried LA: Factitious disorders in a teaching hospital. Ann Intern Med 99:240–247, 1983.

tious disorders have been associated with severe personality disorders, such as borderline or antisocial personality. In one study, the majority of patients had worked in medically related occupations, including medicine, nursing, and medical technology. Most had a variety of abnormal personality traits, but none was diagnosed as having a major mental disorder (i.e., Axis I disorder). Ninety-three percent were women.

Some experts believe that the patient with a factitious disorder consciously produces the signs or symptoms of physical illness to obtain medical care. Although patients are aware of their role in producing signs and symptoms of illness, they are typically unaware of their motivation for having done so. Only psychological inference may give us clues as to what these motivations are. Some investigators believe that these patients may have a personal history of emotional deprivation coupled with absent or inattentive parents, but find love and caring from health care givers. Therefore, by producing genuine illness, patients may recreate the nurturing atmosphere that they had experienced earlier. However, not all patients with factitious disorders have a background of deprivation, so these theories can apply to only a minority of patients.

The differentiation of factitious disorder from somatoform disorders and malingering, based on presumed psychological mechanisms, is presented in Table 12–10.

Diagnosis of factitious illnesses requires almost as much inventiveness as is displayed by the patient in producing symptoms. Clues to the diagnosis will include a long and involved medical history that does not correspond to the patient's apparent health and vigor, a clinical presentation that too closely resembles textbook descriptions, a sophisticated medical vocabulary, demands for specific medications or treatments, and a history of excessive surgeries. When

Table 12–10. Differentiating among the somatoform disorders, factitious disorders, and malingering

Disorder	Mechanism of illness production	Motivation for illness production
Somatization disorder	Unconscious	Unconscious
Conversion disorder	Unconscious	Unconscious
Hypochondriasis	Unconscious	Unconscious
Pain disorder	Unconscious	Unconscious
Factitious disorder	Conscious	Unconscious
Malingering	Conscious	Conscious

Source.   Adapted from Eisendrath SJ: Factitious illness: a clarification. Psychosomatics 25:110-117, 1984.

factitious disorder is suspected, previous hospital charts should be gathered and prior clinicians spoken to. In one case reported in the literature, the authors were able to document at least 15 different hospitalizations in a 2-year period before admission, and they learned that the medical evaluations had led to repeated cardiac catheterizations and angiograms and had also resulted in the complication of the loss of a limb. In this particular patient, clues to the diagnosis included the manner in which the patient presented his story, the absence of family or friends at the hospital, the presence of multiple surgical scars, and the absence of distress despite complaints of crushing retrosternal pain.

Treatment of patients with factitious disorder is difficult and frustrating. The first task in treatment is identifying the illness as factitious, so that additional and potentially harmful procedures are avoided. Because most of these patients are hospitalized on medical and surgical wards, a psychiatric consultation should be sought. The psychiatrist can assist with the diagnosis and help to educate the physicians and nurses about the nature of factitious disorders. Once sufficient evidence has been gathered to support the diagnosis, the patient should be confronted, preferably in a nonthreatening manner by the attending physician and the psychiatrist. In a follow-up of 42 patients, 33 patients were confronted; none signed out of the hospital or became suicidal, and although only 13 patients acknowledged causing their disorders, most improved after the confrontation, and 4 became asymptomatic. It is difficult to know, however, how extensive the improvement was or how long it lasted. The authors reported that their lawyers had advised that room searches could be justified legally and ethically in their pursuit of a diagnosis, just as a search would be justified in the case of the patient who was thought to be suicidal. In either situation, the condition could be life threatening.

Malingering

DSM-IV classifies malingering with the V-code conditions, which are not attributable to mental illness but are a focus of attention or treatment. Malingering is defined as the intentional production of false or grossly exaggerated physical or psychological symptoms, motivated by external incentives, such as avoiding military conscription or duty, avoiding work, obtaining financial compensation, evading criminal prosecution, obtaining drugs, or securing better living conditions.

Unlike factitious disorder, where symptoms are produced for presumably unconscious reasons, malingering is produced intentionally for reasons that are generally apparent to the malingerer. Although the prevalence of malingering is not known, most malingerers are likely to be male, and most have obvious reasons to feign illness, such as prisoners, factory workers, or persons in other unpleasant settings where illness may provide a temporary escape from harsh responsibilities.

Malingering should be strongly suspected if any combination of the following is noted: medicolegal context of presentation (e.g., the person is being referred by his or her attorney for examination), a marked discrepancy between the person's claimed disability and the objective findings, lack of cooperation during the diagnostic evaluation and noncompliance with the treatment regimen, or the presence of antisocial personality disorder. The patient suspected of malingering should be thoroughly evaluated because most symptoms that patients report will be vague and unverifiable.

There is some debate about the correct approach to the malingerer. Some experts believe that the malingerer should be confronted after sufficient evidence has been collected to confirm the diagnosis, whereas others feel that confrontations will simply disrupt the doctor-patient relationship and make the patient even more vigilant to possible detection. Clinicians who take the second position believe that it is best to approach the patient as though the symptoms are real; the symptoms can then be given up in response to treatment without the patient losing face.

Compensation Neurosis

Compensation or accident neurosis consists of psychologically motivated physical or mental symptoms occurring in situations in which the patient is the subject of an unsettled claim for compensation. Material incentive seems to increase or prolong the symptoms, which, according to clinical lore, improve when a single final payment is negotiated (the "greenback poultice"). Thus, as long as a claim is unsettled, or if compensation depends on regular review of the continued disability, symptoms are believed likely to persist.

In these situations, it is almost impossible to determine to what extent the patient is producing the symptoms consciously or experiencing the result of an unconscious process. In most cases, physical symptoms (e.g., chronic low back pain) occur without demonstrable pathology.

A follow-up study of 35 claimants with accident neurosis revealed that few had recovered, and the recovery that took place was unrelated to the time of compensation. Overprotection by relatives appeared to be the most important factor in prolonging the symptoms.

Bibliography

Andreasen NC, Bardach J: Dysmorphophobia: symptom or disease? Am J Psychiatry 134:673–676, 1977

Bash IY, Alpert M: The determination of malingering. Ann NY Acad Sci 347:86–99, 1980

Black DW: Somatoform disorders. Prim Care 14:711–723, 1987

Blumer D, Heilbronn M: Antidepressant treatment for chronic pain—treatment outcome of 1,000 patients with the pain prone disorders. Psychiatric Annals 14:796–800, 1984

Coryell W, Norten SG: Briquet's syndrome (somatization disorder) and primary depression: comparison of background and outcome. Compr Psychiatry 22:249–256, 1981

Dickes RA: Brief therapy of conversion reactions: an in-hospital technique. Am J Psychiatry 131:584–586, 1974

Eisendrath SJ: Factitious illness: a clarification. Psychosomatics 25:110–117, 1984

Fallon BA, Klein BW, Liebowitz MR: Hypochondriasis: treatment strategies. Psychiatric Annals 23:374–381, 1993

Hollander E, Liebowitz MR, Winchel R, et al: Treatment of body dysmorphic disorder with serotonin reuptake blockers. Am J Psychiatry 146:768–770, 1989

Katon W, Ries RK, Kleinman A: The prevalence of somatization in primary care. Compr Psychiatry 25:208–214, 1984

Kellner R: Hypochondriasis and somatization. JAMA 258:2718–2722, 1987

Kenyon FF: Hypochondriacal states. Br J Psychiatry 129:1–14, 1976

Lilienfeld SO, VanValkenberg C, Larntz K, et al: The relationship of histrionic personality disorder to antisocial personality and somatization disorders. Am J Psychiatry 143:718–722, 1986

Morrison J: Childhood sexual histories of women with somatization disorder. Am J Psychiatry 146:239–241, 1989

Murphy GE: The clinical management of hysteria. JAMA 247:2559–2564, 1982

Noyes R, Kathol RG, Fisher MM, et al: The validity of DSM-III-R hypochondriasis. Arch Gen Psychiatry 50:961–970, 1993

Noyes R, Reich J, Clancy J, et al: Reduction in hypochondriasis with treatment of panic disorder. Br J Psychiatry 149:631–635, 1986

Perley MJ, Guze SB: Hysteria—the stability and usefulness of clinical criteria. N Engl J Med 266:421–426, 1962

Phillips KA: Body dysmorphic disorder: the distress of imagined ugliness. Am J Psychiatry 148:1138–1149, 1991

Pope HG, Jonas JM, Jones B: Factitious psychosis: phenomenology, family history, and long-term outcome of nine patients. Am J Psychiatry 139:1480–1483, 1982

Quill TE: Somatization disorder—one of medicine's blind spots. JAMA 254:3075–3079, 1985

Reich P, Gottfried LA: Factitious disorders in a teaching hospital. Ann Intern Med 99:240–247, 1983

Rosenblatt RM, Reich J, Dehring D: Tricyclic antidepressants in treatment of depression and chronic pain—analysis and supporting evidence. Anesth Analg 63:1025–1032, 1984

Shah KA, Forman MB, Freedman HS: Munchausen's syndrome and cardiac catheterization—a case of a pernicious interaction. JAMA 248:3008–3009, 1982

Simon GE, Von Korff M: Somatization and psychiatric disorder in the NIMH Epidemiologic Catchment Area study. Am J Psychiatry 148:1494–1500, 1991

Slater ETO, Glithero E: A follow-up of patients diagnosed as suffering from "hysteria." J Psychosom Res 9:9–13, 1965

Smith GR, Monson RA, Ray DC: Psychiatric consultation in somatization disorder. N Engl J Med 314:1407–1413, 1986

Tarsh MJ, Roysten C: A follow-up study of accident neurosis. Br J Psychiatry 146:18–25, 1985

Wesner RB, Noyes R: Imipramine, an effective treatment for illness phobia. J Affect Disord 22:43–48, 1991

Self-Assessment Questions

1. What is the origin or the terms *hysteria* and *hypochondriasis?*
2. How is somatization disorder diagnosed?
3. What do family studies of somatization disorder show?
4. Explain conversion as an ego-defense mechanism.
5. What are the risk factors for conversion disorder?
6. What is the natural history of the different somatoform disorders?
7. How does somatization disorder differ from hypochondriasis?
8. How are the somatoform disorders managed?
9. How do the somatoform disorders, factitious disorders, and malingering differ?
10. Explain compensation neurosis.

Chapter 13

Dissociative Disorders

In a bright, unfamiliar voice that sparkled, the woman said
"Hi, there, Doc!"

The Three Faces of Eve, 1957

The history of dissociation parallels that of hysteria and hypnosis. Charcot at the Salpêtrière in Paris had recognized somnambulism, fugue, and multiple personality as manifestations of *la grande hysterie*. Janet, Charcot's disciple, believed that dissociation of mental processes was the basis of all hysterical phenomena.

According to Janet, dissociation is a defect of mental integration in which one or more groups of mental processes have become separated from consciousness and function independently. Freud, who also visited Charcot at the Salpêtrière, identified among the hysterical disorders those disorders due to dissociation, which included altered states of consciousness (e.g., somnambulism, fugue, and multiple personality), and those due to conversion, which encompass sensory and motor phenomena (e.g., hysterical paraplegia and anesthesia). This distinction has proved useful and has been adopted in DSM-IV, the former comprising the dissociative disorders and the latter comprising the somatoform disorders.

In the twentieth century, interest in the dissociative disorders, particularly multiple personality, has waxed and waned. In the early part of the century, the syndrome of multiple personality fell into disrepute, as many psychiatrists came to believe that it was caused by hypnosis and that they were being duped by patients. However, cases continued to accumulate in the literature, and in the last decade, interest in the disorder has been revived. Hollywood and the popular press have never lost interest in dissociative disorders, especially amnestic states and multiple personality, because these disorders have continued to fascinate the public for more than 50 years as the subjects of movies and books.

According to DSM-IV, dissociative disorders are characterized by a disturbance or alteration in the normally integrative functions of identity, memory, and consciousness. The disturbance may have a sudden or gradual onset, and its course may be transient or chronic. These disorders range from manifesting additional personalities to developing disturbances in memory to developing a feeling that one's own reality is lost.

These disorders tend to present in colorful ways. Their dramatic quality and presumed rarity have probably contributed to the skepticism found among many mental health professionals about the validity of these disorders, particularly multiple personality. Recent reports suggest that these disorders may be more common than once thought and that over 10% of the population meet criteria for some form of dissociative disorder. The dissociative disorders include the amnestic states, dissociative identity disorder (multiple personality disorder), and depersonalization disorder. A residual category exists for dissociative disorders that do not meet the criteria for a more specific disorder (Table 13–1).

Amnestic States

Memory loss from psychological causes is called *dissociative amnesia* (Table 13–2). It is defined as one or more episodes of inability to recall important personal information, usually of a traumatic or stressful nature—a loss too extensive to be explained by ordinary forgetfulness. The prevalence of dissociative amnesia is unknown, but it has been reported to occur after severe physical or psychosocial stressors (e.g., natural disasters, war). In a study of combat veterans, between 5% and 20% were amnestic for combat experiences; an estimated 5%–14% of all military psychiatric casualties experience amnesia.

Table 13–1.   Dissociative disorders

Amnestic states
   Dissociative amnesia
   Dissociative fugue
Dissociative identity disorder (multiple personality disorder)
Depersonalization disorder
Dissociative disorder not otherwise specified

Typically, perplexity, confusion, and disorientation occur, followed by an awareness that the subject does not recall significant personal information or even his or her own identity. Amnesia typically comes on suddenly and last from minutes to days, or in some cases even longer. In one series of cases, 79% of amnestic episodes lasted less than a week.

Although the cause of dissociative amnesia is unknown, Freud explained it as the result of the repression of unacceptable thoughts and wishes that would otherwise cause distress. An alternate explanation is that amnesia is an innate ability to enter altered states in response to stressful stimuli.

Dissociative fugue is characterized by amnesia with inability to recall one's past and the assumption of a new identity, which may be partial or complete (Table 13–3). The fugue usually involves sudden, unexpected travel away from home or from one's customary place of work and by definition is not due to dissociative identity disorder or the direct effects of a substance or general medical condition, such as temporal lobe epilepsy. Fugue states, like dissociative amnesia, have been reported to occur in situations associated with severe psychological stress, such as war and natural disasters. Personal rejections, losses, or financial

---

Table 13–2.   DSM-IV criteria for dissociative amnesia

A. The predominant disturbance is one or more episodes of inability to recall important personal information, usually of a traumatic or stressful nature, that is too extensive to be explained by ordinary forgetfulness.

B. The disturbance does not occur exclusively during the course of dissociative identity disorder, dissociative fugue, posttraumatic stress disorder, acute stress disorder, or somatization disorder and is not due to the direct physiological effects of a substance (e.g., a drug of abuse, medication) or a general medical condition (e.g., amnestic disorder due to head trauma).

C. The symptoms cause clinically significant distress or impairment in social, occupational, or other important areas of functioning.

Table 13–3.   DSM-IV criteria for dissociative fugue (psychogenic fugue)

A. The predominant disturbance is sudden, unexpected travel away from home or one's customary place of work, with inability to recall one's past.

B. Confusion about personal identity or assumption of new identity (partial or complete).

C. The disturbance does not occur exclusively during the course of dissociative identity disorder and is not due to the direct physiological effects of a substance (e.g., a drug of abuse, medication) or a general medical condition (e.g., temporal lobe epilepsy).

D. The symptoms cause clinically significant distress or impairment in social, occupational, or other important areas of functioning.

pressures may precede the fugue in some persons. A fugue can last for months and develop into a complicated pattern of travel and identity formation.

Recovery from dissociative amnesia or fugue tends to be spontaneous; in fugue states, recovery of past memories and the resumption of the former identity may occur abruptly over several hours, but can take longer. These conditions may recur, particularly if the precipitating stressors remain or return. Hypnosis and interviews assisted by the administration of intravenous amobarbital sodium (Amytal) both have been reported to help patients recover missing memories. (See Chapter 26 for a discussion of the "Amytal interview.") Once the memories have returned, it may be helpful to assist patients in understanding the motivation behind their memory loss.

A case example of a woman who had a fugue state follows.

Carrie, a 31-year-old attorney from a small midwestern town, was reported to the police as missing for 4 days under mysterious circumstances. Normally dedicated and dependable, Carrie was known to have finished her day at work, exercised at a health spa, and then failed to return home to her husband. Her car was later found abandoned in town. A search was mounted, and it was assumed that she had been abducted or even murdered, especially after a headless corpse had turned up. Candlelight vigils were held, psychics were consulted, and friends blanketed the community with posters offering rewards for help in locating Carrie.

One month after her disappearance, Carrie called her father from Las Vegas, where she said she had been the entire time. She claimed to have had amnesia, had been admitted to a mental hospital, and was regaining her memory with the help of a psychologist. There was no history of mental illness, although she had been described by friends as a free spirit.

Carrie stated that after jogging on the night of her disappearance, she had been physically assaulted, which prompted the amnesia, and she had been unable to recall her past. An assailant had forced her toward an alley, and an altercation ensued. Carrie said that during the struggle she was "struck in the head" and knocked unconscious. "When I came to, I was dazed, confused, and disoriented." Afterwards she had obtained transportation to Las Vegas and assumed a new name. Her condition soon became known to the police, who helped her receive medical care and treatment.

Carrie quickly recovered her memory and her identity. She returned home and resumed her legal practice.

The differential diagnosis of dissociative amnesia or fugue includes a variety of medical and neurological conditions that can cause memory impairment (e.g., a brain tumor, closed head trauma, dementia), as well as the effects of a substance (e.g., alcohol-induced blackouts). Therefore, alternative explanations need to be ruled out before assuming that the amnesia or fugue is psychologically motivated.

A workup should include a thorough physical examination, mental status examination, toxicological studies, an electroencephalogram, and other measures when indicated. (The complete medical workup is listed in Table 6–7 in Chapter 6.)

The chief differential will be among the different dissociative disorders, medical or neurological conditions, the direct effects of a substance, and malingering. If the amnesia develops into a period characterized by separate identity and experiences, dissociative fugue and dissociative identity disorder must be considered.

As a general rule, amnestic and fugue states due to medical or neurological conditions or the effects of a substance are unlikely to have sudden onset and termination related to psychological stressors; memory impairments are more likely to be severe for recent than for remote events, to resolve slowly if at all, and rarely to be followed by full return of memory. Additionally, a labile affect, disorientation, or disturbances in attention are characteristic of many brain disorders (e.g., dementia), but are unlikely in dissociative amnesia. Memory loss from alcohol intoxication (blackouts) is distinguished by the failure of full short-term recall and evidence of heavy substance abuse. Malingering involves the simulation of inability to recall one's past or representing oneself as having amnesia for behaviors that are alleged to be out of character (e.g., claiming amnesia for a crime). (Malingering is further discussed in Chapter 12.) Careful observation in a hospital setting will be helpful in clarifying the diagnosis.

Dissociative Identity Disorder (Multiple Personality Disorder)

Dissociative identity disorder is characterized by the development of two or more distinct identities or personality states (Table 13–4), each with its own relatively enduring pattern of perceiving, relating to, and thinking about the environment and self. In this context, a personality state is not as well developed, or as well integrated in both thinking and behavior, as an identity. In some cases of dissociative identity disorder, there may be at least two fully developed identities, whereas in other cases there may be only one distinct identity and one or more personality states. According to DSM-IV, at least two of these identities or personality states recurrently take full control of the person's behavior.

Although dissociative identity disorders have been described for centuries, most lay conceptions are based on media depictions. The most famous portrayals are found in *The Three Faces of Eve* and *Sybil*, both of which provide detailed accounts of women with many strikingly different personalities. Although the prevalence of dissociative identity disorder is unknown, it is reportedly rare. In the past decade the number of reported cases has been growing, and some experts suggest that it is actually quite common in both inpatient and outpatient settings.

The alleged increase in the incidence of dissociative identity disorder during recent years has led others to question whether the disorder is actually the creation of certain therapists who unwittingly contribute to the phenomenon. These experts contend that through attention, suggestion, and the process of hypnosis itself (often used in therapy), multiple personalities can be created, or at the very least encouraged. These experts recommend that the personalities not be given undue attention; the unwanted symptoms will subside, they believe, because they no longer gain the attention they are designed to generate.

Between 75% and 90% of patients with dissociative identity disorder are female, and the disorder is believed to have its onset in childhood, usually before age 9 years. Dissociative identity disorder has been described as occurring in multiple generations and in siblings within families. It apparently runs a chronic course.

The cause of dissociative identity disorder is unknown, although severe abuse during early childhood has been implicated. A current etiological model holds that dissociative identity disorder is the result of self-induced hypnosis, in which individuals overwhelmed by abuse, psychological mistreatment, or neglect develop different personalities to deal with different aspects of trauma. As a result, some experts have compared dissociative identity disorder with posttraumatic stress disorder, a condition induced by life-threatening traumatic situations.

Table 13–4.　DSM-IV criteria for dissociative identity disorder (multiple personality disorder)

A. The presence of two or more distinct identities or personality states (each with its own relatively enduring pattern of perceiving, relating to, and thinking about the environment and self).

B. At least two of these identities or personality states recurrently take control of the person's behavior.

C. Inability to recall important personal information that is too extensive to be explained by ordinary forgetfulness.

D. The disturbance is not due to the direct physiological effects of a substance (e.g., blackouts or chaotic behavior during alcohol intoxication) or a general medical condition (e.g., complex partial seizures). **Note:** In children, the symptoms are not attributable to imaginary playmates or other fantasy play.

According to one large case series, the average number of personalities in the dissociative identity disorder patient is 7, although approximately half of the patients had more than 10 personalities. Over the course of the disorder, different personalities may vary in the percentage of the time that they control a person's behavior.

The transition from one personality to another usually occurs suddenly, although it may be gradual. The switches are thought to be brought on by stressful situations, conflict among the personalities, or deep-seated psychological conflicts. The personalities may or may not be aware of the other personalities.

Common symptoms reported by patients with dissociative identity disorder, as well as characteristics of their alternate personalities, are presented in Table 13–5.

A case example of a relatively typical patient with dissociative identity disorder follows.

Cindy, a 24-year-old, was transferred from a hospital in another state to facilitate arrangements for placement in the community. At the other hospital, Cindy had received a diagnosis of multiple personality disorder, although in the past she had received diagnoses of chronic schizophrenia, borderline personality disorder, schizoaffective disorder, and bipolar affective disorder.

Table 13–5. Common symptoms in dissociative identity disorder (multiple personality disorder) and characteristics of alternate personalities in 50 patients

Symptoms	%	Alternate personality characteristics	%
Markedly different moods	94	Amnestic personalities	100
Exhibiting an alternate personality	84	Personalities with proper names (e.g., Nick, Sally)	98
Different accents	68		
Inability to remember angry outbursts	58	Angry alternate personality	80
		Depressed alternate personality	74
Inner conversations	58	Personalities of different ages	66
Different handwriting	34	Suicidal alternate personality	62
Different dress or makeup	32	Protector alternate personality	30
Unfamiliar people know them well	18	Self-abusive alternate personality	30
Amnesia for a previously learned subject	14	Opposite-sexed alternate personality	26
		Personality with non-proper names	
Discovery of unfamiliar possessions	14	(e.g., "observer," "teacher")	24
Different handedness	14	Unnamed alternate personality	18

Source. Adapted from Coons PM, Bowman ES, Milstein V: Multiple personality disorder: a clinical investigation of 50 cases. J Nerv Ment Dis 176:519–527, 1988.

Cindy had been well until 3 years before admission, when she developed "voices." She also developed other symptoms, including multiple somatic complaints, periods of amnesia, and self-abusive behaviors. Her family and friends noticed abrupt changes in personality and mood and thought that Cindy had become a pathological liar because she would do or say things that she would later deny. She became chronically ill, was in and out of hospitals, and was puzzling to her doctors. She had received trials of antipsychotic medications, antidepressants, lithium carbonate, and anxiolytics with little or no benefit. Cindy continued to get worse.

Cindy was a friendly, diminutive young woman, who was clean and neatly groomed. There was no evidence of a formal thought disorder, but Cindy carefully described the voices that she had heard for many years. She reported that these voices were from nine separate personalities that, with the help of a therapist, she had learned about during her prior hospitalization. The personalities ranged in age from 2 to 48 years, and two of the personalities were masculine. Her problem, she said, was her inability to control the switches among the personalities, which made her feel out of control. Cindy reported that she had been sexually abused by her father as a child and was made to perform unspeakable acts. She also reported visual hallucinations consisting of visions of her father coming at her with a knife. Although we were not able to confirm the history of sexual abuse, it was felt to be likely, on the basis of what we had learned about her father.

Cindy cooperated well with the ward routine and looked forward to placement in the community. The nurses recorded several episodes of acting out, which occurred when Cindy switched to one of her troublesome personalities. The nurses noted that at these times her voice would change in inflection and tone. Cindy would become childlike and appear bewildered. Cindy told us that her alternate personality, Joy, an 8-year-old, was responsible for the acting-out behaviors. Arrangements were made for individual psychotherapy, and the patient was discharged to the community.

Three years later, a follow-up showed that Cindy still had multiple personalities but was functioning better, had fewer switches, and lived independently. She continued to see a therapist frequently and hoped to one day integrate all of her personalities.

Patients with dissociative identity disorder often have multiple physical complaints and may fulfill criteria for somatization disorder; headaches are particularly common. Patients may report time lapses (losing time), hearing voices, and being told of behaviors for which they have no memory. Their symptoms and level of function may fluctuate, and multiple prior diagnoses are common.

These patients usually meet criteria for other disorders, including somatization disorder, borderline personality, and major depression. The differentiation from borderline personality is particularly difficult because the two disorders coexist in proportions ranging up to 70%, and many symptoms overlap, including mood instability, identity disturbance, and self-abusive behaviors. Many patients report psychotic symptoms, such as auditory hallucinations, and may have a prior diagnosis of schizophrenia, schizoaffective disorder, or mood disorder with psychotic features, all of which need to be ruled out.

The careful clinician will observe that patients with dissociative identity disorder usually report that voices originate within their heads, are not experienced with the ears or as a percept, and are not associated with mood changes; insight is generally preserved. Patients with psychotic disorders usually report that auditory hallucinations "come from the outside," have the quality of a percept (as opposed to one's own thoughts), and often result in changes in mood or affect; they often have minimal insight. The hallucinations reported by persons with dissociative identity disorder are best considered *pseudohallucinations*, that is, hallucinations brought about by the exercise of the imagination and accompanied by the realization that the experience is due to illness and is not real.

Many experts believe that long-term psychotherapy is of value in helping patients to integrate their personalities, although there is little objective evidence to support this recommendation. Other aspects of treatment remain controversial. Some experts use hypnosis or intravenous amobarbital sodium, or both, to help access the different personalities in the course of psychotherapy. Some therapists are now using cognitive therapy to help patients achieve reintegration. All experts seem to agree that therapy is lengthy and difficult, but at least one study has shown that motivated patients treated by experienced therapists achieved integration of their personalities and remission of symptoms.

No medication has proven benefit in treatment of dissociative identity disorder. Antidepressants may be effective for coexisting depression, although their role in these patients has not been systematically evaluated. Some clinicians claim that different personalities require different medications. Although this belief may have some theoretical value, it runs counter to known pathophysiological mechanisms of the major disorders. As with any patient, polypharmacy should be avoided.

Depersonalization Disorder

Depersonalization disorder is characterized by periods in which persons may feel detached from their own mental processes or bodies and feel that they are outside observers, or they may describe a dreamlike state. The criteria are presented in Table 13–6. This experience often makes the patient feel mechanical and separated from his or her thoughts, emotions, or identity. Some patients, for instance, describe themselves as feeling like robots or automatons. Depersonaliza-

Table 13–6.   DSM-IV criteria for depersonalization disorder

A. Persistent or recurrent experiences of feeling detached from, and as if one is an outside observer of, one's mental processes or body (e.g., feeling like one is in a dream).

B. During the depersonalization experience, reality testing remains intact.

C. The depersonalization causes clinically significant distress or impairment in social, occupational, or other important areas of functioning.

D. The depersonalization experience is not better accounted for by another disorder such as schizophrenia, panic disorder, acute stress disorder, or another dissociative disorder, and is not due to the direct effects of a substance (e.g., a drug of abuse, a medication) or a general medical condition (e.g., temporal lobe epilepsy).

---

tion may be accompanied by *derealization,* a sense of detachment, unreality, and altered relationship to the outside world.

The prevalence of depersonalization disorder is unknown, but it is apparently common in mild forms, and many psychiatrically normal persons have transiently experienced this phenomenon. Transient depersonalization may occur under conditions such as sleep deprivation, travel to unfamiliar places, or acute intoxication with hallucinogens, marijuana, or alcohol. In a study of college students, between one-third and one-half reported having experienced depersonalization. A similarly high frequency has been reported in persons who had been exposed to life-threatening situations, such as serious accidents. Therefore, depersonalization disorder is only diagnosed when it is severe and persistent and causes marked subjective distress.

The disorder typically begins in adolescence or early adult life, and rarely after age 40. Many persons will vividly recall their first episode of depersonalization, the beginning of which was abrupt and without a precipitating stressor. Others may report a precipitating event, such as smoking marijuana. The duration of the episodes is highly variable from person to person; they can last hours, days, or weeks. The course of depersonalization disorder is reportedly chronic; some will experience remissions and exacerbations, and others will have an unremitting course with nearly continuous depersonalization. Exacerbations may follow psychologically stressful situations, such as the breakup of a relationship.

The cause of depersonalization is unknown, but Freud postulated that depersonalization allowed a person to deny one's painful or unacceptable feelings by denying one's experience of self. On the other hand, episodes that have an onset after serious accidents suggest that depersonalization may be an adaptive response to overwhelming stress. More recently, a biological basis has been suggested, particularly because it has become clear that depersonalization frequently accompanies a number of central nervous system disturbances (e.g., temporal lobe epilepsy, tumors, encephalitis, migraine). Depersonalization has also been

---

Recommendations for treatment of dissociative disorders

1. Be sure that medical causes of amnesia or dissociation are completely ruled out.

2. Be patient and supportive. In most cases of amnesia, return of memory is rapid and complete.

3. The amobarbital sodium interview ("Amytal interview") (see Chapter 26) may be helpful both diagnostically and therapeutically.
   - The interview will help many patients to recover missing memories.
   - The interview can be helpful diagnostically in separating psychological from medical causes of amnesia, because the patient with psychologically motivated amnesia may experience a return of memory, and the patient with medically induced amnesia will tend to become more confused.

4. Dissociative identity disorder patients are especially problematic, and therapy may be long term. You may want to refer the patient to a therapist who has experience with these patients.
   - It may be useful to help patients gradually learn about the number and nature of their personalities.
   - A goal with these patients should be to help them learn how to control their switches and accept responsibility for their actions.

5. Medications have no proven value in the treatment of dissociative disorders; an exception is that depersonalization disorder may respond to serotonin reuptake inhibitors (e.g., fluoxetine).

---

linked to obsessive-compulsive disorder by some investigators; they point out that patients may be preoccupied by their depersonalization symptoms and may repetitively scrutinize themselves to check out feelings of unreality.

There is no proven treatment for this disorder, but benzodiazepines (e.g., diazepam, alprazolam) may be of help in managing the accompanying anxiety. A report that six patients responded to a serotonin reuptake inhibitor (e.g., fluoxetine, fluvoxamine) suggests that these medications may hold promise for treating this otherwise-refractory condition. Patients have also been reported to benefit from hypnotherapy or behavioral techniques to help control their episodes of depersonalization.

It is important to rule out other disorders that may be associated with depersonalization, such as schizophrenia, major depression, specific phobias, panic disorder, obsessive-compulsive disorder, drug abuse, sleep deprivation, partial complex seizures, and migraine.

Bibliography

Andreasen PJ, Seidel JA: Behavioral techniques in the treatment of patients with multiple personality disorder. Annals of Clinical Psychiatry 4:29–32, 1992

Bliss EL: Multiple Personality, Allied Disorders, and Hypnosis. New York, Oxford UNiversity Press, 1986

Fahy TA: The diagnosis of multiple personality disorder: a critical review. Br J Psychiatry 153:597–600, 1988

Hollander E, Liebowitz MR, DeCaria C, et al: Treatment of depersonalization with serotonin reuptake blockers. J Clin Psychopharmacol 10:200–203, 1990

Kluft RP: Personality unification in multiple personality disorder: a follow-up study, in The Treatment of Multiple Personality Disorder. Edited by Braun BG. Washington, DC, American Psychiatric Press, 1986, pp 29–60

Lauer J, Black DW, Keen P: Multiple personality disorder and borderline personality disorder—distinct entities or variations on a common theme? Annals of Clinical Psychiatry 5:129–134, 1993

Mersky H: The manufacture of personalities—the production of multiple personality disorder. Br J Psychiatry 160:327–340, 1992

Putnam FW, Guroff JJ: A clinical phenomenology of multiple personality disorder: review of 100 recent cases. J Clin Psychiatry 47:285–293, 1986

Ross CA, Miller SD, Reagor P, et al: Structured interview data on 102 cases of multiple personality disorder from four centers. Am J Psychiatry 147:596–601, 1990

Saxe GN, Vander Kolk BA, Berkowitz R, et al: Dissociative disorders in psychiatric inpatients. Am J Psychiatry 150:1037–1042, 1993

Schenk L, Bear D: Multiple personality and related dissociative phenomena in patients with temporal lobe epilepsy. Am J Psychiatry 138:1311–1315, 1981

Schreiber FR: Sybil. Chicago, IL, Henry Regnery, 1973

Simeon D, Hollander E: Depersonalization disorder. Psychiatric Annals 23:382–388, 1993

Thigpen CH, Cleckley HM: The Three Faces of Eve. New York, McGraw-Hill, 1957

Self-Assessment Questions

1. What is dissociation?
2. How does dissociative amnesia differ from dissociative fugue?
3. What is the differential diagnosis of the dissociative disorders?
4. What is a current popular etiological theory of dissociative identity disorder?
5. What is depersonalization? How common is it?

Chapter 14

Alcohol-Related Disorders

At such gruesome moments, I would solace myself with thoughts of the wondrous gifts of alcohol, the manna that mankind so seldom appreciates.

W. C. Fields

Persons in virtually all cultures have consumed alcoholic beverages for medicinal purposes, for religious ceremony, and for recreation. It is likely that since the days when cave dwellers first drank beverages made from fermented juices and grains, alcohol has also led to trouble. Drunkenness was condemned in the Old Testament as early as the story of Noah and in later years was thought to represent Satan's influence. Despite these associations, production of all types of liquors, wine, and beer has flourished over the centuries. Apart from failed attempts at controlling alcohol production and distribution, such as during the Prohibition era in the United States, attempts at control have largely been unsuccessful. Only Islamic countries specifically proscribe the use of alcohol.

A change has slowly taken place in how American society perceives the alcoholic person. The disease concept of alcoholism gradually took root, starting with the work of the American physician Benjamin Rush and the British physician Thomas Trotter. By the turn of the century, institutions had opened for the treatment of alcoholism, and societies and journals devoted to the study of alcoholism were established.

The disease concept lost popularity during Prohibition, but it was revived after World War II, due in part to the influence of Jellinek's *Disease Concept of*

Alcoholism, published in 1960, and in part to the number of returning veterans with alcohol-related problems. Although the debate on whether alcoholism is a disease is ongoing, the American Medical Association and American Psychiatric Association have both endorsed the disease model. The model's value has been that it encourages problem drinkers to seek help in a humane, nonjudgmental way. The drawback of the disease model is that it tends to excuse drinkers from responsibility for an essentially voluntary behavior: no one forces the alcoholic person to drink.

Definition

According to DSM-IV, all substance use disorders follow the same set of criteria, including alcohol abuse and dependence (Tables 14–1 and 14–2). The definition of substance abuse requires a maladaptive pattern of substance use leading to significant impairment and distress, as manifested in at least one of four problem areas (e.g., job, physical hazard, legal, interpersonal) occurring during a 12-month period. Further, the person has never met criteria for substance dependence.

The definition of dependence requires that the person exhibit at least three of seven behaviors at any time during a 12-month period. The criteria focus on drinking behavior, impairment caused by drinking, and the development of tolerance or withdrawal symptoms. Further, substance dependence is subtyped as occurring with or without physiological dependence (i.e., evidence of either

Table 14–1.   DSM-IV criteria for substance abuse

A. A maladaptive pattern of substance use leading to clinically significant impairment or distress as manifested by one (or more) of the following occurring within a 12-month period:

  1. Recurrent substance use resulting in a failure to fulfill major role obligations at work, school, or home (e.g., repeated absences or poor work performance related to substance use; substance-related absences, suspensions, or expulsions from school; neglect of children or household)

  2. Recurrent substance use in situations in which it is physically hazardous (e.g., driving an automobile or operating a machine when impaired by substance use)

  3. Recurrent substance-related legal problems (e.g., arrests for substance-related disorderly conduct)

  4. Continued substance use despite having persistent or recurrent social or interpersonal problems caused or exacerbated by the effects of the substance (e.g., arguments with spouse about consequences of intoxication, physical fights)

B. Has never met the criteria for substance dependence for this class of substance withdrawal or tolerance). The concept of a general drug-dependent syndrome, introduced in DSM-III-R in 1987, has been endorsed by the World Health Organization.

Epidemiology

About two-thirds of American adults drink alcoholic beverages occasionally, whereas 12% are heavy drinkers—that is, they drink almost every day and become intoxicated several times a month. Drinkers tend to be young, relatively prosperous, well educated, and urban. According to the Epidemiologic Catchment Area study, the lifetime prevalence for alcohol dependence is almost 14%;

Table 14–2. DSM-IV criteria for substance dependence

A maladaptive pattern of substance use leading to clinically significant impairment or distress, as manifested by three (or more) of the following, occurring at any time in the same 12-month period:

1. Tolerance, as defined by either of the following:
   a. Need for markedly increased amounts of the substance to achieve intoxication or desired effect
   b. Markedly diminished effect with continued use of the same amount of the substance
2. Withdrawal, as manifested by either of the following:
   a. The characteristic withdrawal syndrome for the substance
   b. The same (or closely related) substance is taken to relieve or avoid withdrawal symptoms
3. The substance is often taken in larger amounts or over a longer period than was intended
4. There is a persistent desire or unsuccessful efforts to cut down or control substance use
5. A great deal of time is spent in activities necessary to obtain the substance (e.g., visiting multiple doctors or driving long distances), use the substance (e.g., chain-smoking), or recover from its effects
6. Important social, occupational, or recreational activities are given up or reduced because of substance use
7. The substance use is continued despite knowledge of having a persistent or recurrent physical or psychological problem that is likely to have been caused or exacerbated by the substance (e.g., current cocaine use despite the recognition of cocaine-induced depression, or continued drinking despite recognition that an ulcer was made worse by alcohol consumption)

Specify if:

   With physiological dependence: evidence of tolerance or withdrawal (i.e., either item 1 or 2 is present)

   Without physiological dependence: no evidence of tolerance or withdrawal (i.e., neither item 1 nor 2 is present) in any given 6-month period, 5% of persons will meet criteria for alcohol dependence. In hospitals, however, the prevalence is far greater. Between 25% and 50% of medical-surgical patients in general hospitals are alcoholic, and an estimated 50%–60% of psychiatric inpatients in some settings have coexisting alcoholism or other substance abuse. Alcoholism is the third leading cause of death in the United States.

There are about four alcoholic men to each alcoholic woman, and the typical age at onset is between 16 and 30 years. Onset in men occurs earlier than it does in women, although alcoholism in women progresses more rapidly.

Rates of alcoholism tend to be very high in certain countries, including Russia, France, Ireland, and Korea, and very low in other countries, such as China. Islamic nations (e.g., Saudi Arabia, Syria) have among the lowest rates in the world. Certain professions are prone to alcoholism, including waiters, bartenders, longshoremen, and writers. Other groups that are predisposed to alcoholism include patients with antisocial personality disorder, patients with anxiety or mood disorders, and homosexual persons.

Based on epidemiological distinctions, a simple classification for alcoholism has been developed. Type I alcoholic patients are characterized by an adult onset; gradually increasing consumption; personality characteristics of guilt, worry, dependency, and introversion; a lack of (or modest) family history of drinking; equal prevalence in males and females; and a better response to treatment than Type II alcoholic patients. About 75% of all alcoholic patients meet this description.

Type II alcoholic patients are characterized by early onset; personality characteristics of impulsivity, distractibility, and recklessness; presence of antisocial personality disorder; a positive family history for alcoholism; being male; and poor treatment response. Nearly 25% of alcoholic patients meet this description.

Clinical Findings

No general picture applies to the alcoholic person. Patterns of drinking and symptoms vary widely. In its earliest stages, alcoholism may be hard to identify. Symptoms may be minimal, and the patient will probably deny drinking excessively. Family members and co-workers are the most likely candidates to identify early symptoms in the alcoholic person, which may include an insidious change in work habits or productivity, lateness or unexplained absences, or minor personality disturbances, such as irritability or moodiness.

As alcoholism progresses, minor physical changes may occur, such as acne rosacea (i.e., the large red nose that develops in some alcoholic persons); palmar erythema (i.e., the red palms associated with higher levels of estrogen circulating in the blood of alcoholic persons); or painless enlargement of the liver consistent with fatty infiltration, the earliest form of liver involvement in alcoholism. Other symptoms may include cigarette-burned fingers, an increasing number of minor respiratory or other infections, blackouts, minor accidents and bruises, complaints by others about the drinker's driving skills, and perhaps an arrest or accident due to drunk driving. Increasing signs of liver disease may develop, such as jaundice or ascites. Additional physical changes may occur, including testicular atrophy, gynecomastia, and the development of Dupuytren's contractures. At this stage, jobs may be lost, marriages forfeited, and families estranged due to the toll that alcohol takes.

The following case example illustrates many of the clinical symptoms and findings of alcoholism and represents an example of the Type I alcoholic patient.

John, a 66-year-old attorney, was brought to an alcohol rehabilitation unit by his wife and son. When he arrived, he smelled of alcohol and had a boozy appearance and slurred speech. In a loud, belligerent manner, he said that he would not stay and attempted to leave. His wife intervened, and told him that she would divorce him if he did not stay and get help. He stayed.

John had a 20-year history of excessive drinking. He had started drinking when in the Army during the Korean War, and he enjoyed drinking with his friends, mostly on social occasions. He had grown up in a house where alcohol had been prohibited for religious reasons. After his military service, he married, attended law school, and established a successful career as a trial attorney. Although he sometimes enjoyed a single beer or martini after work, the drinking never led anywhere. Then, in his mid-40s, his alcohol consumption began to increase, at first imperceptibly, and then noticeably. John would drink several beers or cocktails in the evening and usually fall asleep afterward. He and his wife began to fight, mostly about his drinking, which he denied was a problem. He was occasionally belligerent with his four children, whom he generally ignored. He preferred to drink his beer and watch television.

A series of personal crises followed. John had an affair with a divorced woman, separated from his wife, and eventually divorced. He had a falling out with his law partners, left the firm, and seemed to withdraw from his longtime friends. His drinking took a more serious turn. Although he was still able to practice law, his case load dried up as lawyers in the small town became increasingly aware of his impairment. He began to drink in the morning (to calm his nerves, he said), took advantage of the three-martini lunch, and drank in the evening, usually passing out in a chair. He continued to deny his alcoholism, even when confronted by his new wife and his four children. He pointed out that he was still able to work and was not a skid row bum.

His doctor also became concerned. John had become overweight and hypertensive, and he had developed the stigmata of alcoholism: spider angiomata, acne rosacea, palmar erythema, and testicular atrophy. The progression of the alcoholism was so gradual that by the time of hospital admission, no one could remember what John was truly like. All that people remembered was his boozy appearance, his occasional belligerence, and his social withdrawal.

The inpatient program consisted of individual, group, and family therapy sessions after a period of alcohol withdrawal that was uneventful. By the end of his 30-day stay, he was noted by his family to be happier, optimistic, more talkative, and motivated. He had new ideas for improving his law practice and looked forward to the future. At 3-year follow-up, he had remained sober, had developed a satisfying relationship with his wife and children, and had a growing law practice.

Complications

Complications of alcoholism, summarized in Table 14–3, are medical, emotional, and social. Medical problems can range from benign fatty infiltration of the liver to death from an alcohol overdose. Almost all organ systems can be affected by heavy use of alcohol, the gastrointestinal tract perhaps most of all. Minor problems include gastritis and diarrhea. Peptic ulcers may develop or be worsened by the direct toxic effect that alcohol has on the mucosa. Fatty infiltration of the liver occurs in almost all alcoholic persons, whereas Laennec's cirrhosis occurs in 10% of heavy drinkers. Pancreatitis may develop and lead to impaired glucose control and impaired digestion or frank diabetes mellitus. Other possible complications include cardiomyopathy, thrombocytopenia, anemia, and myopathy.

The central and peripheral nervous systems may be damaged by the direct and indirect effects of alcohol. Peripheral neuropathy commonly occurs in a stocking-and-glove distribution, probably from alcohol-induced vitamin B deficiency. Cerebellar damage may occur, leading to dysarthria and ataxia. The *Wernicke-Korsakoff syndrome* may develop as a result of thiamine deficiency; the Wernicke stage of this syndrome consists of the triad of nystagmus, ataxia, and mental confusion, which readily reverses with an injection of thiamine. This stage may lead to *Korsakoff's psychosis*, which involves an anterograde amnesia characterized by the presence of *confabulation*, which occurs when patients invent stories to fill in memory gaps. The syndrome is associated with necrotic lesions of the mamillary bodies, thalamus, and other brain stem areas. Korsakoff's syndrome is not always permanent and may be reversible in up to one-third of patients. A mild dementia may occur, due either to vitamin deficiency or to the direct effect of alcohol, although the exact cause is hotly debated. Alcoholism

Table 14–3. Medical and psychosocial hazards associated with alcoholism

• **Drug interactions**	• **Alcohol withdrawal syndromes**
• **Gastrointestinal**	"The shakes"
Esophageal bleeding	Withdrawal seizures
Mallory-Weiss tear	Alcohol hallucinosis
Gastritis	Alcohol withdrawal delirium ("delirium
Intestinal malabsorption	tremens")
• **Pancreatitis**	• **Infectious disease**
• **Liver disease**	Pneumonia
Fatty infiltration	Tuberculosis
Alcoholic hepatitis	• **Cardiovascular**
Cirrhosis	Cardiomyopathy
• **Nutritional deficiency**	Hypertension
Malnutrition	• **Cancer**
Vitamin B deficiency	Oral cavity
• **Neuropsychiatric**	Esophagus
Wernicke-Korsakoff syndrome	Large intestine/rectum
Cortical atrophy/ventricular dilation	Liver
Alcohol-induced dementia	Pancreas
Peripheral neuropathy	• **Birth defects**
Myopathy	Fetal alcohol syndrome
Depression	• **Psychosocial**
Suicide	Accidents
• **Endocrine system**	Crime
Testicular atrophy	Spouse and child abuse
Increased estrogen levels	Job loss
	Divorce, separation
	Legal entanglements

has also been found to enlarge the cerebral ventricles and widen cortical sulci, effects that are partly reversible. Careful neuropsychological testing of alcoholic patients generally reveals mild to moderate cognitive impairment, primarily in conceptual shifting. Many of these deficits are reversible, particularly as the period of sobriety lengthens.

A *fetal alcohol syndrome* has been described. This syndrome is induced by excessive maternal consumption of alcohol during pregnancy, especially when it produces sudden, large increases in blood alcohol levels, as during binge drinking. Abnormalities associated with alcohol teratogenicity include a characteristic facial appearance (i.e., small head circumference and/or flattening of the facial features), low IQ, behavioral problems, and minor malformations. This syndrome occurs with a frequency between 1 and 2 per 100,000 live births. Women should probably be instructed to avoid alcohol altogether during pregnancy.

Traumatic injuries are common in alcoholic persons. Alcohol contributes to over one-half of all motor vehicle deaths each year. Minor household injuries are also frequent, as the alcoholic person may stumble and fall, sustaining bruises, fractures, and lacerations. The highly publicized deaths of actor William Holden and actress Natalie Wood testify to the lethal nature of these accidents. Subdural hematomas occur in many elderly alcoholics who fall, hitting their heads and tearing the bridging veins within the skull.

Cancer rates of the mouth, tongue, larynx, esophagus, stomach, liver, and pancreas are increased in persons with alcoholism. The etiological role that alcohol has in these cancers is confounded by the effects of smoking and tobacco use. Alcohol interferes with male sexual function; it can cause impotence and affect fertility through its direct effects on testosterone levels and testicular atrophy. Increased circulating levels of female hormones (e.g., estrogen) can lead to breast enlargement and a female pubic hair pattern in the alcoholic man.

The direct psychiatric complications of alcoholism include acute intoxication, alcohol withdrawal disorders (i.e., "the shakes"), amnestic syndromes such as Korsakoff's psychosis, and dementia. Depression commonly occurs in up to 60% of patients with alcoholism; in fact, alcohol itself can cause depression by its direct effects on the brain. The depression may lead to an increased risk of suicide, which occurs in 2%–3% of alcoholic persons, although alcoholic persons may commit suicide in the absence of depression. Alcoholic persons at greatest risk for suicide include those with a history of interpersonal loss within the past year, best defined as loss of a sexual partner.

Other problems associated with alcoholism are largely social and occupational. Alcoholic persons commonly have marital problems leading to spouse abuse, separation, and divorce; frequent job problems, including absenteeism and job loss; and legal entanglements due to their public intoxication, drunk driving, and bar fights. Alcoholism also increases the risk that persons have for abuse or dependence of other substances.

Etiology

Although the cause of alcoholism is unknown, strong evidence has supported a role for genetics. Family studies of alcoholism have consistently shown high rates of the disorder among first-degree relatives of alcoholic persons. In fact, about 25% of the fathers and brothers of alcoholic persons are themselves alcoholic. Compared with control subjects, the relatives of alcoholic persons have higher rates of depression, criminal behavior, and antisocial personality disorder. Typically, depression occurs in the female relatives of alcoholic persons, and alcoholism or antisocial personality disorder occurs in the male relatives.

Monozygotic twins have a higher concordance rate for alcoholism than dizygotic twins. Adoption studies have shown that the biological relatives of alcoholic probands are significantly more likely to become alcoholic than the relatives of control adoptees. Males and females exhibit different patterns of genetic transmission. Male alcoholism is likely to be familial, whereas alcoholism in females is likely to be sporadic.

Molecular genetic techniques have recently been used to search for an alcoholism gene. An association between the D_2 receptor gene and alcoholism was reported, but the evidence remains inconclusive. As with the study of other disorders using the techniques of molecular biology, strategies that employ polygenic and multifactorial models will probably be most fruitful over the long run.

Social and environmental factors are also important factors in the development of alcoholism. Among adult adoptees, alcoholism is related not only to the biological background of the proband, but also to the environment in which the proband was reared.

Neurobiological theories of alcoholism are compatible with genetic theories; a stress-diathesis model has been suggested in which an environmental stressor will lead to alcoholism in persons who have inherited a vulnerability to alcoholism. Various explanations for that vulnerability have been hypothesized: that alcohol leads to increased activity of endorphins (i.e., morphinelike substances), creating an increased desire for alcohol; that alcohol may, at least initially, increase relaxation in susceptible individuals (e.g., sons of alcoholic persons), as evidenced by slow-wave alpha activity on an electroencephalogram; that the sons of alcoholic persons may be particularly prone to high tolerance in early stages of alcoholism; and that unpleasant physiological reactions, such as the *oriental flush*, might protect certain ethnic groups from alcoholism.

Behaviorists suggest that learning may play a role in alcoholism. Children tend to follow their parents' drinking patterns. Boys are encouraged to drink more than girls. Learning processes may contribute to the development of alcohol dependence through repeated experience with withdrawal symptoms, in that relief of withdrawal symptoms by alcohol may reinforce further drinking.

Psychodynamically oriented clinicians suggest that overindulgent mothering and overprotection encourage infantile oral demands that may lead to adult alcoholism. Marital conflict between such a parent and her spouse, or paternal attitudes that are alternately severe and overindulgent, lead to inconsistency. Bewildered, the child evolves into a passive-dependent adult who turns to alcohol as a release from painful internalized emotions. Thus, the dynamically oriented physician would argue that alcoholic persons may have been psychologically traumatized early in life and their personality fixated in the oral stage of development, a stage characterized by overindulgence, a need for instant gratification, and selfishness. No characteristic personality pattern (except antisocial personality disorder) or family constellation has been consistently identified in alcoholism research, however.

Course and Outcome

Alcoholism is associated with a variety of outcomes. Authors of a 1983 review of 10 major follow-up studies concluded that despite methodological differences, the results were remarkably similar in showing that 2%–3% of alcoholic persons become abstinent each year and 1% return to asymptomatic or controlled drinking. These findings were true for both treated and untreated groups of alcoholic persons, supporting the hypothesis that for some persons, alcoholism is self-limiting. In the 10 studies, 46%–87% of the subjects remained alcoholic at follow-up, 8%–39% had achieved abstinence, and 0%–33% were asymptomatic drinkers.

Diagnosis

The diagnosis of alcoholism can usually be made on the basis of a careful history and mental status examination. However, because alcoholic persons are notorious for denying their illness and tend to grossly underestimate the extent of their drinking, it is usually necessary to gather information from family members or other informants when alcoholism is suspected. Blood alcohol levels are often useful. A level of 150 mg/dl in a nonintoxicated person is strong evidence for alcoholism. Further, blood alcohol levels can be roughly correlated to level of intoxication:

0–100 mg/dl	A sense of well-being, sedation, and tranquility
100–150 mg/dl	Incoordination and irritability
150–250 mg/dl	Slurred speech and ataxia
>250 mg/dl	Passing out or unconsciousness

Other laboratory measures may be useful, but none is diagnostic. Alcoholic patients may develop increased high-density-lipoprotein cholesterol, increased lactate dehydrogenase, decreased low-density-lipoprotein cholesterol, decreased blood urea nitrogen, decreased red blood cell volume, and increased uric acid.

Mean corpuscular volume is increased in up to 95% of alcoholic patients. Thirty percent of alcoholic patients have evidence of an old rib or vertebral fracture on chest X ray (versus 1% of control subjects). Liver enzymes are often abnormal. γ-Glutamyltransferase (GGT) may be increased in 75% of alcoholic patients and is often the earliest laboratory sign of alcoholism. Transaminases (serum glutamic-oxaloacetic transaminase [SGOT] and serum glutamic pyruvic transaminase [SGPT]) are also increased. Mathematical models have been developed that combine the results of different laboratory tests, allowing high sensitivity and specificity in the identification of the alcoholic patient. For example, one study showed that a combination of elevated serum GGT and elevated erythrocyte mean corpuscular volume identified 90% of alcoholic patients. However, these methods of diagnosis have not had wide clinical use and at present are primarily used in research settings.

Clinical Management

Alcohol-induced disorders often require medical intervention. Intoxication is the most common disorder needing treatment; it rarely requires more than simple supportive measures, such as decreasing external stimuli and removing the source of alcohol (see Table 14–4 for the DSM-IV criteria). In cases of excessive intake of alcohol in which respiratory compromise is present or likely, intensive care may be required.

Treatment of alcohol withdrawal depends on the syndrome exhibited (Table

Table 14–4. DSM-IV criteria for alcohol intoxication

A. Recent ingestion of alcohol.

B. Clinically significant maladaptive behavioral or psychological changes (e.g., inappropriate sexual or aggressive behavior, mood lability, impaired judgment, impaired social or occupational functioning) that developed during or shortly after alcohol ingestion.

C. One (or more) of the following signs, developing during or shortly after use:
1. Slurred speech
2. Incoordination
3. Unsteady gate
4. Nystagmus
5. Impairment in attention or memory
6. Stupor or coma

D. The symptoms are not due to a general medical condition and are not better accounted for by another mental disorder.

14–5). These syndromes are usually precipitated by abrupt withdrawal from alcohol, but they may be seen in alcoholic persons who simply reduce their usual intake. Uncomplicated *alcohol withdrawal* ("the shakes") (Table 14–6) begins 12–18 hours after the cessation of drinking and peaks between 24 and 48 hours. Untreated, uncomplicated alcohol withdrawal subsides within 5–7 days, but may linger. It is characterized by tremors, nausea and vomiting, and signs of autonomic hyperactivity such as increased heart rate and blood pressure.

Alcoholic seizures ("rum fits") occur 7–38 hours after cessation of drinking and peak between 24 and 48 hours. These seizures consist of a burst of between one and six generalized seizures, but they rarely lead to status epilepticus. Alcoholic seizures occur primarily in chronic, long-term alcoholic patients and generally precede delirium tremens in about 30% of cases.

Alcoholic hallucinosis, characterized by vivid, unpleasant auditory hallucinations, has an onset within 48 hours of cessation of drinking and may last 1 week

Table 14–5.   Alcohol withdrawal syndromes

Minor withdrawal ("the shakes")
Alcoholic seizures ("rum fits")
Alcoholic hallucinosis
Alcoholic withdrawal delirium (delirium tremens)

Table 14–6.   DSM-IV criteria for alcohol withdrawal

A. Cessation of (or reduction in) alcohol use that has been heavy and prolonged.
B. Two (or more) of the following, developing within several hours to a few days after criterion A:
  1. Autonomic hyperactivity (e.g., sweating or pulse rate greater than 100)
  2. Increased hand tremor
  3. Insomnia
  4. Nausea or vomiting
  5. Transient visual, tactile, or auditory hallucinations or illusions
  6. Psychomotor agitation
  7. Anxiety
  8. Grand mal seizures
C. The symptoms in criterion B cause significant distress or impairment in social, occupational, or other important areas of functioning.
D. The symptoms are not due to a general medical condition and are not better accounted for by another mental disorder.
Specify if:
  With perceptual disturbances

or more. In rare cases the hallucinations may become chronic. These hallucinations occur in the presence of a clear sensorium.

The most dramatic withdrawal syndrome is the *alcohol withdrawal delirium* (delirium tremens). Delirium tremens occurs in only 5% of hospitalized alcoholic patients, but in about one-third of those who have had alcoholic seizures. Symptoms include the development of delirium (confusion and disorientation, perceptual disturbances, sleep cycle disturbance, agitation), mild fever, and autonomic hyperarousal. The withdrawal delirium may begin 2–3 days after the drinking stops or after a significant reduction of intake, and symptoms peak on days 4 and 5. On average, the syndrome typically lasts 3 days, but it can persist for weeks. In the past, mortality rates of up to 15% were reported, although with good supportive care, deaths should now be rare. The following case illustrates the diagnosis and management of alcohol withdrawal delirium.

Dave, a 34-year-old unemployed veteran, had a 10-year history of chronic alcoholism, including a history of delirium tremens, alcoholic blackouts, and rum fits. He was also well known at the hospital for his unpleasant and critical attitude. He had been admitted multiple times for alcohol withdrawal and rehabilitation services, which seemed to have little impact on his drinking.

Dave came to the hospital requesting treatment for alcohol withdrawal. He stated that he had been drinking heavily since his last inpatient stay 3 months earlier, particularly during the week before seeking help. He had been drinking at least a quart, and probably more, of distilled liquor daily. He was tremulous, hypertensive, and diaphoretic. A tapering Librium protocol (i.e., chlordiazepoxide taper, see below) was instituted, but the next morning Dave insisted on leaving the hospital against medical advice. He stated that he had more important things to do than letting the doctors "fool with him." During the prior evening, he had been mildly intrusive and had wandered around looking into other person's rooms, much to the annoyance of the nurses. They were happy to see him discharged.

Dave was brought back to the hospital the following day by the police after he had been found wandering around town acting strangely. At the hospital, he was noticeably paranoid about people plotting against him, but he also appeared to be confused. Although he knew where he was, he was unable to give the date or the year. By the next morning, he was floridly delirious and agitated. He was loud, aggressive, and disoriented to place, date, and situation. In addition, he was febrile, had very high diastolic blood pressure, and was diaphoretic. Because of his belligerence and physical restlessness, he was placed in seclusion, and restraints were required. Over the next 2 days, he was given nearly 1,200 mg of chlordiazepoxide, which was still not enough to quiet him. He remained loud and agitated, and intravenous hydration was required because of his poor oral intake. The nurses noted that on one of the days he played an imaginary game of chess with imaginary playmates. He seemed to be in a world of his own, having a variety of hallucinatory experiences.

On the third day, Dave awakened fully oriented. He was no longer hallucinating, but he was mildly suspicious. Over the next few days he returned to his normal baseline behavior and was eventually discharged to the community.

The management of alcohol withdrawal consists of 1) supportive measures (i.e., adequate food and hydration, careful medical monitoring), 2) nutritional supplementation, 3) benzodiazepines, and 4) anticonvulsants in selected patients.

Patients who have a history of uncomplicated withdrawal and a physician who is familiar with them can usually be managed as outpatients. Treatment may include 25–50 mg of chlordiazepoxide four times daily, tapered slowly over the next 5 days, combined with daily visits to the physician to assess symptoms.

Alcoholic patients with medical or psychiatric comorbidity, poor ability to follow instructions, poor social support, or a history of severe withdrawal symptoms should receive inpatient care. Nutritional supplementation should include oral thiamine (100 mg) and folic acid (1 mg) plus multivitamins and an adequate diet. Thiamine (100–200 mg im) may be administered if oral intake is not possible and should be given before any situation in which glucose loading is required, because glucose can deplete thiamine stores. Chlordiazepoxide may be administered in doses ranging from 25 to 100 mg orally four times daily on the first day with a 20% per day decrease in dose over 5–7 days. A specific protocol is recommended in Table 14–7. Additional doses may be given for breakthrough signs or symptoms (e.g., tremors, diaphoresis). Chlordiazepoxide and other benzodiazepines are the preferred drugs to treat withdrawal because of their safety and cross-tolerance with alcohol. However, chlordiazepoxide is most often recommended because of its long half-life and low cost. Other benzodiazepines probably work as well. Intermediate- or short-acting benzodiazepines, such as lorazepam or oxazepam, are generally preferred in patients with substantial liver damage and in elderly patients, because these benzodiazepines lack metabolites and are renally excreted.

Patients with a history of alcohol withdrawal seizures should receive low doses of phenytoin (100 mg orally three times daily for 5 days). Although this dosage produces low blood levels, it has been shown to reduce the risk of seizures. Diazepam may be used to interrupt the seizures if status epilepticus occurs. Other agents have been used for treating withdrawal, including carbamazepine, clonidine, and propranolol, but their role in the treatment of withdrawal is not yet clear.

Delirious patients require additional care, which may include seclusion and restraints. To facilitate medical and nursing care, diazepam 10 mg iv (or lorazepam 2–4 mg) may be given, followed by 5-mg doses every 5 minutes thereafter

Table 14–7.   Management of alcohol withdrawal syndromes

1. Chlordiazepoxide protocol
   - 50 mg q 4 hours × 24 hours, then
   - 50 mg q 6 hours × 24 hours, then
   - 25 mg q 4 hours × 24 hours, then
   - 25 mg q 6 hours × 24 hours, then discontinue

   The protocol should be started if three of seven parameters are met: systolic blood pressure >160, diastolic blood pressure >100, pulse >110, temperature >38.3°C, nausea, vomiting, or tremors. The dose should be held if any of the following signs are present: nystagmus, sedation, ataxia, slurred speech, or the patient is asleep.

2. Thiamine: 50–100 mg po or im × 1; folic acid: 1 mg po daily

3. Phenytoin: 100 mg tid × 5 days, in patients with a history of withdrawal seizures

4. Haloperidol: 2–5 mg bid for patients with alcoholic hallucinosis

5. For delirium tremens:
   - Intravenous diazepam 10 mg (or lorazepam 2–4 mg), followed by 5-mg doses every 5 minutes until calm. Once the patient is stabilized, the dose may be tapered slowly over 4 or 5 days
   - Seclusion and restraints as necessary
   - Adequate hydration and nutrition

until the patient is calm. Once the patient has stabilized, the benzodiazepine dose should be tapered slowly over the next 4 or 5 days. Intravenous hydration may also be necessary, although most alcoholic patients are overhydrated, not dehydrated as is commonly believed. Electrolyte disturbances should be corrected, and the patient should be examined for injuries and evidence of major physical illnesses, such as pneumonia.

Alcoholic hallucinosis may be treated with antipsychotic medication. A small dose of haloperidol (2–5 mg orally twice daily) may be beneficial in relieving the frightening auditory hallucinations. The medications are usually discontinued when the hallucinations cease.

Rehabilitation

Once alcohol detoxification has been accomplished, efforts at rehabilitation can begin. Rehabilitation has two goals: 1) that the patient remain sober and 2) that coexisting disorders be identified and treated. Perhaps two-thirds of alcoholic patients have other psychiatric diagnoses (including mood or anxiety disorders) that may require treatment. Because alcoholism itself can cause depression and most depressions lift with sobriety, antidepressants should be prescribed only to abstinent alcoholic patients who remain depressed after 2–4 weeks of sobriety.

The first step toward rehabilitation is for the physician to diagnose alcohol abuse or dependence when it is present. Patients should be told that they have a significant alcohol problem and that treatment is recommended. Although a diagnosis may not produce change, in some patients it may be the single most important step toward precipitating change.

Alcoholic patients should be encouraged to attend Alcoholics Anonymous (AA), a worldwide self-help group for recovering alcoholic persons founded in 1935. The meetings provide members with acceptance, understanding, forgiveness, and confrontation. Using a program of 12 steps, new members are asked to admit their problems, give up a sense of personal control over the disease, make personal amends, and help others to achieve sobriety.

For the hospitalized alcoholic patient, a team approach is used. Group therapy enables patients to see their own problems mirrored in others and to learn better coping skills. Family therapy is often important, because the family system that changes to accommodate the patient's drinking may often reinforce it. The issue of *codependency* is now popular—that is, the notion that the alcoholic person's drinking is maintained (or enabled) by his or her spouse, family, or close friends. In family therapy, such issues can be addressed. Inpatient programs provide education about the harmful effects of alcohol on the mind and body.

Disulfiram (Antabuse) may be a helpful adjunct in maintaining abstinence in some patients. Antabuse inhibits aldehyde dehydrogenase, an enzyme necessary for the metabolism of alcohol. Inhibiting this enzyme leads to the accumulation of acetaldehyde if alcohol is consumed. Acetaldehyde is toxic and induces unpleasant symptoms, such as nausea, vomiting, palpitations, and hypotension. Because the effects may be fatal in rare cases, disulfiram should be prescribed only after careful consideration and with the full cooperation of the patient. The usual dose is 250 mg once daily. Interestingly, the deterrent effect of antabuse is psychological and is not dose dependent.

Aversive conditioning has been used in the past. This conditioning has involved a variety of chemicals used to induce either vomiting (e.g., emetine, apomorphine) or apnea (e.g., succinylcholine), or electrical stimulation to produce pain. Although the treatment effectiveness has been found to equal or exceed that of other modalities, the relatively greater risks of medical complications from these methods and their unpleasantness have not made them popular.

Lithium carbonate has been used experimentally to treat alcoholism. Lithium appears to enhance abstinence and to antagonize the effects of alcohol intoxication, independent of its effect on mood. The opiate antagonist naltrexone has also been used to treat alcoholism, mainly by decreasing craving and relapse rates. Further study is needed to learn which alcoholic patients are most likely to benefit from lithium or naltrexone therapy.

Recommendations for management of alcoholism

1. The alcoholic person needs acceptance, not blame.
2. Although it is tempting to refuse treatment to the chronic alcoholic person because of his or her history of failure, it is always possible that the next rehabilitation may work. Don't give up!
3. Treatment of withdrawal syndromes should take place in an inpatient setting if the patient has a history of severe "shakes," hallucinations, seizures, or delirium tremens. Other patients (the majority) can be handled as outpatients.
   - Chlordiazepoxide is standard treatment, but other benzodiazepines (e.g., lorazepam) work just as well.
4. Be sure to manage the patient's other emotional problems as well (e.g., panic disorder, depression), because if untreated, they may lead to a resumption of drinking.
5. Refer the patient to Alcoholics Anonymous to provide ongoing support and encouragement from persons similarly affected.
6. Be sure to include the family in the treatment process.
   - Alcoholism affects every member of the family, and unresolved issues may lead to relapse.
   - Family members should be encouraged to attend Al-Anon, a support group for relatives of alcoholic persons.

Although inpatient rehabilitation programs have become increasingly popular, it is difficult to determine their effectiveness. Although many outcome studies have shown that the programs benefit patients, the studies are not comparable in terms of patient population or treatment interventions used. In general, factors that have been associated with a good outcome include having a stable marriage and home life, a stable job, less psychopathology (especially antisocial personality disorder), and a family history negative for alcoholism. The length of the inpatient program does not appear to be an important factor. Patients sent involuntarily to rehabilitation programs probably benefit as much as voluntary patients. Nearly half of treated alcoholic persons will relapse, most commonly during the first 6 months after hospital discharge.

Bibliography

Cadoret RJ, O'Gorman TW, Troughton E, et al: Alcoholism and antisocial personality—interrelationships, genetic and environmental factors. Arch Gen Psychiatry 42:162–167, 1985

Clancy J, Vanderhuth E, Campbell P: Evaluation of an aversive technique as a treatment for alcoholism—control trial with succinylcholine induced apnea. J Stud Alcohol 28:476–485, 1967

Cloninger CR: Neurogenic adaptive mechanisms in alcoholism. Science 236:410–416, 1987

Eckardt MJ, Harford TC, Kaelber CT, et al: Health hazards associated with alcohol consumption. JAMA 246:648–666, 1981

Fawcett J, Clark DC, Aagesen CA, et al: A double-blind, placebo controlled trial of lithium carbonate therapy for alcoholism. Arch Gen Psychiatry 44:248–258, 1986

Frances RJ, Bucke S, Alexopoulous GS: Outcome study of familial and non-familial alcoholism. Am J Psychiatry 141:1469–1471, 1984

Fuller RK, Branchey L, Brightwell DR, et al: Disulfiram treatment of alcoholism—a Veterans Administration cooperative study. JAMA 256:1449–1455, 1986

Gelernter J, Goldman D, Risch N: The A1 allele at the D2 dopamine receptor gene and alcoholism: a reappraisal. JAMA 269:1673–1677, 1993

Goodwin DW: Alcoholism and genetics. Arch Gen Psychiatry 42:171–174, 1985

Grant I, Adams KM, Reed R: Aging, abstinence, and medical risk factors in the prediction of neuropsychologic deficit among long-term alcoholics. Arch Gen Psychiatry 41:710–718, 1984

Helzer JE, Pryzbeck TR: The co-occurrence of alcoholism with other psychiatric disorders in the general population and its impact on treatment. J Stud Alcohol 49:219–224, 1988

Helzer JE, Robins LN, Taylor JR, et al: The extent of long-term moderate drinking among alcoholics discharged from medical and psychiatric treatment facilities. N Engl J Med 312:1678–1682, 1985

Holden C: Is alcoholism treatment effective? Science 236:20–22, 1987

Irwin M, Schuckit M, Smith TL: Clinical importance of age at onset in type I and type II primary alcoholics. Arch Gen Psychiatry 47:320–324, 1990

Jellinek EM: The Disease Concept of Alcoholism. New Haven, CT, College and University Press, 1960

Malcolm R, Ballenger JC, Sturgis ET, et al: Double-blind controlled trial comparing carbamazepine to oxazepam treatment of alcohol withdrawal. Am J Psychiatry 146:617–621, 1989

Morse RM, Flavin DK: The definition of alcoholism. JAMA 268:1012–1014, 1992

Pickins RW, Hatsukami DK, Spicer JW, et al: Relapse by alcohol abusers. Alcohol Clin Exp Res 9:244–247, 1985

Schuckit MA, Smith TL, Anthenelli R, et al: Clinical course of alcoholism in 646 male inpatients. Am J Psychiatry 150:786–792, 1993

Streissguth AP, Clarren SK, Jones KL: Natural history of the fetal alcohol syndrome: a 10 year follow up of 11 patients. Lancet 2:85–91, 1985

Stein LI, Newton JR, Bowman RS: Duration of hospitalization for alcoholism. Arch Gen Psychiatry 32:247–252, 1975

Vaillant GE: The Natural History of Alcoholism—Causes, Patterns, and Paths to Recovery. Cambridge, MA, Harvard University Press, 1983

Volpicelli JR, Alterman AI, Hayashida M, et al: Naltrexone in the treatment of alcohol dependence. Arch Gen Psychiatry 49:876–880, 1992

Self-Assessment Questions

1. Who originated the disease concept of alcoholism?
2. How is alcohol dependence diagnosed?
3. How do Type I and Type II alcoholic patients differ?
4. What are the clinical findings in alcoholism's earliest stage? middle stage? late stage?
5. List the medical complications of alcoholism.
6. What are the purported psychodynamic causes of alcoholism?
7. What laboratory abnormalities are associated with alcoholism?
8. What are the major withdrawal syndromes, and how are they treated?
9. Discuss the role of disulfiram in the treatment of alcoholism.
10. What are the predictors of good outcome for alcohol rehabilitation efforts?

Chapter 15

Other Substance-Related Disorders

O true apothecary! Thy drugs are quick.

William Shakespeare, Romeo and Juliet

Psychoactive substances are compounds that can alter one's state of mind. Alcohol, the most important psychoactive substance, is discussed in Chapter 14. Other agents have also been around since antiquity, although some new ones are the product of modern organic chemistry techniques. A cornucopia of psychoactive substances is available in the United States, and these drugs have been subject to both appropriate and inappropriate use.

The problems resulting from substance abuse appear to be more extensive today than before, probably due to the increased availability and number of agents that are subject to experimentation and use. Drug problems cut across all social and economic boundaries. All age groups—but particularly adolescents and young adults—are affected. Due to the near epidemic nature of illicit drug use and growing public concern, the government has acted to increase funding for research in the area of drug abuse, presidential commissions have been appointed, and since 1989, a "drug czar" has been in place to coordinate drug containment efforts.

In this chapter, we review the major categories of psychoactive substance use disorders, as well as related syndromes that may occur secondary to them. The major categories include sedative-hypnotic or anxiolytic substance use disorders, opioid use disorders, central nervous system (CNS) stimulants and their associated disorders, cannabis (e.g., marijuana) use disorders, and the disorders associated with hallucinogen and arylcyclohexylamine use. Other substance use disorders (e.g., caffeine, nicotine) are also discussed. See Table 15–1 for a list of the categories and substances of abuse.

Definition

As pointed out in Chapter 14, DSM-IV uses generic criteria for substance abuse and dependence, a concept endorsed by the World Health Organization. *Substance dependence* involves a maladaptive pattern of substance use as manifested by at least three significant behaviors from a seven-item list occurring at any time in the same 12-month period. These include evidence of physiological tolerance or withdrawal, as well as psychosocial problems that indicate a serious degree of involvement with the drug (see Table 14–2).

Substance abuse is a category for persons who continue to abuse substances despite problems caused by the use, but who fail to meet criteria for dependence. The criteria are geared toward separating individuals whose use of a substance is *hazardous* from those whose use is merely harmful. Clearly, overlap exists between the abuse and dependence, and the disorders are probably better thought of as lying along a continuum, because either the abuse of or dependence on any substance can result in a similar array of problems. Criteria for substance abuse appear in Table 14–1.

Additionally, DSM-IV identifies specific substance-induced mental disor-

Table 15–1.   Categories of drug use disorders

• **Sedatives, hypnotics, and anxiolytics**	• **Hallucinogens**
Barbiturates	• **Arylcyclohexylamines**
Nonbarbiturates (e.g., meprobamate)	Phencyclidine
Benzodiazepines	• **Cannabis**
• **Opiates**	• **Inhalants**
Heroin	• **Other substances**
Meperidine	Nicotine
Codeine	Caffeine
Hydromorphone (Dilaudid)	Anabolic steroids
• **Stimulants**	Nitrate inhalants
Amphetamines	Nitrous oxide
Methylphenidate	
Cocaine	

ders (e.g., sedative, hypnotic, or anxiolytic withdrawal; delirium; opioid withdrawal) resulting from acute or chronic effects of various substances on the CNS.

Epidemiology

Substance use and abuse are widespread in the United States. It is probably impossible to know the true extent of this use and abuse because drug abusers may not readily cooperate with surveys and because much use is recreational and not necessarily accompanied by signs or symptoms of abuse or dependence. The Epidemiologic Catchment Area survey in the early 1980s found that the combined category of drug abuse/dependence had a lifetime prevalence ranging from 5.5% to 5.8% in three urban centers. Among the respondents, drug abuse or dependence was more common in young persons, especially those ages 18–24, men, blacks, and persons in urban settings.

Those statistics do not reveal the true extent of illicit drug use, however. For example, surveys show that marijuana has been used by over one quarter of Americans and is regularly smoked by about 20 million persons. Cocaine achieved great popularity in the 1980s, particularly among yuppies (i.e., young urban professionals), and nearly one quarter of young Americans have used it, including nearly 7% of high school seniors. In a 1990 household survey, over 6 million Americans admitted to cocaine use in the year before the survey. Patterns of use change, however, reflecting the fluctuating popularity of drugs, their availability, and their cost. Opiates and barbiturates, for example, peaked in popularity long ago, but the estimated number of heroin addicts has remained stable at about 500,000 for some time. Cocaine is widely available and less expensive than in the past. A freebased derivative of cocaine, crack, is even cheaper, and its use has become epidemic in inner cities and elsewhere. Another factor in drug use is the introduction of new substances to the black market. Many are easily synthesized in basement laboratories and are available at low prices. Methcathinone (cat) is the latest example. A stimulant that is inhaled or injected, methcathinone can be synthesized from battery acid, drain cleaner, paint thinner, and ephedrine, an over-the-counter cold remedy.

Among the worrisome trends in abuse is the use of multiple agents. In fact, the use of one substance greatly increases the chance of a person using another. Some compounds are deliberately combined to produce a desired effect (e.g., a speedball, consisting of a combination of cocaine and heroin). The extent of combined drug use is only now becoming apparent. In DSM-IV, such use is classified as polysubstance dependence, that is, three or more compounds have been repeatedly used, but no single agent has predominated.

Etiology

Understanding substance use involves knowledge of the user, his or her environment, and the drug itself. None of these variables works in isolation, and it is probably the interaction of the three that leads to drug use disorders.

Some users probably have an inherited vulnerability to drug use. Family studies show that dependence on certain substances (e.g., tobacco, narcotics, alcohol) is familial; adoptees born to substance-abusing parents and placed in drug-free homes also show an increased tendency to use drugs, suggesting that the tendency to use drugs is not only familial, but also genetic to some extent.

Although no one personality pattern has been found to predict drug abuse, the frequency of personality disorders among drug abusers is very high. Certain personality characteristics appear to predispose persons to illicit drug use, including antisocial and borderline traits. Narcissistic traits have been identified as a possible risk factor in cocaine abusers. Other psychological characteristics are also seen in drug abusers, including hostility, low frustration tolerance, inflexibility, and low self-esteem. Although these traits may have led to the drug abuse, it is also likely that they may have resulted from their use.

Other physical and psychiatric conditions have been linked with drug abuse, including chronic pain, anxiety disorders, and depression. It is not hard to see how these disturbances could lead to substance abuse. Several longitudinal studies have shown that many traits precede and predict the use of psychoactive substances. Some predictive factors can be identified long before drug use begins, such as aggressiveness and rebelliousness manifested in childhood.

Neurobiological factors may be important in predisposing to abuse, such as the presence of opiate receptors in several brain regions, including the limbic system. Opiates interact directly with these brain receptors. Benzodiazepine receptors have been identified in the brain and may play a role in sedative, hypnotic, or anxiolytic abuse. Knowledge of these neurotransmitter systems helps us to understand why drug abusers can become increasingly reliant on drugs while progressively ignoring other means to enjoy life (e.g., food, work, sex, family, friends).

The pharmacological properties of the drug itself may contribute to abuse. Some compounds (e.g., opiates, sedatives, hypnotics, and anxiolytics) can produce rapid relief of anxiety. Stimulants generally relieve boredom and fatigue and provide a sensation of energy and increased mental alertness. Hallucinogens provide a temporary escape from reality. These properties all contribute to their abuse. Substances that do not provide such pleasurable sensations (e.g., phenothiazines) are rarely abused. In general, drugs with rapid onset and briefer action (e.g., heroin, cocaine) are preferred. Methods of administration that enhance the rapidity of onset are often exploited to provide an added kick, for example, sniffing, smoking, and intravenous use. Tolerance and withdrawal phenomena also contribute to abuse, because users quickly learn that higher doses of some substances are needed to get the same effect and that the drug itself can be used to prevent uncomfortable withdrawal symptoms.

Societal and family values also influence the use of illicit drugs. For example, if parents smoke, drink alcoholic beverages, or use psychoactive substances, their offspring are more prone to use illicit drugs, perhaps through modeling. Persons whose friends use drugs are more likely to use them, too, which suggests the influence of one friend on another. However, a person may simply seek out friends who share similar values and interests, hence leading to drug abuse. Susceptibility to the influence of friends has been associated with lack of a close relationship with parents, a large amount of time spent away from home, and increased reliance on peers as opposed to parents.

Drug laws can also have an effect. Antidrug laws have been tried for centuries (e.g., alcohol, tobacco, opium). Their success has been mixed, but laws have tended to be more successful in totalitarian (e.g., China, the former Soviet Union) than in democratic (e.g., Western Europe, United States) regimes. In some countries (e.g., Islamic countries), drug use is proscribed for religious reasons and has severe consequences; drug abuse in these countries is uncommon.

The following case example illustrates many of the problems that beset substance abusers, as well as some of the factors that lead to the abuse.

Laura was referred to the hospital for drug rehabilitation. The 21-year-old Native American worked as a nursing assistant in a care center.

Laura was adopted at an early age into a middle-class family and had several adopted brothers and sisters. Her adoptive parents made sure she was adequately clothed and fed, but they provided little emotional nurturing or stability. As a child, she was sexually abused by one of her adoptive brothers and forced to have intercourse with him on a regular basis for several years. At age 12, she became pregnant, carried the baby to term, and gave it up for adoption.

Laura reported an extensive history of antisocial and delinquent behaviors, and she admitted to using a variety of psychoactive substances, including marijuana, alcohol, amphetamines, cocaine, and most recently crack. To pay for her drug use, she had become a drug dealer at age 14 and later moved on to prostitution. Laura reported that she started smoking marijuana and drinking alcoholic beverages at about age 12 and had used the two substances on a regular basis since then. Several years later, she started to use amphetamines and later added cocaine and crack. She also admitted to having tried an assortment of other drugs, including phencyclidine (PCP), LSD, and heroin.

In the 6 months before her hospitalization, she had graduated from snorting co-caine to injecting it intravenously, sometimes in combination with heroin. She re-ported that she enjoyed the "orgasmic" feeling that she received from the injections and had actually lost interest in sexual activity with her boyfriend as a result. The two would use drugs together, and she admitted that she used unclean needles despite knowing that they could transmit the human immunodeficiency virus (HIV). Her boyfriend, as described by Laura, was an unsavory character who was a drug dealer, had an extensive prison record, and worked as her pimp.

Laura had had prior psychiatric hospitalizations for depression and had had sev-eral for drug detoxification, one occurring after a suicide attempt. She had never remained in the hospital very long and usually left against medical advice.

Although Laura had been referred to our hospital under a court order for evalua-tion of substance abuse, she told us that despite her heavy use of drugs, she did not plan to give them up. Despite her resistance, she was transferred involuntarily to a drug rehabilitation center. Because of her chronic drug use, Laura had became a menace to the community, and the referral was based on our hope that at some point the treatment would "take." The alternative was to do nothing.

Sedative, Hypnotic, and Anxiolytic Substance Use Disorders

Sedatives, hypnotics, and anxiolytics have been used to provide sedation, in-duce sleep, relieve anxiety, prevent seizures, relax muscles, and induce general anesthesia. All sedatives, hypnotics, and anxiolytics are cross-tolerant with one another and with alcohol. They are also all capable of producing physical and psychological dependence and withdrawal syndromes. Classes of these com-pounds include the barbiturates, the nonbarbiturate sedative-hypnotics (e.g., meprobamate), and the benzodiazepines.

The history of sedative-hypnotics dates to 1903, when barbital, the first bar-biturate, was introduced. Later, other sedative-hypnotics (e.g., meprobamate) were synthesized; benzodiazepines first became available in the 1960s. Because of their wide margin of safety, the benzodiazepines have largely displaced barbi-turates and the earlier nonbarbiturate sedative-hypnotics from the market. Al-though an overdose of barbiturates is potentially fatal, the benzodiazepines produce almost no respiratory depression, and the ratio of lethal to effective dos-age is extraordinarily high. Although the barbiturate and nonbarbiturate seda-tive-hypnotics are effective in providing both sedation and hypnosis (e.g., sleep induction), they are rarely used today. The main indication for phenobarbital now is as an anticonvulsant. Methaqualone, a nonbarbiturate sedative-hypnotic, no longer has any accepted medical use and is not manufactured in the United States, although it is readily available on the black market. The benzodiazepines are among the most widely prescribed medications in the United States, and about 15% of the general population is prescribed a benzodiazepine in any given year. Research has shown that most prescriptions for benzodiazepines are appropriate, and only a small minority of patients abuse the drugs. Further information about the rational use of sedative-hypnotics is found in Chapter 26.

Sedative-hypnotic abuse involves a maladaptive pattern of use leading to clinically significant impairment, as indicated by one or more independent indications of inappropriate use or problems directly attributable to the substance at any time during a 12-month period. Dependence requires the presence of three or more behaviors out of seven at any time in the same 12-month period, including manifestations of tolerance and withdrawal. (Please refer to Tables 14–1 and 14–2.)

There may be two distinct groups of sedative, hypnotic, and anxiolytic abusers. The first group includes men and women in their teens or 20s who obtain the drugs illegally and use them for recreational purposes. Similar to persons with Type II alcoholism, this group is likely to have coexisting psychopathology, such as antisocial personality disorder. The other group consists of middle-aged women who obtain the drug from their physician for complaints of nervousness and become physically dependent. Although in the past it was believed that there might be an addictive personality that is more prone to abusing these agents, no consistent personality profile has emerged.

Sedative, hypnotic, and anxiolytic dependence may eventually lead to both physical and social problems, occupational difficulties (e.g., job loss), and problems with relationships. Dependent persons sometimes turn to crime to obtain their drug. Not much is known about the natural history of sedative, hypnotic, and anxiolytic dependence, but like alcoholism, the course probably is chronic and relapsing.

Sedative, hypnotic, and anxiolytic use is associated with intoxication, withdrawal, and withdrawal delirium. These syndromes vary little from drug to drug, although the withdrawal phenomena may be worse with the shorter-acting drugs and more prolonged with the longer-acting ones. The syndromes are similar to those seen with alcoholism, which is not surprising because these agents are cross-tolerant.

The symptoms of sedative, hypnotic, and anxiolytic intoxication are dose related. The intoxicated patient may show lethargy, impaired mental functioning, poor memory, irritability, self-neglect, and emotional disinhibition. As intoxication progresses, slurred speech, ataxia, and impaired coordination develop. With higher doses, death may occur due to respiratory depression (although this complication does not occur with the benzodiazepines). The criteria for sedative, hypnotic, or anxiolytic intoxication are found in Table 15–2.

Table 15–2.   DSM-IV criteria for sedative, hypnotic, or anxiolytic intoxication

A. Recent use of a sedative, hypnotic, or anxiolytic.

B. Clinically significant maladaptive behavioral or psychological changes (e.g., inappropriate sexual or aggressive behavior, mood lability, impaired judgment, impaired social or occupational functioning) that developed during, or shortly after, sedative, hypnotic, or anxiolytic use:

C. One (or more) of the following signs, developing during, or shortly after, sedative, hypnotic, or anxiolytic use:

   1. Slurred speech

   2. Incoordination

   3. Unsteady gait

   4. Nystagmus

   5. Impairment in attention or memory

   6. Stupor or coma

D. The symptoms are not due to a general medical condition and are not better accounted for by another mental disorder.

Withdrawal from barbiturates can be dangerous, unlike the withdrawal from other sedatives, hypnotics, and anxiolytics, which is merely uncomfortable. Withdrawal symptoms can occur when the substance is abruptly withdrawn or when the dose is reduced. Symptoms of the barbiturate withdrawal syndrome are presented in Table 15–3. During the first 24 hours of withdrawal, the patient becomes anxious, restless, and apprehensive. Coarse tremors develop, and deep tendon reflexes become hyperactive. Weakness, nausea and vomiting, orthostatic hypotension, sweating, and other signs of autonomic hyperarousal occur. On the second or third day of withdrawal, grand mal seizures can occur. The seizures generally consist of a single convulsion or burst of several convulsions, although status epilepticus rarely develops. A withdrawal delirium—associated with confusion, disorientation, and visual and somatic hallucinations—sometimes develops at this stage. Withdrawal symptoms in patients using longer-acting substances (e.g., phenobarbital, diazepam) tend to come on later and last longer than the symptoms from short-acting agents (e.g., amobarbital, lorazepam). The DSM-IV criteria for sedative, hypnotic or anxiolytic withdrawal are listed in Table 15–4.

Patients addicted to sedatives, hypnotics, or anxiolytics should undergo withdrawal in the hospital due to the severity of the withdrawal symptoms. Before a tapering withdrawal schedule is initiated, a tolerance test should be administered with either pentobarbital or diazepam (see Table 15–5). The test should be administered to a patient who is not intoxicated.

Once the level of tolerance has been established, the patient is withdrawn

Table 15–3.   Barbiturate withdrawal syndrome

Severity	Symptoms	Onset	Duration
Minor	Postural hypotension; nausea, vomiting, anorexia; tremors; sleeplessness; agitation/anxiety	12–24 hours	Up to 14 days
Moderate	Status epilepticus; seizures; myoclonic jerking	2–3 days	Up to 8 days
Dangerous	Death; hyperpyrexia; delirium tremens; hallucinosis	3–4 days	Up to 14 days

Table 15–4.   DSM-IV criteria for sedative, hypnotic, or anxiolytic withdrawal

A. Cessation of (or reduction in) sedative, hypnotic, or anxiolytic use that has been heavy and prolonged.

B. Two (or more) of the following, developing within several hours to a few days after criterion A:

1. Autonomic hyperactivity (e.g., sweating or pulse rate greater than 100)
2. Increased hand tremor
3. Insomnia
4. Nausea or vomiting
5. Transient visual, tactile, or auditory hallucinations or illusions
6. Psychomotor agitation
7. Anxiety
8. Grand mal seizures

C. The symptoms in criterion B cause clinically significant distress or impairment in social, occupational, or other important areas of functioning.

D. The symptoms are not due to a general medical condition and are not better accounted for by another mental disorder.

Specify if:

With perceptual disturbances

by using phenobarbital or diazepam. The initial dose is determined by substituting 30 mg of phenobarbital for every 100 mg of pentobarbital administered during the tolerance test. During withdrawal, the daily requirement of phenobarbital is decreased by 30 mg. The daily requirement of diazepam is decreased by 10 mg from an initial level equal to the intoxicating dose. On this schedule, the patient will be somewhat uncomfortable. If signs of withdrawal worsen or if the patient becomes somnolent or intoxicated, the schedule may need to be adjusted. Some patients will present at the hospital already experiencing withdrawal symptoms, in which case pentobarbital or diazepam should be administered in sufficient doses to make them comfortable before the withdrawal procedure is initiated.

Table 15–5.   Pentobarbital-diazepam tolerance test

1. Pentobarbital 200 mg (or diazepam 20 mg) is administered orally. Evaluate in 2 hours.
   - No tolerance—the patient is asleep but arousable
   - Tolerance to 400–500 mg of pentobarbital (or 40–50 mg of diazepam)—the patient is grossly ataxic and has a coarse tremor or lateral nystagmus
   - Tolerance to 600 mg of pentobarbital (or 60 mg of diazepam)—the patient is mildly ataxic
   - Tolerance to 800 mg of pentobarbital (or 80 mg of diazepam)—the patient has slight nystagmus
   - Tolerance to 1,000 mg of pentobarbital (or 100 mg of diazepam)—the patient is asymptomatic
2. If the patient remains asymptomatic, an additional oral dose of pentobarbital 200 mg (or diazepam 20 mg) is given.
   - Failure to become symptomatic at this dose suggests a daily tolerance of >1,600 mg of pentobarbital (or 160 mg of diazepam)

Although few patients who obtain legitimate prescriptions for sedatives, hypnotics, or anxiolytics abuse these agents, certain general rules should apply to all patients. These medications should be targeted to specific symptoms or syndromes (e.g., generalized anxiety disorder), and their use should be limited if at all possible (e.g., weeks or months only). In addition, the drug should be prescribed in the minimum necessary dose to control the patient's symptoms, and prescriptions should generally be nonrefillable. Some patients, however, may benefit from chronic administration of benzodiazepines. Because of the proven safety and efficacy of benzodiazepines, there is no reason to prescribe the more dangerous barbiturates, except for their use as anticonvulsants, or the other non-barbiturate sedative-hypnotics.

Opioid Use Disorders

The opiates include morphine, heroin, hydromorphone (Dilaudid), codeine, and meperidine. Meperidine is a synthetic opiate pharmacologically similar to morphine. The opiates are commonly used for pain control, and heroin is the only one of these substances not available in the United States for medical use. It is difficult to know how widespread opiate abuse is, but there are probably a half million opiate addicts in the United States, a number that has been relatively stable over the years despite growing public concern and increased efforts at rehabilitation.

Opiate abuse is more common in urban settings, males, and blacks. Addiction is also more common among physicians and other health care professionals, probably due to their easy access to the opiates. Many opiate addicts have other psychiatric disorders as well, particularly the other substance use disorders, antisocial and borderline personality disorders, and mood disorders.

The natural history of opiate addiction probably varies depending on the setting, suggesting that circumstances of exposure and availability are important factors in maintaining use. In a 12-year follow-up of opiate addicts treated by a U.S. government-operated treatment center, 98% had returned to the use of opiates within 12 months of release. A follow-up study in London found a relapse rate of 53% within 6 months. A 24-year follow-up of narcotic addicts in California confirmed that substance use and criminal involvement continued over the years and that cessation of abuse was uncommon. However, a study of Vietnam veterans who had used opiates in Vietnam found that fewer than 2% continued to use the substances after returning home. These discrepant findings suggest that there may be more than one type of user.

Like other drugs of abuse, opiates may lead to both abuse and dependence. It is likely that opiate addiction leads to more crime than addiction to other compounds due to its relatively high cost. Opiate addiction is associated with high fatality rates because inadvertent fatal overdoses, deaths from accidents, and suicide are common in abusers. Opiate addicts are also at high risk for developing medical problems due to their poor nutrition and use of dirty needles for injecting the substance (e.g., heroin). Among the medical problems that plague opiate addicts are serum hepatitis, HIV infection, pneumonia, and cellulitis. Although it is not likely that addicts will outgrow their habit over the years, the death rate is high, so there are relatively few older abusers.

When the opiate users are brought to medical attention, they need to be carefully evaluated because they are likely to have comorbid medical problems and to be in poor physical condition. Opiate intoxication and withdrawal are the most probable reasons for the patient being brought to medical attention, because both can lead to life-threatening complications.

Most heroin or morphine addicts take opiates intravenously, which produces flushing and an orgasmic sensation. This sensation is followed by euphoria and a sense of well-being. Drowsiness and inactivity, psychomotor retardation, and impaired concentration then develop. Physical signs that occur after a heroin addict shoots up (which may occur three or more times a day) include pupillary constriction, slurred speech, respiratory depression, hypotension, hypothermia, and bradycardia. Constipation, nausea, and vomiting are also common. Skin ulcers may develop at injection sites. The DSM-IV criteria for opioid intoxication are presented in Table 15–6.

Eventually, tolerance develops to most of the opiate effects, including the euphoria. Sexual interest diminishes, and in women, menstruation may cease.

Table 15–6.   DSM-IV criteria for opioid intoxication

A. Recent use of an opioid.

B. Clinically significant maladaptive behavioral or psychological changes (e.g., initial euphoria followed by apathy, dysphoria, psychomotor agitation or retardation, impaired judgment, or impaired social or occupational functioning) that developed during, or shortly after, opioid use.

C. Pupillary constriction (or pupillary dilation due to anoxia from severe overdose) and one (or more) of the following signs, developing during, or shortly after, opioid use:

   1. Drowsiness or coma

   2. Slurred speech

   3. Impairment in attention or memory

D. The symptoms are not due to a general medical condition and are not better accounted for by another mental disorder.

Specify if:

With perceptual disturbances

Daily use of opiates over days to weeks, depending on the dose and drug potency, will produce opiate withdrawal symptoms starting approximately 10 hours after the last dose with short-acting opioids (e.g., morphine, heroin), or after a longer period with longer-acting substances (e.g., meperidine). Mild withdrawal symptoms include lacrimation, rhinorrhea, sweating, yawning, piloerection, hypertension, and tachycardia. More severe symptoms include hot and cold flashes, muscle and joint pain, nausea, vomiting, and abdominal cramps. Seizures may occur during meperidine withdrawal. All of these withdrawal symptoms have been seen in babies born to addicted mothers. In addition to the physical symptoms, psychological symptoms include severe anxiety and restlessness, irritability, insomnia, and decreased appetite. Patients may be extremely demanding and manipulative. The DSM-IV criteria for opioid withdrawal are found in Table 15–7.

Patients addicted to opiates should be gradually withdrawn by using methadone. First, tolerance to opiates must be established by the development of symptoms of withdrawal. The initial methadone dose is determined by the presenting signs and symptoms (see Table 15–8). The dose is then repeated in 12 hours, and supplemental doses are provided if necessary. Once the 24-hour dose is determined, the dose is tapered at the rate of 20% per day for a short-acting opiate or 20% every other day for long-acting opiates. After the patient has stabilized, the methadone should be given two to three times daily, with the patient's vital signs recorded before each dose. Most withdrawals from short-acting substances (e.g., heroin, morphine) take 7–10 days, and withdrawal from longer-acting substances (e.g., methadone) will proceed more slowly (e.g., 2–3 weeks).

Table 15–7. DSM-IV criteria for opioid withdrawal

A. Either of the following:
   1. Cessation of (or reduction in) opioid use that has been heavy and prolonged (several weeks or longer)
   2. Administration of an opioid antagonist after a period of opioid use

B. Three (or more) of the following within minutes to several days after criterion A:
   1. Dysphoric mood
   2. Nausea or vomiting
   3. Muscle aches
   4. Lacrimation or rhinorrhea
   5. Pupillary dilation, piloerection, or sweating
   6. Diarrhea
   7. Yawning
   8. Fever
   9. Insomnia

C. The symptoms in criterion B cause clinically significant distress or impairment in social, occupational, or other important areas of functioning.

D. The symptoms are not due to a general medical condition and are not better accounted for by another mental disorder.

Table 15–8. Methadone withdrawal dosing schedule

Signs and symptoms	Initial methadone dose (mg)
Lacrimation, rhinorrhea, diaphoresis, yawning, restlessness, insomnia	5
Dilated pupils, piloerection, muscle twitching, myalgias, arthralgias, abdominal pain	10
Tachycardia, hypertension, tachypnea, fever, anorexia, extreme restlessness, nausea	15
Diarrhea, vomiting, dehydration, hyperglycemia, hypotension	20

Source. Adapted from Perry PJ, Alexander B, Liskow BI: Psychotropic Drug Handbook, 6th Edition. Cincinnati, OH, Harvey Whitney Books, 1991.

An alternative method for withdrawing patients from opiates is the use of clonidine, which provides good suppression of the autonomic signs of withdrawal. Patients do better with an abrupt switch to clonidine when the methadone dosage is first stabilized at 20 mg or less daily. At the first sign of withdrawal, the patient is given 0.3–0.5 mg of clonidine (0.006 mg/kg), which is repeated at bedtime. For the next 4 days the patient should receive 0.9–1.5 mg of clonidine per day in three to four divided doses. The dose should be withheld if the diastolic blood pressure falls below 60 mmHg or marked sedation occurs.

On days 6–8, the clonidine dose can be decreased by 50%, and on day 9, it can be discontinued altogether. For long-acting opiates, reduction of the clonidine dose should occur on days 11–14, with discontinuation on day 15.

A combination of clonidine and the long-acting opiate antagonist naltrexone has also been recommended. Naltrexone may act to "reset" or desensitize opiate receptors, facilitating withdrawal. With this approach, the withdrawal period may be shortened to as little as 3–4 days. Buprenorphine, a mixed opiate agonist-antagonist, is also being studied for use in both opiate withdrawal and maintenance treatment. These newer approaches appear promising, but they need additional study before they can be recommended.

It is not uncommon to find patients tolerant to different substances (e.g., both a sedative-hypnotic and an opiate). In these cases it is safest to stabilize the patient on a dose of methadone and withdraw the sedative-hypnotic first, because sedative-hypnotic withdrawal is potentially the more dangerous syndrome.

Methadone maintenance treatment continues to be a major alternative in managing persons addicted to opiates. In this approach, methadone, a long-acting opiate, is administered orally once daily (e.g., 60–100 mg). Because of its long half-life (between 22 and 56 hours in methadone-maintained subjects) and its wide distribution in the body, the drug creates few subjective effects or withdrawal symptoms. The rationale of methadone maintenance is that when addicts are switched to methadone, their drug hunger is alleviated so that they are less preoccupied with drug-seeking behavior. For the most part this approach has been successful. The majority of patients in these well-regulated programs show significant decreases in opiate and nonopiate drug use, criminal activity, and depressive symptoms. They also show increases in gainful employment and stability in social relationships. Programs now espouse the view that methadone is a transitional treatment leading to total abstinence. Methadone programs also emphasize ongoing individual and group psychotherapy to help addicts stay in the program and cope with day-to-day problems without using drugs.

A methadone alternative now available, levo-α-acetylmethadol (LAAM), a long-acting form of methadone, offers a more subtle and prolonged clinical effect. Its main advantage over methadone is that it can be administered three times weekly instead of daily; it also appears to have less abuse potential than methadone.

Central Nervous System Stimulant Use Disorders

CNS stimulants include dextroamphetamine, methylphenidate, methamphetamine, phenmetrazine, and cocaine. The action of these agents is to elevate mood, increase energy and alertness, decrease appetite, and slightly improve task performance. These drugs also cause autonomic hyperarousal, leading to tachycardia, elevated blood pressure, and pupillary dilation. Amphetamines were first used in the 1930s and have been prescribed for many conditions over the years, including depression, obesity, narcolepsy, and childhood attention-deficit disorder. Their rational use in the treatment of attention-deficit hyperactivity disorder is discussed in Chapter 26.

The abuse potential of stimulants was recognized relatively early, and illicit use of the drugs has become widespread. Because of their overuse in the 1970s (e.g., as diet pills), changes in the regulation of their legitimate distribution were made in an attempt to stem the tide of abuse. Unfortunately, many of these compounds are easy to synthesize, and although their legal use has declined, their illegal use continues to grow. One of the newest drugs to hit the black market, "ice," is a crystallized form of the easily synthesized methamphetamine.

Cocaine is included with these other drugs because it has similar stimulant effects, although it differs structurally from the amphetamines. Derived from the coca plant, which is indigenous to certain countries in South America, cocaine has legitimate medical use as a local anesthetic. Because of its pleasurable stimulant effects, cocaine has always had a following in the United States. In fact, it was used in the late nineteenth century in a variety of elixirs and tonics, including the original Coca-Cola formulation. Early researchers, including Sigmund Freud, became advocates of its use. However, cocaine became increasingly associated with sudden death, emotional and domestic problems, and addiction, and it was finally declared an illegal narcotic in the Harrison Act of 1914. Cocaine has continued to be very popular as a recreational drug, although until recently its use was restricted to affluent groups because of its high cost. A low-cost derivative, crack, became available for smoking in the 1980s.

The clinical syndromes produced by the CNS stimulants include those of abuse and dependence, intoxication, delirium, psychosis, mood disorders, and withdrawal. Amphetamine intoxication and cocaine intoxication are quite similar and are diagnosed on the basis of recent use of these agents, maladaptive behavior (e.g., grandiosity, hypervigilance), and signs of autonomic hyperarousal (e.g., tachycardia or pupillary dilation). The DSM-IV criteria for amphetamine intoxication are presented in Table 15–9.

Unlike intoxication with the other stimulants, cocaine intoxication tends to cause tactile hallucinations (e.g., "coke bugs"). Psychological symptoms may include euphoria, disinhibition, an enhanced sense of mastery, sexual arousal, and improved self-esteem. Depending on how it is administered (e.g., intranasally, intravenously), users may also report a rush (i.e., rapid onset of euphoria). By smoking a purified cocaine base that has been "freed" from its salts and cut-

Table 15–9.   DSM-IV criteria for amphetamine intoxication

A. Recent use of amphetamine or a related substance (e.g.,methylphenidate).

B. Clinically significant maladaptive behavioral or psychological changes (e.g., euphoria or affective blunting; changes in sociability; hypervigilance; interpersonal sensitivity; anxiety, tension, or anger; stereotyped behaviors; impaired judgment; or impaired social or occupational functioning) that developed during, or shortly after, use of amphetamine or a related substance.

C. Two (or more) of the following, developing during, or shortly after, use of amphetamine or a related substance:

1. Tachycardia or bradycardia
2. Pupillary dilation
3. Elevated or lowered blood pressure
4. Perspiration or chills
5. Nausea or vomiting
6. Evidence of weight loss
7. Psychomotor agitation or retardation
8. Muscular weakness, respiratory depression, chest pain, or cardiac arrhythmias
9. Confusion, seizures, dyskinesias, or coma

D. The symptoms are not due to a general medical condition and are not better accounted for by another mental disorder.

Specify if:

With perceptual disturbances

---

ting agents by a chemical process (i.e., freebasing), users report an even more rapid but short-lived high. The DSM-IV criteria for cocaine intoxication are essentially identical to those for amphetamine intoxication. Common psychological and physical symptoms seen in 32 freebase cocaine abusers are presented in Table 15–10.

Stimulant intoxication can lead to aggression, agitation, impaired judgment, and transient psychosis. The psychosis may resemble the persecutory delusions seen in patients with paranoid schizophrenia, but it usually subsides 1 or 2 weeks after the drug use stops. If a stimulant-induced psychosis persists, a diagnosis of schizophrenia should be considered, as long as it is clear that there is no continuing source of the drug. Antipsychotics have been used to treat the symptoms of stimulant-induced psychosis, although they may not be needed because the psychosis is short lived once the offending drugs have been stopped. Occasionally, patients who use stimulants develop a delirium, usually shortly after taking the drug, which resolves as the blood stimulant level drops. In some patients, binge-crash cycles may develop from psychostimulant abuse.

Cocaine has also been associated with serious medical complications such as acute myocardial infarction due to coronary artery constriction and anoxic brain damage due to cocaine-induced seizures.

Table 15–10.   Common psychological and physical symptoms in 32 freebase cocaine abusers

Psychological symptoms	%	Physical symptoms	%
Paranoia	63	Blurred vision	34
Visual hallucinations	50	Coughing	34
Craving	47	Muscle aches	34
Asocial behavior	41	Dry skin	28
Impaired concentration	38	Tremors	28
Irritability	31	Weight loss	25
Bad dreams	31	Chest pains	22
Hyperexcitability	28	Episodic unconsciousness	16
Violence	28	Difficult urination	16
Auditory hallucinations	25	Respiratory problems	9
Lethargy	25	Edema	9
Depression	25	Seizures	3

Source.   Adapted from Vereby K, Gold MS: From coca leaves to crack: the effects of dose and routes of administration in abuse liability. Psychiatric Annals 18:513–520, 1988.

Cessation or reduction of amphetamine or cocaine use may lead to a characteristic withdrawal syndrome often called a crash. Symptoms may include fatigue and depression, nightmares, headache, profuse sweating, muscle cramps, and hunger. (See Table 15–11 for the amphetamine withdrawal criteria.) Withdrawal symptoms usually peak in 2–4 days. Depression may occur, peaking between 48 and 72 hours after the last dose of the stimulant. DSM-IV criteria for cocaine withdrawal are essentially identical to those of amphetamine withdrawal.

Amphetamine intoxication and amphetamine psychotic disorder are generally self-limiting, so no specific treatment is required. Antipsychotics may be prescribed for the psychosis, particularly if the person is agitated or dangerous. Elimination of the drug may be accelerated by acidifying the urine with ammonium chloride. A withdrawal depression that persists longer than 2 weeks can be treated with tricyclic antidepressants, although their use in these cases has not been systematically evaluated. Desipramine is now being recommended for use in treating cocaine withdrawal and is reported to be helpful in reducing the craving for cocaine that many addicted persons experience on withdrawal. Bromocriptine and amantadine have also been used experimentally to facilitate cocaine withdrawal. Flupenthixol, an antipsychotic not available in the United States, is reported to produce similar benefits for the crack cocaine user. Although these approaches to treating cocaine withdrawal show promise, their routine use in these patients is premature.

Table 15–11. DSM-IV criteria for amphetamine withdrawal

A. Cessation of (or reduction in) amphetamine (or a related substance) use that has been heavy and prolonged.

B. Dysphoric mood and two (or more) of the following physiological changes, developing within a few hours to several days after criterion A:
   1. Fatigue
   2. Vivid, unpleasant dreams
   3. Insomnia or hypersomnia
   4. Increased appetite
   5. Psychomotor retardation or agitation

C. The symptoms in criterion B cause clinically significant distress or impairment in social, occupational, or other important areas of functioning.

D. The symptoms are not due to a general medical condition and are not better accounted for by another mental disorder.

Hallucinogen Use Disorders

Hallucinogens are agents that induce psychotic-like experiences, such as hallucinations, perceptual disturbances, and feelings of unreality. Some persons believe that hallucinogens will bring them closer to God or expand their minds. The drugs became very popular in the late 1960s and early 1970s when psychedelic substances were romanticized and self-styled drug gurus (e.g., Timothy Leary) advocated their use. Their use continues, although they are probably not as popular now.

Hallucinogens are a diverse group of mostly synthetic compounds, and two (i.e., peyote, mescaline) are of botanical origin. Newer hallucinogens such as 3,4-methylenedioxymethamphetamine (MDMA) appear to cause less disorientation and perceptual distortion than older hallucinogens such as D-lysergic acid diethylamide (LSD) and have been popularized as mood drugs.

Hallucinogens are sympathomimetics and can cause tachycardia, hypertension, sweating, blurry vision, pupillary dilation, and tremors. They affect multiple neurotransmitter systems, including dopamine, serotonin, acetylcholine, and γ-aminobutyric acid (GABA). Tolerance can develop to some hallucinogens (e.g., LSD) but not others (e.g., phencyclidine). These compounds are probably not physically addicting, but many persons have become psychologically dependent on them.

Although the different hallucinogens differ in quality and duration of subjective effects, LSD can be taken as a prototype. The drug is short acting and rapidly absorbed. Onset occurs within an hour of ingestion, and the effects last from 8–12 hours. In addition to autonomic hyperarousal, the drug causes varied psychological reactions, including profound alterations in perception (e.g., colors may be experienced as brighter and more intense, colors may be heard or sounds seen), and senses appear to be heightened. Emotions may become intense and labile. Religious feelings, introspection, and philosophical insight are reported to occur. In fact, these properties led psychiatrists to experiment with LSD and other hallucinogens for therapeutic purposes, such as to facilitate therapeutic communication, improve insight, and increase self-esteem. DSM-IV has termed this reaction *hallucinogen intoxication*. See Table 15–12 for the complete list of criteria for this disorder.

Although many effects of hallucinogens are reported as pleasant, bad trips can occur during which patients develop marked anxiety or paranoia. Another common undesirable effect is the flashback, a brief reoccurrence of a drug-induced experience that occurs in situations unrelated to taking the drug. Flashbacks may consist of visual distortion, geometric hallucinations, and misperceptions. This symptom leads to a DSM-IV diagnosis of hallucinogen persisting perception disorder if the flashbacks cause marked distress (see Table 15–13 for the criteria). The disorder is usually self-limiting, but it may become chronic.

Chronic psychosis has been reported in a minority of hallucinogen users, and it was once thought that these drugs could induce schizophrenia. Although these agents may possibly precipitate psychotic episodes in vulnerable persons, it is

Table 15–12. DSM-IV criteria for hallucinogen intoxication

A. Recent use of a hallucinogen.

B. Clinically significant maladaptive behavioral or psychological changes (e.g., marked anxiety or depression, ideas of reference, fear of losing one's mind, paranoid ideation, impaired judgment, or impaired social or occupational functioning) that developed during, or shortly after, hallucinogen use.

C. Perceptual changes occurring in a state of full wakefulness and alertness (e.g., subjective intensification of perceptions, depersonalization, derealization, illusions, hallucinations, synesthesias) that developed during, or shortly after, hallucinogen use.

D. Two (or more) of the following signs, developing during or shortly after hallucinogen use:
   1. Pupillary dilation
   2. Tachycardia
   3. Sweating
   4. Palpitations
   5. Blurring of vision
   6. Tremors
   7. Incoordination

E. The symptoms are not due to a general medical condition and are not better accounted for by another mental disorder.

Table 15–13. DSM-IV criteria for hallucinogen persisting perception disorder (flashbacks)

A. The reexperiencing, following cessation of use of a hallucinogen, of one or more of the perceptual symptoms that were experienced while intoxicated with the hallucinogen (e.g., geometric hallucinations, false perceptions of movement in the peripheral visual fields, flashes of color, intensified colors, trails of images of moving objects, positive afterimages, halos around objects, macropsia, and micropsia).

B. The symptoms in criterion A cause clinically significant distress or impairment in social, occupational, or other important areas of functioning.

C. The symptoms are not due to a general medical condition (e.g., anatomic lesions and infections of the brain, visual epilepsies) and are not better accounted for by another mental disorder (e.g., delirium, dementia, schizophrenia), entopic imagery, or hypnopompic hallucinations.

likely that users who develop schizophrenia would have developed the illness regardless of their hallucinogen use.

Arylcyclohexylamine Use Disorders

Phencyclidine (PCP) has also become a significant drug of abuse since the late 1960s and may be taken in a variety of ways (e.g., orally, intravenously, intranasally). Common street terms for the drug include *angel dust* and *crystal*. PCP was originally developed as an anesthetic agent for animals, and although it affects several neurotransmitter systems, its mechanism of action is still unknown. The drug may produce intoxication, delirium, and delusional and mood disorders, and it has been known to cause flashbacks.

Because of variation in doses available on the streets, PCP's effects can vary widely. It is easy to manufacture and relatively cheap; as a result, it is often used to adulterate other illicit compounds. Onset of action may occur in only 5 minutes and generally peaks in 30 minutes. Users report feelings of euphoria, warmth, tingling, and derealization. With moderate doses, bizarre behavior may develop, accompanied by a blank stare and myoclonic jerks, confusion, and disorientation. With higher doses, users can become comatose and have convulsions. Death may occur as a result of respiratory depression. Unlike users of hallucinogens that tend to dilate pupils, users of PCP have normal or small pupils. Chronic psychotic episodes have been reported to follow its use, and unlike other hallucinogens, PCP apparently can lead to long-term neuropsychological damage. DSM-IV criteria for phencyclidine intoxication are found in Table 15–14.

Adverse reactions may require treatment. Diazepam has been used to reduce agitation, but severe behavioral disturbances may require short-term use of an

Table 15–14. DSM-IV criteria for phencyclidine intoxication

A. Recent use of phencyclidine (or a related substance).

B. Clinically significant maladaptive behavioral changes (e.g., belligerence, assaultiveness, impulsiveness, unpredictability, psychomotor agitation, impaired judgment, or impaired social or occupational functioning) that developed during, or shortly after, phencyclidine use.

C. Within an hour (less when smoked, "snorted," or used intravenously), two (or more) of the following signs:
   1. Vertical or horizontal nystagmus
   2. Hypertension or tachycardia
   3. Numbness or diminished responsiveness to pain
   4. Ataxia
   5. Dysarthria
   6. Muscle rigidity
   7. Seizures or coma
   8. Hyperacusis

D. The symptoms are not due to a general medical condition and are not better accounted for by another mental disorder.

Specify if:

   With perceptual disturbances

antipsychotic, preferably haloperidol because of its relative absence of anticholinergic side effects. Phentolamine or other antihypertensive agents may be needed to reduce elevated blood pressure. Ammonium chloride can be used to acidify the urine to promote the drug's elimination.

Cannabis Use Disorders

The active ingredient in marijuana is believed to be Δ-9-tetrahydrocannabinol (THC). Marijuana, or *Cannabis sativa*, is a hemp plant that has been used for centuries for medicinal purposes. The plant itself contains varying amounts of THC; plants used today tend to have much higher THC content than was available in the past. Although marijuana has long been used for recreational purposes, it became popular among the drug subculture in the 1960s and 1970s and is probably less popular today. Nonetheless, of the illicit psychoactive compounds, marijuana is still probably the most widely used.

The substance is generally smoked in a cigarette (often called a joint), leading to intoxication in 10–30 minutes. THC and its metabolites are highly lipid soluble and accumulate in fat cells, having a half-life of approximately 50 hours. Intoxication may last 2–4 hours depending on the dose, although behavioral changes may continue for many hours. Oral ingestion (usually from adding marijuana to baked goods) produces a slower onset of intoxication and more powerful effects.

Psychological effects of marijuana include euphoria, drowsiness, and a feeling of calm. Users also report feeling that time has slowed, develop increased appetite and thirst, feel that their senses are heightened, and report improved self-confidence. Physical symptoms include a conjunctivitis (red eyes), a strong odor, pupillary dilation, tachycardia, dry mouth (cotton mouth), and coughing fits. Many effects reported by marijuana users are similar to those reported by LSD users, such as the development of perceptual distortions, sensitivity to sound, and a feeling of oneness with the environment. Unwanted effects include anxiety and paranoia (e.g., suspiciousness, hyperalertness), impaired attention, and decreased motor coordination. Marijuana rarely causes severe reactions. DSM-IV criteria for cannabis intoxication are found in Table 15–15.

Users often report a morning hangover that can interfere with functioning. Marijuana has been shown to impair the transfer of material from immediate to long-term memory, and electroencephalogram studies show both a decrease and increase in alpha rhythm patterns. Chronic use has been associated with an *amotivational syndrome* characterized by impersistence at schoolwork or any task that requires a prolonged attention period. Patients may seem apathetic or inert and become unproductive; in fact, these symptoms resemble the apathy and amotivation seen in schizophrenia (e.g., Bleuler's fundamental symptoms). Many users develop cannabis abuse or dependence, as well as the social, psychological, and medical problems attributable to marijuana. Often it is difficult to isolate the effects of marijuana because many of its regular users also take other drugs.

Table 15–15.   DSM-IV criteria for cannabis intoxication

A. Recent use of cannabis.

B. Clinically significant maladaptive behavioral or psychological changes (e.g., impaired motor coordination, euphoria, anxiety, sensation of slowed time, impaired judgment, social withdrawal) that developed during, or shortly after, cannabis use.

C. Two (or more) of the following signs, developing within 2 hours of cannabis use:
    1. Conjunctival injection
    2. Increased appetite
    3. Dry mouth
    4. Tachycardia

D. The symptoms are not due to a general medical condition and are not better accounted for by another mental disorder.

Specify if:

With perceptual disturbances

Adverse effects of marijuana usually do not require professional help. Occasionally, anxiolytics (e.g., diazepam) are needed to calm the highly anxious user. Because there is no characteristic withdrawal syndrome, detoxification is unnecessary.

Inhalant Use Disorders

Inhalants are a group of chemicals that produce psychoactive vapors. Popular inhalants include airplane glue, paint thinner, nail polish remover, gasoline, and many other substances in aerosol cans including hair spray and room deodorizers. The active substances in the inhalants include toluene, acetone, benzene, and other organic hydrocarbons. Methods of inhalation may vary, but commonly a substance is sprayed into a plastic bag and inhaled. DSM-IV criteria for inhalant intoxication are presented in Table 15–16.

The use of volatile solvents is widespread, and it is estimated that 1 in 10 persons under 17 years of age has experimented with them. Because they are widely available and cheap, inhalants are mostly used by young persons who may have trouble gaining access to other psychoactive substances.

Inhalants act as CNS depressants and produce an intoxication that is similar to that of alcohol but of shorter duration. Effects may last from 5 to 45 minutes after cessation of sniffing and include excitation, disinhibition, and a sense of euphoria. Less desirable symptoms include dizziness, slurred speech, and ataxia. Inhalants may also cause symptoms of an acute delirium (e.g., impaired concentration, disorientation). Hallucinations and delusions have been reported with their use. Other effects include loss of appetite, lateral nystagmus, hypoactive reflexes, and double vision. At higher doses, patients may become stuporous or comatose.

Most users of inhalants are male. Hispanics and Native Americans seem to be overrepresented among inhalant users. Although experimentation with inhalants is extremely common, regular use is found primarily among lower socioeconomic groups, children of alcoholic parents, and children from abusive or disruptive homes.

There is no characteristic withdrawal syndrome from inhalants. Because inhalants often contain high concentrations of heavy metals, permanent neuromuscular and brain damage has occurred with their use, and serious risk of irreversible damage to the kidneys, liver, and other organs from benzene and other hydrocarbons is possible.

Table 15–16.   DSM-IV criteria for inhalant intoxication

A. Recent intentional use of short-term, high-dose exposure to volatile inhalants (excluding anesthetic gases and short-acting vasodilators).

B. Clinically significant maladaptive behavioral or psychological changes (e.g., belligerence, assaultiveness, apathy, impaired judgment, impaired social or occupational functioning) that developed during, or shortly after, use of or exposure to volatile inhalants.

C. Two (or more) of the following signs, developing during, or shortly after, inhalant use or exposure:
   1. Dizziness
   2. Nystagmus
   3. Incoordination
   4. Slurred speech
   5. Unsteady gait
   6. Lethargy
   7. Depressed reflexes
   8. Psychomotor retardation
   9. Tremor
   10. Generalized muscle weakness
   11. Blurred vision or diplopia
   12. Stupor or coma
   13. Euphoria

D. The symptoms are not due to a general medical condition and are not better accounted for by another mental disorder.

Other Substance Use Disorders

A variety of other substances have been subject to abuse. Nicotine and caffeine are the most commonly used substances worldwide. Others are anabolic steroids, nitrate inhalants, and nitrous oxide.

Nicotine

Nicotine is a highly addictive compound found in cigarettes, chewing tobacco and snuff, and other tobacco products. Currently, about 25% of Americans smoke, although smoking is even more prevalent in certain groups (e.g., minority groups, persons with low socioeconomic status, less-educated persons). Rates among psychiatric patients are also very high; for example, up to 90% of patients with schizophrenia smoke.

Smoking has been implicated as a cause of lung cancer, emphysema, and cardiovascular disease. Snuff and chewing tobacco have been associated with oropharyngeal cancers. Secondary smoke has been associated with respiratory and cardiovascular diseases.

Dependence on nicotine develops quickly and is often reinforced by peer pressure. However, society has clearly changed its views on smoking, and in recent years, smokers' rights have been increasingly limited.

Nicotine withdrawal usually begins within 1 hour after the last cigarette is smoked and peaks within 24 hours. Withdrawal may last weeks or months and consists of craving for nicotine, anger and irritability, anxiety, restlessness, and decreased heart rate. Weight gain often follows smoking cessation.

Relapse is common for former smokers, especially during the first year. Nicotine transdermal patches and nicotine-containing gum are helpful in assisting motivated persons to quit, but even with these aids, relapse rates remain distressingly high. Because the potential consequences of tobacco use are so harmful, all physicians have a responsibility to urge their patients, particularly young patients, not to smoke or to use tobacco products and to assist patients who do use them to quit.

Caffeine

Caffeine is found in coffee, tea, chocolate, cola drinks, and many over-the-counter pain and cold remedies. Except for certain groups that proscribe its use (e.g., Mormons), use of caffeine is nearly universal.

The mild stimulant effects of caffeine occur at doses of 50–150 mg (i.e., one cup of coffee) and are readily appreciated. These effects include increased alertness, a sense of well-being, and improved verbal and motor performance. At higher doses, unless tolerance has been achieved, signs of intoxication will occur, such as restlessness, irritability, and insomnia. High doses (e.g., >1 g/day) can lead to seizures and coma. Withdrawal from caffeine can lead to headaches, lethargy, irritability, and depression. Higher daily doses are more likely to lead to withdrawal.

Chronic use of caffeine can lead to excess gastric acidity and aggravate esophageal and gastric disorders, can exacerbate fibrocystic breast disease in women, and can exacerbate anxiety disorders, such as panic disorder or generalized anxiety disorder. Chronic use can itself lead to excessive anxiety; in DSM-IV this condition is termed a *caffeine anxiety disorder*. Once the caffeine anxiety disorder is identified, the treatment consists of reducing or eliminating caffeine from the diet. Decaffeinated cola drinks, tea, and coffee are now widely available.

Anabolic Steroids

These compounds are now widely abused by athletes who believe that their performance and muscle mass will be improved by their use. Although they may initially produce an enhanced sense of well-being, this feeling is later replaced by lack of energy, dysphoria, and irritability. Frank psychosis can develop, as can serious physical problems, such as liver disease.

Nitrate Inhalants

These compounds (poppers) produce an intoxicated state characterized by a feeling of fullness in the head, mild euphoria, a change in time perception, relaxation of the smooth muscles, and possibly an increase in sexual (i.e., orgasmic) feeling. These drugs carry the possible risk of immune system impairment, respiratory system irritation, and a toxic reaction that may lead to vomiting, severe headaches, and hypotension. They are commonly abused by the gay community, and at least initially they were thought to be a risk factor for the acquired immunodeficiency syndrome (AIDS).

Nitrous Oxide

Nitrous oxide (laughing gas) can cause intoxication characterized by lightheadedness and a floating sensation that quickly clears once the administration of the gas ceases. Temporary confusion or paranoia may be induced when this substance is used regularly.

Clinical Management of the Psychoactive Substance User

Although specific treatment approaches will differ depending on the primary agent of abuse, the pattern of abuse, and the characteristic of the abuser, general guidelines apply to all psychoactive substance abusers. These guidelines are similar to those applied to alcoholic patients and are summarized in Chapter 14.

Treatment can be thought of as having two phases—an acute phase and a chronic phase. In the acute phase, detoxification is the major goal. This goal may be difficult to achieve in some patients, for example, those with potentially serious withdrawal syndromes (e.g., barbiturate or opiate abusers). It may be easier to achieve in other patients (e.g., marijuana abusers) in whom there is no specific withdrawal syndrome. Hospitalization is necessary for safe detoxification in some patients so that tolerance can be determined and a slow, tapering withdrawal can be monitored under medical supervision. Other patients, like alcoholic persons, may be able to stop their drug use after having a physician make a diagnosis and explain its significance. In any event, the circumstances of detoxification should be determined by the patient and physician working together.

Clearly, many drug addicts have serious medical conditions that the physician will also need to address during this phase of treatment. For example, a heroin addict may have antecubital cellulitis and be seropositive for HIV; a cocaine addict may have an eroded nasal septum from sniffing the drug that has become secondarily infected.

Psychiatric comorbidity is also important to assess during the initial phase of treatment. Many, if not most, psychoactive substance abusers have additional psychiatric diagnoses that can have a profound impact on their treatment outcome. Abuse of other substances is the most common comorbidity, followed by mood disorders and personality disorders. Comorbidity always complicates treatment efforts and reduces the likelihood of success. Examples include the amphetamine abuser who develops a suicidal depression during withdrawal, as well as the heroin addict with an antisocial personality disorder whose use seems, in part, motivated by his membership in a street gang that celebrates drug use.

The second phase of treatment consists of efforts to rehabilitate the patient and to prevent future use of psychoactive substances. The success of this phase depends almost completely on the motivation of the patient, because there is no way to truly assess or enforce compliance (except, of course, by frequent and random drug screening tests and threats of punishment for noncompliance). Except in the military, among certain professions (e.g., pilots), and in totalitarian societies, such strict enforcement is neither possible nor desirable.

Multimodal approaches to patients are needed for their rehabilitation. Individual psychotherapy may be important in helping patients to learn about their motivation for using drugs and to learn alternative methods of handling stressors. Group approaches, especially in the hospital, are useful in confronting patients with the seriousness of their problem and how it significantly affects their lives. Peer groups seem unequalled in their ability to achieve confrontation. Behav-

---

Recommendations for management of psychoactive substance abuse

1. Do not let your personal beliefs and attitudes about drug abuse interfere with your care of the addict.
   - Patients need consistent yet firm handling.
   - Neither condemn addicts nor condone their behavior.
2. Be sure to consider both medical and psychiatric comorbidity. Many addicts have potentially serious medical problems that require treatment, significant addictions to other substances, mood disorders, or personality disorders.
3. Be prepared for relapses during the rehabilitation phase of treatment. Relapse is almost inevitable, but it does not represent failure of the treatment program. Be there to help the patient get back on the wagon.
4. Support groups can be very helpful to the patient, and referral to community-based organizations is essential.

ioral or cognitive approaches may be needed to help the patient to reverse habits that lead to or exacerbate drug use, or to help the patient to correct cognitive distortions (e.g., "If I don't use drugs, I won't be popular with my friends"). Social skills training may be needed for some patients to help them break a cycle of getting in with the wrong crowd and learn to meet and be accepted by more appropriate peers.

Family therapy and marital counseling are necessary adjuncts in other patients. Examples include the teenager whose inhalant use has led to considerable disruption of her family life and the young man whose marriage is falling apart due to his cocaine addiction.

Medical approaches for the rehabilitation or maintenance phase of treatment are important for some patients. Methadone maintenance in opiate addicts has been popular for years and seems to have an established role in the treatment of at least some opiate addicts. Methadone maintenance provides a carefully monitored substitute addiction that allows the patient to function in the community. Patients with comorbid psychiatric disorders may, of course, benefit from ongoing somatic treatment for anxiety, depression, or psychosis. It is probably wise to avoid the use of benzodiazepines in these patients due to their abuse potential. The use of desipramine or flupenthixol in cocaine abusers, discussed earlier in the chapter, can only be considered experimental.

Self-help groups have become an integral part of a comprehensive treatment approach to drug use disorders. Alcoholics Anonymous (AA) has led the way for the creation of sister groups, such as Cocaine Anonymous (CA), Narcotics Anonymous (NA), and Drugs Anonymous (DA). These groups are organized along the same lines as AA, following a 12-step program to provide an atmosphere in which recovering addicts can share their experiences. These programs are now available in many parts of the country.

Bibliography

Breslau N, Kilbey M, Andreski P: Nicotine withdrawal symptoms and psychiatric disorders: findings from an epidemiologic study of young adults. Am J Psychiatry 149:464–469, 1992

Busto U, Sellers EM, Naranjo CA, et al: Withdrawal reaction after long-term therapeutic use of benzodiazepines. N Engl J Med 315:854–859, 1986

Cadoret RJ, Troughton E, O'Gorman TW, et al: An adoption study of genetic and environmental factors in drug abuse. Arch Gen Psychiatry 43:1131–1136, 1986

Charney DS, Henninger GR, Kleber HD: A combined use of clonidine and naltrexone as a rapid, safe, and effective treatment of abrupt withdrawal from methadone. Am J Psychiatry 143:831–837, 1986

Council on Scientific Affairs: Marijuana—its health hazards and therapeutic potentials. JAMA 246:1823–1827, 1981

Council on Scientific Affairs: Methaqualone—abuse limits its usefulness. JAMA 250:3052, 1983

Cregler LL, Mark H: Medical complications of cocaine abuse. N Engl J Med 315:1495–1500, 1986

Dinwiddie SH, Zorumski CF, Rubin EH: Psychiatric correlates of chronic solvent abuse. J Clin Psychiatry 48:334–337, 1987

Fishbain DA, Rosomoff HL, Cutler R, et al: Opiate detoxification protocols—a clinical manual. Annals of Clinical Psychiatry 5:53–65, 1993

Gawin FH, Allen D, Humblestone B: Outpatient treatment of "crack" cocaine smoking with flupenthixol decanoate. Arch Gen Psychiatry 46:322–325, 1989

Gawin FH, Kleber HD: Cocaine abuse treatment. Arch Gen Psychiatry 41:903–909, 1984

Gawin FH, Kleber HD, Byck R, et al: Desipramine facilitation of initial cocaine abstinence. Arch Gen Psychiatry 46:117–121, 1989

Gossop M, Green L, Phillips G, et al: What happens to opiate addicts immediately after treatment: a prospective follow-up study. Br Med J 294:1377–1380, 1987

Gossop M, Johns A, Green L: Opiate withdrawal: inpatient versus outpatient programmes and preferred versus random assignment. Br Med J 293:103–104, 1986

Group for the Advancement of Psychiatry Committee on Alcoholism and Addictions: Substance use disorders: a psychiatric minority. Am J Psychiatry 148:1291–1300, 1991

Halikas JA, Weller RA, Morse CL, et al: Regular marijuana use and its effect on psychosocial variables: a longitudinal study. Compr Psychiatry 24:229–235, 1983

Hser YI, Anglin MD, Powers K: A 24 year follow-up of California narcotic addicts. Arch Gen Psychiatry 50:577–584, 1993

Khantzian EJ, McKenna GJ: Acute toxic and withdrawal reactions associated with drug use and abuse. Ann Intern Med 90:361–372, 1979

Kozel NJ, Adams EH: Epidemiology of drug abuse: an overview. Science 234:970–974, 1986

McNagney SE, Parker RM: High prevalence of recent cocaine use and the unreliability of patient self-report in an inner city walk-in clinic. JAMA 267:1106–1108, 1992

Millman RB: Drug abuse and drug dependence, in Psychiatric Update. American Psychiatric Association Annual Review, Vol 5. Edited by Frances AJ, Hales RE. Washington, DC, American Psychiatric Press, 1986, pp 120–232

Nicholi AM: The non-therapeutic use of psychoactive drugs—a modern epidemic. N Engl J Med 308:925–933, 1983

O'Brien CP, Woody GE, McLellan AT: Psychiatric disorders in opioid dependent patients. J Clin Psychiatry 45:9–13, 1984

Perry P, Anderson K, Yates W: Illicit anabolic steroid use in athletes: a case series analysis. Am J Sports Med 184:422–428, 1990

Strain EC, Stitzer ML, Liebson IA: Comparison of buprenorphine and methadone in the treatment of opioid dependence. Am J Pspychiatry 151:1025–1030, 1994

Vaillant GE: A 12-year follow-up of New York narcotic addicts. Arch Gen Psychiatry 15:599–609, 1966

Vardy M, Kay S: LSD psychosis or LSD induced schizophrenia? Arch Gen Psychiatry 40:877–883, 1983

Vereby K, Gold MS: From coca leaves to crack: the effects of doses and routes of administration in abuse liability. Psychiatric Annals 18:513–520, 1988

Warner EA: Cocaine abuse. Ann Intern Med 119:226–235, 1993

Woody GE, McLellan AT, Luborsky L, et al: A 12-month follow-up of psychotherapy for opiate dependence. Am J Psychiatry 144:590–596, 1987

Yates WR, Fulton AI, Gabel J, et al: Personality risk factors for cocaine abuse. Am J Public Health 79:891–892, 1989

Self-Assessment Questions

1. How widespread is substance abuse and dependence, and what are their risk factors?
2. What appear to be the two types of sedative-hypnotic abusers?
3. Describe the withdrawal syndrome from sedatives, hypnotics, and anxiolytics.
4. Why are barbiturates especially dangerous?
5. Describe the pentobarbital/diazepam tolerance test.
6. Describe the opiate withdrawal syndrome and how it differs from sedative-hypnotic withdrawal.
7. What are the pharmacokinetics of cocaine?
8. Does use of LSD lead to schizophrenia?
9. What are the symptoms of PCP intoxication?
10. What is the amotivational syndrome in association with marijuana?
11. Why are the inhalants dangerous substances of abuse?
12. Why do athletes abuse anabolic steroids?

Chapter 16

Personality Disorders

All is caprice, they love without measure those whom they will soon hate without reason.

Thomas Sydenham, 1682

Maladaptive character traits have been part of humans' makeup since the dawn of time; their recognition as a mental illness termed *personality disorder* is relatively recent. The ancient Greeks, for example, observed and classified many of the mental illnesses that are recognized today, including mania, paranoia, and melancholia. Although they did not recognize personality disorders, they did elaborate a system of four temperaments—sanguine, choleric, melancholic, and phlegmatic—to describe variations of personality type. The ancients felt that these temperaments were the embodiments of the four elements: earth, air, fire, and water. These four temperaments continued to be recognized through the nineteenth century. In fact, Kraepelin characterized the personalities often found in manic-depressive patients and their relatives as *depressive, hypomanic,* or *irritable,* terms that corresponded to the Greek temperaments of melancholic, sanguine, and choleric. These terms are still useful descriptively.

In the early nineteenth century, descriptive psychiatrists working in Europe and the United States began to describe abnormal personality traits. The French psychiatrist Pinel used the term *manie sans délire* to describe patients who were prone to unexplained outbursts of rage and violence, but who were not insane. This group of patients probably included many who would now be regarded as having antisocial personality disorder. Prichard, a Scottish physician, used the term *moral insanity* to describe persons who violated social norms, but who were neither intellectually impaired nor psychotic. The concept of moral insanity has persisted; the closest modern equivalent is antisocial personality disorder. Later, Freud and other leaders of the psychoanalytic movement attempted to describe character along the lines of psychosexual development (e.g., oral, anal, phallic, and genital). These stages of development are discussed later in the chapter.

More recently, attempts have been made to describe the variety of personality types important to clinicians. In DSM-IV, 10 personality types are described. This manual uses a polythetic schema, in which a combination of four or five of eight or nine items can trigger the corresponding diagnosis. An advantage of polythetic schemata is their greater coverage, which occurs at the expense of diminished specificity. For example, a person may receive a diagnosis of borderline personality disorder, even in the absence of impulsivity, undue anger, or unstable interpersonal relationships, as long as five other items are present.

Although this approach offers more rigorously defined subtypes than were available before, the subtypes are not perfect. Normal personality variants and the way they shade into more dysfunctional types are left out. Additionally, few persons with personality disorders show exclusively the traits of the diagnosed personality disorder; they usually manifest traits belonging to several of the defined types. As a result, many clinicians prefer a dimensional approach to the diagnosis of personality disorder, in which scales are used to measure different qualities, such as obsessionality or narcissism.

Most clinicians probably think along both dimensional and categorical lines simultaneously. For example, a patient may be diagnosed as having obsessive-compulsive personality disorder with avoidant and narcissistic features, meaning that the person's symptoms satisfy the criteria for obsessive-compulsive personality disorder, but also that there are symptoms consistent with both avoidant and narcissistic personality disorders.

Ten distinct personality disorders are listed in DSM-IV, in addition to a residual category for the disorders with mixed or atypical traits that do not fit into the better-defined categories (personality disorder not otherwise specified). Further, the 10 disorders are grouped into three separate personality clusters according to their clinical similarity. These include cluster A (the eccentric disorders), cluster B (the dramatic disorders), and cluster C (the anxious disorders). See Table 16–1 for the list of personality disorders.

In DSM-III-R, 11 personality disorders were listed. Passive-aggressive personality disorder was omitted from DSM-IV because it was thought that passive-aggressive traits are common to almost all patients with a personality disorder, and therefore the disorder does not stand alone. Passive-aggressive behavior, however, is worth mentioning because it is so common among the general pop-

Table 16–1. DSM-IV personality disorders

Cluster A (the eccentric disorders)	• Histrionic
• Paranoid	• Narcissistic
• Schizoid	**Cluster C (the anxious disorders)**
• Schizotypal	• Avoidant
Cluster B (the dramatic disorders)	• Dependent
• Antisocial	• Obsessive-compulsive
• Borderline	

ulation as well as psychiatric patients. This behavior is manifested by dawdling, procrastination, and forgetting. Persons with passive-aggressive behavior tend to be complaining and whiny, argumentative, discontented, and disgruntled. They tend to express their anger indirectly through resistant and negativistic behavior.

Definition

Personality disorders are coded on Axis II in an attempt to separate them from the major mental disorders, which are coded on Axis I. Theoretically, a person may have both Axis I and Axis II disorders, with some exceptions. For example, personality disorders are not diagnosed in persons with chronic psychotic disorders (e.g., schizophrenia) that are so devastating to the personality that the concept of personality disorder becomes meaningless. In fact, many persons with personality disorders meet criteria for Axis I diagnoses, most often major depressive disorder.

Personality disorders are defined in DSM-IV as behaviors or traits that are characteristic of a person's recent and long-term functioning (i.e, generally since adolescence or early adulthood). The constellation of character traits must cause either significant impairment in social or occupational functioning or subjective distress. It is important to note that these behaviors or traits are not limited to episodes of illness, but represent long-term functioning. A personality disorder would not be diagnosed, for instance, in a person who develops transient personality changes during an episode of depression.

The term *personality disorder* is sometimes considered pejorative, because many patients who receive this diagnosis have undesirable or unpleasant qualities, such as being defensive, overdramatic, or even criminal. These qualities lead to trouble getting along with other people, as well as difficulties in other domains of life. Conversely, many patients with personality disorders, probably the majority, are not unpleasant or difficult to work with. These patients tend to be lonely, isolated, anxious, or dependent. Persons with these qualities also tend to develop interpersonal difficulties and experience unhappiness. What unites all patients with personality disorders, despite their heterogeneous character traits, is the way in which the disorder causes pervasive problems in their social and occupational adjustment.

Many patients with personality disorders tend either to be untroubled by their maladaptive traits or to be unaware of them. Other patients are acutely aware of their personality problems but seem powerless to change them. It is not surprising that patients with personality disorders seek help for a variety of problems that may occur in their lives, including marital or work-related problems, depression, and substance abuse. Thus, it is rarely the personality disorder per se that leads the patient to seek professional help, although it may be the underlying problem. It is the task of the clinician to help patients recognize the maladaptive character traits as the source of their ongoing troubles and to help patients modify them if possible.

Because many character traits of these patients are unpleasant, patients with personality disorders have a bad reputation among clinicians. Many mental health professionals dislike working with these patients or refuse to treat them, and view treatment as necessarily long-term, complicated, and only minimally effective. Fortunately, most patients with personality disorders are not difficult to work with, treatment is not always long-term, and treatment results are often rewarding. Personality disorders themselves are heterogeneous, so that it is rarely useful to make generalizations about all patients with personality disorders based on one's experience with a particular type (e.g., borderline personality disorder).

Epidemiology

Surveys show that from 10% to 20% of the general population may meet criteria for one or more personality disorders. The prevalence is far greater, however, in psychiatric populations (see Table 16–2, which is based on data collected at our hospital). In this table, the prevalence of personality disorder diagnosed with a self-report instrument (the Personality Diagnostic Questionnaire) is compared in four groups: control subjects who had been screened to exclude those with Axis I disorders, persons with major depression, persons with obsessive-compulsive disorder, and persons with panic disorder. Although the prevalence of specific personality disorders differed among the four groups, and no particular personality disorder was specific to Axis I pathology, the prevalence of personality disorder was high in all three patient groups with psychiatric disorders. In fact, more than 50% of hospitalized patients with major depression had a person-

Table 16–2. Prevalence of DSM-III personality disorders among psychiatric patients and screened control subjects

Disorder	Screened control subjects (*n* = 35)	Major depression (*n* = 78)	Obsessive-compulsive disorder (*n* = 37)	Panic disorder (*n* = 83)
Cluster A				
Paranoid	0	1	19	6
Schizoid	0	1	0	0
Schizotypal	3	9	19	0
Cluster B				
Histrionic	3	18	11	10
Narcissistic	3	0	5	0
Antisocial	0	1	0	1
Borderline	0	23	19	7
Cluster C				
Avoidant	0	15	27	20
Dependent	0	17	46	18
Compulsive	3	6	30	8
Passive-aggressive	9	4	49	2

Source. Adapted from Pfohl B, Black DW, Noyes R, et al: Axis I and Axis II comorbidity findings: implications for validity, in Personality Disorders: New Perspectives on Diagnostic Validity. Edited by Oldham JM. Washington, DC, American Psychiatric Press, 1991, pp 145–161.

ality disorder. There is great overlap among personality disorders as well, and most patients with a personality disorder will meet criteria for more than one disorder.

Abnormal character traits are even more prevalent than specific personality disorders. Epidemiological data from Iowa show that nearly 30% of the general population, 20% of subjects screened to exclude those with Axis I disorders, and nearly two-thirds of psychiatric outpatients have maladaptive personality traits (see Table 16–3).

Attention has recently been focused on the importance of the comorbidity of personality disorders and Axis I disorders, because there are many differences between patients who have personality disorders and those who do not. For example, patients with both depression and personality disorders tend to be younger and are more likely to be female, to have a history of marital instability, to report precipitating stressors, and to have a history of nonserious suicide attempts. Depressed patients with personality disorders are also less likely to have

Table 16–3.   Prevalence (in percentages) of DSM-III personality traits in a community sample, psychiatric outpatients, and screened subjects

Traits	Community sample ($n = 235$)	Outpatient sample ($n = 82$)	Screened psychiatrically normal subjects ($n = 40$)
Any	29	67	8
Cluster A	13	32	7
Paranoid	1	1	5
Schizoid	1	4	3
Schizotypal	13	30	8
Cluster B	6	42	5
Narcissistic	0	0	0
Histrionic	4	28	5
Borderline	0	5	0
Antisocial	1	30	3
Cluster C	26	53	18
Avoidant	0	16	8
Dependent	15	43	10
Compulsive	15	26	5
Passive-aggressive	0	4	0

Note.   The numbers are not additive, because many patients have traits of several different disorders.
Source.   Adapted from Reich J, Yates W, Nguaguba M: Prevalence of DSM-III personality disorders in the community. Social Psychiatry and Psychiatric Epidemiology 24:12–16, 1989.

an abnormal dexamethasone suppression test and are more likely to have a family history of alcoholism and antisocial personality disorder. These findings suggest that depressed patients with personality disorders may form an important subgroup that differs genetically and biochemically from depressed patients with primary depressive illness. The presence of a personality disorder also predicts a poor response to somatic treatments, including antidepressant medication and electroconvulsive therapy. These interesting findings also seem to be true, to some extent, for patients with panic disorder or obsessive-compulsive disorder and probably for other diagnostic groups as well.

Age at onset of personality disorder tends to be in adolescence, and the disorder is established by young adulthood. (By definition, antisocial personality disorder is established before age 15 years.) In general, late-onset personality changes suggest the presence of a major mental illness (e.g., the prodrome of schizophrenia) or a disorder caused by a general medical condition or the effects of a substance (e.g., dementia). Gender distribution differs among the 10 personality disorders. Some personality disorders (e.g., antisocial, schizoid, and obsessive-compulsive personality disorders) are seen preponderantly in men, whereas others (e.g., avoidant and dependent personality disorders) are seen preponderantly in women. Other personality disorders (e.g., borderline and schizotypal personality disorders) have a more equal distribution.

Personality disorders tend to be stable and enduring. There have been few long-term follow-up studies, which is not surprising because many of the different personality disorders have only recently been defined. Apparently, schizotypal, borderline, and antisocial personality disorders are all stable on follow-up.

Etiology

Freud believed that fixation at certain stages of development led to certain personality types. Several of the DSM-IV disorders derive from his oral, anal, and phallic character types. Fixation at the oral stage was felt to result in a personality characterized by demanding and dependent behavior (i.e., dependent personality disorder). Fixation of the anal stage led to a personality characterized by obsessionality, rigidity, and emotional aloofness (i.e., obsessive-compulsive personality disorder). Fixation of the phallic stage was believed to lead to shallowness and an inability to engage in intimate relationships (i.e., histrionic personality). These broad character types have, in fact, been supported by factor analytic studies, but there is little evidence that early childhood events or fixation at certain stages of development leads to specific personality patterns. An exception may be a growing body of evidence linking childhood molestation with borderline personality disorder; the resulting trauma is thought to cause difficulty in developing trust and intimacy.

To a limited extent, genetic factors appear to help explain some of the personality disorders. Family, twin, and adoption studies suggest that schizotypal personality may be genetically related to schizophrenia. Family and adoption studies have also confirmed a strong genetic factor in the etiology of antisocial and borderline personality disorders. There is less evidence available for the heritability of the other DSM-IV personality disorders. On the other hand, there is some evidence that basic dimensions of personality (e.g., callousness, intimacy problems) are inherited along a continuum with normality.

Neurobiological models have also been applied to personality disorders. Schizotypal personality has been associated with low platelet monoamine oxidase activity and impaired smooth pursuit eye movement. Among borderline patients, low cerebrospinal fluid 5-hydroxyindoleacetic acid (5-HIAA) has been negatively correlated with measures of aggression and a past history of suicide attempts. Depressed patients with personality disorders are less likely to have an abnormal dexamethasone suppression test than patients with depression alone.

Electroencephalographic (EEG) abnormalities have been reported in persons with antisocial personality disorder for many years. The most widely reported abnormality is an increase in slow-wave activity. A study of patients with borderline personality disorder reported that 38% had at least marginal EEG abnormalities, compared with 19% of control subjects. Based on this evidence, it has been suggested that some patients with borderline or antisocial personality disorder might actually be manifesting characterological changes resulting from a subtle brain injury or defect.

Diagnosis

As with most mental disorders, the diagnosis of personality disorder rests on a thorough personal and social history and a careful mental status examination. There are currently no tests to aid in the diagnosis of personality disorder, although several structured interviews (e.g., the Structured Interview for DSM-IV Personality Disorders) and self-report instruments (e.g., the Personality Diagnostic Questionnaire) can be helpful. (These interviews and questionnaires are further described in Chapter 4.) Patients with personality disorders generally present for evaluation of an Axis I disorder, not for their characterological problems. When a personality disorder is suspected, the clinician should carefully inquire about typical problems and behaviors that can result. One of our colleagues has recently put together a series of six questions that can be used to screen for the presence of a personality disorder. A "yes" answer on two or more items suggests a better than 80% chance of a personality disorder being present. These questions appear in Table 16–4. We have often found that when the patient's immediate problem (e.g., depression, relationship issues) intertwines with the past history, it is highly likely that a personality disorder is present.

Interviewing informants such as friends and family members is probably more important for the diagnosis of a personality disorder than it is for the diagnosis of other psychiatric disorders. Patients may be unaware of the extent to which their abnormal character traits disrupt their lives. For example, a patient with borderline personality disorder may not feel that his or her relationships are characterized by overidealization and devaluation, but it is extremely likely that a close friend or family member will have witnessed the behavior firsthand.

Collateral information is also important when a personality disorder is suspected but the patient denies having the trait. A person with antisocial person-

Table 16–4. Screening questions for the presence of a DSM-IV personality disorder

I'd like to ask you a few questions about some of your thoughts and feelings. Your answers will help me better understand what you are usually like. If the way you have been in recent weeks or months is different from the way you usually are, please look back to when you were your usual self when you answer these questions.

1. **Experiences marked shifts in mood: throughout the course of a typical day, experiences sudden spells of depression, irritability, anxiety, or anger**

   Y N

   How often do you have days when your mood is constantly changing—days when you shift back and forth from feeling as you usually do to feeling angry or depressed or anxious? **(IF PRESENT):** How long has this been going on?

2. **Feels inadequate and uncomfortable in situations where he or she is not the center of attention**

   Y N

   Some people prefer to be the center of attention, while others are content to remain on the edge of things. How would you describe yourself? **(IF CENTER):** How do you feel when you're not the center of attention?

3. **Actions usually directed toward obtaining immediate satisfaction; difficulty persisting with long-term goals**

   Y N

   Do you frequently insist on having what you want right now, even when waiting a little longer would get you something much better? Do you get excited by a new project or job, but then lose interest before it's done?

4. **Is reluctant to confide in others because of unwarranted fear that the information will be used against him or her**

   Y N

   Do you think it's best if other people don't get to know you too well? **(IF YES):** What are the reasons for this?

   Are you concerned that certain friends or co-workers are not really loyal or trustworthy? **(IF YES):** What has caused you concern?

5. **Excessive social anxiety, e.g., extreme discomfort in social situations involving unfamiliar people**

   Y N

   Are you concerned about saying the wrong thing in front of other people? **(IF YES):** Does this keep you from speaking up?

   How would you feel at a gathering where you didn't know many people? **(IF UNCOMFORTABLE):** Even if you're uncomfortable at first, do you relax after a while and enjoy yourself? How often would you make the first move in starting a conversation with someone?

6. **Unwilling to get involved with people unless certain of being liked, such that the number of friends has been limited**

   Y N

   How often do you avoid getting to know someone because you are worried they may not like you? **(IF OFTEN):** How has this affected the number of friends you have?

Source. Used with permission of Bruce Pfohl, M.D.

ality disorder may deny criminal activity or trivialize its significance. Information from the police or a parole officer can be enormously helpful in confirming the extent of the antisocial behavior. An informant can also be helpful in determining whether a personality disorder is present when a patient seems unconcerned with the trait or behavior. For example, a person suspected of having a schizoid personality disorder may be comfortable with his or her seclusiveness and not identify that trait as a problem.

Another concern about the diagnosis of personality disorder is that it may be made prematurely. Patients with major depression are frequently socially anxious and dependent on others, traits that may recede or disappear when the depression is successfully treated. Therefore, caution needs to be exercised in making the diagnosis, particularly when the patient is in the throes of an Axis I disorder, such as major depression.

Long-term observation is often necessary to confirm the diagnosis of personality disorder. Frequently, the clinician will defer diagnosis of a personality disorder, even if it is suspected, until he or she has seen the patient a number of times and has had the opportunity to gather more information from informants.

The DSM-IV Disorders

DSM-IV divides the 10 personality disorders among three clusters, each characterized by disorders that are similar phenomenologically or whose criteria tend to overlap. Another purpose of the division into clusters is to facilitate teaching.

Cluster A consists of the eccentric disorders: the schizoid, schizotypal, and paranoid personality disorders. These disorders are characterized by a pervasive pattern of abnormal cognition (e.g., suspiciousness), self-expression (e.g., odd speech), and relating to others (i.e., seclusiveness).

Cluster B consists of the dramatic disorders: the antisocial, borderline, histrionic, and narcissistic personality disorders. These disorders are characterized by a pervasive pattern of violating social norms (e.g., criminal behavior), impulsive behavior, excessive emotionality, and grandiosity. The Cluster B disorders tend to give all patients with personality disorders a bad reputation because these disorders often involve acting out (i.e., outward expression of their traits), leading to tantrums, self-abusive behavior, and angry outbursts. Patients in clusters A and C tend to have disorders that are more likely to be directed inward.

Cluster C consists of the anxious disorders: the avoidant, dependent, and obsessive-compulsive personality disorders. These disorders are characterized by a pervasive pattern of abnormal fears involving social relations, separation, and need for control.

Cluster A Disorders

Paranoid Personality Disorder

Although paranoid personality was first described by Adolph Meyer in the early twentieth century, it has rarely been researched. Psychoanalysts have associated paranoid traits with the anal character and a reaction formation to and projection of homosexual impulses. However, there is no evidence that homosexual persons are differentially affected with paranoid personalities. Patients with paranoid personality disorder have a pervasive distrust and suspiciousness of others and interpret others' motives as malevolent. This misperception occurs in a variety of contexts and may be indicated by a variety of behaviors. These behaviors and the full criteria are listed in Table 16–5.

Some researchers have hypothesized that paranoid personality disorder may lie along the spectrum of schizophrenic disorders, providing a manifestation of a common genetic predisposition. Paranoid features have been noted to occur premorbidly in persons with delusional disorder. A behavioral model has been suggested in which suspiciousness and mistrust are learned, leading to withdrawal, testing of others, and ruminative suspiciousness. Paranoid patients tend to fulfill their suspicious prophecies by inducing in others a tendency to be overcautious and deceptive.

Table 16–5. DSM-IV criteria for paranoid personality disorder

A. A pervasive distrust and suspiciousness of others such that their motives are interpreted as malevolent, beginning by early adulthood are present in a variety of contexts, as indicated by four (or more) of the following:
   1. Suspects, without sufficient basis, that others are exploiting or deceiving him or her
   2. Is preoccupied with unjustified doubts about the loyalty or trustworthiness of friends or associates
   3. Is reluctant to confide in others because of unwarranted fear that the information will be used maliciously against him or her
   4. Reads hidden demeaning or threatening meanings into benign remarks or events
   5. Persistently bears grudges, i.e., is unforgiving of insults, injuries, or slights
   6. Perceives attacks on his or her character or reputation that are not apparent to others and is quick to react angrily or to counterattack
   7. Has recurrent suspicions, without justification, regarding fidelity of spouse or sexual partner

B. Does not occur exclusively during the course of schizophrenia, a mood disorder with psychotic features, or another psychotic disorder, and is not due to the direct physiological effects of a general medical condition.

Note: If criteria are met prior to the onset of schizophrenia, add "premorbid," e.g., "paranoid personality disorder (premorbid)."

Patients with paranoid personality disorder rarely seek treatment, probably due to their suspiciousness of everyone, including therapists. With these patients it is probably best to use a supportive approach, listening patiently to their accusations and complaints, while at the same time being open, honest, and respectful. Once rapport has been established, alternative explanations of the patient's misperceptions might be suggested. Group therapy should probably be avoided, because patients with paranoid personality disorders tend to misinterpret what is said. Although suspiciousness may suggest to the clinician that antipsychotic medication is indicated, the usefulness of antipsychotics has not been studied in this disorder.

Schizoid Personality Disorder

Schizoid personality disorder was originally described to characterize the premorbid seclusiveness of schizophrenic patients and the eccentricity of their relatives. Over the years, the term was used to include almost all persons with problems in achieving intimacy. The concept was narrowed in 1980 in DSM-III, when odd, eccentric persons were placed in a new diagnostic category, *schizotypal personality*, and persons who were isolated due to an unwillingness to confront rejection were placed in another new diagnostic category, *avoidant personality*. Schizoid personality disorder is now restricted to persons with a profound defect in the ability to form personal relationships and respond to others in a meaningful way. The diagnostic criteria for schizoid personality disorder are listed in Table 16–6. The following case example illustrates the disorder.

Table 16–6.   DSM-IV criteria for schizoid personality disorder

A. A pervasive pattern of detachment from social relationships and a restricted range of expression of emotions in interpersonal settings, beginning by early adulthood and present in a variety of contexts, as indicated by four (or more) of the following:
   1. Neither desires nor enjoys close relationships, including being part of a family
   2. Almost always chooses solitary activities
   3. Has little, if any, interest in having sexual experiences with another person
   4. Takes pleasure in few, if any, activities
   5. Lacks close friends or confidants other than first-degree relatives
   6. Appears indifferent to the praise or criticism of others
   7. Shows emotional coldness, detachment, or flattened affectivity

B. Does not occur exclusively during the course of schizophrenia, a mood disorder with psychotic features, another psychotic disorder, or a pervasive developmental disorder, and is not due to the direct physiological effects of a general medical condition.

Note: If criteria are met prior to the onset of schizophrenia, add "premorbid," e.g., "schizoid personality disorder (premorbid)."

Michael, a 24-year-old, was transferred to the psychiatric ward after receiving treatment for a superficial gunshot wound to the head in a suicide attempt. Michael had had spells of depression in the past and, according to his family, had been depressed for several weeks before shooting himself. On transfer, however, it was apparent that Michael was no longer depressed, and he believed there was no reason to remain in the hospital.

According to his family, Michael had always been considered shy, was isolative, and had no friends that the family was aware of. He had not done well in school and had dropped out before graduating from high school. He had never dated and admitted having no interest in sexual activity with boys or girls, preferring solitary masturbation. Michael admitted that he was not particularly close to any of his family members, and although he lived with his elderly father, he showed no interest or emotion in describing their relationship. Despite adequate intelligence, Michael had never been able to persist with a job; as a result, he had never had significant employment. He preferred to stay home and watch television or play computer games. In fact, Michael was so unmotivated and so isolated from the community that he had never bothered to obtain a driver's license.

Despite his seclusive nature and emotional aloofness, Michael believed that his only problem was his occasional bouts of depression. He neither complained about his social isolation and emotional aloofness nor accepted the fact that these symptoms could be part of his underlying problem. He had no interest in changing his ways and refused referral for psychotherapy.

Patients with schizoid personality disorder are characterized by the absence of close relationships (including with their family of origin), choosing solitary activities, rarely experiencing strong emotions, having little desire for sexual experience with another person, showing indifference to praise or criticism, having no close friends or confidants other than first-degree relatives, and displaying constricted affect. The diagnosis is not made in persons with schizophrenia or other psychotic disorders, although patients with these conditions may have had schizoid traits premorbidly.

Schizoid personality disorder tends to be rare in clinical settings, although schizoid traits are relatively common. Little is known about the treatment of the disorder. Most persons with this condition probably do not seek professional help except for depression, substance abuse, or other problems. Most persons with the disorder lack the insight or motivation for individual psychotherapy and would probably find the intimacy of group therapy too threatening. If the patient is motivated to change, simple behavioral techniques may be helpful, such as graded exposure to a variety of social tasks. For example, the clinician might encourage social activity by having the patient start with attending a concert, then join a bridge club, and eventually enter a dance class.

Schizotypal Personality Disorder

Schizotypal personality disorder was created in the development of DSM-III based on its presumed genetic relatedness to schizophrenia. The Danish Adoption Study had revealed that relatives of schizophrenic patients often had a cluster of schizophrenic-like traits, a fact noted much earlier by both Kraepelin and Bleuler. Antecedents for this disorder include Bleuler's *simple* and *latent* schizophrenia. These diagnoses were applied to persons who displayed mild or attenuated symptoms of schizophrenia but who were nonpsychotic. Schizotypal personality disorder is now considered part of the schizophrenia spectrum, along with schizophreniform disorder, schizoaffective disorder, and perhaps mood disorder with mood-incongruent psychotic features.

Schizotypal personality disorder is characterized by a pattern of peculiar behavior, odd speech and thinking, and unusual perceptual experiences. Schizotypal patients tend to be socially isolated and to have idiosyncratic speech, unusual (i.e., "magical") beliefs, mild paranoid tendencies, inappropriate or constricted affect, and undue social anxiety. The criteria are found in Table 16–7.

Because the disorder is relatively new, there is limited information about its distribution, natural history, and treatment. Community surveys suggest that

Table 16–7. DSM-IV criteria for schizotypal personality disorder

A. A pervasive pattern of social and interpersonal deficits marked by acute discomfort with, and reduced capacity for, close relationships as well as by cognitive or perceptual distortions and eccentricities of behavior, beginning by early adulthood and present in a variety of contexts, as indicated by five (or more) of the following:

　1. Ideas of reference (excluding delusions of reference)
　2. Odd beliefs or magical thinking that influences behavior and is inconsistent with subcultural norms (e.g., superstitiousness, belief in clairvoyance, telepathy, or "sixth sense"; in children and adolescents, bizarre fantasies or preoccupations)
　3. Unusual perceptual experiences, including bodily illusions
　4. Odd thinking and speech (e.g., vague, circumstantial, metaphorical, overelaborate, or stereotyped)
　5. Suspiciousness or paranoid ideation
　6. Inappropriate or constructed affect
　7. Behavior or appearance that is odd, eccentric, or peculiar
　8. Lack of close friends or confidants other than first-degree relatives
　9. Excessive social anxiety that does not diminish with familiarity and tends to be associated with paranoid fears rather than negative judgments about self

B. Does not occur exclusively during the course of schizophrenia, a mood disorder with psychotic features, another psychotic disorder, or a pervasive developmental disorder.

Note: If criteria are met prior to the onset of schizophrenia, add "premorbid," e.g., schizotypal personality disorder "(premorbid)."

schizotypal personality disorder has a prevalence of between 3% and 5% of the population and is one of the more common personality disorders. As noted in Table 16–3, up to 30% of psychiatric outpatients have schizotypal traits. The gender distribution is about equal, and there is frequent comorbidity with mood, substance use, and anxiety disorders.

Treatment of patients with schizotypal personality disorders will often center on issues that led the person to seek treatment. These problems may include feelings of alienation or isolation, mild feelings of paranoia or suspiciousness, or feelings of alienation due to paranoid ideation or ideas of reference. A supportive approach is recommended, because exploratory and group psychotherapies tend to be too threatening for these patients. Social skills training may be useful in helping eccentric, odd persons to feel more comfortable with others.

More commonly, a person with a schizotypal personality will present seeking help for a mood or an anxiety disorder. These conditions should be treated in the usual manner with medication. Unfortunately, schizotypal personality disorder has been identified as a predictor of poor response to treatment of obsessive-compulsive disorder.

Some evidence suggests that low-dose antipsychotics will help alleviate the intense anxiety, odd speech, and unusual perceptual experiences that are often found in patients with schizotypal personality. However, any enthusiasm for using these medications must be tempered by the knowledge of their tendency to induce troublesome and potentially irreversible side effects. Antipsychotics should not routinely be used in these patients.

Cluster B Disorders

Antisocial Personality Disorder

Antisocial personality is the oldest and best validated of the 10 personality disorders and was first recognized in the nineteenth century as *manie sans délire* and *moral insanity*. These terms were used to describe manipulative behavior unaccompanied by impairments in reasoning. More frequently used terms include *psychopathic personality* and *sociopathic personality*. The disorder is characterized by a pattern of socially irresponsible, exploitative, and guiltless behavior, as evidenced by failure to conform to the law, failure to sustain consistent employment, exploitation and manipulation of others for personal gain, deception, and failure to develop stable relationships. One of the best descriptions of this disorder appears in the classic book *The Mask of Sanity*, by Hervey Cleckley, originally published in 1941.

Although the diagnostic criteria for antisocial personality have been criticized for their "Chinese menu" approach and their failure to include psychological traits such as guiltlessness, egocentricity, incapacity for love, lack of remorse, and failure to learn from past experience, they have proved to be both reliable and valid. In fact, lack of remorse is now included as a criterion. The criteria are listed in Table 16–8.

In a recent study at the University of Iowa, antisocial males admitted to our hospital between 1945 and 1970 were interviewed an average of 29 years after admission. The following case was unfortunately typical and illustrates the personal and interpersonal difficulties that arise from the disorder:

> In 1958, at age 18, Douglas was admitted for evaluation of antisocial behavior. Douglas had had a chaotic childhood. His father was alcoholic, had married five times, and had abandoned his family when Douglas was 6 years old. Because his mother had a history of incarceration and was unable to care for him, Douglas had lived in a series of foster homes until he was adopted at age 8. His adoptive father was a university professor, and his mother was described as a compulsive woman with strict standards.
>
> Since early childhood, Douglas had stolen various articles, had shoplifted, had burglarized churches, and later had stolen automobiles. His school performance was poor, and he was frequently in detention for breaking rules. Because of continued lawbreaking, Douglas was sent to a juvenile reformatory for 2 years at age 16. While in the reformatory, he slashed another boy with a razor blade in a fight.
>
> Douglas reported first having sexual intercourse at age 15, and since leaving the

Table 16–8.   DSM-IV criteria for antisocial personality disorder

A. Current age at least 18 years.

B. Evidence of conduct disorder with onset before age 15.

C. A pervasive pattern of disregard for and violation of the rights of others occurring since age 15, as indicated by at least three of the following:
   1. Failure to conform to social norms with respect to lawful behaviors, as indicated by repeatedly performing acts that are grounds for arrest
   2. Deceitfulness, as indicated by repeated lying, use of aliases, or conning others for personal profit or pleasure
   3. Impulsivity or failure to plan ahead
   4. Irritability and aggressiveness, as indicated by repeated physical fights or assaults
   5. Reckless disregard for safety of self or others
   6. Consistent irresponsibility, as indicated by repeated failure to sustain consistent work behavior or honor financial obligations
   7. Lack of remorse, as indicated by being indifferent to or rationalizing having hurt, mistreated, or stolen from another

D. Occurrence of antisocial behavior is not exclusively during the course of schizophrenia or a manic episode.

reformatory, he claimed to have had intercourse with many different partners. At the time of admission, he was living off of girls he had charmed into supporting him. He chain-smoked and admitted to considerable drinking since age 16.

An electroencephalogram was normal, and his IQ was measured at 112. He was discharged after a 16-day stay.

Douglas was found after we had learned that he was using an alias. The follow-up occurred in November 1988, when he was 48 years old. His home, in an impoverished area of a midsized Midwestern community, was badly deteriorated and had a collapsing roof. At interview, Douglas was thin, gaunt, and poorly groomed. He appeared nervous and tremulous. His home was dark and cold; he admitted that the furnace did not work. He proceeded to talk about his troubled life in a meaningless way.

Douglas acknowledged more than 20 arrests and more than five felony convictions for various reasons, including attempted murder, armed robbery, receiving stolen goods, using aliases, burglary, and driving while intoxicated. Since his hospitalization, he had spent more than 17 years in prison, including the period from 1958 to 1974. He had escaped from prison, but he was returned 2 months later. Interestingly, he escaped with the help of his biological mother, with whom he then had a sexual relationship. His most recent arrest occurred within the past year and was for public intoxication and assault.

Douglas reported at least nine hospitalizations for alcohol detoxification, with the latest being earlier that year. He admitted to having used marijuana, amphetamines, tranquilizers, cocaine, and heroin in the past.

He told us that he had never held a full-time job in his life and that the longest job he had held lasted 60 days. He reported doing paint and body work on cars in his own garage to earn a living, but he had not done any work for several months. He estimated that he had held about 150 jobs in the past 10 years. His family was currently receiving public assistance.

Douglas reported that nine persons lived in his home, including his four children. He had met his common-law wife in a psychiatric hospital. He told us that she required tranquilizers for emotional problems and that the marriage was unsatisfactory.

He had lived in six different states, and in the last 10 years had moved more than 20 times. He reported occasionally attending Alcoholics Anonymous at a local church, but otherwise he did not socialize outside his family.

He reported being afraid of closed places, which he related to graphic memories of prison life. He claimed to have witnessed several murders of "snitches" and to have committed murder himself during a prison riot. He admitted that he had not yet settled down and told us that he was still spending money foolishly, was frequently reckless, and was getting into frequent fights and arguments. He said that he got a "charge out of doing dangerous things."

Thirty years after his hospitalization, Douglas remained unrepentant, and he clearly lacked remorse for past crimes. He remained actively antisocial and was still being arrested with some frequency, albeit for less significant charges. His alcoholism was uncontrolled, and he had an unstable work record and an impoverished life.

Family, twin, and adoption studies suggest that the disorder has a hereditary basis. Nearly one quarter of first-degree relatives of patients with antisocial personality have the disorder themselves. Antisocial personality disorder also appears to be genetically related to alcoholism, which is not surprising because the disorder is frequently complicated by alcohol abuse. It has been hypothesized that low cortical arousal and a reduced level of inhibitory anxiety may contribute to an impulsive, sensation-seeking life-style.

Patients with antisocial personality disorder have substantial comorbidity; nearly one quarter develop major depression, and three quarters develop alcoholism and/or other substance abuse. They are also prone to making suicide attempts, engaging in felonious behavior, and having accidents. These problems present an ongoing challenge to the therapist charged with caring for them. Unfortunately, long-term follow-up studies, including the one at the University of Iowa, show that the disorder is stable and enduring—even into the 60s and 70s. A common myth is that the disorder "burns out" or attenuates by age 40. Generally, after age 40, people with antisocial personality disorder have fewer legal problems and are less troublesome to the community. Other characteristics of the disorder often persist, however, including marital instability, substance abuse, impulsiveness, poor temper control, and failure to honor financial obligations. About 5% of persons with antisocial personality disorder commit suicide, and deaths from accidents (e.g., motor vehicle accidents) are common.

According to the Epidemiologic Catchment Area study, about 3% of men and 1% of women in the general population have antisocial personality disorder. By definition, onset occurs before age 15; in fact, most persons with antisocial personality will have manifested deviant behavior by age 5. Prevalence varies with the setting, and in jails and prisons the prevalence may reach 75%. Common symptoms of antisocial personality both before age 15 and after age 18 are shown in Table 16–9.

Treatment of antisocial patients is extremely difficult due to their lack of empathy and insight. Long-term behaviorally oriented inpatient programs have been recommended, although there are few supporting data. Correctional facilities may be the best means of controlling antisocial persons who engage in criminal activity. Lithium carbonate, carbamazepine, or propranolol is occasionally prescribed for the rage attacks or poorly controlled episodes of anger that many antisocial persons have. These medications have not been systematically studied for this indication, however. Antisocial personality disorder has been linked with poor outcome of formal alcohol and drug rehabilitation programs.

Table 16–9. Common antisocial behaviors in 71 males, currently adults, with antisocial personality disorder (assessed at baseline, mean age 26 years)

Behavior before age 15 years	%	Behavior after age 18 years	%
Violates rules	85	Multiple arrests	75
Fights	47	Repeated fights	61
Drunkenness	42	Frequent job changes	54
Poor school performance	37	Promiscuity	48
Truancy	28	Felony conviction	48
Expulsion/suspension	27	Significant unemployment	47
Running away	24	Lying	41
Persistent lying	24	Wanderlust	34
		Two or more divorces	21
		Spouse/child abuse	20
		Repeated thefts	17
		Walking off jobs	16
		Nonpayment of child support	13
		Bad debts	10
		Lack of fixed address	9
		Conning others	6

Source.   Adapted from Black DW, Baumgard CH, Bell SE: A 16- to 45-year follow-up of 71 males with antisocial personality disorder. Comprehensive Psychiatry (in press).

Borderline Personality Disorder

Borderline personality disorder was introduced in DSM-III, although the concept has a much longer history. It was created to characterize persons with instability in a number of areas, including their self-identity, interpersonal relationships, and mood. Many of these features would have been included in the DSM-II disorder *emotionally unstable personality*. Early conceptualizations of borderline personality considered it to be a variant of schizophrenia, and the term *borderline schizophrenia* was created to describe persons who had transient episodes of psychosis during periods of regression or during psychotherapy. These patients were later separated from patients with schizotypal personality disorder on the basis of a factor analytic study.

The disorder is of great interest to psychoanalysts. Kernberg, for example, uses the term *borderline personality organization* to describe his broad diagnostic concept and diagnoses borderline personality on the basis of the presence of identity diffusion, primitive defense mechanisms such as splitting (e.g., exaggerated dichotomies of good and evil, black and white), and the maintenance of reality testing except in the perception of self and others. Unfortunately, reliable diagnosis is very difficult to achieve with these psychological criteria.

As currently conceptualized, the disorder represents a pervasive pattern of mood instability, unstable and intense interpersonal relationships, impulsivity, inappropriate or intense anger, lack of control of anger, recurrent suicidal threats and gestures, self-mutilating behavior, marked and persistent identity disturbance, chronic feelings of emptiness or boredom, and frantic efforts to avoid real or imagined abandonment. Patients may also experience transient paranoid ideation or dissociative symptoms. Thomas Sydenham, an English physician best known for describing Saint Vitus' dance, captures the essence of borderline personality in the quotation at the beginning of this chapter. See Table 16–10 for the criteria.

The diagnosis identifies a large group of patients and tends to overlap with many other personality disorders, especially the histrionic, antisocial, and schizotypal types. One of the more common personality disorders among psychiatric patients, as indicated in Table 16–2, its frequency in the general population has been estimated at 1%–2%. Borderline personality disorder, which is relatively stable in long-term follow-up studies, is associated with poor outcome and a suicide rate exceeding 5%. Good long-term outcome has been associated with high intelligence, self-discipline, and social support from friends and relatives.

Table 16–10. DSM-IV criteria for borderline personality disorder

A pervasive pattern of instability of interpersonal relationships, self-image, and affects, and marked impulsivity beginning by early adulthood and present in a variety of contexts, as indicated by five (or more) of the following:

1. Frantic efforts to avoid real or imagined abandonment. **Note:** Do not include suicidal or self-mutilating behavior covered in criterion 5.

2. A pattern of unstable and intense interpersonal relationships characterized by alternating between extremes of idealization and devaluation

3. Identity disturbance: persistent and markedly disturbed, distorted, or unstable self-image or sense of self

4. Impulsivity in at least two areas that are potentially self-damaging (e.g., spending, sex, substance abuse, reckless driving, binge eating). **Note:** Do not include suicidal or self-mutilating behavior covered in criterion 5.

5. Recurrent suicidal behavior, gestures, or threats, or self-mutilating behavior

6. Affective instability due to a marked reactivity of mood (e.g., intense episodic dysphoria, irritability, or anxiety usually lasting a few hours and only rarely more than a few days)

7. Chronic feelings of emptiness

8. Inappropriate, intense anger or lack of control of anger (e.g., frequent displays of temper, constant anger, recurrent physical fights)

9. Transient, stress-related paranoid ideation or severe dissociative symptoms

Anger, antisocial behavior, suspiciousness, and vanity are associated with poor outcome.

Family studies have shown that the disorder is common in the first-degree relatives of patients with borderline personality, and many relatives also have major depression, substance use disorder, or antisocial personality disorder. Borderline personality disorder has also been associated with certain biochemical and psychophysiological abnormalities, such as shortened rapid eye movement latency, abnormal dexamethasone suppression, and an abnormal thyrotropin-releasing hormone test—abnormalities often found in major depression.

Some researchers have argued that borderline personality is a variant of affective disorder, as evidenced by its association with depression in family studies, follow-up studies showing that most patient with borderline personality develop depression, and response to antidepressant medication. In their view, the chronic mood instability creates a personality disturbance, not vice versa. On the other hand, it can be argued that patients with borderline personality disorder may simply be sensitive to developing depressions either because of a psychosocial predisposition (e.g., history of verbal and sexual abuse during childhood) or a biological vulnerability.

The treatment of borderline patients is controversial. It ranges from Kernberg's recommendation for intensive, interpretive, and confrontational psychotherapy focusing on the transference relationship to an emphasis on a more practical, supportive, and problem-solving approach. Borderline patients are reported to form an intense transference, and countertransference itself can be a problem, because these patients tend to stimulate intense feelings of frustration, guilt, or anger in their therapists. Family or group psychotherapy may help to dilute the transference. Cognitive restructuring techniques may be effective in correcting dysfunctional attitudes and ambivalent perceptions of others and oneself. Behavioral techniques, particularly in the inpatient setting, may also be useful in managing self-mutilating and other impulses (e.g., impulsive behaviors will result in reduced privileges).

Pharmacological approaches have also been recommended, but no one treatment has emerged as superior to another. Low-dose antipsychotics may be helpful in treating perceptual distortions, lithium carbonate may be useful in treating mood swings, and monoamine oxidase inhibitors (MAOIs) may be useful in treating dysphoria secondary to interpersonal rejection. In one study, four treatments were compared, including an antipsychotic (trifluoperazine), carbamazepine, alprazolam, and a MAOI (phenelzine). All treatments were somewhat effective, except for alprazolam, which caused behavioral disinhibition and anger dyscontrol. Serotonin reuptake inhibitors (SRIs), such as fluoxetine, may also be helpful in reducing depressive symptoms and suicidal ideations and behavior. The fact that overdoses of these agents are not fatal is an important consideration in patients known for impulsive suicide attempts. Because self-mutilating behavior and frequent suicide attempts are a problem in borderline patients, physicians need to be cautious about prescribing any medication that can be potentially fatal in overdose. The long-term value of any of these medications is unknown.

Histrionic Personality Disorder

Histrionic personality takes its name from hysteria, a disorder first characterized in the nineteenth century and associated with conversion, phobias, anxiety, and somatization. Hysterical features (e.g., a self-dramatizing, attention-seeking nature) were felt to be associated with hysteria. *Hysterical personality* was included in DSM-II and was renamed *histrionic personality* in DSM-III, so as not to be confused with hysteria (renamed *somatization disorder*). Many persons with somatization disorder do have histrionic personality disorder, although there is not a one-to-one relationship.

According to DSM-IV, persons with histrionic personality exhibit a pattern of excessive emotionality and attention-seeking behavior. Typical behaviors include excessive concern with appearance and wanting to be the center of attention. The full set of criteria are listed in Table 16–11. These persons are often gregarious and superficially charming, but they can be manipulative, vain, and demanding.

Results from the Epidemiologic Catchment Area study show histrionic personality disorder to have a prevalence of about 2% in the general population, affecting men and women equally. The study also found that persons with this

Table 16–11. DSM-IV criteria for histrionic personality disorder

A pervasive pattern of excessive emotionality and attention seeking, beginning by early adulthood and present in a variety of contexts, as indicated by five (or more) of the following:

1. Is uncomfortable in situations in which he or she is not the center of attention
2. Interaction with others is often characterized by inappropriate sexually seductive or provocative behavior
3. Displays rapidly shifting and shallow expression of emotions
4. Consistently uses physical appearance to draw attention to self
5. Has a style of speech that is excessively impressionistic and lacking in detail
6. Shows self-dramatization, theatricality, and exaggerated expression of emotion
7. Is suggestible, i.e., easily influenced by others or circumstances
8. Considers relationships to be more intimate than they actually are

disorder tend to seek out medical attention and to make frequent use of available health services. The picture that emerges is of a person who has much difficulty in sustaining interpersonal relationships; frequently has depression, occasionally expressed in suicide attempts; and makes frequent use of medical and mental health services.

Although the cause of histrionic personality is unknown, the disorder has been linked through family studies to somatization disorder and antisocial personality disorder. It has also been suggested that histrionic personality is a gender-biased diagnosis that merely describes a caricature of stereotypic femininity, because it is frequently diagnosed among females in clinical samples.

Interventions have not been well studied; however, psychodynamic psychotherapy, which has a long tradition in the treatment of this and related syndromes, is considered by some to be the treatment of choice. However, others advocate a more supportive, problem-solving approach or a cognitive approach to deal with distorted thinking, such as the inflated self-image many histrionic patients have. An interpersonal approach may focus on conscious (or unconscious) motivations for seeking out disappointing lovers and being unable to commit oneself to a stable, meaningful relationship. Group therapy may be useful in addressing provocative and attention-seeking behavior. As patients may not be aware of their behaviors, it may be helpful to have others point these traits out to them. A condition that may be related, *hysteroid dysphoria*, described in depressed women who have a history of sensitivity to rejection in relationships, is reportedly responsive to MAOIs (e.g., phenelzine).

Narcissistic Personality Disorder

The category *narcissistic personality*, created during the development of DSM-III, has long been of interest to psychoanalysts. This disorder is characterized by grandiosity, lack of empathy, and hypersensitivity to evaluation by others. The criteria are listed in Table 16–12.

This relatively new disorder has met with various criticisms. First, its prevalence in surveys is very low; in one community survey no cases were found among a sample of nearly 800. Next, some experts argue that it is not a distinctive syndrome, because narcissistic traits are common in varying degrees in most patients with personality disorders; that the criteria tend to ignore more subtle and indirect manifestations (e.g., dependency conflicts); and that the overlap with other disorders, such as borderline personality disorder, adds to its lack of distinctiveness. Some clinicians believe that the diagnosis can be made only on the basis of the emerging transferential relationship in psychoanalytic psychotherapy.

Little is known about the treatment of this condition, although some experts

Table 16–12.   DSM-IV criteria for narcissistic personality disorder

A pervasive pattern of grandiosity (in fantasy or behavior), need for admiration, and lack of empathy, beginning by early adulthood and present in a variety of contexts, as indicated by five (or more) of the following:

1. Has a grandiose sense of self-importance (e.g., exaggerates achievements and talents, expects to be recognized as superior without commensurate achievements)
2. Is preoccupied with fantasies of unlimited success, power, brilliance, beauty, or ideal love
3. Believes that he or she is "special" and unique and can only be understood by, or should associate with, other special or high-status people (or institutions)
4. Requires excessive admiration
5. Has a sense of entitlement, i.e., unreasonable expectations of especially favorable treatment or automatic compliance with his or her expectations
6. Is interpersonally exploitative, i.e., takes advantage of others to achieve his or her own ends
7. Lack of empathy: unwilling to recognize or identify with the feelings and needs of others
8. Is often envious of others or believes that others are envious of him or her
9. Shows arrogant, haughty behaviors or attitudes

have recommended insight-oriented psychotherapy. Others have recommended interpersonal or cognitive behavioral psychotherapy. Narcissistic patients are often very difficult to work with, tend to devalue the therapist, and may abruptly terminate therapy.

Cluster C Disorders

Avoidant Personality Disorder

Avoidant personality disorder was also introduced in DSM-III and represents a variant of what had previously been termed *schizoid personality*. Another predecessor was *inadequate personality*, a term used to describe persons who had experienced failure in a number of spheres of life (e.g., interpersonal relations, occupation).

Avoidant behavior is characterized as inhibited, introverted, and anxious. Persons with avoidant personality disorder tend to have low self-esteem, hypersensitivity to rejection, apprehension and mistrust, social awkwardness, timidity, social discomfort, and self-conscious fears of being embarrassed or acting foolish. Table 16–13 lists the criteria.

A current issue is whether avoidant personality disorder represents a dimension along a spectrum of anxiety disorders, similar to the way borderline person-

Table 16–13. DSM-IV criteria for avoidant personality disorder

A pervasive pattern of social inhibition, feelings of inadequacy, and hypersensitivity to negative evaluation, beginning by early adulthood and present in a variety of contexts, as indicated by four (or more) of the following:

1. Avoids occupational activities that involve significant interpersonal contact because of fears of criticism, disapproval, or rejection
2. Is unwilling to get involved with people unless certain of being liked
3. Shows restraint within intimate relationships because of the fear of being shamed or ridiculed
4. Is preoccupied with being criticized or rejected in social situations
5. Is inhibited in new interpersonal situations because of feelings of inadequacy
6. Views self as socially inept, personally unappealing, or inferior to others
7. Is unusually reluctant to take personal risks or to engage in any new activities because they may prove embarrassing

ality disorder has been linked to mood disorders and schizotypal personality disorder to schizophrenia. Clearly, many features of avoidant personality disorder are indistinguishable from social phobia, and the two frequently overlap. It is possible that avoidant personality disorder involves a genetic predisposition to chronic anxiety.

Several psychotherapeutic strategies have evolved for the treatment of avoidant personality disorder. Group therapy may help avoidant patients to learn to overcome social anxiety and to develop interpersonal trust. Assertiveness and social skills training may be useful, as well as systematic desensitization to treat anxiety symptoms, shyness, and introversion. Cognitive therapy has been recommended to help correct dysfunctional thinking (e.g., "I had better not open my mouth, because I'll probably say something stupid"). Benzodiazepines are often helpful during periods in which the patient is attempting to reverse previously avoided behavior. It is best to limit the use these agents to short periods (i.e., weeks or months), although some patients will benefit from long-term use.

Because tricyclic antidepressants, MAOIs, SRIs, and alprazolam have all been shown to be helpful in treating social phobia, they might also be helpful in treating avoidant personality, because the two conditions seem to overlap. However, the use of these medications to treat avoidant personality has not been subjected to systematic study.

Dependent Personality Disorder

Dependent personality was a subtype of the DSM-I passive-aggressive personality, was not included in DSM-II, but was reintroduced in DSM-III. Psychoanalysts have suggested that dependent personality results from fixation at the oral stage of development. The disorder is a pattern of relying excessively on others for emotional support. Typical behaviors are listed in the criteria (Table 16–14), and a case is described below.

Bob, a 45-year-old farm laborer, presented for evaluation of depression, which had been chronic for several years. He also reported a long-standing eating disorder, which had resulted in significant weight loss. For 10 years, Bob had feared becoming fat like his father, who had died unexpectedly of a myocardial infarction.

In addition to these problems, Bob described a dull, passive life-style. The third of eight children, he was reared on a farm and taken out of school after the 8th grade to work, as the other children had been. The family remained close, because there were few opportunities for friendships outside the family. Bob reported that he had rarely dated and had once been "sweet on a girl." He denied any current interest in developing a relationship.

Bob lived with his mother until she insisted he move out at age 44, which he did reluctantly. Although he lived alone, he remained in close contact with his mother, eating meals with her twice daily and phoning her between 10 and 20 times daily. He relied on her to make decisions for him, even trivial ones about his day-to-day activities.

Bob had no interests or hobbies apart from his farm chores. He admitted to us that he was uncomfortable being alone in his mobile home, which prompted him to phone his mother. He cried when he was asked how he would handle his mother's eventual death. (She was then more than 80 years old.)

Table 16–14. DSM-IV criteria for dependent personality disorder

A pervasive and excessive need to be taken care of, leading to submissive and clinging behavior and fears of separation, beginning by early adulthood and present in a variety of contexts, as indicated by five (or more) of the following:

1. Is unable to make everyday decisions without an excessive amount of advice and reassurance from others

2. Needs others to assume responsibility for most major areas of his or her life

3. Has difficulty expressing disagreement with others because of fear of loss of support of approval. **Note:** Do not include realistic fears of retribution.

4. Has difficulty initiating projects or doing things on his or her own (because of a lack of self-confidence in judgment or abilities rather than a lack of motivation or energy)

5. Goes to excessive lengths to obtain nurturance and support from others, to the point of volunteering to do things that are unpleasant

6. Feels uncomfortable or helpless when alone because of exaggerated fears of being unable to care for himself or herself

7. Urgently seeks another relationship as a source of care and support when a close relationship ends

8. Is unrealistically preoccupied with fears of being left to take care of himself or herself

Although Bob gained weight steadily on a refeeding protocol, it became clear that he would need supervision outside the hospital. Because his mother was too old to help (and her supervision would only worsen his dependency on her), a decision was made by his family to place Bob in a care facility.

Dependent personality disorder has not been well studied, and it has been questioned whether it is sufficiently distinctive from other disorders, such as avoidant personality, to stand alone. Additionally, dependent personality appears to be diagnosed more frequently in women, suggesting a gender bias. Finally, chronic illnesses (both psychiatric and physical) may lead to dependent behavior.

Recommended treatment includes insight-oriented psychotherapy, group therapy, and marital counseling when it is clear that the patient is overdependent on his or her spouse. A problem frequently encountered with these patients is their tendency to have the therapist take responsibility for all decisions. Assertiveness training, social skills training, cognitive-behavior psychotherapy, and other approaches may be helpful in selected patients.

Obsessive-Compulsive Personality Disorder

Obsessive-compulsive personality is thought by psychoanalysts to represent a fixation at the anal stage of development, characterized by the triad of obstinacy, parsimony, and orderliness. It was originally thought that this disorder predisposed patients to obsessive-compulsive disorder. Although early studies showed that some patients with obsessive-compulsive disorder were likely to have a premorbid obsessional personality, it became apparent that obsessive-compulsive personality and obsessive-compulsive disorder do not have a one-to-one relationship. The relationship between obsessive-compulsive personality disorder and obsessive-compulsive disorder is more fully explored in Chapter 11.

Obsessive-compulsive personality disorder represents a lifelong pattern of perfectionism and inflexibility typically associated with overconscientiousness and constricted emotions. The diagnostic criteria are listed in Table 16–15. Patients with obsessive-compulsive personality are prone to develop depression, particularly as they get older. Commonalities exist with the Type A personality described by Rosenman (characterized by intense ambition and competitiveness), which has been identified as a risk factor for cardiovascular disease.

Obsessive-compulsive personality disorder is relatively difficult to treat. Some experts recommend psychodynamic psychotherapy; however, patients tend to intellectualize and may be insightful, but they develop little feeling or affect. Paradoxical strategies have been recommended, such as suggesting that

Table 16–15. DSM-IV criteria for obsessive-compulsive personality disorder

A pervasive pattern of preoccupation with orderliness, perfectionism, and mental and interpersonal control, at the expense of flexibility, openness, and efficiency, beginning by early adulthood and present in a variety of contexts, as indicated by four (or more) of the following:

1. Is preoccupied with details, rules, lists, order, organization, or schedules to the extent that the major point of the activity is lost
2. Shows perfectionism that interferes with task completion (e.g., is unable to complete a project because his or her own overly strict standards are not met)
3. Is excessively devoted to work and productivity to the exclusion of leisure activities and friendships (not accounted for by obvious economic necessity)
4. Is overconscientious, scrupulous, and inflexible about matters of morality, ethics, or values (not accounted for by cultural or religious identification)
5. Is unable to discard worn-out or worthless objects even when they have no sentimental value
6. Is reluctant to delegate tasks or to work with others unless they submit to exactly his or her way of doing things
7. Adopts a miserly spending style toward both self and others; money is viewed as something to be hoarded for future catastrophes
8. Shows rigidity and stubbornness

Recommendations for management of personality disorders

1. Some patients with personality disorders can be difficult, unpleasant, and manipulative. You should not let this fact interfere with or color your understanding of *all* patients with personality disorders.
2. Patients have enduring, long-term problems, and therapy may be long-term as well. Decades of maladaptive behavior cannot be easily understood or reversed.
3. Maintain a professional distance from the patient. You are not a friend or collaborator; you are a therapist.
   - Avoid becoming overinvolved with patients, doing favors (e.g., giving out home telephone number), or relating your problems. These "boundary" issues can create enormous problems if not dealt with from the outset.
4. Establish ground rules for therapy (e.g., that you are willing to see the person regularly, at a specified time).
   - Spell out what the patient should do or who is to be called in a crisis (e.g., who is on call).
   - Spell out consequences of self-damaging acts (e.g., hospitalization, referral to another therapist).
5. Avoid fantasies of becoming a "savior" to your patient. If the personality disorder is chronic, the patient has undoubtedly seen other therapists without success. Why should you be the exception?
6. Seek support for yourself from peers or supervisors. Patients with personality disorders can be a handful, and you will probably need advice or consultation now and then.

the patient become even more perfectionistic or rigid. Cognitive techniques may be helpful in addressing the illogic of the obsessive-compulsive patient's rigid beliefs and moral standards. Thought stopping may be helpful for ruminations.

Bibliography

Akhtar S, Thompson JA: Full review: narcissistic personality disorder. Am J Psychiatry 139:12–20, 1982

Beck A: Cognitive Therapy of Personality Disorders. New York, Guilford, 1990

Black DW, Baumgard CH, Bell SE: A 16- to 45-year follow-up of 71 males with antisocial personality disorder. Comprehensive Psychiatry (in press)

Black DW, Bell S, Hulbert J, et al: The importance of Axis II in patients with major depression—a controlled study. J Affect Disord 14:115–122, 1988

Cadoret RJ, O'Gorman TW, Troughton E, et al: Alcoholism and antisocial personality. Arch Gen Psychiatry 42:161–167, 1985

Cleckley H: The Mask of Sanity. St. Louis, MO, Mosby, 1941

Cornelius JR, Soloff PH, Perel JM, et al: A preliminary trial of fluoxetine in refractory borderline patients. J Clin Psychopharmacol 11:116–120, 1991

Cornelius JR, Soloff PH, Perel JM, et al: Continuum pharmacotherapy of borderline personality disorder with haloperidol and phenelzine. Am J Psychiatry 150:1843–1848, 1993

Cowdry RW, Gardner D: Pharmacotherapy of borderline personality disorder. Arch Gen Psychiatry 45:111–119, 1988

Fulton M, Winokur G: A comparative study of paranoid and schizoid personality disorders. Am J Psychiatry 150:1363–1367, 1993

Goldman SJ, D'Angelo EJ, De Maso DR: Psychopathology in the families of children and adolescents with borderline personality disorder. Am J Psychiatry 150:1832–1835, 1993

Kernberg O: Severe Personality Disorders. New Haven, CT, Yale University Press, 1984

Lewis G, Appleby L: Personality disorders: the patients psychiatrists dislike. Br J Psychiatry 153:44–49, 1988

Liebowitz M, Stone M, Turkat I: Treatment of personality disorders, in Psychiatry Update: American Psychiatric Association Annual Review, Vol 5. Edited by Frances AJ, Hales RE. Washington, DC, American Psychiatric Press, 1986, pp 356–393

Livesley WJ, Jang LL, Jackson DN, et al: Genetic and environmental contributions to dimensions of personality disorder. Am J Psychiatry 150:1826–1831, 1993

McGlashan TH: Schizotypal personality disorder. Arch Gen Psychiatry 43:329–334, 1986

Nestadt G, Romanoski AJ, Chahal R, et al: An epidemiological study of histrionic personality disorder. Psychol Med 20:413–422, 1990

Pfohl B, Stangl D, Zimmerman M: The implication of DSM-III personality disorders for patients with major depression. J Affect Disord 7:309–319, 1984

Pollack J: Obsessive-compulsive personality. Journal of Personality Disorders 1:248–262, 1987

Pope HG, Hudson JI, Zubenko GS, et al: Schizoid personality disorder among psychiatric inpatients. McLean Hospital Journal 9:1–9, 1986

Pope HG, Jonas JM, Hudson JI, et al: The validity of DSM-III borderline personality disorder. Arch Gen Psychiatry 40:23–30, 1983

Reich J: Sex distribution of DSM-III personality disorders in psychiatric outpatients. Am J Psychiatry 144:485–488, 1987

Reich JH, Green AI: Effect of personality disorders on outcome of treatment. J Nerv Ment Dis 179:74–82, 1991

Siever LJ, Davis KL: A psychobiological perspective on the personality disorders. Am J Psychiatry 148:1647–1658, 1991

Stone MH: Long term outcome in personality disorders. Br J Psychiatry 162:299–313, 1993

Tarnepolsky A, Berelowitz M: Borderline personality—a review of recent research. Br J Psychiatry 151:724–734, 1987

Thompson DJ, Goldberg D: Hysterical personality disorder. Br J Psychiatry 150:241–245, 1987

Torgerson S: The oral, obsessive, and hysterical personality syndromes: a study of hereditary and environmental factors by means of the twin method. Arch Gen Psychiatry 37:1272–1277, 1980

Torgerson S: Genetic and nosologic aspects of schizotypal and borderline personality disorders: a twin study. Arch Gen Psychiatry 41:546–554, 1984

Tucker L, Bauer S, Wagner S, et al: Long-term hospital treatment of borderline patients. Am J Psychiatry 144:1443–1448, 1987

Widiger TA, Frances A, Spitzer RL, et al: The DSM-III-R personality disorders: an overview. Am J Psychiatry 145:786–795, 1988

Zimmerman M, Coryell W: DSM-III personality disorder diagnosis in a nonpatient sample. Arch Gen Psychiatry 46:682–689, 1989

Self-Assessment Questions

1. What are the Greek temperaments, and why are they still useful descriptively?
2. How are the personality disorders defined? What is the difference between trait and disorder?
3. Why is the term *personality disorder* considered pejorative?
4. How common are personality disorders? Which ones are more common in

men? Which ones are more common in women? Are these disorders stable?

5. What are Freud's character types? How well do they correspond to present-day categories?

6. What evidence is there for genetic or biological origin for the personality disorders? Which personality disorders?

7. Describe the three personality disorder clusters.

8. How do schizoid and schizotypal personality disorders differ? How do these two categories differ from avoidant personality disorder?

9. Are medications useful in treating cluster A disorders? Which medications?

10. For which disorders might social skills training or assertiveness training be useful?

11. What is the polythetic approach to diagnosis? Why has it been criticized, using antisocial personality as an example?

12. What are the antecedents of borderline personality? What biological abnormalities have been found in these patients? Why is transference a problem with treatment of patients with borderline personality disorder? Are medications of any value?

13. What features characterize the cluster C disorders? What are the general treatment recommendations for these disorders? How does obsessive-compulsive personality differ from obsessive-compulsive disorder?

Chapter 17

Sexual and Gender
Identity Disorders

Lolita, light of my life, fire of my loins. My sin, my soul.
Lo-lee-ta.

Vladimir Nabokov, Lolita

The three categories of sexual disorders include *sexual dysfunctions*, which involve either a disturbance of sexual arousal or a disturbance of psychophysiological performance; *paraphilias*, which involve culturally inappropriate or dangerous patterns of sexual arousal, such as exhibitionism; and *gender identity disorders* (e.g., transsexualism), which involve dissatisfaction with one's biological sex and a desire to become a member of the opposite sex. Sexual dysfunction is probably very common, although its full extent is unknown due to the sensitive and private nature of sexual relations. Paraphilias are less common but more problematic, because they may lead to public arrest and incarceration. Gender identity disorders are relatively rare, but remain of interest to psychiatrists and other mental health professionals because of the distress and unhappiness they create. The sexual disorders are listed in Table 17–1.

Sexual Dysfunction

DSM-IV identifies four major categories of sexual dysfunction: sexual desire disorders, sexual arousal disorders, orgasm disorders, and sexual pain disorders.

457

Table 17–1.   Sexual and gender identity disorders

Sexual Disorders

Sexual dysfunctions	**Sexual dysfunction not otherwise specified**
Sexual desire disorders	**Paraphilias**
• Hypoactive sexual desire disorder	• Exhibitionism
• Sexual aversion disorder	• Fetishism
Sexual arousal disorders	• Frotteurism
• Female sexual arousal disorder	• Pedophilia
• Male erectile disorder	• Sexual masochism
Orgasm disorders	• Sexual sadism
• Female orgasmic disorder	• Transvestic fetishism
• Male orgasmic disorder	• Voyeurism
• Premature ejaculation	• Paraphilia not otherwise specified
Sexual pain disorders	**Other sexual disorders**
• Dyspareunia	• Sexual disorder not otherwise specified
• Vaginismus	

Gender Identity Disorders

- Gender identity disorder
- Gender identity disorder not otherwise specified

There are two residual categories, sexual dysfunction not otherwise specified and sexual disorder not otherwise specified; these categories may be used to diagnose sexual disorders that are not classifiable as any one of the more specific disorders.

The four categories tend to correspond with the different phases of the sexual response cycle (see Table 17–2). All of the sexual dysfunctions may be classified as due either to psychological factors or to a combination of psychological factors and a general medical condition.

According to DSM-IV, the normal human sexual response cycle consists of four stages:

Stage 1—an appetitive phase lasting minutes to hours characterized by sexual fantasies and the desire for sexual intimacy.

Stage 2—an excitement phase (foreplay) consisting of 1) an early phase lasting minutes to hours characterized by physiological arousal, penile erection in males, and vaginal lubrication, nipple erection, and vasocongestion of the external genitalia in females; and 2) a late phase lasting seconds to minutes characterized by the appearance of drops of fluid at the head of the penis in males and a tightening of the outer one-third of the vagina and breast engorgement in females.

Table 17–2.   Relationship of sexual dysfunction to stage of the sexual response
cycle

Stage	Disorders
Appetitive	Hypoactive sexual desire disorder
	Sexual aversion disorder
Excitement	Male erectile disorder (impotence)
	Female sexual arousal disorder
Orgasm	Female orgasmic disorder
	Male orgasmic disorder
	Premature ejaculation

Stage 3—orgasm, typically lasting 5–15 seconds, accompanied in males by
ejaculation and involuntary muscular contractions of the pelvis and in females
by contractions of the outer one-third of the vagina and involuntary pelvic
thrusting. Females may have multiple orgasms, but the male has an obligatory
refractory period before another orgasm is possible.

Stage 4—the resolution phase, consisting of relaxation, detumescence, and
a sense of well-being.

Disorders of the Appetitive Phase

DSM-IV recognizes *hypoactive sexual desire disorder* and *sexual aversion disorder*,
which correspond to the appetitive phase of the sexual response cycle.

In *hypoactive sexual desire disorder*, there is a persistent or recurrent deficiency
or absence of sexual fantasy and desire, which is not due to major depression or
another major Axis I disorder, such as schizophrenia (because these disorders are
commonly associated with low sex drive), or to the direct effects of a substance
or a general medical condition (e.g., diabetes mellitus). Many persons with this
disorder have problems with social uneasiness, lack of self-confidence, and avoidance of social situations. The disorder is common among married couples, and
more women are affected than men. In one study, 35% of women and 16% of
men reported having no desire for sexual activity at least for some temporary
period. (See Table 17–3 for additional findings from this study.) In a community
survey of women, 17% reported having little sexual interest; among women
treated for sexual disorders, the frequency may exceed 75%.

The disorder may be primary or due to stressful situations that are temporary.
In the latter case, low sex drive may result from overwork, lack of privacy, lack
of opportunity for sex, lack of proper education about sex, or religious taboos.
Before making a diagnosis of hypoactive sexual desire disorder, a clinician must

Table 17–3. Frequency of self-reported sexual problems in "normal couples"

Problem	Percent	
	Women	Men
Sexual dysfunctions—women		
Difficulty getting excited	48	
Difficulty in reaching orgasm	46	
Difficulty maintaining excitement	33	
Inability to have an orgasm	15	
Reaching orgasm too quickly	11	
Sexual dysfunctions—men		
Ejaculating too quickly		36
Difficulty maintaining an erection		9
Difficulty getting an erection		7
Difficulty in ejaculating		4
Inability to ejaculate		0

Source. Adapted from Frank E, Anderson C, Rubenstien D: Frequency of sexual dysfunction in "normal couples." N Engl J Med 229:111–115, 1978.

take into account factors that affect sexual functioning, including age, gender, and the context of a person's life (e.g., it may be culturally appropriate for a nun to report a lack of sexual desire).

Sexual aversion disorder, on the other hand, represents a persistent and recurrent aversion to and avoidance of genital contact with a sexual partner and is not due to obsessive-compulsive disorder, major depression, or another serious Axis I disorder. Many investigators believe that persons with this disorder have been sexually victimized in the past and harbor unpleasant memories and beliefs about sexual activity.

Disorders in the Excitement Phase

The sexual arousal disorders include *male erectile disorder* (impotence) and *female sexual arousal disorder*.

Primary impotence occurs when a man has never been able to achieve an erection sufficient for vaginal insertion. With *secondary impotence*, the man has successfully achieved vaginal penetration at some time during his life, but is later unable to do so. Primary impotence is rare, but secondary impotence is reported in up to one quarter of all men. Among men treated for sexual disorders, more than 50% report this problem.

Female sexual arousal disorder occurs in up to one-third of all married women and leads to partial or complete failure to attain or maintain the lubrication-swelling response characteristic of the excitement phase, or to the total lack of sexual excitement and pleasure. The disorder may be due to physical factors, such as dyspareunia, and may be associated with anorgasmia.

Disorders of Orgasm

The disorders of orgasm include *female orgasmic disorder* (anorgasmia) and *male orgasmic disorder*. In women, this disorder is manifested by the delay in or absence of orgasm after a normal sexual excitement phase, when the clinician judges the woman's orgasmic capability to be less than expected for her age, sexual experience, and the degree of sexual stimulation received. *Male orgasmic disorder*, or inhibited male orgasm, occurs when a man achieves ejaculation during intercourse only with great difficulty, if at all. Again, the clinician must take into account the man's age, sexual experience, and the degree of sexual stimulation received.

Premature ejaculation, a common disorder reported by more than one quarter of married males, is the second most frequent complaint among men seeking help for sexual disorders. The diagnosis is made when the man has persistent or recurrent ejaculation either with minimal sexual stimulation, or before, on, or shortly after vaginal penetration; and before the man wants to ejaculate. Because women can experience multiple orgasms in a short time, there is no corresponding disorder in women.

Sexual Pain Disorders

The sexual pain disorders include *dyspareunia*, or painful intercourse in men or women, and *vaginismus* in women, in which involuntary muscle contractions sufficient to prevent penile insertion occur in the outer one-third of the vagina. Dyspareunia should not be diagnosed when it is better accounted for by an Axis I disorder, such as somatization disorder, or when it is thought to be due to the direct effects of a substance or a general medical condition. Further, it is not diagnosed if it is caused exclusively by vaginismus or lack of lubrication. Although dyspareunia is uncommon among men, it is a frequent complaint of women evaluated for sexual therapy and is common, at least temporarily, among women who have had pelvic surgery or who have recently undergone childbirth.

Other Sexual Dysfunctions

Less common sexual dysfunctions include *postcoital headaches* (i.e., headaches that occur immediately after intercourse); *orgasmic anhedonia*, a condition in which there is no physical sensation of orgasm even though ejaculation may have occurred; and *masturbatory pain,* in which pain is experienced with masturbation in the absence of physical abnormality. The latter disorder is usually caused by a small vaginal tear, Peyronie's disease of the penis, or some other physical disorder.

Etiology of Sexual Dysfunction Disorders

Sexual dysfunction may be caused by psychological or physical factors, or a combination of the two. For example, lack of desire can result from chronic stress, anxiety, or depression or may result from medications that either depress the central nervous system or decrease testosterone production. Prolonged abstinence itself may suppress sexual desire. Major physical stresses, such as illness or surgery, especially when they alter body image (e.g., mastectomy, ileostomy), may also depress sexual desire.

Impotence may be caused by both physical and psychological conditions (see Table 17–4 for a list of conditions associated with impotence). Recent studies have shown that up to 75% of men evaluated in medical clinics for impotence have a physical cause, including cardiovascular disease (e.g., atherosclerotic disease), renal disorders (e.g., chronic renal failure), liver disease (e.g., cirrhosis), malnutrition, diabetes mellitus, multiple sclerosis, traumatic spinal cord injury, abuse of alcohol and other addictive drugs, psychotropic medication, prostate surgery, and pelvic irradiation.

In determining the origin of impotence, it is important to obtain a record of spontaneous erections at times when the man does not plan to have intercourse (e.g., morning erections or erections with masturbation). If erections occur at these times, a psychological cause is likely. Evaluation of possible physical causes of impotence may include 1) recording of nocturnal penile tumescence, 2) measuring blood pressure in the penis with a penile plethysmograph or Doppler flow meter, and 3) measuring pudendal nerve latency time. Other laboratory tests used in the evaluation may include a glucose tolerance test, thyroid and liver function tests, serum prolactin, luteinizing hormone, and follicle-stimulating hormone measures to rule out metabolic or endocrinological causes of impotence, such as diabetes mellitus. Invasive tests (e.g., penile arteriography, infusion cavernosography, radioactive xenon penography) are used in evaluating the rare patient who is a candidate for vascular reconstructive surgery. The most common surgical treatment for impotence involves the insertion of a penile prosthesis; these devices are generally either semirigid or inflatable. Each type has its advantages and disadvantages, although most implant recipients report satisfaction with the results.

Table 17–4.   Causes of male erectile disorder (impotence)

Medical illness	Psychiatric illness
Acromegaly	Anxiety disorders
Addison's disease	Dementia
Diabetes mellitus	Major depression
Hyperthyroidism	Schizophrenia
Hypothyroidism	**Drugs**
Klinefelter's syndrome	Alcohol
Multiple sclerosis	Antiandrogens
Parkinson's disease	Anticholinergics
Pelvic surgery or irradiation	Antidepressants
Peripheral vascular disease	Antihypertensives (especially centrally
Pituitary adenoma	acting ones)
Spinal cord injury	Antipsychotics
Syphilis	Barbiturates
Temporal lobe epilepsy	Benzodiazepines
	Marijuana
	Opiates
	Stimulants

Anorgasmia may result from physical causes, such as medication or surgery, but it may also be associated with psychological factors. Psychological factors may include fears of impregnation, rejection by the sex partner, depression, and cultural factors. For example, in Victorian times, girls were commonly told by their mothers that sex was not to be enjoyed, but endured!

Male orgasmic disorder (i.e., inhibited male orgasm) is relatively uncommon and must be differentiated from *retrograde ejaculation,* in which ejaculation occurs, but the seminal fluid passes backward into the bladder. Both inhibited male orgasm and retrograde ejaculation most likely have a physiological cause, such as medication, genitourinary surgery (e.g., prostatectomy), or neurological disorders involving the lumbosacral section of the spinal cord. Medications that may be responsible include centrally acting antihypertensives (e.g., guanethidine, α-methyldopa), tricyclic antidepressants (e.g., amitriptyline), and antipsychotics, particularly the phenothiazines (e.g., chlorpromazine, thioridazine). The serotonin reuptake inhibitor antidepressants (e.g., fluoxetine, paroxetine) are frequent offenders as well. Age itself is an important factor; older men may not ejaculate at every sexual encounter, but perhaps only every second or third time.

Clinical Management of Sexual Dysfunction Disorders

The most widely used approach for the treatment of sexual dysfunction disorders was pioneered by Masters and Johnson in the 1970s. Their "dual" sex therapy includes both partners, because the sexual problem affects both persons in a relationship; the principles apply equally to heterosexual and homosexual couples. With this approach, therapy may begin with a review of the psychological and physiological aspects of sexual functioning and an evaluation of the couple's attitudes about sexual behavior and of their ability to communicate. After the sexual disturbance is diagnosed (e.g., male erectile disorder), suggestions are made for specific sexual activity that the couple is expected to carry out in private. Sexual relations are emphasized as natural and healthy behaviors that enhance a couple's relationship. The relatively brief sex therapy (i.e., 8–12 sessions) focuses on correcting dysfunctional behavior, not on interpreting presumed underlying psychodynamics. These methods are used for a variety of disorders, and they can be modified depending on whether the sexual problem represents a disorder of the appetitive, excitement, or orgasmic stage of the sexual response cycle.

As an example of sex therapy for male erectile disorder, the couple is prohibited from engaging in sexual activity other than that prescribed by the therapist. Exercises may focus on increasing sensory awareness of erogenous zones, so that couples can learn to give and receive bodily pleasure (i.e., "sensate focus"). Sensate focus exercises are a technique in which the patient engages initially in nongenital, nondemanding caressing with his or her partner with the focus on the patient's own pleasure and concentration on sexual feelings. At this stage, intercourse is prohibited so that couples can learn to separate sexual pleasure from intercourse.

Genital stimulation is eventually included in the exercises; couples are instructed to try various positions for intercourse but not to worry about completing the act. In time, the couples gain confidence, improve their communication skills, and learn to give and receive pleasure without the pressure of intercourse. Without that pressure, the man gradually is able to have erections, to successfully complete vaginal intercourse, and to have a satisfactory orgasm.

Specific instructions are altered depending on the couple's presenting complaint. For example, in cases of male orgasmic disorder, the female may be instructed to insert her partner's penis herself. In anorgasmia, therapy may first involve training the woman partner to have an orgasm by masturbation before treating the couple. Vaginismus may require individual therapy, relaxation techniques (e.g., progressive muscle relaxation), or the use of Hegar's dilators, which are inserted into the vagina. The size of the dilators is slowly increased over 3–5 days to gradually enlarge the vaginal opening. The "squeeze method" has been advocated for treating premature ejaculation. The woman is instructed to squeeze the head of her partner's glans penis before ejaculation. This action effectively aborts the ejaculation so that the couple may prolong the excitement phase (i.e., foreplay). Alternatively, males may benefit from 1% dibucaine (Nupercaine) ointment applied to the coronal ridge and frenulum of the penis to reduce stimulation. A case example of inhibited male orgasm and its treatment is illustrated below.

Robert, a 34-year-old bank officer, had been happily married for 6 months, but he reported that he was now having trouble achieving orgasm. Although he had had no sexual experience before marriage, he and his more experienced wife quickly developed a satisfying sexual relationship. They both had versatile sexual interests and were both able to achieve orgasm with adequate stimulation.

Robert reported that for the past month he had been having difficulty achieving orgasm even though foreplay was mutually stimulating and he readily became erect. Although he was able to reach orgasm through masturbation, he was unable to achieve orgasm with vaginal intercourse, despite trying a variety of positions.

An evaluation found no evidence of an anxiety disorder or major depression or of a physical disorder. Although Robert had denied any recent change in his marital relationship, he disclosed to the therapist a deep-seated fear that he was unworthy of his new mate and felt that he could not satisfy her sexually. The therapist met with the couple, recommended that Robert abstain from masturbation, prescribed sensate focus exercises to be tried initially without intercourse, and suggested that, as intercourse was attempted, the wife take a dominant role. Learning that he could give and receive pleasure without the pressure of intercourse apparently allowed Robert and his wife to experience intercourse and each to achieve a satisfactory orgasm.

Recommendations for treatment of the sexual dysfunction disorders

1. Learn to take a sexual history without shame or embarrassment. Patients will detect your anxiety, which will only serve to increase their own.

2. Don't apologize for asking intimate questions. How couples behave sexually is important to assess.
   - Most couples will be surprisingly forthcoming in describing their sex life.

3. Both members of the couple need to participate in the therapy, which may be used with equal success in heterosexual and homosexual couples.

4. The principles of dual sex therapy are relatively simple to learn and emphasize education about sexual functioning, assisting couples to communicate better, and correcting dysfunctional attitudes about sex that one or both partners may hold.

5. Therapy involves homework assignments, which assist the couple in learning to increase sensory awareness. Techniques may include self-masturbation, sensate focus exercises, special coital techniques, and learning to separate pleasure from physiological response (e.g., erection).

Paraphilias (Sexual Deviations)

The paraphilias are disorders characterized by a disturbance in the object of sexual gratification or in the expression of sexual gratification. Common paraphilias include *exhibitionism*, in which there is repeated exposing of the genitals to unprepared strangers for the purpose of achieving sexual gratification; *fetishism*, in which inanimate objects are the preferred or only means of achieving sexual excitement; *pedophilia*, in which repeated sexual activity with prepubertal children is the preferred or exclusive method of obtaining sexual release (e.g., the character Humbert Humbert in Nabokov's *Lolita*); *transvestitism*, in which a person experiences sexual excitement while dressed in the clothes of the opposite sex; and *voyeurism*, in which observing the sexual activity of others is the preferred means of sexual arousal. There are other paraphilias as well, although they are much less common, such as sexual sadism, sexual masochism, frotteurism, and necrophilia. Various paraphilias are listed in Table 17–5.

Paraphilias have been known throughout recorded time, but they have been

Table 17–5.   Paraphilias (sexual deviations)

Preferential sex act	Behavior of gratification
Exhibitionism	Exposing self to others
Fetishism	Use of inanimate object (e.g., shoe)
Frotteurism	Rubbing against nonconsenting persons
Pedophilia	Preferring prepubertal children
Sexual masochism	Enjoying pain and humiliation
Sexual sadism	Inflicting pain on others
Transvestic fetishism	Cross-dressing
Voyeurism	Window peeping
Paraphilia not otherwise specified	
Telephone scatologia	Obscene phone calls
Necrophilia	Dead persons
Partialism	Focusing on one part of the body (e.g., feet) to the exclusion of all else
Zoophilia (bestiality)	Animal contacts
Coprophilia	Feces
Klismania	Enemas
Urophilia	Urine
Hypoxophilia	Desire to achieve altered state of consciousness secondary to hypoxia
Oralism	Focusing on oral-genital contact to the exclusion of intercourse

subject to classification and study only in recent years. DSM-IV provides specific criteria for eight paraphilias and a residual category for other disorders. For a person to be considered paraphilic, sexual activity must be characterized by a preference for the use of nonhuman objects in achieving sexual arousal, by imposed sexual humiliation or suffering, or by the sexual involvement of nonconsenting partners, such as children.

Sexual deviations are currently viewed as having three aspects. First, the behavior does not conform to the generally accepted views of what is normal, although the accepted view of normality is not identical in each society, nor has it been during each period in history. Second, the behavior may cause harm to another person involved in the sexual behavior, for example, intercourse with young children and extreme forms of sexual sadism. Third, the behavior may result in the suffering of the individual. This suffering may result from societal attitudes, as a result of which persons see their sexual urges to be at odds with their moral standards, and from their awareness that their sexual practices cause distress to another person. A relatively typical example of a patient with a paraphilia treated in our hospital follows.

Frank, a 38-year-old mechanic, presented to the emergency room requesting help. He had left his wife 3 days earlier, fearing that another arrest for indecent exposure would humiliate his family and friends. His story soon unfolded.

At age 10, he lost a testicle in an accident—a fact that was known to his classmates. He was teased endlessly, leading to feelings of insecurity and inadequacy. He began to masturbate at age 12 and was soon masturbating up to five times daily. Although he could not remember when, he began to masturbate in public settings— not out in the open, but in areas where he might be discovered. He found the challenge of avoiding detection sexually exciting. He would usually masturbate where he could observe women, such as in shopping centers, libraries, or even in his parked car where he could watch women walk by. Although he denied genital exposure, he admitted that occasionally women would "accidentally" observe him masturbating, adding to his excitement. His masturbation had a compulsive quality, and he felt powerless to stop.

The behavior continued over a 25-year period, leading to several arrests for indecent exposure. Feeling guilty and wanting to make amends, Frank sought psychotherapy after each arrest, but he would soon drop out. One psychiatrist prescribed thioridazine to dampen his sex drive, but it only caused retrograde ejaculation. Another physician recommended that he read pornography and masturbate in private.

Although he denied other paraphilic behaviors and called pedophilia "disgusting," he admitted to two episodes of exhibitionism, first at age 18 to a girl sitting next to him in class and again during his honeymoon. Although he was socially awkward with women and did not date until age 21, Frank married at age 23 and had a stable marriage and a satisfying sexual relationship with his wife. He admitted, however, that he preferred public masturbation to sexual intercourse with his wife.

Frank was admitted to the hospital for further evaluation. Physical examination confirmed the absence of the right testicle, but results of the examination were otherwise normal. Serum testosterone was 288 ng/dl (normal serum levels, 200–800 ng/dl). Treatment was started with medroxyprogesterone acetate (Depo-provera). At a follow-up visit 1 month later, his serum testosterone had fallen to 41 ng/dl. He had been able to resist masturbating in public and no longer had spontaneous erections. He felt that he could control his behavior. Six months later, he chose to discontinue the medication and within 1 month had returned to his old ways.

A follow-up 10 years later showed that his paraphilia had persisted unchanged. No treatment had been sought in the interim.

Epidemiology of Paraphilias

The paraphilias are relatively uncommon in psychiatric practice, probably due to the furtiveness and secrecy surrounding most of them. Most cases are noted only if treatment is sought or if there are legal entanglements. Their true prevalence is unknown due to lack of adequate information. The best available statistics are legal, not medical. About 80,000 persons are arrested annually on sexually related charges in the United States, excluding forcible rape, and nearly 90,000 are in state and federal prisons; the perpetrators are overwhelmingly male. These estimates are biased toward impulsive individuals and paraphilias that are considered to be dangerous or a public nuisance.

Of legally identified cases, pedophilia is the most common paraphilia, probably because of its unsavory nature and the greater societal effort spent in apprehending pedophiles. Exhibitionism is commonly reported, possibly because it may involve repeated public display to young girls. Sexual masochism and sadism are underrepresented in crime statistics, because it is unlikely that these disorders would come to public attention unless a tragedy occurred (e.g., autoerotic suffocation). Many of these disorders, such as fetishism, would scarcely be reported at all, because the activity takes place between consenting adults or is done by a lone individual. Furthermore, many individuals who are comfortable with their paraphilias are completely underrepresented in all samples.

Etiology of Paraphilias

For centuries, variations of the sexual act were regarded as offenses against nature, God, or the law rather than disorders that doctors should study and treat. The systematic study of the paraphilias began in the 1870s with the work of Krafft-Ebing, Hirschfeld, Ellis, and others. In 1886, Krafft-Ebing, a Viennese psychiatrist, compiled the first systematic account of sexual deviations in his book *Psychopathia Sexualis*. Krafft-Ebing considered the sexual deviations to be due mainly to heredity, and he believed they could be modified by social and psychological factors. Freud, also active at this time, attempted to explain sexual deviations as failures of the developmental processes during childhood. Psychoanalysts have devoted much attention to sexual deviations, and recent psychoanalytic literature follows this tradition.

Much of the recent work on paraphilias has focused on learning theory in both initiating and maintaining the disorder. In this model, persons with paraphilias learn that their fantasies and urges are inappropriate. Attempting to suppress these desires, they inadvertently use paraphilic fantasies during masturbation, which intensifies their interest and pairs the fantasy with the positive experience of orgasm. The paraphilic arousal strengthens, control breaks down, and the fantasy is acted on. Once this process becomes entrenched, it is likely to reoccur. Learning theory does not explain all cases of paraphilia, but behavioral techniques have proven valuable in the treatment of paraphilias, regardless of etiology.

Paraphilic acts may also represent poor impulse control resulting from a major mental disorder, such as schizophrenia, dementia, or delirium. Persons with antisocial personality disorder sometimes commit paraphilic acts to gratify their immediate needs, although a true paraphilia may not exist. Many antisocial persons do have paraphilias, however.

A small body of research has accumulated implicating possible neurobiological roots for sexually deviant behavior. The evidence includes the finding of an increased frequency of neuropsychological impairment and electroencephalogram abnormalities in sex offenders. Computed tomography has shown abnormal brain scans in pedophiles and other sexually aggressive men; dilation of the temporal horns, especially the right horn, is the major finding. Familial transmission and hypothalamic-pituitary-gonadal axis dysfunction have been reported in pedophilia. Clearly, more research is needed, but these results suggest that there may be a biological substrate for many sexually deviant behaviors.

Clinical Description, Course, and Outcome of Specific Paraphilias

Paraphilias are generally established in adolescence and occur almost exclusively among men, although cases are described in women. Most paraphilic patients are heterosexual, not homosexual, contrary to popular belief. These features appear to be true for fetishists, pedophiles, exhibitionists, and voyeurs. Most patients with paraphilias have a variety of sexual behaviors and may meet criteria for several paraphilias simultaneously; many have other psychiatric disorders as well (e.g., substance abuse, mood disorders, personality disorders).

The *fetishist* often uses objects of gratification such as rubber garments, women's underclothing, and high-heeled shoes. Contact with the object causes sexual arousal, which is usually followed by masturbation. Fetishists may spend considerable time seeking their desired objects. There are no reliable follow-up data, but the disorder appears to start in adolescence or young adulthood for most patients and may diminish when satisfying heterosexual relationships are established. A case example of fetishism follows.

> A 41-year-old attorney had his law license suspended after admitting to breaking into and entering more than 100 homes in his small town to obtain women's underwear for sexual gratification. He would generally enter houses through unlocked doors or would jimmy a lock with a credit card or knife. Once inside the house, he would search for the undergarments to use later in solitary acts of masturbation. He was finally caught at a neighbor's home after he had entered an unlocked back door and was found searching for the neighbor's underwear. He was discovered by the woman's husband, who reported him to the police. He was charged with criminal trespass, convicted, and put on probation. A follow-up 5 years later showed that although he denied subsequent episodes of stealing undergarments, he admitted that the interest was still there. A renewed interest in religion was responsible for his self-control, he reported.

Transvestic fetishism often begins at puberty. Persons may start by putting on only a few garments. In time, the individual may dress entirely in the clothes of the opposite sex. Transvestites experience erections when cross-dressing and may masturbate. As they gain confidence, the clothes may be worn in public. Although data are limited, the disorder may continue for years but become less severe as the sexual drive declines.

The *pedophile* chooses a child of the same or opposite sex as a sexual partner. Although the condition may begin at any age, most pedophiles seen by physicians are middle-aged; the preference, however, probably starts much earlier. Prognosis has not been reliably studied, but it probably depends on the length of the history of the pedophilic behavior, the frequency of the behavior, the presence or absence of other social and sexual relationships, and the individual's underlying personality.

Exhibitionists make up about one-third of the sexual offenders referred for treatment and generally involve two groups of men—those with an inhibited temperament who struggle with their urges and often expose a flaccid penis and those with aggressive traits who often expose an erect penis and masturbate. If the behavior begins in middle or advanced age, the behavior may be an indication of a dementia. Exhibitionists who repeat their behavior are likely to persist for years, according to evidence from the courts. In keeping with clinical impression, the evidence suggests that the reconviction rate for indecent exposure is low after the first conviction but high after a second conviction.

Voyeurism in adolescence is often an expression of sexual curiosity. The behavior is often replaced by direct sexual experience, although voyeurism may persist. A typical case of voyeurism was reported in a local paper:

> A 27-year-old law student pleaded guilty to five counts of criminal trespass after admitting that he had spied on women in dormitory showers several times over a 6-month period. He had been arrested near the dormitory one morning after students had caught him spying on the women's shower. He had been seen lying on the floor outside the shower looking through the ventilation grate and was chased out of the dormitory by women who had found him there.
>
> Residents of the dorm had banded together and would watch for him daily from 5 to 9 A.M., believing that he would repeat his act. The "peeper" was well known at the dorm for his voyeurism and for making a nuisance of himself.

Although *homosexuality* has traditionally been included with the sexual deviations, most psychiatrists now believe it to be an alternate form of sexual behavior that should be of little concern to physicians, other than as a risk factor for various diseases such as herpes or the acquired immunodeficiency syndrome (AIDS). In fact, members of the American Psychiatric Association voted in 1973 to delete homosexuality from its list of mental disorders. Currently, homosexuality is not considered a mental disorder, unless the patient is chronically distressed by it (i.e., ego-dystonic homosexuality), although most homosexuals will experience a transient phase during which they are disturbed or distressed by their sexual orientation. Ego-dystonic homosexuality is classified in DSM-IV as a *sexual disorder not otherwise specified*.

Clinical Management of the Paraphilias

In the last two decades, behavioral interventions have become the mainstay of treatment of the paraphilias. Methods have been developed both to reduce deviant arousal patterns through masturbatory satiation (i.e., satiating or boring the patient with his own deviant fantasies) or covert sensitization (i.e., replacing fantasies with unpleasant images) and to generate arousal in response to nondeviant themes through masturbatory conditioning. Social skills training is used to help the patient learn to communicate more effectively with appropriate adult partners. Cognitive techniques are used to help the paraphiliac patient to restructure faulty cognitions used to justify behavior (e.g., the pedophile erroneously interprets a child's docility as an expression of desire). Relaxation training may help reduce the anxiety and stress that frequently precede paraphilic behavior. A follow-up study of 194 child molesters treated with behavior modification techniques indicated an 82% success rate (defined as no recidivism) at 12 months posttreatment. Although these results are encouraging, it is not known whether they may be generalized to the other paraphilias and to persons not motivated by threats of arrest or imprisonment.

Reports on the use of antiandrogen medications, such as medroxyprogesterone (Provera) or cyproterone (not available in the United States), indicate promising results for the treatment of repeat offenders—for example our patient Frank, whose care is described in the first part of this section. These medications work peripherally to reduce serum testosterone levels and centrally to reduce sexual drive. The goal is to decrease paraphilic fantasies and their associated behavior, while avoiding (particularly in married persons) erectile difficulties. Medroxyprogesterone is given orally starting with doses of 100–200 mg daily; some patients will need up to 400 mg daily. A long-acting preparation (Depo-Provera) may be given intramuscularly at doses of 200–400 mg every 7–10 days.

These medications are primarily useful in carefully selected patients whose hypersexuality is uncontrolled or dangerous. Unfortunately, sustained use is necessary, as relapse generally follows discontinuation of the medication. The long-term risk of these medications has not been adequately studied; as there may be a risk of liver disease or cancer, they should be used with caution and the patient's health should be carefully monitored. Other drug therapy, including

---

Recommendations for treatment of the paraphilic patient

1. The history is of utmost importance in treating the paraphilic patient. The therapist must learn where and when the behavior occurs, who or what the desired object is, and what occurs in the presence of the object.
   - Most paraphilic patients have a variety of abnormal behaviors, and the therapist is safe in assuming that more are present than are initially disclosed by the patient.
2. Paraphilic patients are notoriously difficult to treat, but behavior therapy techniques may offer the best hope for success. The purpose of these techniques is to reduce deviant arousal patterns and to generate new arousal in response to nondeviant themes.
   - Methods may include masturbatory satiation and conditioning, social skills training, and cognitive restructuring.
3. Antiandrogens are promising treatments for severe repeat offenders whose actions are uncontrolled or dangerous. Do not casually prescribe these medications.
4. You may want to refer difficult cases to therapists who have experience in treating these disorders.

antipsychotic or antidepressant medication, is indicated for treatment of accompanying schizophrenia or major depression if the paraphilia is associated with those disorders.

Gender Identity Disorders

Gender identity disorders are relatively rare and usually have their onset in childhood and adolescence. A residual category, *gender identity disorder not otherwise specified*, exists for disorders that do not meet the full syndrome criteria (e.g., a person preoccupied with castration, in the absence of a desire to acquire the sex characteristics of the opposite gender).

The essential feature of gender identity disorder (i.e., transsexualism) is the desire to become a member of the opposite sex. According to DSM-IV, transsexual persons typically manifest a strong and persistent cross-gender identification and a sense of inappropriateness about their assigned sex. In adults, these feelings often lead to a persistent preoccupation with getting rid of their primary and secondary sex characteristics and acquiring the sex characteristics of the opposite gender. In children, these feelings may be manifested in a boy, for instance, by an assertion that his penis or testes are disgusting. The diagnostic criteria for transsexualism are listed in Table 17–6.

The prevalence of the disorder is not known, but is estimated at 1 in 30,000 men and 1 in 100,000 women. A case example of transsexualism follows.

William, a 25-year-old convict, was referred to our hospital for evaluation of gender dysphoria. He had recently filed a lawsuit requesting that the state pay for his sex reassignment surgery, as well as allow him to wear women's clothing, transfer to a women's prison, and have hormone injections—all of which the corrections officials had refused.

William reported that he had never felt comfortable with his gender and had decided years earlier that he needed an operation. As a child, he was effeminate, enjoyed playing house, and when playing house assumed feminine roles such as the mother or sister. He also liked games typically associated with girls, such as hopscotch and jump rope, and was not very good at team sports. He began to cross-dress at age 9 and said that he felt more comfortable and natural dressed as a girl. He wished he had been born a girl and told us that he was unhappy with his male genitals, stating: "I can't stand them. I don't consider them mine."

In his early 20s, William began to cross-dress full-time and for a 5-month period lived as a woman, calling himself Julie. William had never had a desire for heterosexual relations, although he had experimented. He was able to perform sexually with a woman and have an orgasm, but he "didn't like it." While experiencing sexual intercourse, William would fantasize about himself being made love to as a woman. He had had considerable homosexual experience, with over 100 different partners by his count, and reported having had several long-term relationships (5–6 months in duration). He would generally assume a passive role, for example, performing oral sex on others or being the receptive partner of anal sex. He refused to allow any of his partners to touch his genitals and would not allow mutual masturbation.

William had read widely about transsexualism and had written to many different medical centers for information. Imprisonment had been difficult for him, because

Table 17–6. DSM-IV criteria for gender identity disorder

A. A strong and persistent cross-gender identification (not merely a desire for any perceived cultural advantages of being the other sex).

In children, manifested by four (or more) of the following:

1. Repeatedly stated desire to be, or insistence that he or she is, the other sex
2. In boys, preference for cross-dressing or simulating female attire; in girls, insistence on wearing only stereotypical masculine clothing
3. Strong and persistent preferences for cross-sex roles in make-believe play or persistent fantasies of being the other sex
4. Intense desire to participate in the stereotypical games and pastimes of the other sex
5. Strong preference for playmates of the other sex

In adolescents and adults, manifested by symptoms such as a stated desire to be the other sex, frequent passing as the other sex, desire to live or be treated as the other sex, or the conviction that one has the typical feelings and reactions of the other sex.

B. Persistent discomfort with one's sex or sense of inappropriateness in the gender role of that sex.

In children, manifested by any of the following: in boys, assertion that his penis or testes are disgusting or will disappear or assertion that it would be better not to have a penis, or aversion toward rough-and-tumble play and rejection of male stereotypical toys, games, and activities; in girls, rejection of urinating in a sitting position, assertion that she has or will grow a penis or assertion that she does not want to grow breasts or menstruate, or marked aversion towards normative feminine clothing.

In adolescents and adults, manifested by symptoms such as preoccupation with getting rid of one's primary and secondary sex characteristics (e.g., request for hormones, surgery, or other procedures to physically alter sexual characteristics to simulate the other sex) or belief that one was born the wrong sex.

C. The disturbance is not concurrent with a physical intersex condition.

D. The disturbance causes clinically significant distress or impairment in social, occupational, or other important areas of functioning.

Code based on current age:

Gender identity disorder in children
Gender identity disorder in adolescents or adults

Specify if (for sexually mature individuals):

Sexually attracted to males
Sexually attracted to females
Sexually attracted to both
Sexually attracted to neither

he claimed that other inmates would make fun of his personal habits, including shaving his chest, arms, legs, and axilla. He had attempted to mutilate his genitals on three occasions, and several months before his evaluation, he had managed to lacerate his penis with a piece of glass and had required sutures.

In addition to his gender dysphoria, William had a lifelong history of disciplinary and behavioral problems and as a young boy had been placed in detention for a period of time. He also had a history of abusing both alcohol and marijuana and had many run-ins with the law for shoplifting, theft, and writing bad checks. He had had many psychiatric hospitalizations, mostly for depression or after suicide attempts. None of his suicide attempts had been medically serious, however.

At the time of evaluation, William was noted to cross his legs in an effeminate manner, was limp-wristed, and had long, greasy hair parted down the middle, covering half of his face in a Veronica Lake sort of way. There was no evidence of mood disturbance, but he exhibited a nervous giggle. He had no formal thought disorder, hallucinations, or delusions, and although somewhat guarded during the interview, he summarized everything with the words, "It's all a confused mess."

Although the diagnosis of transsexualism is easily made, it is important to rule out schizophrenia, transvestism, and effeminate homosexuality. In schizophrenia, a desire to change one's anatomic sex is generally part of a complex delusional system, for example, the belief that the FBI is conspiring to change the patient's sex. Transvestites who cross-dress may occasionally come to feel that sex change surgery is a natural extension of their cross-dressing. Effeminate homosexuals, on the other hand, might request a sex change to make themselves more appealing to potential sex partners.

Transsexualism generally begins in childhood, when gender identity is usually established. In boys, early features of transsexualism typically include over-identification with the mother, overtly feminine behavior (e.g., plays with dolls), little interest in usual male pursuits (e.g., dislikes sports), and peer relationships primarily with girls. Tomboyishness, on the other hand, will be found in young transsexual females, but the behavior is more acceptable in our society than feminine behavior in boys and tends to draw less attention.

DSM-IV subtypes transsexual persons according to their attraction to men or women. Those not attracted to either gender generally have a history of either no sexual activity or limited pleasure derived from the genitals. The homosexual transsexual person reports sexual arousal from same-sex partners. The heterosexual transsexual person reports arousal from opposite-sex partners. Transsexual men and women generally deny any interest in homosexuality because they believe themselves to be members of the opposite sex.

Depression is a frequent complication among transsexual persons, as is substance abuse and personality disorder. Many transsexual persons meet criteria for borderline personality disorder, as evidenced by their frequently unstable mood, persistent identity problems, self-mutilation, and angry outbursts. Self-mutilation may include damage to their genitals, including autocastration in extreme cases. These acts are generally not suicide attempts, because they are aimed at forcing physicians to deal with the transsexualism.

As transsexual persons age, many will seek medical help and request hormonal therapy and sex reassignment surgery. A new birth certificate designating the new sexual status will be sought after surgery. By the time they present for surgery, many transsexual persons will have been living as a member of the opposite sex for years. In fact, many clinics offering surgery will demand that the patients have lived as members of the opposite sex for more than 1 year before surgery.

Treatment of transsexualism presents a vexing problem to the psychiatrist. Transsexual persons will plead for surgery, yet studies suggest that the outcome in terms of social and occupational adjustment is no better with surgery than with psychotherapy. Regardless, many transsexual persons will pursue surgery and seek treatment from one of many sex-reassignment clinics around the United States and elsewhere. The male-to-female transsexual patient is prescribed hormones (e.g., estradiol, progesterone) to create breasts and feminine contours, undergoes electrolysis to remove hair, and has surgery to remove the testes and penis and to create an artificial vagina. The female-to-male transsexual patient undergoes mastectomy, hysterectomy, and oophorectomy; is prescribed testosterone to help develop muscle mass and deepen the voice; and may have an artificial penis constructed. Clearly, the male-to-female sex reassignment surgery is more successful, because a penis capable of erection and ejaculation has yet to be constructed. Male-to-female transsexual persons have good cosmetic results, and many are able to achieve orgasm.

Transsexual patients who adjust well after surgery tend to have had a lifelong cross-gender identification, were able to pass convincingly as a member of the opposite sex before surgery, have good social support, have a college education, and have a steady job. Patients without these characteristics tend to do poorly after surgery.

For patients who do not seek surgery, psychotherapeutic strategies include individual and group sessions aimed at helping patients to accept their anatomic sex, assisting them to develop an ability to experience pleasure from their genitals, and helping them to make a successful adjustment in other domains of life, including social and occupational functioning.

Of patients who undergo sexual reassignment surgery, 70%–80% are pleased with the outcome of surgery and their new anatomical contours; however, psychological problems, such as an underlying personality disorder, endure for many patients. The patient who was emotionally unstable before surgery is the same person after surgery, despite the physical changes. Therefore, many patients will continue to benefit from psychotherapy after surgery to assist them in handling day-to-day problems, as well as adjusting to their new gender role.

Bibliography

Abel GG, Blanchard EB: The role of fantasy in the treatment of sexual deviation. Arch Gen Psychiatry 30:467–475, 1974

Abel GG, Osborn C: Stopping sexual violence. Psychiatric Annals 22:301–306, 1992

Black DW, Goldstein RB, Blum N, et al: Personality characteristics in 60 subjects with psychosexual dysfunction: a non-patient sample. Journal of Personality Disorders (in press)

Brown GR: A review of clinical approaches to gender dysphoria. J Clin Psychiatry 51:57–64, 1990

Fagan PJ, Wise TN, Derogatis LR, et al: Distressed transvestites—psychometric characteristics. J Nerv Ment Dis 176:626–632, 1988

Frank E, Anderson C, Rubinstein D: Frequency of sexual dysfunction in "normal couples." N Engl J Med 229:111–115, 1978

Fuller AK: Child molestation and pedophilia—an overview for the physician. JAMA 261:602–606, 1989

Gaffney GR, Berlin FS: Is there a gonadal dysfunction in pedophilia? A pilot study. Br J Psychiatry 145:657–660, 1984

Gaffney GR, Lurie SF, Berlin FS: Is there familial transmission of pedophilia? J Nerv Ment Dis 172:546–548, 1984

Gottesman HG, Schubert DSP: Low-dose medroxyprogesterone acetate in the management of paraphilias. J Clin Psychiatry 54:182–188, 1993

Green R: Gender identity in childhood and later sexual orientation: follow-up of 78 males. Am J Psychiatry 142:339–341, 1985

Grob CS: Female exhibitionism. J Nerv Ment Dis 173:253–256, 1985

Hawton K: Sex Therapy, A Practical Guide. New York, Oxford University Press, 1985

Herman J, LoPiccolo J: Clinical outcome of sex therapy. Arch Gen Psychiatry 40:443, 1983

Langevin R: Biological factors contributing to paraphilic behavior. Psychiatric Annals 22:307–314, 1992

Masters WH, Johnson VE: Human Sexual Inadequacy. Boston, MA, Little, Brown, 1970

Meyer JK, Reter DJ: Sex reassignment follow-up. Arch Gen Psychiatry 36:1010–1015, 1979

Osborn M, Hawton K, Gath D: Sexual dysfunction among middle-aged women in the community. Br Med J 296:959–962, 1988

Rooth G: Exhibitionism, sexual violence, and pedophilia. Br J Psychiatry 122:705–710, 1973

Schiavi RC, Schreiner-Engel P, Mandeli J, et al: Healthy aging and male sexual function. Am J Psychiatry 147:766–771, 1990

Segraves RJ: Effects of psychotropic drugs on human erection and ejaculation. Arch Gen Psychiatry 46:275–284, 1989

Seidman SN, Rieder RO: A review of sexual behavior in the United States. Am J Psychiatry 151:330–341, 1994

Smith RS: Voyeurism: a review of the literature. Arch Sex Behav 5:585–609, 1975

Spector KR, Boyle M: The prevalence and perceived aetiology of male sexual problems in a non-clinical sample. Br J Med Psychol 59:351–358, 1986

Wise TN: Fetishism, etiology and treatment: a review from multiple perspectives. Compr Psychiatry 26:249–256, 1985

Self-Assessment Questions

1. What are the three types of sexual disorders?
2. What are the stages of the sexual response cycle?
3. What are the disorders of the appetitive phase?
4. What are the causes of male erectile disorder (impotence)?
5. Describe dual sex therapy.
6. How common are paraphilias?
7. How can learning experiences lead to paraphilic behavior?
8. Is homosexuality a sexual deviation?
9. What are the antecedent behavioral characteristics of transsexuals?
10. What are the treatments for transsexuals?

Chapter 18

Eating Disorders

O! that this too too solid flesh would melt.

William Shakespeare, Hamlet

Many persons believe that the eating disorders are relatively new, brought on by the stress of modern society and its near obsession with youth, beauty, and slimness. Nonetheless, the eating disorders have ancient roots. Bulimia, generally a cycle of excessive bingeing and purging, has as its precursor the banquets of Roman Sybarites. At these banquets, guests ate with gluttonous abandon and then vomited so that they could eat more. Many early Christian saints were observed to have episodes of severe starvation and bingeing. Saint Catherine of Siena was one of the so-called fasting saints. However, it was not until 1868 that William Gull, an English physician, formally described anorexia nervosa as a disorder involving starvation in the pursuit of thinness.

The eating disorders now share the limelight with the news of the day, as the media appear to be fascinated by them. Perhaps this attention is due to the association between eating disorders and celebrity; for example, singer Karen Carpenter died tragically from the complications of anorexia nervosa, and actress Jane Fonda has admitted to a decades-long problem with bulimia.

Definition

Anorexia nervosa and bulimia nervosa comprise the two major eating disorders, according to DSM-IV. Another category, *eating disorder not otherwise specified*, exists for patients who do not meet the criteria for a more specific eating disor-

479

der. A woman who has symptoms of anorexia nervosa but who still menstruates would fit this category.

Anorexia nervosa is characterized by a refusal to maintain body weight and weight loss leading to maintenance of body weight less than 85% of that expected; intense fear of gaining weight or becoming fat even though underweight; a disturbance in the way in which one's body shape is experienced; and, in women, absence of a least three consecutive menstrual cycles (Table 18–1). The clinician should specify whether the disorder is restricting type (i.e., no bingeing or purging) or the binge-eating/purging type.

Bulimia nervosa consists of recurrent episodes of binge eating; a feeling of lack of control over eating during the binges; recurrent inappropriate compensatory behaviors to prevent weight gain, such as vomiting, use of laxatives or diuretics, strict dieting or fasting, and vigorous exercise; an average of two binge episodes weekly for 3 months; and persistent overconcern with body shape and weight. Further, the disturbance does not occur exclusively in the course of anorexia nervosa. The clinician should specify whether the disorder is the purging type (e.g., self-induced vomiting) or the nonpurging type. The complete set of criteria are found in Table 18–2.

Although the two disorders differ, patients with either one share an intense preoccupation with body weight and shape. Additionally, there is considerable diagnostic overlap between the two disorders, and their natural histories tend to intertwine.

Table 18–1.   DSM-IV criteria for anorexia nervosa

A. Refusal to maintain body weight at or above a minimally normal weight for age and height (e.g., weight loss leading to maintenance of body weight less than 85% of that expected; or failure to make expected weight gain during period of growth, leading to body weight less than 85% of that expected).

B. Intense fear of gaining weight or becoming fat, even though underweight.

C. Disturbance in the way in which one's body weight or shape is experienced; undue influence of body weight or shape on self-evaluation, or denial of the seriousness of the current low body weight.

D. In postmenopausal females, amenorrhea, i.e., the absence of at least three consecutive menstrual cycles. (A women is considered to have amenorrhea if her periods occur only following hormone, e.g., estrogen, administration.)

Specify if:

   Restricting type: during the current episode of anorexia nervosa, the person has not regularly engaged in binge-eating or purging behavior (i.e., self-induced vomiting or the misuse of laxatives, diuretics, or enemas)

   Binge-eating/purging type: During the current episode of anorexia nervosa, the person has regularly engaged in binge-eating or purging behavior (i.e., self-induced vomiting or the misuse of laxatives, diuretics, or enemas)

The discrepancy between weight and perceived body image is key to the diagnosis of anorexia nervosa. Underweight persons, who are normally concerned about their weight, recognize that their weight is low and possibly harmful and express a desire to gain weight. Anorexic persons, on the other hand, take delight in their weight loss and express a fear of gaining weight. The requirement that the anorexic person be 15% underweight for body height emphasizes severity, and amenorrhea (in women) adds to the specificity of the diagnosis. Bulimic patients are generally able to hide their binge-eating and purging behaviors and often have normal weight.

Epidemiology

There has been some concern that eating disorders are increasing in prevalence, and several investigators have suggested that anorexia nervosa is more common than it was just 20 years ago. It seems more likely, however, that increasing public awareness has simply led to the recognition of the disorder. Also, because treatments have become available, patients may be more likely to seek help. Estimates from high school and college-age populations yield a prevalence rate

Table 18–2. DSM-IV criteria for bulimia nervosa

A. Recurrent episodes of binge eating. An episode of binge eating is characterized by both of the following:
   1. Eating, in a discrete period of time (e.g., within any 2-hour period), an amount of food that is definitely larger than most people would eat during a similar period of time and under similar circumstances
   2. A sense of lack of control over eating during the episode (e.g., a feeling that one cannot stop eating or control what or how much one is eating)

B. Recurrent inappropriate compensatory behavior to prevent weight gain, such as self-induced vomiting; misuse of laxatives, diuretics, enemas, or other medications; fasting; or excessive exercise.

C. The binge eating and inappropriate compensatory behaviors both occur, on average, at least twice a week for 3 months.

D. Self-evaluation is unduly influenced by body shape and weight.

E. The disturbance does not occur exclusively during episodes of anorexia nervosa.

Specify if:
   Purging type: during the current episode of bulimia nervosa, the person has regularly engaged in self-induced vomiting or the misuse of laxatives, diuretics, or enemas
   Nonpurging type: during the current episode of bulimia nervosa, the person has used other inappropriate compensatory behaviors, such as fasting or excessive exercise, but has not regularly engaged in self-induced vomiting or the misuse of laxatives, diuretics, or enemas

among women of approximately 1% for anorexia nervosa and up to 4% for bulimia nervosa. For both disorders, the frequency for men is about one-tenth that for women. Individual symptoms characteristic of eating disorder, such as binge-ing, purging, or fasting, are far more common than the disorders themselves. It is not known why women are more likely to be affected than men, but the differences are probably not artifactual, because population surveys confirm what clinicians have noted.

The typical age at onset of eating disorders is adolescence or young adulthood. Studies comparing anorexia and bulimia generally find an earlier age at onset among anorexic persons (early teens) compared with bulimic persons (late teens, early 20s). Eating disorders are believed to be more prevalent in the higher socioeconomic groups. Anorexia nervosa, in particular, is uncommon in nonindustrialized countries. Eating disorders tend to be overrepresented in certain occupations that require rigorous control of body shape (e.g., modeling, ballet).

The following case example describes a patient who developed anorexia nervosa first and later achieved normal weight complicated by bulimia nervosa.

Mary, a 36-year-old registered nurse, has a 16-year history of abnormal eating behaviors. Now at normal weight and having regular periods, she has frequent binge episodes followed by spontaneous vomiting.

Mary grew up in a competitive, upper-middle-class family. The middle child of five children, Mary always felt unloved and ignored by her parents, whom she felt favored the other children. There were frequent temper outbursts during her childhood and teen years. Despite these problems, she performed well in school, was active in clubs, was a cheerleader, and had many friends. Still, Mary felt insecure and unattractive and dated little.

At age 20, she and a friend toured Europe together and would skip meals to save money. In fact, both felt they could afford to lose some weight, although Mary then weighed about 120 pounds (height 5 feet, 3 inches). On her return from Europe, she weighed less than 85 pounds. Her family was concerned about her scarecrowlike appearance, but Mary was pleased with her weight loss, because she felt she now was attractive. In fact, she believed she still weighed too much and could afford to lose more weight.

Over the next 5 years, her weight fluctuated, but she remained considerably underweight. Family members had become concerned about her eating habits. She refused to eat meals with her family, adopted a vegetarian diet, and was constantly found in the kitchen preparing high-calorie snacks of sugar, condensed milk, or other sweets. Her mother noted that cakes, cookies, and other desserts prepared for the family would mysteriously disappear, or a cake might be found with all the frosting removed. Mary eventually moved into her own apartment. Her brother remembers running into her at a grocery store and finding in her shopping cart only diet soda, a single head of lettuce, and several bags of candy.

Her family had noticed purging behaviors. Early on, Mary had learned how to induce vomiting with her fingers, but later vomiting became spontaneous. She would keep empty jars in her room to hold her emesis. After she had moved out, several jars were found under her bed, some of them moldy. Also, she made frequent trips to the bathroom to vomit and rarely cleaned up, leaving a visible trail of emesis in the unflushed toilet.

Always active, she became obsessed with exercise. She took up jogging before it had become popular and eventually was jogging 10 miles daily. She took great pride in her running and was able to place high in several marathons. The running continued at a high level until bone spurs and an old back injury flared up, which led her to cut back on her running. She developed a new routine involving a reduced amount of running, followed by biking 10 miles, and then swimming for 45 minutes. Mary was so busy with her exercise routine that her social life became very constricted. She had little time for friends and seemed to have lost interest in dating. Despite her routine, she lived independently, maintained a full-time job, and attended school part-time, eventually obtaining a bachelor's degree in nursing.

When Mary was 25, her mother talked her into seeing a physician for evaluation of her thinness, but the physician, who was not familiar with distorted eating behavior, told her mother that Mary's thinness and abnormal behaviors were an idiosyncrasy. Mary later sought help from a counselor for relationship problems, but she had not sought help specifically for an eating disorder.

At follow-up 6 years later, Mary still had occasional bingeing and purging, but maintained normal weight. She continued to work part-time, had married, and had two children.

Etiology and Pathophysiology

Psychological, genetic, and biological mechanisms have been used to explain the etiology of eating disorders. Psychological theories, which stress the importance of phobic mechanisms, have suggested that anorexia nervosa represents a phobic response to food resulting from the sexual tensions generated during puberty. Psychodynamic formulations have suggested that anorexic patients have fantasies of oral impregnation. It is unclear how bulimia nervosa fits either of these models, and some researchers have compared bulimia to alcohol addiction or obsessive-compulsive disorder. Social theories stress the importance of conforming to the American ideal of youth, beauty, and slimness; it is thought that this preoccupation with body shape and image may lead to the development of eating disorders in vulnerable persons.

Studies of hereditary influences have shown that anorexia nervosa tends to run in families (e.g., 6%–10% of female relatives of anorexic patients have the condition), as do mood disorders and substance abuse. Twin studies also tend to confirm a genetic predisposition. For example, in one study of 34 twin pairs and 1 set of triplets, 9 of 16 monozygotic twin pairs but only 1 of 14 dizygotic twin pairs were concordant for anorexia nervosa.

Biological theories tend to focus on the role of the hypothalamus, a region of the brain concerned with the regulation of essential body functions, such as appetite, weight, temperature regulation, and general homeostasis. Evidence supporting a primary hypothalamic disturbance comes from neurotransmitter studies, which show increased corticotropin-releasing factor in the cerebrospinal fluid of patients with anorexia nervosa. The occurrence of amenorrhea before weight loss also suggests a hypothalamic disturbance. Further, there is evidence of central neurotransmitter system dysregulation affecting dopamine, serotonin, and norepinephrine. The most consistent finding in patients with anorexia or bulimia is reduced norepinephrine activity and turnover. Further research is needed to pin down the disturbances.

Clinical Findings

The anorexic person quickly develops a repertoire of behaviors in the pursuit of weight loss. These behaviors can include extreme dieting, adoption of special diets or vegetarianism, and refusal to eat meals with family members or to eat in public. Anorexic persons often show an unusual interest in food that belies their fear of gaining weight. This interest may be manifested by collecting and clipping recipes, preparing elaborate meals for friends and relatives, and developing an interest in nutrition. Friends and relatives may become concerned about persons with weight loss, but they will insist that their weight is not abnormal and, in fact, that they are still overweight. Many patients begin to abuse laxatives, diuretics, or stimulants in an effort to enhance their weight loss.

Anorexic persons frequently develop an intense, almost obsessive interest in physical exercise and develop elaborate workout routines. In fact, many ballet dancers and women athletes (e.g., marathon runners) have anorexia nervosa. Eating disorders also occur in male athletes, particularly wrestlers urged by their coaches to meet strict weight criteria. This situation has led some states to set regulations governing the amount of weight loss allowed before wrestling competitions.

Anorexic persons with bulimic behavior and persons with bulimia tend to carry out their binge eating and purging in private. They may consume enormous amounts of food in a short period, for example, an entire cake, a quart of ice cream, *and* a box of cookies. Although families may be unaware of the bingeing, they may observe that their food bill is increasing or that special foods, such as those high in calories or carbohydrates, seem to disappear. The binge may initially bring the patient some relief from tension; however, this relief is invariably followed by guilt and feelings of disgust. The patient then induces vomiting, often at first by placing her fingers in the throat; later, she may be able to vomit at will. Some patients abuse emetics, such as ipecac. Many bulimic persons, perhaps as many as 10%, steal food by shoplifting or other means.

Other unusual food-related habits may develop. Patients may be observed to play with the food on their plate at mealtime, cut meat into tiny pieces, or buy large amounts of candy at stores. When these behaviors are pointed out to patients, they tend to deny them.

According to clinical lore, persons with anorexia nervosa tend to have above-average scholastic achievement, are highly perfectionistic, and come from families that are achievement oriented. Many have relatively poor sexual adjustment, which has suggested to some clinicians that anorexia nervosa represents an attempt to prolong childhood and escape the responsibilities of adulthood. In fact, many anorexic persons have delayed sexual development and show a diminished interest in sex, which accompanies the onset of their illness. Amenorrhea precedes the onset of obvious weight loss in one-fifth of cases.

Physical symptoms of these disorders tend to center around the eating behaviors manifested by the patient. Anorexic persons may develop profound weight loss that may make them look emaciated or cadaverous. Other physical changes can occur with severe weight loss, including hypothermia, dependent edema, bradycardia, hypotension, and the growth of lanugo hair. The anorexic person may complain of sensitivity to cold weather and chronic constipation. Hormonal abnormalities may occur in persons with anorexia nervosa; these include elevated growth hormone levels, increased plasma cortisol, and reduced gonadotropin levels. Although thyroxin and thyroid-stimulating hormone are usually normal, triiodothyronine (T_3) may be reduced.

Bulimic persons, on the other hand, may develop calluses on the dorsal surface of their hands (resulting from the irritation caused by placing fingers down the throat), dental erosion and numerous caries, and in some cases, esophageal erosion—all complications of frequent vomiting.

Medical complications may include hypocalcemia or hypokalemic alkalosis in persons who engage in self-induced vomiting or who abuse laxatives and diuretics. Electrolyte disturbances may result in weakness, lethargy, or cardiac arrhythmias. Serum transaminases may become elevated, reflecting fatty degeneration of the liver. Elevated serum cholesterol and carotenemia may develop, both a reflection of malnutrition. Parotid gland enlargement and elevated serum amylase levels may develop in persons with bulimia. Esophageal tears may develop from repeated vomiting in severely ill bulimic patients and can be life threatening. The medical complications of the eating disorders are summarized in Table 18–3.

Course and Outcome

The prognosis for eating disorders varies from full recovery to malignant weight loss and rapid death. One study of anorexic patients showed a death rate of 11% after a 12-year follow-up, which is significantly higher than expected. Additionally, long-term studies show that although some anorexic patients may be much improved, many continue to display characteristic symptoms of the illness, such as a distorted body image. From 25% to 40% of these patients have a good outcome, meaning that there are no abnormal eating behaviors and that the person

Table 18–3. Medical complications of the eating disorders

Physical manifestations

• Amenorrhea	• Hair loss
• Sensitivity to cold	• Petechia
• Constipation	• Carotenemic skin
• Low blood pressure	• Parotid gland enlargement[a]
• Bradycardia	• Dental erosion, caries[a]
• Hypothermia	• Pedal edema
• Lanugo hair	• Dry skin

Endocrine abnormalities

- Increased growth hormone levels
- plasma cortisol and loss of diurnal variation
- Reduced gonadotropin levels (LH, FSH, impaired response to LHRH)
- Low T_3, high T_3RU impaired TRH responsiveness[a]
- Abnormal glucose tolerance test
- Abnormal dexamethasone suppression test[a]

Laboratory abnormalities

• Dehydration[a]	• Elevated transaminases
• Hypokalemia[a]	• Elevated serum cholesterol
• Hypochloremia[a]	• Carotenemia
• Alkalosis	• Elevated BUN[a]
• Leukopenia	• Elevated amylase levels[a]

Note. LH = luteinizing hormone. FSH = follicle-stimulating hormone. LHRH = luteinizing hormone–releasing hormone. T_3 = triiodothyronine. T_3RU = triiodothyronine reuptake. TRH = thyrotropin-releasing hormone. BUN = blood urea nitrogen.
[a]Seen in patients who binge and purge.

is emotionally and socially well adjusted. Poor outcome is generally associated with longer duration of illness, older age at onset, prior psychiatric hospitalizations, poor premorbid adjustment, and the presence of a comorbid personality disorder.

Differential Diagnosis and Evaluation

Before making a diagnosis of either anorexia or bulimia, other major psychiatric disorders must be ruled out. Schizophrenia may be accompanied by bizarre eating habits, but they are usually related to psychosis. Major depressive disorder may be accompanied by poor appetite and significant weight loss, but the weight loss is not associated with a distorted body image. Obsessive-compulsive disorder may be characterized by ritualistic eating behaviors resulting in weight loss, but the weight loss is not accompanied by a distorted body image or fear of gaining weight. The majority of patients with anorexia or bulimia also fulfill criteria for another psychiatric disorder, most commonly major depressive disorder, an anxiety disorder, or a personality disorder, such as borderline personality. Obsessive-compulsive disorder, specific phobias, and agoraphobia are the most common anxiety disorders in patients with anorexia nervosa.

Medical disorders also need to be ruled out as the cause of an eating disturbance and significant weight loss. Gastrointestinal disorders (e.g., a malabsorption syndrome) can lead to severe weight loss, as can endocrine disorders (e.g., hyperthyroidism). Neoplasms, particularly midline tumors in the brain, may be associated with anorexia nervosa and weight loss in the absence of localizing neurological abnormalities. Therefore, patients who present for evaluation of an eating disorder need to have physical explanations ruled out.

In addition to a careful history, a thorough physical examination should be performed, paying particular attention to vital signs, weight, skin, and the cardiovascular system. Laboratory studies should be individualized based on the patient's condition to rule out alternate diagnoses. These tests should include a complete blood count, urinalysis, blood urea nitrogen, and serum electrolytes. For malnourished and severely symptomatic patients, other tests are indicated, including serum cholesterol and lipids, serum calcium, magnesium, phosphorus, amylase, liver enzymes, and an electrocardiogram. Brain imaging with magnetic resonance imaging or computed tomography is indicated in some patients to rule out a mass lesion. Thyroid function tests are indicated if hyperthyroidism is suspected as a cause of weight loss. Bone mineral densitometry will be helpful in assessing and monitoring osteoporosis in patients with anorexia nervosa.

Clinical Management

There are two fundamental goals in the treatment of the patient with an eating disorder. The first and most important goal is to restore the patient's nutritional state. In anorexic patients, this goal means restoring their weight to within a normal range; in bulimic patients, it means insuring that metabolic balance is achieved. The second goal is to modify patients' distorted eating behavior. This modification will help patients to maintain their weight within a normal range and to reverse (or at least attenuate) binge eating, purging, and other abnormal eating behaviors. Treatment can usually be conducted on an outpatient basis, but many patients will need hospitalization. Indications for hospitalization include starvation and severe weight loss or the presence of hypotension, hypothermia, or electrolyte imbalance. The depressed patient with suicidal ideations or psychosis will also need to be hospitalized. Other reasons for hospitalization include failure of outpatient treatment, as indicated by failure to gain weight, or failure to reverse severe binge/purge cycles.

Treatment of patients with eating disorders generally involves behavioral modification combined with individual psychotherapy. The purpose of behavioral therapy is to restore normal eating behavior. In the hospital, this goal is accomplished through strict protocols in which specific weight goals for anorexic patients are set (e.g., expectations for daily average weight gain) and certain abnormal behaviors are targeted for correction (e.g., reducing the number of vomiting episodes for bulimic patients). Positive reinforcement is used to help patients achieve the specific goals outlined in a treatment contract that is agreed to by the patient. For example, patients who are able to achieve their weight goals are rewarded with special privileges, such as a pass with a family member. Patients who do not achieve their targeted goals have their privileges reduced.

Patients should be weighed daily, early in the morning after emptying the bladder and while wearing only a hospital gown. Daily fluid intake and output should be recorded. Patients should be observed for at least 2 hours after meals to prevent vomiting, even if attendants must accompany them to the bathroom. Generally, it is advisable to start patients on a diet providing about 500 calories more than the amount required to maintain their present weight and to increase their caloric intake slowly. At first, to prevent discomfort at meals, it may be helpful to spread meals out over six feedings during the day. Patients who are significantly underweight or who are having trouble gaining weight may need tube feedings.

Medication may be indicated in the treatment of selected patients. Tricyclic antidepressants, monoamine oxidase inhibitors, trazodone, and fluoxetine have been shown to decrease both bingeing and purging behaviors, although they have no specific role in treating anorexia nervosa. An antidepressant may be useful in anorexic patients with a superimposed major depression, although the role of antidepressants in treating depressed anorexic patients has not specifically been studied. Some success has been demonstrated with cyproheptadine (Periactin) in helping patients to gain weight, particularly patients with anorexia nervosa who have no history of bulimia. Phenothiazines (e.g., chlorpromazine) and benzodiazepines (e.g., lorazepam) have sometimes been used to reduce the anxiety that accompanies early refeeding efforts, especially when tube feedings are needed. An example of how these medications can be helpful follows.

Allan, a 25-year-old, presented for treatment of anorexia nervosa weighing 85 pounds. A behavioral program was instituted with a primary emphasis on refeeding.

Allan made slow but steady progress. When his weight exceeded 100 pounds, he began to vomit his food. This behavior gradually became more frequent. Allan told us that he "hated" the foods given him and that they made him "gag."

Because there was no medical explanation for the vomiting and because it interfered with refeeding efforts, chlorpromazine 25 mg before meals was prescribed. Allan soon ceased vomiting and told us how much more relaxed he was at mealtime. Although he still did not like his food, he was able to keep it down and gain needed weight.

Practical and goal-oriented psychotherapy is probably the best approach to follow with an eating disorder patient, particularly during the acute phase of illness. Efforts to alter abnormal eating behavior in patients with insight-oriented therapy are generally not helpful. After initial symptom control, however, psychodynamic approaches may help the patient to resolve problems and conflicts that may have contributed to (or reinforced) the abnormal eating behavior. Family therapy may be helpful, particularly when the patient is living at home and the eating behavior has been perpetuated by disturbed family interactions or the disturbed eating behavior has created problems among the family members.

Group psychotherapy has emerged as an effective treatment for bulimia nervosa. Intensive programs that emphasize a behavioral approach include nutritional education, cognitive restructuring techniques, and psychosocial support seem to be the most effective.

Many patients with eating disorders will not seek treatment on their own and deny their illness. Patients may be brought unwillingly to a physician by their family or friends, and they may resist hospitalization or leave the hospital against medical advice. In the hospital, anorexic and bulimic patients have a reputation for being critical and manipulative; the eating disorder protocol is usually the focus of their criticism. Typically, these patients make repeated requests to get the physician to modify the protocol. A vicious cycle can develop; as soon as one modification is agreed to, requests for other changes follow. The safest approach is to refuse any modifications once the behavioral contract has been set.

Recommendations for treatment of eating disorders

1. An empathic relationship should be encouraged. This goal may be difficult to achieve, as anorexic patients may be manipulative and unmotivated and lack insight.

2. A commonsense approach is probably best for outpatients.
   - Develop simple targets for behavioral modification.
   - Use antidepressants in the patient with bingeing and vomiting who does not respond to behavioral measures.

3. Use a strict, vigorous behavioral protocol with inpatients.
   - Set the goals and then do not change them. Trivial changes in the protocol will open a Pandora's box.

4. Look carefully for comorbidity. Eating disorder patients are highly likely to have comorbid major depression, anxiety disorders, substance abuse, or a personality disorder.
   - Remember, the presence of a personality disorder complicates treatment of almost all psychiatric disorders, including eating disorders.

5. Family therapy is especially helpful with patients who still live at home or whose behavior has created problems within the family.

Bibliography

American Psychiatric Association: Practice guidelines for eating disorders. Am J Psychiatry 150:212–228, 1993

Andersen AE: Practical Comprehensive Treatment of Anorexia Nervosa and Bulimia. Baltimore, MD, Johns Hopkins University Press, 1985

Crisp AH, Hsu LKG, Harding B, Hartshorn J: Clinical features of anorexia nervosa: a study of 102 cases. J Psychosom Res 24:179–191, 1980

Deter HC, Herzog W: Anorexia nervosa in a long-term perspective: results of the Heidelberg-Mannheim Study. Psychosom Med 56:20–27, 1994

Drewnowski A, Hopkins SA, Kessler RC: Prevalence of bulimia nervosa in the U.S. college student population. Am J Public Health 78:1322–1325, 1988

Fairburn CG, Jones R, Peveler RC, et al: Psychotherapy and bulimia nervosa—long-term effects of interpersonal psychotherapy, behavior therapy, and cognitive behavior therapy. Arch Gen Psychiatry 50:419–428, 1993

Fava M, Copeland PM, Schweiger U, et al: Neurochemical abnormalities of anorexia nervosa and bulimia nervosa. Am J Psychiatry 146:963–971, 1989

Fluoxetine Bulimia Nervosa Collaborative Study Group: Fluoxetine in the treatment of bulimia nervosa: a multicenter, placebo-controlled, double-blind trial. Arch Gen Psychiatry 49:139–147, 1992

Halmi KA, Eckert E, LaDeut J, et al: Anorexia nervosa: treatment efficacy of cyproheptadine and amitriptyline. Arch Gen Psychiatry 43:177–181, 1986

Halmi KA, Eckert E, Marchi P, et al: Comorbidity of psychiatric diagnoses in anorexia nervosa. Arch Gen Psychiatry 48:712–718, 1991

Holland AJ, Hall A, Murray R, et al: Anorexia nervosa study of 34 twin pairs and one set of triplets. Br J Psychiatry 145:414–419, 1984

Hughes TL, Wells LA, Cunningham CJ, et al: Treating bulimia with desipramine. Arch Gen Psychiatry 43:182–186, 1986

Logue CM, Crowe RR, Bean JA: A family study of anorexia nervosa and bulimia. Compr Psychiatry 30:179–188, 1989

Mitchell JE, Pyle RL, Eckert ED, et al: A comparison study of antidepressants and structured intensive group psychotherapy in the treatment of bulimia nervosa. Arch Gen Psychiatry 47:149–157, 1990

Pope HG, Hudson JI, Jonas JM, et al: Bulimia treated with imipramine: a placebo controlled double blind study. Am J Psychiatry 140:554–558, 1983

Pope HG, Keck PE, McElroy S, et al: A placebo controlled study of trazodone in bulimia nervosa. J Clin Psychopharmacol 9:254–259, 1989

Sharp CW, Freeman CPL: The medical complications of anorexia nervosa. Br J Psychiatry 162:452–463,1993

Yates WR, Sieleni B, Reich J, et al: Comorbidity of bulimia nervosa and personality disorder. J Clin Psychiatry 50:57–59, 1989

Self-Assessment Questions

1. How do bulimia nervosa and anorexia nervosa differ? How do they overlap?
2. What are the sociodemographic characteristics of eating disorder patients?
3. What are some of the theories about the cause of anorexia nervosa?
4. What are typical clinical findings in anorexia and bulimia?
5. What potential medical complications may result from anorexia nervosa? From bulimia nervosa?
6. What are the major goals in the treatment of eating disorders?

Chapter 19

Adjustment Disorders and Disorders of Impulse Control

. . . Whether 'tis nobler in the mind to suffer the slings
and arrows of outrageous fortune or to take arms against a
sea of troubles, and, by opposing, end them.

William Shakespeare, Hamlet

Adjustment Disorders

Stressful situations are a regular occurrence for all of us. Whether one is a home-maker caring for small children or is a bank president, stressful situations arise nearly daily. The homemaker may need to calm a colicky child and clean up the spilled ice cream cone her other child accidentally dropped on the new living room carpet. The bank president may have to reprimand an errant employee or handle the consequences of learning about her husband's surreptitious love affair with his secretary. In these examples, the people involved and the circumstances differ tremendously, but they illustrate the universality of stressful events.

Most of us learn to handle stressful situations. Some people, however, feel overwhelmed by these situations and develop symptoms of emotional distress, such as depression, anxiety, or impaired work ability. These symptoms may be sufficiently severe to require brief periods of psychiatric care, usually on an out-patient basis. People with these problems often represent the walking wounded—the wife of an abusive alcoholic person, the person rejected by a lover or spouse, or the teenager failing in school.

The term *adjustment disorder* was introduced in DSM-III to describe condi-

493

tions in which a person develops psychological symptoms in reaction to stressful events, such as the situations noted above. The concept of adjustment disorders was included in DSM-I under *transient situational personality disorders* and in DSM-II under *transient situational disturbances*. These categories were used to describe superficial maladjustment to difficult situations or to newly experienced environmental factors in the absence of serious underlying personality defects. These disorders could be of any severity, including those of psychotic proportions.

In DSM-III, specific criteria for adjustment disorders were enumerated. The maladaptive reaction had to occur within 3 months of the psychosocial stressor. The diagnosis could be made in addition to another mental disorder, but could not be part of a characterological pattern, and the disturbance could not be an exacerbation of an existing mental disorder, such as major depression. DSM-III also prohibited psychotic disturbances from being categorized as adjustment disorders. The definition is the same in DSM-IV as it was in DSM-III-R, except that it is now specified that a maladaptive reaction cannot persist for more than 6 months after the termination of the stressor or its consequences (see Table 19–1).

Depending on the predominant symptoms that develop in response to the stressor, five subtypes of adjustment disorder are specified: depressed mood, anxiety, disturbance of conduct, mixed disturbance of emotions and conduct, or mixed anxiety and depressed mood. An unspecified subtype exists for reactions that do not fit into any specific categories, such as a patient responding to a new diagnosis of acquired immunodeficiency syndrome (AIDS) with denial and noncompliance with the treatment regimen.

Epidemiology

Because the definition of adjustment disorder keeps changing and because the diagnosis is often flexibly applied, it is difficult to know how widespread it is. Adjustment disorders are probably quite common; according to one report, nearly 5% of the psychiatric patients in Monroe County, New York, in 1971 had received a diagnosis of adjustment reaction of adult life. Data from our own hospital show that about 5% of psychiatric inpatients receive a diagnosis of adjustment disorder. It is likely that the percentage of psychiatric outpatients receiving this diagnosis may be closer to 10%. On consultation services at general hospitals, the frequency of this diagnosis may exceed 20%; one study of newly hospitalized cancer patients reported a prevalence of 32%.

The diagnosis appears to be more common in women, unmarried persons, and young persons. Among adolescents, common symptoms include behavioral

Table 19–1.   DSM-IV criteria for adjustment disorder

A. The development of emotional or behavioral symptoms in response to an identifiable stressor(s) occurring within 3 months of the onset of the stressor(s).

B. These symptoms or behaviors are clinically significant as evidenced by either of the following:

   1. Marked distress that is in excess of what would be expected from exposure to the stressor

   2. Significant impairment in social or occupational (academic) functioning

C. The stress-related disturbance does not meet the criteria for any specific Axis I disorder and is not merely an exacerbation of a preexisting Axis I or Axis II disorder.

D. Does not represent bereavement.

E. Once the stressor (or its consequences) have terminated, the symptoms do not persist for more than an additional 6 months.

Specify if:

   Acute: if the symptoms have persisted for less than 6 months

   Chronic: if the symptoms have persisted for 6 months or longer

Code based on type:

   With depressed mood

   With anxiety

   With mixed anxiety and depressed mood

   With disturbance of conduct

   With mixed disturbance of emotions and conduct

   Unspecified

changes or acting out, whereas adults typically manifest mood or anxiety symptoms. Although adjustment disorders may occur at any age, the average age for patients is in the mid-20s.

In one study of patients with adjustment disorders seen on a consultation service, medical illness was the identified stressor in more than two-thirds of cases. These patients, who were largely free of preexisting psychiatric illness, had experienced prolonged hospitalizations for serious physical illnesses, such as cancer or diabetes. The one-third of patients in whom medical illness was not the stressor were more likely to have established psychiatric histories and recurrent problems with relationships or finances.

Etiology

According to DSM-IV, adjustment disorders must occur in reaction to identifiable psychosocial stressors within 3 months of their onset. As a result of this definition, adjustment disorder is one of the few psychiatric diagnoses in which a cause-and-effect relationship is presumed. Posttraumatic stress disorder is another example. Clearly, most persons who experience stressful events do not develop psychiatric symptoms, which suggests that individuals who develop an adjustment disorder may have an underlying vulnerability.

Psychodynamic explanations are sometimes used to infer why stressful situations produce illness in some persons and not in others; for example, unpleasant childhood experiences could lead to fixation at certain stages of development, which later triggers a regression when sufficient stress is applied. Thus, each person has his or her own breaking point, depending on the amount of stress applied and the person's underlying constitution, personality structure, and temperament. To draw an analogy, if enough pressure is applied to a bone, it will fracture. However, the amount of pressure required to fracture the bone will differ from person to person depending on age, gender, and physical well-being. To carry the analogy a bit further, adjustment disorders can occur in psychiatrically normal people, just as healthy bones will break if subjected to sufficient stress. At the other end of the continuum, people with fragile personalities, like bones with osteoporosis, will break more readily.

Clinical Findings

Different subtypes of adjustment disorder reflect the varied symptoms that can occur, which typically include *depressed mood*, manifested by dysphoria, tearfulness, and hopelessness; *anxiety*, manifested by psychic anxiety, palpitations, jitteriness, or hyperventilation; *disturbance of conduct*, in which rights of others are violated or age-appropriate societal norms and rules are disregarded, as in vandalism, reckless driving, or fighting; and *mixed disturbance of emotions and conduct*, manifested by emotional symptoms such as depression or anxiety, in addition to a disturbance of conduct such as truancy or vandalism. Other examples not listed in DSM-IV include work disturbance (or academic inhibition), manifested by difficulty functioning on the job or in school, and withdrawal, manifested by socially withdrawn behavior that is not typical for the person.

In one study of adjustment disorders, the frequency of various psychosocial stressors considered to have provoked the patient's symptoms was determined. The results are listed in Table 19–2. Few of the listed stressors can be considered overwhelming, and in many cases, the stressors were multiple, recurrent, or continuous. Among adolescents, school problems were the most common stressor. Parental rejection, alcohol and drug problems, and parental separation or divorce were also quite common. Among adults, the most common stressors were marital problems, separation or divorce, moving, and financial problems. Many of the stressors were chronic. For example, among the adolescents, nearly 60% of the stressors had been present for a year or more, and only 9% had been present for 3 months or less. Among adults, stressors showed more variation, but 36% had

Table 19–2. Precipitants occurring in adolescents and adults with adjustment disorder

Adolescents		Adults	
Stressor	**%**	**Stressor**	**%**
School problems	60	Marital problems	25
Parental rejection	27	Separation or divorce	23
Alcohol and/or drug problems	26	Move	17
Parental separation or divorce	25	Financial problems	14
Girlfriend or boyfriend problems	20	School problems	14
Marital problems in parents	18	Work problems	9
Move	16	Alcohol and/or drug problems	8
Legal problem	12	Illness	6
Work problem	8	Legal problems	6
Other	60.2	Other	81.3

Source. Adapted from Andreasen NC, Wasek P: Adjustment disorders in adolescents and adults. Arch Gen Psychiatry 37:1166–1170, 1980.

been present for a year or more and nearly 40% had been present for 3 months or less.

A relatively typical patient who developed an adjustment disorder with depressed mood is described below.

Carol, a 34-year-old housewife, was admitted to the hospital after a tricyclic antidepressant overdose. According to Carol, she had felt well until earlier that day, when she learned that she had lost a battle for custody of her 13-year-old daughter to her ex-husband. After the ruling, Carol became upset, anxious, sad, and tearful. That evening, feeling desperate, Carol gulped a handful of nortriptyline tablets, prescribed months earlier for migraine, from her medicine chest. When her husband returned home from work, Carol told him what she had done. He called an ambulance, which brought her to the hospital emergency room, where she underwent charcoal lavage. Carol had no history that suggested emotional instability.

As the story unfolded, Carol explained that her current husband had been accused of sexually molesting her daughter, an allegation that had been reported to local social service agencies, bringing about her daughter's placement in foster care. Although the patient denied that her husband had ever touched her daughter inappropriately, she conceded that such an allegation was serious and would be taken into account by a judge in determining custody. After thinking through her situation, the patient reported that she was no longer depressed or suicidal and that she was in an appropriate frame of mind to work with her lawyer in an attempt to regain custody of her child.

Course and Outcome

Although most adjustment disorders are relatively transient, lasting days or weeks, some are more chronic (e.g., as in a woman with an alcoholic husband). By definition, however, adjustment disorders persist no longer than 6 months after termination of the stressor or its consequences. If a disturbance lasts longer, it will presumably meet criteria for another disorder, such as generalized anxiety disorder, major depression, or dysthymia.

In a 5-year follow-up of 100 patients with adjustment disorder, 79% of the adults were well at follow-up, with 8% having had an intervening problem. The rest (21%) had a current mental illness (e.g., schizoaffective disorder, major depression, alcoholism). Comparable figures for adolescents were 57% well at follow-up, with 13% having had an intervening problem. An additional 43% had a current mental illness (e.g., schizophrenia, major depression, schizoaffective disorder, bipolar disorder, antisocial personality, alcoholism, drug abuse). Two adults and one adolescent had committed suicide. These findings suggest that adults with adjustment disorders have a relatively good outcome, but that the diagnosis may be less useful in adolescents, because they tend to have a variety of outcomes. The diagnosis of adjustment disorder is relatively nonpejorative; it avoids stereotyping patients with a harsher, more severe diagnosis that may lead to self-fulfilling prophecies. Therefore, some clinicians consider it particularly useful for younger patients.

In another follow-up study, adjustment disorders were associated with increased risk of suicide, perhaps reflecting the tendency of some persons to become severely dysphoric or to develop frank major depression.

Differential Diagnosis

The variety of symptoms possible in adjustment disorders makes the differential diagnosis of adjustment disorders necessarily broad. The differential diagnosis includes mood disorders such as major depression, anxiety disorders such as panic disorder or generalized anxiety disorder, or conduct disorders in the child or adolescent. Personality disorders should also be considered because they are frequently associated with mood instability and behavioral problems. Patients with personality disorders typically react to stressful situations in maladaptive ways; therefore, an additional diagnosis of adjustment disorder cannot be justified unless the new reaction differs from their usual maladaptive pattern. Schizophrenic disorders are often preceded by the development of social withdrawal, work or academic inhibition, and dysphoria and need to be differentiated from adjustment disorders. Other psychiatric disorders believed to occur in reaction to a stressor must also be considered, including brief psychotic disorder, in which a person develops psychotic symptoms in response to a stressor, and posttraumatic stress disorder, which develops after a traumatic event that involves actual or threatened death or serious injury (e.g., wartime experiences).

As with the assessment of any mental disorder, the patient being evaluated for an adjustment disorder needs to have a thorough physical examination and mental status examination to rule out alternate diagnoses.

Clinical Management

The treatment of adjustment disorders has not been systematically evaluated, but psychotherapy is probably the most widely used treatment. Individual psychotherapy may give the patient an opportunity to review the meaning and significance of the psychosocial stressor that led to the disturbance. The therapist can assist the patient to adapt to the stressor if it is ongoing, or to better understand the stressor if it has passed. Group approaches can provide a supportive atmosphere for persons who have experienced similar stressors, such as patients who have received a diagnosis of AIDS.

Pharmacological interventions may also be helpful when somatic symptoms, such as insomnia, are prominent. A patient with an adjustment disorder with depressed mood who has initial insomnia may benefit from a hypnotic (e.g., flurazepam 15–30 mg) at bedtime for a few days. A patient experiencing anxiety may benefit from a brief course (e.g., days to weeks) of diazepam (e.g., 5 mg three times a day). If the disorder persists, it is worthwhile reviewing the diagnosis. At some point, an adjustment disorder with depressed mood, for

---

Recommendations for management of adjustment disorders

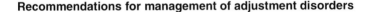

1. Adjustment disorders frequently evolve into other, better-defined disorders, such as major depression.
   - Be alert to changes in mental status and in symptoms.
2. Most adjustment disorders are transient. Tincture of time and supportive psychotherapy are usually all that is necessary.
   - In some cases, the disorder may be chronic, and ongoing supportive psychotherapy may be helpful.
3. Patients with common psychosocial stressors (e.g., a diagnosis of cancer or AIDS, chronic back pain, breakup of a relationship) often benefit from attending support groups with others who have experienced the same stressor.
4. Benzodiazepines are short-term solutions only and should be prescribed with the idea of making the patient more comfortable.
   - If long-term therapy is needed, the patient may have another disorder (e.g., generalized anxiety disorder), which will need recognition and treatment.

example, may develop into a major depressive disorder, which would best respond to antidepressant medication.

Disorders of Impulse Control

Five types of impulse-control disorders are listed in DSM-IV: intermittent explosive disorder, kleptomania, pyromania, pathological gambling, and trichotillomania. Another category exists for impulse-control disorders that do not meet criteria for a more specific disorder, for example, compulsive spending or buying. (See Table 19–3 for a list of these disorders.)

Disorders of impulse control are frequently underdiagnosed and underappreciated. In fact, some, such as pathological gambling, are quite common. They can all lead to considerable emotional distress, as well as social or occupational impairment. For these reasons, they are important to diagnose and treat. All are unified by the presence of irresistible urges or impulses to carry out potentially harmful or self-destructive behaviors.

Intermittent Explosive Disorder

Intermittent explosive disorder is characterized by the presence of several discrete episodes of losing control over one's aggressive impulses that are out of proportion to any stressor; these episodes may involve assaultive acts or destruction of property. The diagnosis is used in persons in whom the loss of control is out of character and not merely part of a pattern of overreacting to life's problems. Therefore, psychiatric conditions in which assaultive behaviors may occur as a matter of course need to be ruled out, such as antisocial or borderline personality disorders, psychotic disorders, mania, and alcohol or drug intoxication. A sudden behavioral change accompanied by outbursts in an otherwise healthy

Table 19–3.   Impulse-control disorders

Disorder	Uncontrolled behavior
Intermittent explosive disorder	Aggression
Kleptomania	Stealing
Pyromania	Fire setting
Pathological gambling	Gaming
Trichotillomania	Hair pulling
Impulse-control disorder not otherwise specified	

person suggests a brain disorder, which needs to be ruled out; these conditions are discussed in Chapter 6.

This condition, which was formally recognized in DSM-III, has been little studied. Patients who receive the diagnosis tend to be young males with relatively low frustration tolerance. Pure cases of intermittent explosive disorder—which occur in the absence of any indication of a brain disorder, such as an abnormal electroencephalogram, neurological soft signs, or the presence of abnormal personality traits—are rare.

The clinical management of intermittent explosive disorder is empiric, because treatments have not been well studied. Individual psychotherapy may be helpful in teaching patients how to recognize when they are becoming angry and in identifying typical stressors that lead to aggressive outbursts. At that point, patients can be taught alternate ways to grapple with the stimuli that would otherwise trigger rages, which then can be defused.

Medication to reduce or eliminate aggressive impulses may be useful in selected cases. Lithium carbonate, carbamazepine, and β-blockers (e.g., propranolol) have all been tried. Benzodiazepines may be helpful in treating the unbearable tension that some patients describe as leading to outbursts, although they may cause behavioral disinhibition. These compounds should be used with caution, and their use should be carefully monitored.

Kleptomania

Kleptomania produces an irresistible impulse to steal unneeded objects. A typical person with this disorder is a 35-year-old married woman apprehended for shoplifting items she could easily afford and does not need. DSM-IV defines kleptomania as 1) recurrent failure to resist impulses to steal objects not needed for personal use or for their monetary value; 2) an increasing sense of tension immediately before committing the theft; 3) pleasure, gratification, or relief at the time of the theft; 4) the stealing is not committed to express anger or vengeance and is not in response to hallucinations or delusions; and 5) the stealing is not better accounted for by antisocial personality disorder, a conduct disorder, or a manic episode.

Most of our knowledge about kleptomania comes from police records on shoplifting, which causes an estimated $40 billion in losses annually. The prevalence of kleptomania has been estimated at 6 per 1000, which may be an underestimate, because most persons with this disorder are ashamed of their behavior and may not report it to physicians. Most persons with kleptomania are women.

Although the cause of kleptomania is unknown, psychoanalysts have suggested that stolen items may be symbolic of psychosexual fixations and therefore are used to gratify primitive needs. More recently, kleptomania has been likened to obsessive-compulsive disorder (OCD) because both conditions are characterized by irresistible urges, and in some situations, stealing may resemble a compulsive ritual. However, there is no evidence that persons with kleptomania are differentially affected with OCD.

There are few reports in the literature about treatment. Behavioral techniques such as covert sensitization may be helpful, for example, coupling images of nausea and vomiting with a desire to steal. Antidepressants, particularly the newer serotonin-selective antidepressants (e.g., fluoxetine), have been reported to produce at least partial relief of urges and behaviors in some patients. Perhaps the best and easiest method to stop the stealing is to urge the patient to accept a self-imposed ban on all shopping unless accompanied by a friend or family member.

Pyromania

Pyromania as defined in DSM-IV is relatively rare. The disorder is characterized by deliberate and purposeful fire setting on more than one occasion; tension or affective arousal before the act; fascination with, interest in, curiosity about, or attraction to fire, its contents, and its characteristics; and pleasure, gratification, or relief when setting fires or witnessing or participating in their aftermath. By this definition, the typical arsonist who sets fires for monetary gain or for political or criminal purposes does not qualify for the diagnosis. Persons with antisocial personality disorder, a conduct disorder, or mania may set fires, but they generally do not share the sense of fascination with fire or experience the associated tension and relief with fire setting. Most deliberate fire setting seems to be motivated by anger or revenge.

Fire setting is more common among psychiatrically ill children (mostly boys) from large families of low social status. They usually have a history of serious delinquent behavior. Fire setting is considered a poor prognostic sign for children with conduct disorders.

Treatment of pyromania begins with the identification of other treatable psychiatric disorders that may be present (e.g., attention-deficit/hyperactivity disorder). Treatment of the coexisting disorder may itself reduce fire-setting behavior. Next, the parents need to be taught consistent but nonpunitive methods of discipline. Family therapy may help in dealing with the broader issue of family dysfunction often found in the families of patients with pyromania. Further, the patient needs to understand the dangerousness and significance of the fire setting. A visit to a burn unit or scene of a fire may help to make patients aware of the consequences of their behavior. Last, patients need to learn alternative ways of coping with stressful situations to decrease reliance on fire setting as an outlet.

Pathological Gambling

Pathological gambling is a progressive disorder characterized by a continuous or periodic loss of control over gambling. Other aspects of the definition are shown in Table 19–4. First included in DSM-III, the criteria are patterned after those used for substance dependencies, because there are so many superficial similarities (e.g., preoccupation with gambling [or using a substance], repeated efforts to stop gambling [or to control substance use]). For this reason, many persons consider gambling an *addiction*. The disorder is easily diagnosed, particularly in advanced cases, despite the patient's usual denial, which is also typical of the substance abuser.

Pathological gambling affects up to 2%–3% of the general population. The prevalence is less in places with limited wagering opportunities. With many states now dependent on tax revenues accrued from gambling, the disorder is likely to become even more widespread. The disorder typically begins in adolescence, and a few people become hooked almost from their first bet. Others may have a more insidious onset, after years of social gambling. About one-third of

Table 19–4. DSM-IV criteria for pathological gambling

A. Persistent and recurrent maladaptive gambling behavior as indicated by at least five of the following:

1. Preoccupation with gambling (e.g., preoccupied with reliving past gambling experiences, handicapping or planning the next venture, or thinking of ways to get money with which to gamble)
2. Needs to gamble with increasing amounts of money in order to achieve the desired excitement
3. Has repeated unsuccessful efforts to control, cut back, or stop gambling
4. Is restless or irritable when attempting to cut down or stop gambling
5. Gambles as a way of escaping from problems or of relieving a dysphoric mood (e.g., feelings of helplessness, guilt, anxiety, depression)
6. After losing money gambling, often returns another day to get even (chasing one's losses)
7. Lies to family members, therapist, or others to conceal the extent of involvement with gambling
8. Has committed illegal acts such as forgery, fraud, theft, or embezzlement to finance gambling
9. Has jeopardized or lost a significant relationship, job, or education or career opportunity because of gambling
10. Relies on others to provide money to relieve a desperate financial situation caused by gambling

B. Is not better accounted for by a manic episode.

gamblers are women, who generally start gambling later in life. Although women are more apt to experience comorbid depression, men are likely to experience alcoholism or other drug dependence. More men who present for help have had the problem for decades, although women usually have been ill for only a few years.

Although the cause of pathological gambling is unknown, family studies have shown a high prevalence of mood and substance use disorders among first-degree relatives of gamblers. Psychoanalysts believe that the compulsive gambler's certainty of winning stems from a childhood sense of omnipotence and an unconscious need for punishment. Behaviorists focus on the positive reinforcement gained from winning, as well as the other exciting stimuli, such as those found in typically garish Las Vegas casinos. There is some evidence that pathological gambling is associated with a functional disturbance of the noradrenergic system, which may underlie risk-taking behavior in general; thus, the disorder may be biologically mediated as well.

The treatment of pathological gambling begins with total abstinence. For many, Gamblers Anonymous, a 12-step program similar to Alcoholics Anonymous (discussed in Chapter 14), is sufficient. Others benefit from individual psychotherapy geared toward helping them to understand why they gamble and to assist them in dealing with feelings of helplessness, depression, and guilt. Relapse prevention needs to focus on knowledge of specific triggers that lead to gambling and how to deal more appropriately with these triggers.

Family therapy is often crucial, because family relationships are often severely disrupted by financial problems and chronic abuse and mistrust. Therapy sessions offer the gambler an opportunity to make amends, to learn better communication skills, and to repair the rifts that gambling inevitably creates in families.

Trichotillomania

Trichotillomania is defined in DSM-IV as 1) recurrent pulling out of one's hair resulting in noticeable hair loss; 2) an increasing sense of tension before pulling out the hair; 3) pleasure, gratification, or relief when pulling out the hair; 4) the absence of another mental disorder (e.g., schizophrenia) or a dermatological condition (e.g., alopecia areata) that could explain the symptom; and 5) clinically significant distress or impairment caused by the disturbance.

This disorder is generally chronic and can affect any site where hair grows, including the scalp, eyelids, eyebrows, and pubic regions. Among clinical populations, 70%–90% of hair pullers are female, and most report a childhood onset.

Compulsive hair pullers frequently have accompanying depression, anxiety disorders, or personality disorders. There seems to be some overlap with OCD, in that many hair pullers will meet criteria for OCD and vice versa. Pedigrees have been described in which both OCD and trichotillomania are found.

After alternate diagnoses and medical conditions are ruled out, the diagnosis should be easily made. Most patients do not have obvious balding, but they may have small, easily disguised bald spots or patches or missing eyebrows and eyelashes. A typical patient seen in our clinic is described below.

Shirley, a 42-year-old married homemaker, presented to our clinic for evaluation of compulsive hair pulling. She had recently learned of a new medication that might be helpful and wanted to try it.

Shirley grew up in a small midwestern farming community. Her childhood was relatively happy, and her family life was harmonious. As a young girl, she began to twist and twirl her hair and later, before age 10, began to pull out scalp, eyebrow, and eyelash hair.

The amount of hair pulling fluctuated over the years, but she has never been free of it. The pulling is sometimes automatic, as when she is reading or watching television, but at other times it is more deliberate. Shirley reported that she had tried to stop pulling her hair, but her many attempts had all failed.

At her interview, Shirley mentioned that she was wearing a wig. She removed it, revealing an essentially bald scalp except for a fringe around the top. She had no eyebrows or eyelashes, which she disguised with makeup and eyeglasses. She admitted to feeling embarrassed and ashamed by her problem and tearfully remembered how classmates had made fun of her as a child. Over the years, she had received many medical and dermatological evaluations. Ointments and solutions had been prescribed, all without benefit.

She was given clomipramine up to 150 mg per day, which appeared to reduce her urge to pull, but it was not helpful cosmetically. A trial of fluoxetine was unhelpful, and she declined referral for behavior therapy. Supportive psychotherapy was helpful in assisting her to accept her disorder and to develop improved self-esteem. She learned to understand that apart from her hair pulling, her life was generally happy and fulfilling.

Treatment in most cases consists of behavior therapy. Patients learn to identify their hair pulling (it is often automatic) and to substitute other, more benign behaviors; these techniques are often referred to as *habit reversal*. Antiobsessional medication, such as clomipramine, has also been shown to be helpful to some patients. Many will benefit from supportive psychotherapy that aims at upgrading their often low self-esteem, addressing relationship and family issues, and helping to correct faulty cognitions (e.g., "no one likes me because my eyebrows are missing").

Other Disorders

Compulsive buying or shopping is another disorder of impulse control, although is not specifically listed in DSM-IV. It is characterized by an irresistible urge to buy items that are either unneeded or unwanted. Like trichotillomania, there is usually a sense of tension before buying, followed by a sense of gratification or relief when buying. A feeling of guilt or remorse may follow the buying episode.

Most compulsive buyers are young women who spend excessive amounts on clothing, shoes, and makeup. Many have an additional psychiatric disorder, including depression, an anxiety disorder, or an eating disorder. Many have other impulse-control disorders, such as pathological gambling.

Many persons who shop compulsively feel unable to control their behavior, which can lead to considerable debt, personal bankruptcy, and marital and family strife.

Treatment of this condition has not been established, although individual psychotherapy may be helpful in exploring the significance of the compulsive buying and in helping the patient to recognize and learn how to avoid situations that lead to shopping episodes. Case reports suggest that antiobsessional medication may be helpful in reducing the behavior. Family and marital therapy may be helpful in patients whose marriages or family life has been disrupted by this disorder.

Compulsive sexual behavior has achieved recent notoriety, particularly in the mass media. Although there are no formal definitions, most experts feel that compulsive sexual behavior leads to uncontrolled and wanton sexual behavior resulting in impairment in social or occupational functioning. Common manifestations include multiple partners (i.e., the Don Juan syndrome), compulsive masturbation, preoccupation with pornography, unsafe sexual encounters, and telephone sex (e.g., 900 numbers). Most persons with these disorders are male, and many probably meet criteria for specific paraphilias (see Chapter 17).

Bibliography

Andreasen NC, Hoenk PR: The predictive value of adjustment disorders: a follow-up study. Am J Psychiatry 139:584–590, 1982

Andreasen NC, Wasek P: Adjustment disorders in adolescents and adults. Arch Gen Psychiatry 37:1166–1170, 1980

Christenson GA, Mackenzie TB, Mitchell JE: Characteristics of 60 adult chronic hair pullers. Am J Psychiatry 148:365–370, 1991

Derogatis LR, Morrow GR, Fetting J, et al: The prevalence of psychiatric disorders among cancer patients. JAMA 249:751–757, 1983

Fabrega H, Mezzich JE, Mezzich AC: Adjustment disorder as a marginal or transitional illness category in DSM-III. Arch Gen Psychiatry 44:567–572, 1987

Goldman MJ: Kleptomania: making sense of the nonsensical. Am J Psychiatry 148:986–996, 1991

Lion JR: The intermittent explosive disorder. Psychiatric Annals 22:64–66, 1992

Looney JG, Gunderson EKE: Transient situational disturbances: course and outcome. Am J Psychiatry 135:660–663, 1978

McElroy SC, Pope HG, Hudson JI, et al: Kleptomania: a report of 20 cases. Am J Psychiatry 148:652–657, 1991

Popkin MK, Callies AL, Colon EA, et al: Adjustment disorders in medically ill inpatients referred for consultations in a university hospital. Psychosomatics 31:410–414, 1990

Rosenthal RT: Pathological gambling. Psychiatric Annals 22:72–78, 1992

Roy A, Adinoff B, Roehrich L, et al: Pathological gambling—a psychobiological study. Arch Gen Psychiatry 45:369–373, 1988

Schlosser S, Black DW, Blum N, et al: The demography, phenomenology and family history of 22 persons with compulsive hair pulling. Annals of Clinical Psychiatry (in press)

Schlosser S, Black DW, Repertinger S, et al: Compulsive buying: demography, phenomenology and comorbidity in 46 subjects. Gen Hosp Psychiatry 16:205–212, 1994

Soltys SM: Pyromania and firesetting behavior. Psychiatric Annals 22:79–83, 1992

Self-Assessment Questions

1. What is the evolution of the adjustment disorder diagnosis from DSM-I to DSM-IV?
2. How common are adjustment disorders, and what are their typical precipitants and manifestations?
3. What is the differential diagnosis for adjustment disorders?
4. How do the precipitants differ between adolescents and adults?
5. What is the treatment for adjustment disorders?
6. What are the impulse-control disorders?
7. What is pathological gambling? What kind of problems do patients with this problem have?
8. How is trichotillomania treated?
9. What is the differential diagnosis for intermittent explosive disorder?
10. What is compulsive buying?

Section III

Special Topics

Chapter 20

Suicide and Violent Behavior

*The thought of suicide is a great consolation; by means of it
one gets successfully through many a bad night.*

Friedrich Nietzsche

Suicide

Suicide is a serious public health problem that accounts for nearly 30,000 deaths each year in the United States. It is the eighth most frequent cause of death for adults and the second leading cause of death for persons between the ages of 15 and 24 years. The effects of a suicide are devastating; the death affects not only surviving friends and family members, but also the victim's physician, because most people who commit suicide communicate their suicidal intentions to physicians before they die. Thus, suicide is a problem with which clinicians must familiarize themselves. They must be prepared to educate patients and family members about risk for suicide, to assess risk for suicide in their patients, and to act appropriately with interventions to prevent suicides.

Suicide is a self-inflicted death that is intentional rather than accidental. It is a complex human behavior with biological, sociological, and psychological roots. Suicide does not lend itself to simple formulations, such as one suggested in the media after the death of a presidential advisor in the early 1990s. The advisor, a successful small-town attorney, had apparently killed himself after becoming depressed. A suicide note revealed that he had felt hopeless about his future and responsible for the very public problems of the administration. The media reports implied that he had a weak character and could not tolerate the pressure-cooker atmosphere of our nation's capital. Clearly, job pressure may

511

have contributed to the suicide, but little mention was made of other factors, including his depressive illness and the fact that he had only recently sought treatment. The pressure of his job may have been the straw that broke the camel's back, but most people with stressful jobs do not kill themselves; other factors must have also played an important role in his suicide. The tragedy in this story is that his depression was not recognized earlier and treated.

Epidemiology

In the United States, nearly 1% of the general population will commit suicide, a rate of nearly 12.5 suicides per 100,000 persons; suicide rates are specific for age, gender, and race. Rates for men increase steadily with age and peak after age 75 years; rates for women are curvilinear and peak in the late 40s or early 50s. Nearly three times as many men as women take their lives, and whites are more likely than blacks to commit suicide. One alarming trend has been the rise in the suicide rate among young men and women, possibly due to increasing rates of drug abuse or to the cohort effect, which is discussed later. The reason for much of the increase remains a mystery.

Suicide rates differ by geographic region as well. In the United States, rates tend to be the highest in the West and lowest in the mid-Atlantic states. Among European countries, rates are highest in Eastern Europe and Scandinavia; in Hungary, for example, the rate hovers around 40 suicides per 100,000 persons. Rates tend to be low in Mediterranean countries, particularly those with large Catholic or Islamic populations. For reasons of religion, Catholics and Muslims are much less likely than Protestants to commit suicide.

Suicide rates tend to peak during the spring and have a smaller secondary peak in the fall. They are evenly distributed through the week, unlike homicides, which tend to peak on Friday evening or early Saturday morning. Rates are affected by economic conditions and were very high during the Great Depression of the 1930s; they are typically low during wartime. Certain occupations are associated with a high risk for suicide, particularly among the professions. Physicians are at especially high risk; and in contrast to suicide statistics in general, female physicians are at higher risk than male physicians. Married persons are less likely to commit suicide than single, widowed, or divorced persons. It is not clear whether social class affects suicide rates, but some studies suggest that rates are highest in both the highest and the lowest social classes.

Etiology

Several studies have examined the psychological state of suicide completers and have found that more than 90% of completers had a major psychiatric illness, and that half were clinically depressed at the time of the act (Table 20–1).

Nearly one-third of the suicides occurred in persons with chronic alcoholism, whereas schizophrenia, dementia, and other psychiatric conditions were less common. However, the most recent study departs from these conclusions by noting drug abuse in 45% and alcoholism in 54% of the suicide completers. These disconcerting findings may be a reflection of the growing drug and alcohol abuse problem in the United States.

The other findings have also been consistent. About two-thirds of suicide completers are men; most tend to be over age 45, are white, and are separated, widowed, or divorced. Psychiatric diagnosis tends to vary with age. Suicide completers younger than 30 years are more likely to have substance abuse disorders or antisocial personality disorder; suicide completers older than 30 years tend to have mood disorders.

About 5% of suicide completers have serious physical illnesses at the time of suicide; of conditions that have been investigated, suicide rates are elevated in persons who have brain trauma, epilepsy, multiple sclerosis, Huntington's disease, Parkinson's disease, the acquired immunodeficiency syndrome (AIDS), and cancer. A recent study showed that the suicide rate in patients with AIDS in the United States is nearly seven times that of the general population.

Table 20–1. Psychiatric diagnoses (in percentages) in three selected studies of suicides in the general population

Diagnosis	Robins et al.[a] (n = 134)	Barraclough et al.[b] (n = 100)	Rich et al.[c] <30 years (n = 133)	Rich et al.[c] >30 years (n = 150)
Depression	45	80	35	52
Alcohol abuse or dependence	23	15	54	55
Drug abuse or dependence	1	4	66	26
Schizophrenia	2	3	5	2
Dementia	4	1	—	7
Personality disorder	—	—	10	1
Other disorders	19	1	—	—
Not mentally ill	2	7	4	5

[a]*Source.* Adapted from Robins E, Murphy GE, Wilkinson RH, et al: Some clinical considerations in the prevention of suicide based on a study of 134 successful suicides. Am J Public Health 49:888–899, 1959.
[b]*Source.* Adapted from Barraclough B, Bunch J, Nelson B, et al: A hundred cases of suicide: clinical aspects. Br J Psychiatry 125:355–373, 1974.
[c]*Source.* Adapted from Rich CL, Young D, Fowler RL: San Diego suicide study, I: young versus old subjects. Arch Gen Psychiatry 43:577–582, 1986.

In a small number of persons committing suicide, there is no evidence of mental or physical illness. Many have argued that these suicides are rational— that is, based on a logical appraisal of the need for death; for example, an elderly widower with painful terminal cancer may not be clinically depressed but sees no hope for the future and wants to end his physical suffering. It is likely that many of these apparently rational suicides are actually irrational, but information was simply unavailable to confirm the presence of a mental illness because the person who died was socially isolated and informants were not available for interview. It still may be argued that many suicides are logical; philosophers, such as Nietzsche, have argued passionately on behalf of suicide. Of the 900 suicide completers in Jonestown, Guyana, for example, it is unlikely that all were mentally ill. Many probably committed suicide for reasons that had to do with their religious beliefs, not with mental illness.

Research has shown that specific psychiatric disorders are associated with high rates of suicide. Nearly 15% of persons with mood disorders will commit suicide, as will 2%–4% of chronic alcoholic patients and 10% of schizophrenic patients. A few psychiatric disorders, such as obsessive-compulsive disorder, have not been associated with increased rates of suicide. Among psychiatric patients, the risk for suicide is much higher than it is in the general population. Psychiatric illnesses are usually necessary for suicide to occur, but their presence is not a sufficient explanation, because most mentally ill persons do not commit suicide.

Suicide is often familial. Large kindreds, such as the Old Order Amish in Pennsylvania, show that suicide tends to cluster in certain pedigrees and is multigenerational. In these large pedigrees, suicides tend to occur in families filled with unipolar and bipolar affective disorders. Twin studies have demonstrated higher concordance for suicide among monozygotic twins compared with dizygotic twins, suggesting that suicide may be genetic as well as familial. Further, the Danish Adoption Study found a high prevalence of suicide among biological relatives of probands who had killed themselves, providing further evidence of a genetic contribution to suicide.

Methods of Suicide

In the United States, firearms are the most common method for committing suicide, perhaps because firearms are readily available and are generally immediately lethal. Firearms are followed in frequency by poisoning, hanging, and other methods. Men are more likely than women to use violent methods, such as firearms or hanging, a tendency that may explain why men are more successful in killing themselves. Women tend to use less violent means, such as poisoning by overdose. However, women are beginning to choose more lethal methods, a trend that may ultimately lead to higher suicide rates.

Suicide by firearms tends to be rare in societies with strict gun control laws, although other methods, such as use of domestic gas, may be common. In large cities, death by jumping from high places is common; obviously, it is rare in rural areas.

Biology of Suicide

Suicide may be biologically mediated to some extent. Low levels of cerebrospinal fluid 5-hydroxyindoleacetic acid (5-HIAA), a serotonin metabolite, have been measured in suicide completers, particularly those who died by violent means. Decreased imipramine binding in postmortem frontal cortex tissue samples has also been measured in suicide completers. (Imipramine binding tends to correlate highly with plasma serotonin levels.) Follow-up studies have shown that many suicide completers had abnormal dexamethasone suppression tests, suggesting the presence of hypothalamic-pituitary-adrenal axis hyperactivity. Suicide completers have been found to have high levels of urinary metabolites of cortisol and to have enlarged adrenal glands. All of these measures are abnormal in patients with severe depression; therefore, they may indicate depression rather than risk for suicide.

Clinical Findings

Suicide is an act of desperation. Suicidal persons frequently convey their distress to others, and nearly two-thirds communicate their suicidal intentions to others. Their communication may be as direct as reporting their plan and the date they intend to carry it out. Other communications are less obvious, for instance, the statement: "You won't have to put up with me much longer!"

Although depression is the most common psychiatric diagnosis associated with suicide, it is important to understand that suicide can occur during all phases of a depressive episode. It is commonly believed that suicide risk is highest during the recovery phase, when patients have regained sufficient energy to kill themselves. Because the suicidal urge waxes and wanes during the course of a depressive episode, the clinician should not be lulled into a false sense of security by noting the phase of a patient's illness.

Suicide completers tend to be socially isolated. Nearly 30% of suicide completers have a history of suicide attempts, and about one in six leaves a suicide note. Many who plan a suicide prepare wills, give away possessions, and purchase burial plots; therefore, clinicians should be alert to these behaviors. One of the strongest correlates of suicidal behavior is hopelessness, a finding independent of psychiatric diagnosis.

Nearly 40% of suicide completers have alcohol in their bloodstream at the time of death, suggesting that alcohol may have disinhibited them enough to give the courage to complete the act. Nearly 90% of alcoholic suicide completers have alcohol in their bloodstream at the time of death.

Patients remain at high risk for suicide in the posthospitalization period. Although depressed patients may appear to be significantly improved at the time of hospital discharge, a person may relapse quickly and enter another episode of depression. In one study of unipolar and bipolar depressed patients, nearly 42% of 36 suicides during the follow-up occurred within 6 months of hospital discharge, 58% by 1 year, and 70% by 2 years. Therefore, recently discharged patients need close follow-up.

Events that appear to trigger suicide differ by age and diagnostic group. Triggering events in adolescents or young adults often include troubled relationships, whereas in older persons the event may be poor finances or health. Among alcoholic persons who commit suicide, more than 50% have a history of interpersonal loss (usually of a sexual partner) within the year before suicide. This is not the case among depressed persons.

Youth Suicide

Rates have been increasing in men and women between the ages of 15 and 24 years. In fact, studies have shown that recent cohorts (i.e., groups of persons in the population with similar characteristics, such as being born in the same decade) have higher suicide rates than older cohorts. It is difficult to determine why rates should be increasing in this age group, but other data seem to show that the prevalence of depression is increasing in each successive cohort as well. Drug abuse has become a serious problem for society at large and young persons in particular. This problem may be leading to higher rates of suicide. Research has shown that suicide is more frequently associated with drug and alcohol abuse in youthful suicide completers than in adults; however, substance abuse is also associated with depression and behavioral problems.

Teenagers are more prone to the effects of peer pressure than adults, and this may be reflected in suicide clusters. It has been suggested that media depictions of suicide, such as televised movies that create sympathetic portrayals of suicide victims, tend to be followed by an increased rate of both suicide attempts and suicides, usually by the method portrayed.

Suicide Attempters Versus Suicide Completers

Suicide attempts are intentional acts of self-injury that do not result in death. They are easily 5–20 times as frequent as suicides, perhaps more so because most suicide attempts are not reported to authorities, and many attempters do not seek medical attention. Although suicide completers usually have clinical depression or alcoholism, suicide attempters have depression (one-third), alcoholism (one-third), and other disturbances including somatization disorder and antisocial personality, which are relatively uncommon among suicide completers. In fact, up to 40% or more of attempters have personality disorders.

Suicide completers generally plan their act, use effective means (e.g., firearms, hanging), and carry out the suicide in private or make provisions to avoid interruption. Completers are serious about ending their lives. In contrast, suicide attempters, who are three times more likely than suicide completers to be women, are usually younger than 35 years, often act impulsively, make provisions for rescue, and use ineffective or slowly effective means such as drug overdoses. Differences between suicide attempters and completers are summarized in Table 20–2.

The typical picture of a suicide attempter is that of an angry young woman just rejected by her boyfriend after a short-term love affair who rushes to the bathroom, grabs a bottle of pills out of the medicine chest, and gulps the pills in the presence of her boyfriend. With great fanfare, she is taken to the emergency room where her stomach is lavaged. Suicide attempts are often emotionally cathartic, so that the patient may feel a sense of relief afterward. The suicide attempter usually regrets having done such a "stupid" thing. Some will admit that the attempt was an effort to gain attention, to hurt a loved one, or to win back a former lover.

Research has shown that the more serious the attempt, the more closely the suicide attempter resembles the suicide completer in terms of risk factors. Suicide attempters remain at risk for future attempts, and each year thereafter an estimated 1%–2% of those who attempted suicide will complete the act—up to a total of about 10%.

Table 20–2. Differences between suicide completers and attempters

Variable	Completers	Attempters
Gender	Male	Female
Age	Older	Younger
Diagnosis	Depression, alcoholism, schizophrenia	Depression, alcoholism, personality disorder
Planning	Careful	Impulsive
Lethality	High (e.g., firearms)	Low (e.g., poisoning)
Availability of help	Low	High

Assessment of the Suicidal Patient

Assessment of suicide risk begins with recognition of the risk. Because most suicide completers contact their physician in the month before death, it follows that physicians have ample opportunity for intervention, providing that the clues of an impending suicide are observed. Risk factors associated with suicide are presented in Table 20–3.

The accurate assessment of suicide risk must include a thorough psychiatric history, family history, and mental status examination. The clinician must be alert to the possibility of suicide in any psychiatric patient, especially those who are depressed or have a depressed affect. In these patients, the assessment will focus on vegetative signs and cognitive symptoms of depression, death wishes, suicidal ideation, and suicidal plans. Most suicidal patients are willing to discuss their thoughts with a physician if asked, but only one in six clinicians asks his or her patients about suicide! A commonly believed myth is that asking a patient about suicide will give the patient ideas that he or she has not already had. Because suicidal thoughts are common in depression, most depressed patients will have had these thoughts. Patients are often fearful and even feel guilty about having suicidal thoughts, so giving the patient an opportunity to discuss them may provide some relief. Specific questions that should be asked of the patient include the following:

- Are you having any thoughts about harming yourself?
- Are you having any thoughts about taking your life?
- Have you developed a plan for committing suicide? If so, what is your plan?

The physician should also assess the patient's history of suicidal behavior by asking these questions:

Table 20–3. Clinical variables associated with suicide

- Being a psychiatric patient
- Being male, although the gender distinction is less important in psychiatric patients than in the general population
- Age: risk increases as men age, but peaks in the middle years for women
- Race: whites are at higher risk than nonwhites
- Diagnosis: depression, alcoholism, schizophrenia
- History of prior suicide attempts
- Recent interpersonal loss (among alcoholic persons)
- Feelings of hopelessness and low self-esteem
- Timing: early in the post-hospital discharge period
- Adolescents: a history of drug abuse and behavioral problems

- Have you ever had thoughts of killing yourself?
- Have your ever attempted suicide? If so, would you tell me about the attempt?

The physician should approach the subject of suicide in a slow and tactful manner, after having developed rapport with the patient. Because suicidal thoughts may fluctuate, physicians must reassess suicide risk at each contact with the patient. Patients who have developed well-thought-out plans and have the means to carry them out require surveillance, usually in a hospital on a locked psychiatric unit. It may be necessary to obtain a court order for hospitalization if the suicidal patient refuses voluntary hospitalization. Although a suicidal patient may plead with the doctor, family, or friends not to be taken to the hospital, family members and friends are neither sufficiently prepared nor sufficiently educated to handle a suicidal person. Hospitalization is the only way a physician may reasonably ensure the safety of the patient.

Managing the Suicidal Patient

In the hospital, the nursing staff will need to ensure that sharp objects, belts, and other potentially lethal items are taken from the patient and that those patients at risk for elopement are carefully watched. Occasionally, patients require seclusion. The physician will need to document the case carefully in the chart, noting signs and symptoms of depression, risk of suicide, protective measures taken, and treatment interventions provided.

Once the safety of the patient has been ensured, treatment of the underlying illness can begin. Treatment will depend on the diagnosis. Antidepressant medication or electroconvulsive therapy is helpful in the treatment of the depressed patient, although lithium carbonate and antipsychotics are appropriate additions to the treatment of bipolar and psychotically depressed patients, respectively. Antipsychotic medications are helpful in the suicidal schizophrenic patient. Electroconvulsive therapy is often specifically recommended for treatment of the suicidally depressed patient, because it tends to have a quicker onset of action than antidepressant medication. However, there is usually no need for this degree of concern if the patient is in the hospital under constant supervision.

If the patient is treated as an outpatient, close follow-up is absolutely essential. This follow-up must include frequent physician visits for assessment of mood and suicide risk, for psychotherapeutic support, and for frequent refilling of small amounts of prescribed medication to avoid the problem of having a large number of pills on hand for an impulsive suicide attempt. Family members can be helpful in monitoring the medication. Consideration should be given to prescribing one of the newer antidepressants that have a high therapeutic index and are unlikely to be fatal in overdose (e.g., bupropion, fluoxetine, paroxetine). Family members should be instructed to remove all firearms from the home. The lack of a simple, readily available method that is immediately and predictably lethal might dissuade some people from attempting suicide.

Recommendations for management of the suicidal patient

1. Always ask depressed patients about suicidal thoughts and plans. You will not plant ideas that were not there merely by asking.
   - Reassess risk of suicide at every visit with depressed patients.
2. Hospitalize suicidal patients, even if it means hospitalizing them against their will. Patients who do not have suicidal plans and do have supportive families who can monitor them can probably be managed at home.
3. In the hospital, write suicide precautions in the doctors' orders; order one-to-one protection if needed.
   - Document signs and symptoms carefully.
4. In the outpatient, monitor suicide risk frequently, write frequent small prescriptions, and consider using a newer antidepressant that has a higher therapeutic index (e.g., fluoxetine, bupropion).
   - Have the family remove all firearms from the home.
5. Remember that even though the risk factors are known, it is not possible to predict who will commit suicide.
   - One must simply use good clinical judgment, provide close follow-up, and prescribe effective treatments.

Violent Behavior

Violence is an all-too-frequent occurrence in present-day society. The public is bombarded almost daily with news stories about senseless killings and assaults, drive-by shootings, and domestic disputes that end in tragedy. The violence is frequently attributed to psychiatric illness and in some cases may be related (e.g., a psychotically depressed man who kills his wife and children and then takes his own life). More often, the violent acts are not committed by psychiatric patients; in fact, psychiatric patients are no more likely to commit a violent crime than are members of the general population. Certain mental disorders under certain conditions *are* associated with violence, but only 10% of the patients presenting for psychiatric hospitalization have committed a violent act. For this reason, psychiatrists must be able to evaluate the risk of violence and learn to manage violent patients. Violent behavior among chronically mentally ill patients is unfortunately common in psychiatric hospitals and care facilities.

Psychiatrists and other mental health care professionals have no more skill than lay persons in predicting long-term violence. However, mental health care professionals generally have an improved ability to predict violence in clinical settings. Certain elements of the clinical situation, including the patient's diagnosis and past behavior and the ward milieu, can indicate the patient's potential for imminent violence, thereby allowing appropriate interventions to be made. Accurate assessment is improved when dealing with well-defined populations having high base rates for violence, such as very disturbed patients on a locked psychiatric unit.

Etiology of Violence

In clinical settings, the presence of patients with certain psychiatric disorders is the best predictor of violence. Patients with schizophrenia, mania, mental retardation, and brain disorders (including drug and alcohol intoxication) are more likely to become violent than are patients with other conditions. In the hospital, psychotic disorders are more likely to lead to violence than are nonpsychotic disorders.

An example of how these conditions can lead to violence follows.

> Donald, a 71-year-old man with advanced Alzheimer's disease, was admitted to our hospital for violent and unpredictable behavior. His wife and family had cared for him at home during the 7-year illness. As he had become increasingly confused, he had tended to make more frequent misinterpretations of external stimuli. For example, his wife had a deep voice, which led him at times to conclude that a strange man was in the house. This was especially frightening to him, leading him to threaten his wife with a knife.
>
> In the hospital, Donald was disoriented and confused. He required considerable assistance with his grooming and dress. At times, without apparent provocation, he would assault his nurses or would make threatening gestures, such as karate chops. This behavior was frightening due to its apparent unpredictability.

Alcohol has been strongly associated with violence because of its well-known tendency to cause disinhibition, to decrease perceptual and cognitive alertness, and to impair judgment. Other substances of abuse—including amphetamines, cocaine, hallucinogens, phencyclidine (PCP), and the sedative-hypnotics—have also been associated with violent behavior. Of course, much of the violence in society at large is indirectly related to drug abuse, primarily through activities involved in obtaining these compounds.

Other factors are also involved in violence. Being a victim of abuse as a child leads to a greater likelihood of being physically abusive as an adult. Age and maturity level are associated with violent acts in persons with conduct or personality disorders, such as antisocial personality disorder; with advancing age and maturity, persons with these disorders are less likely to act out. Persons with low socioeconomic status are more likely to be both perpetrators and victims of violence, perhaps due to the alienation, discrimination, family breakdown, and general sense of frustration that the poor experience. The presence of readily available firearms in our society has contributed to the general level of violence because they may turn what would be an assault into a murder.

At a more physiological level, aggressive behavior has been related to low cerebrospinal fluid 5-HIAA levels, as has suicidal behavior. It has been hypothesized that low cerebrospinal fluid 5-HIAA may be a marker of impulsivity rather than of a specific type of violent act. In some patients, partial complex seizures have been connected to violence, although violent acts by patients with epilepsy are rare.

Assessing Risk for Violence

Risk assessment involves a review of pertinent clinical variables, including a thorough psychiatric history and careful mental status examination. Some researchers have used a "weather forecast" model, because assessment of the risk of violence, like weather forecasting, becomes progressively less accurate beyond the short term (i.e., 24–48 hours). Therefore, risk assessment, like weather forecasts, should be updated frequently. Clinical variables associated with violence are presented in Table 20–4.

Assessment involves identifying the risk factors associated with violence and making preventive interventions. This assessment must include a careful differential diagnosis because interventions will generally be based on the diagnosis. A violent schizophrenic patient will need treatment with antipsychotic medication, whereas a violent manic patient will probably require a combination of lithium carbonate and an antipsychotic.

Table 20–4. Clinical variables associated with violence

- A history of violent acts
- Inability to control anger
- A history of impulsive behavior (e.g., recklessness)
- Paranoid ideation or frank psychosis
- Command hallucinations in psychotic patients
- The stated desire to hurt or kill another person
- Presence of an acting-out personality disorder (e.g., antisocial personality disorder, borderline personality disorder)
- Presence of dementia, delirium, or alcohol or drug intoxication

When interviewing the patient who has been violent or is threatening violence, one needs to remain calm and speak softly in a nonjudgmental manner. Comments or questions should be nonthreatening, such as "You seem upset; maybe you can tell me why you feel that way." The interviewer should avoid towering over the patient; if possible, both should be seated, allowing personal distance between the interviewer and the patient. Sustained eye contact may be perceived as confrontational and should be avoided. The interviewer should try to project a sense of empathy and concern. Family members, friends, police, and others who have information on the patient should be interviewed to gather additional information about violent behavior and the patient's potential for violence.

Managing the Violent Patient

In the hospital or clinic setting, the violent patient presents an emergency. To ensure the safety of the patient and others, it is important that the staff be sufficient in number and be well trained in seclusion and restraint techniques. Use of tranquilizing medication may be helpful, although the patient may not be cooperative in taking it.

After a decision has been made to restrain or seclude the patient, a staff member, backed up by at least four other team members, should approach the patient, after first clearing the area of other patients. The patient should be told

---

Recommendations for management of the violent patient

1. Approach the patient in a slow and tactful manner.
   - Do not appear threatening or provocative.
   - Use a soft voice, appear passive, and maintain interpersonal distance.
2. Ask the patient what is wrong, or why he or she feels angry.
   - Most patients are willing to disclose their feelings.
3. Violent psychiatric patients need to be in the hospital where their safety, and the safety of others, can be assumed.
4. Write orders for violence precautions and seclusion or restraint orders, if applicable.
   - Monitor the risk of violence and the presence of violent behaviors.
   - Carefully document your assessment and plan.
5. For outpatients, monitor the risk of violent behaviors at each contact; have the patient (or family) rid the house of firearms.
6. Treat the underlying condition vigorously.
7. Remember that predicting violent behavior is difficult, even under the best of circumstances.

in a clear manner that he or she will be secluded or restrained because of uncontrolled behavior. The patient should be asked to walk quietly to the seclusion area and be given a few moments to respond. If the patient does not respond, staff members should each take a limb in a plan agreed to beforehand. At this point, restraints should be applied; or if the patient is taken to the seclusion room, staff members should grab the patient's legs and the arms around the elbow with underarm support.

Once secluded, the patient should be thoroughly searched. Belts, pins, and other items should be removed. Patients should be put in a hospital gown. If medication is needed, it can be injected or given orally (if the patient is cooperative). Patients in seclusion generally receive one-on-one observation by nursing staff.

In most cases, the psychiatrist will not be present when patients are placed in seclusion or restraints. Although the rules differ from hospital to hospital, the clinician will need to carefully document the reasons for seclusion or restraint (e.g., harm to self or others, threatening gestures), the condition of the patient, any laboratory investigations being pursued (e.g., urine drug screen), and the medication being administered.

Bibliography

Barraclough B, Bunch J, Nelson B, et al: A hundred cases of suicide: clinical aspects. Br J Psychiatry 125:355–373, 1974

Beck AT, Steer RA, Kovacs M, et al: Hopelessness and eventual suicide. Am J Psychiatry 142:559–563, 1985

Black DW, Warrack G, Winokur G: The Iowa record-linkage study, I: suicide and accidental death among psychiatric patients. Arch Gen Psychiatry 42:71–75, 1985

Black DW, Winokur G: Suicide and psychiatric diagnosis, in Suicide Over the Life Cycle. Edited by Blumenthal S, Kupfer D. Washington, DC, American Psychiatric Press, 1990, pp 135–153

Coté TR, Biggar RJ, Dannenberg AL: Risk of suicide among persons with AIDS: a national assessment. JAMA 268:2066–2068, 1992

Egeland JA, Sussex JN: Suicide and family loading for affective disorder. JAMA 254:915–918, 1985

Fawcett TJ, Scheftner W, Clark D, et al: Clinical predictors of suicide in patients with major affective disorders: a controlled prospective study. Am J Psychiatry 144:35–40, 1987

Goldstein R, Black DW, Winokur G, et al: The prediction of suicide: sensitivity, specificity, and predictive value of a multivariate model applied to suicide in 1,906 affectively ill patients. Arch Gen Psychiatry 48:418–422, 1991

Key NS, Soreff SM: Psychiatrist role responses and responsibilities when the patient commits suicide. Am J Psychiatry 148:739–743, 1991

Lidz CW, Mulvey EP, Gardner W: The accuracy of prediction of violence to others. JAMA 269:1007–1011, 1993

Marzuk PM, Leon AC, Tardiff K, et al: The effect of access to lethal methods of injury on suicide rates. Arch Gen Psychiatry 49:451–458, 1992

Miller RJ, Zadolinnyj K, Hafner RJ: Profiles and predictors of assaultiveness for different ward populations. Am J Psychiatry 150:1368–1373, 1993

Murphy GE, Wetzel RD, Robins E, et al: Multiple risk factors predict suicide in alcoholism. Arch Gen Psychiatry 49:459–463, 1992

Phillips DP, Carstonson LL: Clustering of teenage suicides after television news stories about suicide. N Engl J Med 55:685–689, 1986

Rich CL, Young D, Fowler RC: San Diego suicide study, I: young versus old subjects. Arch Gen Psychiatry 43:577–582, 1986

Robins E, Murphy GE, Wilkinson RH, et al: Some clinical considerations in the prevention of suicide based on a study of 134 successful suicides. Am J Public Health 49:888–899, 1959

Roy A, Segal NC, Centerwall BS, et al: Suicide in twins. Arch Gen Psychiatry 48:29–32, 1991

Shafii M, Steltz-Lenarsky J, Derrick AM, et al: Comorbidity of mental disorders in the post-mortem diagnoses of completed suicide in children and adolescents. J Affect Disord 15:227–233, 1988

Stanley M, Mann JJ: Biologic factors associated with suicide, in American Psychiatric Press Review of Psychiatry, Vol 7. Edited by Francis AJ, Hales RE. Washington, DC, American Psychiatric Press, 1988, pp 344–352

Tardiff K: The Psychiatric Uses of Seclusion and Restraint. Washington, DC, American Psychiatric Press, 1984

Tardiff K, Sweillam A: Assault, suicide, and mental illness. Arch Gen Psychiatry 37:164–169, 1980

Teplin LA: The criminality of the mentally ill—a dangerous misconception. Am J Psychiatry 142:593–599, 1985

Winokur G, Black DW: Suicide—what can be done? N Engl J Med 327:490–491, 1992

Self-Assessment Questions

1. Why is suicide a major health problem?
2. What are the common risk factors for suicide?

3. How do completed suicides differ from attempted suicides?
4. What is a rational suicide?
5. Are there different risk factors for suicide among youth?
6. How should the suicidal patient be managed in the hospital? As an outpatient?
7. What are the risk factors for violent behavior?
8. How is the violent or potentially violent patient assessed?
9. What are the indications for seclusion and restraint? How are seclusion and restraint orders implemented?

Chapter 21

Psychiatric Aspects of Acquired Immunodeficiency Syndrome

And I looked, and behold a pale horse: and his name that sat on him was Death, and Hell followed with him.

Revelations 6:8

One of the most fascinating (and alarming) stories in medicine during this century has been the development of the acquired immunodeficiency syndrome (AIDS). Although the syndrome was first identified in the early 1980s, there is evidence that it may have existed in the United States for up to two decades before its recognition. From the physician's perspective, a unique aspect of the epidemic is that we have been able to watch a very serious new disease evolve over a short period. Because the disease is nearly always fatal and has such striking social and economic costs, it has gained far more attention than other relatively new epidemics, such as genital herpes. Although by the early 1990s the incidence (i.e., new cases) appeared to have peaked, the prevalence continues to grow as new cases become evident. By 1994, it was estimated that in the United States more than 1.5 million persons had been infected with the virus and that more than 200,000 had died of AIDS. Worldwide, an estimated 15 million persons have been infected, and by the year 2000, that figure may reach 40 million. In the United States, AIDS is now the number-one killer of men between ages 25 and 44 and is straining budgets everywhere, especially because treatments are allowing these patients to live longer.

527

Etiology and Pathophysiology

The disease is transmitted by a slow retrovirus referred to as the human immunodeficiency virus (HIV), which specifically binds to receptors on the surface of cells of the immune system. Once bound, the virus gains entry to the cell, where the enzyme reverse transcriptase copies the viral RNA into DNA, which then inserts itself into the nuclear DNA of the human cell. HIV infects a number of human cells, but its hallmark is the progressive destruction of helper, or CD4$^+$, T lymphocytes. HIV can remain latent for months or years after incorporation into the human cell genome. During this time, these infected cells produce no viral proteins and are able to elude immunological detection. After a period of latency, the virus becomes active, multiplies rapidly, and spreads throughout the body. Infection of various target tissues can take place through cell-to-cell contact or cell fusion, which may be one of the mechanisms by which HIV evades destruction by the immune system.

As CD4$^+$ cell counts fall, the immune system is eventually paralyzed, and patients become progressively more susceptible to opportunistic infections, such as *Pneumocystis carinii*, toxoplasmosis, and certain types of cancer, including Kaposi's sarcoma. Besides devastating the immune system, HIV is neurotropic. Early in the course of the infection, the virus enters the central nervous system (CNS), probably carried there by macrophages, which cross the blood-brain barrier.

The virus is transmitted from person to person through exchange of body fluids such as semen and blood and through intravenous use of contaminated syringes and needles. In the United States, homosexual men comprise the largest risk group and make up about two-thirds of reported cases, although in African countries heterosexual transmission is more common. Intravenous drug abusers account for the next-largest group. Heterosexual persons infected through sexual intercourse, newborns infected via placental transmission, and recipients of HIV-contaminated blood transfusions, including persons with hemophilia, make up the rest. Since 1987, the nature of the epidemic in the United States has shifted as the percentage of cases involving gay and bisexual men has dropped and cases of heterosexual transmission have increased. The virus is not transmitted through the kinds of casual contact that people sharing a home engage in, such as touching, hugging, kissing, or sharing the same dishes.

The serum test used to detect HIV is known as the enzyme-linked immunosorbent assay (ELISA). If the result is positive, the serum is then subjected to the more accurate Western blot test. Because false-positive results may occur with the ELISA, persons should not be notified of a positive result until the

Western blot test has been performed. Both assays test for antibodies to HIV, and many infected patients will have a negative test result until they synthesize antibodies to HIV. A recombinant enzyme immunoassay and/or a radio-immunoprecipitation assay may be used when diagnostic uncertainty persists, and some laboratories use viral cultures as supplemental tests. Positive results are reported to public health authorities in some states, and AIDS registries have been created. In some countries, Cuba for instance, persons with HIV are quarantined.

Clinical Findings

The clinical manifestations of persons infected with HIV are wide-ranging and depend on the stage of illness and organs involved. The *initial* or *acute phase* of infection, the period between infection and the development of detectable anti-bodies, lasts from several weeks to several months, but averages 2 months; some persons may experience a transient flulike syndrome or an acute clinical or sub-clinical meningoencephalitis. Because recently infected patients are not yet im-munocompromised, they are able to recover and contain the virus. The *silent* or *latent phase*, the period between the onset of seropositivity and the onset of clin-ical symptoms, typically lasts from 5 to 7 years; persons are infectious but do not have any AIDS-related medical problems. The *symptomatic phase*, the period be-tween the onset of clinical symptoms and death, lasts from several months to years, depending on the specific complications that develop and their response to treatment.

Patients who have yet to develop an AIDS-defining infection, such as *Pneu-mocystis carinii*, may have persistent lymphadenopathy, fatigue, night sweats, oral candidiasis, and unexplained weight loss. In the past, this condition would have been called *AIDS-related complex (ARC)*, a term no longer used because the dis-tinction between AIDS and ARC is often arbitrary; further, the presence of ARC was not shown to be as predictive of eventual HIV clinical outcome as the $CD4^+$ T-lymphocyte counts.

The diagnosis of AIDS is made when a person who is HIV positive develops an opportunistic infection such as *Pneumocystis carinii*, *Toxoplasma gondii*, or Kaposi's sarcoma (see Table 21–1 for the case definition of AIDS). The case definition was recently expanded to include all HIV-infected persons with $CD4^+$ cell counts of less than 200 cells/mm^3 or a percentage of less than 14%. Pulmo-nary tuberculosis, recurrent pneumonia, and invasive cervical cancer were added to the list of clinical conditions contained in the 1987 definition. *Pneumocystis carinii* pneumonia is the most common initial opportunistic infection disease in

Table 21–1.   Case definition of acquired immunodeficiency syndrome (AIDS)

A case of AIDS is defined as an illness characterized by one or more of the following indicator diseases, depending on the status of laboratory evidence of human immunodeficiency virus (HIV) infection, as shown below.

1. Without laboratory evidence regarding HIV infection (i.e., HIV tests are inconclusive or were not performed) and the patient has no other underlying cause of immunodeficiency (e.g., long-term corticosteroid therapy, certain cancers, congenital immunodeficiency syndrome).
   - Kaposi's sarcoma in patients less than 60 years of age
   - Primary lymphoma of the CNS in patients less than 60 years of age
   - *Pneumocystis carinii* pneumonia
   - Unusually extensive mucocutaneous herpes simplex infection
   - *Cryptosporidium* enterocolitis with diarrhea persisting longer than 1 month
   - Extrapulmonary cryptococcosis
   - Candidiasis of the esophagus, trachea, bronchi, or lungs
   - Cytomegalovirus disease of an organ other than the liver, spleen, or lymph nodes in a patient more than 1 month of age
   - Progressive multifocal leukoencephalopathy
   - Toxoplasmosis of the brain affecting a patient more than 1 month of age
   - Lymphoid interstitial pneumonia and/or pulmonary lymphoid hyperplasia affecting a child younger than 13 years of age
   - *Mycobacterium avium* complex or *M. kansasii* disease, disseminated

2. With laboratory evidence of HIV infection, regardless of the presence of other causes of immunodeficiency, any disease listed above or below (2A or 2B) indicates a case of AIDS.
   A. Indicator disease is diagnosed definitively:
      - Bacterial infections, multiple or recurrent pneumonia, affecting a child younger than 13 years of age (e.g., septicemia, pneumonia, meningitis)
      - Coccidiomycosis, disseminated
      - HIV encephalopathy
      - Histoplasmosis, disseminated
      - Isosporiasis with diarrhea persisting longer than 1 month
      - Kaposi's sarcoma at any age
      - Primary lymphoma of the brain at any age
      - Other non-Hodgkin's lymphoma of B-cell or unknown immunological phenotype and involving certain histological types
      - Any mycobacterial disease, disseminated
      - Disease caused by *M. tuberculosis,* extrapulmonary
      - Salmonella septicemia, recurrent
      - HIV wasting syndrome (e.g., "slim disease")
   B. Indicator disease is diagnosed presumptively:
      - Candidiasis of the esophagus
      - Cytomegalovirus retinitis with loss of vision
      - Kaposi's sarcoma
      - Lymphoid interstitial pneumonia or pulmonary lymphoid hyperplasia affecting a child younger than 13 years of age
      - Mycobacterial disease
      - *Pneumocystis carinii* pneumonia
      - Toxoplasmosis of the brain affecting a patient more than 1 month of age

Table 21–1. Case definition of AIDS *(continued)*

3. With laboratory evidence against HIV infection.
   A. Other causes of immunodeficiency are excluded; and
   B. The patient has had either:
      - *Pneumocystis carinii* pneumonia diagnosed by a definitive method; or
      - Any of the other diseases indicative of AIDS listed in section 1 diagnosed by a definitive method; and a helper/inducer T-lymphocyte count of <400 mm^3.

Source. Centers for Disease Control. MMWR 36:45–65, 1987.

AIDS patients and typically occurs in about 60% of patients. Symptoms include the gradual onset of a nonproductive cough, low-grade fevers, and chest pain. Kaposi's sarcoma, also very common, is diagnosed in up to 30% of AIDS patients and is particularly virulent, leading to rapid spread and death, usually within 2 years.

The Centers for Disease Control has established stages for HIV-related illness. The importance of the CD4$^+$ T-lymphocyte count was recognized in the 1993 revision of these stages, as shown in Table 21–2. Long-term studies, which are now becoming available, suggest that almost all persons who become infected will eventually deteriorate to clinical category C, which indicates a diagnosis of AIDS. Thus, the natural history of HIV disease is a reflection of the ability of HIV to damage the immune system, especially the CD4$^+$ T lymphocyte, which plays a key role in directing the immune system response to foreign invaders, such as viruses, fungi, and protozoa. Although the period between infection and the development of AIDS ranges from about 2 to 15 years or longer, the estimated mean is 9 years.

There are no effective treatments for the underlying immune disturbance of AIDS. Treatment of AIDS patients generally consists of efforts to treat opportunistic infections. Three drugs are currently approved in the United States for use in HIV disease, including azidothymidine (AZT), dideoxyinosine (ddI), and dideoxycytidine (DDC). Each has the ability to inhibit reverse transcriptase, which inhibits HIV replication, diminishing the total viral load. Antiretroviral therapy is routinely used to treat persons with moderate to advanced disease, for example, those with CD4$^+$ cell counts of less than 500 cells/mm^3. AZT was approved based on research that showed its ability to improve longevity and quality of life. However, the duration of the benefit of AZT might be limited, as a clinical study showed no difference in survival at 3 years between patients receiving AZT and patients receiving placebo. AZT has also been shown to ameliorate cognitive impairment in some individuals. ddI and DDC are used in patients unable to tolerate AZT or in whom AZT has failed. Clinical trials with

Table 21–2.   Centers for Disease Control classification of HIV infection

CD4+ T-lymphocyte cell category	Clinical category		
	A[a] (asymptomatic, acute HIV infection or persistent generalized lymphadenopathy)	B[b] (symptomatic, but not with category A or C conditions)	C[c] (AIDS indicator conditions)
≥ 500/mm^3	A1	B1	C1
200–499/mm^3	A2	B2	C2
< 200/mm^3	A3	B3	C3

[a]**Category A.** Category A consists of one or more of the conditions listed below in an adolescent or adult (≥ 13 years) with documented HIV infection. Conditions listed in categories B and C must not have occurred.
• Asymptomatic HIV infection
• Persistent general lymphadenopathy
• Acute (primary) HIV infection with accompanying illness or history of acute HIV infection

[b]**Category B.** Category B consists of symptomatic conditions in an HIV-infected adolescent or adult that are not included among conditions listed in clinical category C and that meet at least one of the following criteria: 1) the conditions are attributed to HIV infection or are indicative of a defect in cell-mediated immunity; or 2) the conditions are considered by physicians to have a clinical course or to require management that is complicated by HIV infection. Examples of conditions in clinical category B include, but are not limited to:
• Bacillary angiomatosis
• Candidiasis, oropharyngeal (thrush)
• Candidiasis, vulvovaginal; persistent, frequent, or poorly responsive to therapy
• Cervical dysplasia (moderate or severe)/cervical carcinoma in situ
• Constitutional symptoms, such as fever (38.5°C) or diarrhea lasting more than 1 month
• Hairy leukoplakia, oral
• Herpes zoster (shingles) involving at least two distinct episodes or more than one dermatome
• Idiopathic thrombocytopenic purpura
• Listeriosis
• Pelvic inflammatory disease, particularly if complicated by tuboovarian abscess
• Peripheral neuropathy
• For classification purposes, category B conditions take precedence over those in category A. For example, someone previously treated for oral or persistent vaginal candidiasis (who has not developed a category C disease) but who is not asymptomatic should be classified in category B.

[c]**Category C.** Category C includes the clinical conditions listed in the AIDS surveillance case definitions. For classification purposes, once a category C condition has developed, the persons will remain in category C.

Source.   Adapted from Centers for Disease Control: 1993 revised classification system for HIV infection and expanded surveillance case definition for AIDS among adolescents and adults. MMWR 41(RR-17):1–19, 1992.

these agents, as well as combination therapy and trials of new agents, continue. Despite these advances, clinical therapy remains mostly palliative.

Neuropsychiatric Manifestations of HIV Disease

Early explanations of psychiatric morbidity among HIV-seropositive and AIDS patients emphasized the emotional repercussions of developing AIDS, but the focus soon turned to the destructive effects of HIV itself, because it became clear that the CNS is a prime target of HIV, particularly areas below and connected to the cerebral cortex. Thus, persons infected with HIV are susceptible to the direct effects of the virus, as well as the effects of opportunistic infections on the CNS.

Postmortem findings seen in HIV-infected patients are variable, reflecting the markedly different clinical presentations from one patient to another. First, there is a relative sparing of the cortex; instead, the most prominent changes are seen in subcortical areas, including the central white matter and the deep gray structures, such as the basal ganglia, thalamus, and brain stem (hence the term *subcortical dementia*). White matter pallor may be accompanied by marked atrophy and an astrocytic reaction. Loss of oligodendrocytes and neurons is not characteristic. The spinal cord may also be involved, showing vacuolation caused by swelling within the layers of the myelin sheath. In about one-third of patients, the presence of HIV is demonstrable in CNS tissue.

Initial symptoms of HIV infection may be subtle; for instance, during the latent phase, before there is any clinical evidence of AIDS, HIV-infected adults may develop a sense of mental slowing or forgetfulness, without significant intellectual decline. In one study, 44% of otherwise asymptomatic persons had some evidence of neuropsychological impairment compared to 87% of persons with full-blown AIDS. Further, HIV-infected children manifest a delay in reaching motor or intellectual milestones, also suggesting the direct effects of HIV on the CNS.

Many persons infected with HIV develop significant CNS involvement, which has been called the *AIDS dementia complex*. Because no single pathological process underlies the dementia and because symptoms may occur before AIDS has developed, it is probably more appropriate to call it *HIV-related brain disease*. The dementia may also result from the sequelae of delirium, as well as from primary infection with HIV, the effects of secondary infections such as cryptococcus, or the effects of treatment.

The early diagnosis of dementia may be difficult, particularly because the symptoms are relatively vague and because the boundary between dementia and neuropsychological impairment is relatively difficult to draw. As the dementia advances, symptoms became more obvious; patients may become aware of their diminishing mental functioning and admit that they are forgetful. They may have trouble concentrating, feel overwhelmed by organizational tasks, and lose their train of thought. A patient may become angry about his or her inability to deal with simple matters, such as balancing a checkbook. Motoric aspects (i.e., the "complex" part of the dementia) include ataxia, leg weakness, tremors, and impaired eye movements. As the dementia progresses, intellectual impairment becomes more severe, affecting nearly all spheres of cognitive functioning, such as further slowing of verbal and motor performance. Late in the illness, patients develop other symptoms of dementia, including muteness, incontinence, incoordination, parkinsonian symptoms, seizures, and coma leading eventually to death. In DSM-IV, HIV dementia is diagnosed on Axis I as *dementia due to HIV disease;* HIV disease should also be coded on Axis III. The variety of clinical manifestations of HIV-related dementia is shown in Table 21–3.

Patients infected with HIV occasionally develop new-onset psychotic symp-

Table 21–3. Clinical manifestations of HIV-related dementia

Cognitive impairments	**Generalized systemic symptoms**
Short-term memory deficit; forgetfulness rather than amnesia	Fatigue, sleep changes (hypersomnia)
Decreased concentration and attention	Anorexia, weight loss
Confusion and disorientation	Enuresis
Overall intellectual ability generally well preserved until late	Hypersensitivity to medications and alcohol
Visuospatial perception deficits	**Cognitive symptoms associated with advanced dementia**
Changes in personality or behavior	Global cognitive impairment
Apathy, decreased interest	Rudimentary social functioning
Impaired judgment, erratic behavior	Disorientation
Social withdrawal	Psychomotor retardation, decreased spontaneity
Rigidity of thought	Agitation, sundowning (e.g., nighttime delusions)
Speech impairment; slowing, dysarthria, hypophonia; difficulty in following other speakers	Mutism, vacant stare
Psychotic symptoms	Coma
Hallucinations	**Motor symptoms associated with advanced dementia**
Suspiciousness and delusions	Ataxia
Agitation and inappropriate behavior	Spastic weakness
Motor symptoms	Paraplegia, quadriparesis
Ataxia, loss of coordination	Hyperreflexia, myoclonus, seizures
Tremors	Bladder and bowel incontinence

toms, such as vivid hallucinations, bizarre delusions, and disorganized speech and behavior. The prevalence of new-onset psychosis in patients with HIV disease may be as high as 15%. In one study, patients had been psychotic from several days to several months before presentation, and the most common symptom was a persecutory, grandiose, or somatic delusion. Auditory hallucinations were also common, as were anxiety, agitation, formal thought disorder, mood disturbance, bizarre behavior, and cognitive impairment. In fact, most patients with new-onset psychosis have substantial mood symptoms, including euphoria, depression, or a mixture of the two. Therefore, patients with new-onset mental status changes who have one or more risk factors for AIDS need to have HIV ruled out as a cause of their illness.

On initial neurological examination, nearly half of HIV-seropositive patients display minor motor disturbances, such as hyperreflexia, increased tone, tremor, and mild ataxia. Cerebrospinal fluid examination tends to be normal unless mental changes are due to treatable CNS tumors or infections (e.g., increased number of cells, positive India ink test for cryptococcus). Brain imaging is normal in most patients at the time of initial evaluation; the remainder have evidence of cortical atrophy or ventricular enlargement on computed tomography or small focal signal hyperintensities or unidentified bright objects on magnetic resonance imaging. An abnormal electroencephalogram consisting of predominantly diffuse cortical slowing may be found, even in patients without clinical evidence of mental changes or neurological impairment. Patients with evidence of CNS involvement follow a more rapidly progressive downhill course.

Psychological Aspects of HIV Disease

Psychological aspects of HIV disease extend to homosexual and bisexual men and persons in other risk groups who have not had symptoms of AIDS but who are at risk for the disease. Many of the worried well develop significant psychological distress, including anxiety, depression, and interpersonal problems. Because of their risk for illness, some persons become preoccupied with their physical condition. Like hypochondriacal persons, these patients tend to misinterpret normal or new bodily sensations. They may demand tests, but the results produce little relief from their anxiety. At this stage, the physician can help most by providing regular contact with patients to examine them for new signs of illness, to explain symptoms, and to offer reassurance. Gay couples may need counseling, and safe sex practices should be discussed at every opportunity, as well as the importance of the proper use of condoms. This is an ideal setting to correct misinformation about AIDS; the appropriateness of HIV testing can be discussed, as can transmission of HIV, including the relative degree of HIV susceptibility associated with various sexual practices (see Table 21–4).

Others at little risk for HIV disease may become unnecessarily fearful or phobic about HIV; these irrational concerns may lead to discrimination against persons with HIV disease or against those in high-risk categories (e.g., homosexual men, drug-addicted persons). The appearance of HIV disease in the early 1980s seems to have led to a backsliding of public opinion about the growing gay-rights movement; many have explained the epidemic as God's retribution for immoral behavior (despite the irony that lesbians are at very low risk for contracting HIV). One recent survey showed, for instance, that 27% of respondents disagreed with the statement that persons with AIDS should be treated with compassion. In another survey, only 19% responded that a group home for AIDS patients would be welcome in their neighborhood; only factories, garbage landfills, and prisons ranked lower in desirability.

The impact of HIV testing can itself be traumatic, because the implications of a positive result are so devastating. In many states, patients must give informed consent before testing and undergo both pre- and posttest counseling. Pretest counseling involves discussion about the different tests, their limitations, and their implications. It also gives the clinician an opportunity to assess the patient's motives for having the test and how he or she might respond to the test results. Posttest counseling is necessary to reinforce the lessons about HIV, the testing procedures, and the implications of positive results, as well as to explain ways to prevent transmission.

Patients who receive negative results will generally express relief; those who learn they are seropositive may experience a variety of emotions; withdrawal, anger, aggression, hysteria, or increased use of drugs or alcohol may result. Some persons will feel guilt about their sexual orientation, drug addiction, or having infected others; others will face the real or perceived loss of support by family, friends, employers, and others. Some persons—particularly those with a preex-

Table 21–4. Relative degree of AIDS susceptibility associated with various sexual practices

Probably safe	Possibly safe	Unsafe
Mutual masturbation	Anal or vaginal intercourse with a condom	Anal or vaginal intercourse without a condom
Social kissing	Fellatio interruptus	Fellatio to orgasm
Body massage, hugging	Mouth-to-mouth kissing	Activities that involve bruising or bleeding
Body-to-body rubbing	Oral-vaginal contact	
Use of own sex toys		

isting personality disorder—may cope with the news with denial and may even increase their self-destructive behavior through unsafe sex practices or intravenous drug use. Most patients eventually adjust, although apathy and denial can persist for many. The risk of depressive episodes and suicidal behavior typically increases after patients adjust to the initial shock of learning that they are HIV positive.

Depression is relatively common in people with HIV disease and serves to worsen the patient's functional capabilities, independent of the underlying medical condition. The degree to which functional impairment is due to depression may be difficult to determine, because many symptoms of major depression are also characteristic of early cognitive defects caused by HIV-related dementia. Depression can interfere with the patient's ability to cope intellectually and emotionally with the complicated information and medical procedures often required to manage the illness. A frequent symptom of depression in patients with HIV disease is social withdrawal, which may result from rejection by others, the patient's growing sense of helplessness, and his or her fear of a rapid and disfiguring death. Regardless of the cause of the patient's depression, treatment should not be delayed. The patient should be counseled to accept the reality of the illness and to work on the issues of social rejection and loss, disfigurement, the specter of declining health, and impending death. Antidepressant medication is helpful for many patients, but careful dosing and close monitoring for adverse effects are imperative.

Although a degree of anxiety is common in persons with HIV disease, the full spectrum of signs and symptoms may occur, including phobias, panic attacks, and generalized anxiety. The most frequent anxiety disorder results from the acute reaction to learning of the diagnosis, which in DSM-IV is termed *adjustment disorder with anxiety*. Depending on the amount of anxiety, the patient may develop a variety of autonomic symptoms (e.g., diarrhea, nausea, vomiting), which could easily be mistaken for evidence of an opportunistic infection or neurological involvement. Proper management of anxiety may include supportive psychotherapy, the use of relaxation training or biofeedback, restricting the intake of caffeine, and the judicious use of benzodiazepines.

Patients with HIV disease are understandably concerned about their physical well-being. This concern may escalate into an unhealthy preoccupation, leading to frequent checking of the body for signs of illness, frequent requests for laboratory tests, obsessive concern about appearance, and other hypochondriacal concerns. Patients need to be reassured that their concerns are being taken seriously and that their symptoms are being carefully monitored. It is helpful for the patient to have a single physician, to avoid the inevitable iatrogenic complications associated with doctor-shopping and unnecessary tests and procedures.

Other disorders in persons with HIV are less common and perhaps no more frequent than in the general population, for example, schizophrenia, bipolar disorder, and antisocial personality disorder. A bizarre aspect of the AIDS epidemic has been reported cases of factitious AIDS, in which persons deliberately fabricate the diagnosis and seek medical attention. (See Chapter 12 on factitious disorders and malingering.) When confronted, patients typically respond angrily and may flee to another hospital or clinic.

The following case example illustrates some of the problems seen in an HIV-seropositive patient treated in our hospital.

Lynn, a 23-year-old man, was admitted after a diazepam overdose. Lynn lived with his parents and after taking the pills told his mother, who brought him to the hospital. At the emergency room, he was alert but lethargic. His stomach was lavaged, and he was admitted to the psychiatric service.

Lynn had grown up in a small midwestern farming community. He had been somewhat effeminate as a boy and was picked on by his peers, but he otherwise developed normally, had friends, and behaved himself in school. Although he had always been attracted to the other boys and had always felt that he was a homosexual, Lynn had come out of the closet only recently. In the past, Lynn had hidden his sexual orientation from his friends and family members and had even dated girls. After his coming out, he tried to fit in with what he thought was a gay lifestyle by dressing colorfully, wearing an earring, and frequenting gay bars in nearby communities. He had had a series of one-night stands and short-lived affairs and an assortment of sexual experiences with dozens of young men.

A year before his hospitalization, Lynn sought HIV testing and was found to be seropositive. He was devastated by this knowledge, became acutely depressed, and felt hopeless about his future. Lynn had sought out individual counseling and saw a therapist on a regular basis. He also joined a local support group for persons with AIDS or AIDS-related illnesses. These measures seemed to help, but he was constantly reminded of what his future held as members of the support group would stop coming, and he and the others would later learn that they had died. He also read widely about AIDS and had learned of its devastating effects on the mind and body. An attractive young man, Lynn had always worked out and felt physically fit. He did not want to think of himself as deformed or debilitated.

On the night before admission, Lynn had been feeling particularly sorry for himself and had been out partying with several of his friends. After returning home, he had started to ruminate about his HIV seropositivity, how alone and isolated he felt, and the devastating complications that he faced in the future. He knew that his mother had been treated for nervous problems in the past, and he located a bottle containing diazepam that had been prescribed for her. Not knowing its effect, but knowing that it was a tranquilizer, he swallowed the contents of the bottle, thinking that it would kill him. Within a few minutes, however, he had a change of mind, informed his parents of what he had done, and he was brought to the hospital.

At the hospital, Lynn admitted that he had adjusted poorly to his HIV seropositivity and that he had initially denied the test result. In fact, to prove that he was healthy, he had engaged in several sexual escapades, which he now regretted, knowing that he had placed these persons at risk for AIDS. He admitted that he had become overly concerned about somatic symptoms and had constantly sought reassurance from his doctors. He also became dysphoric and had spontaneous crying spells. Despite these psychological symptoms, he had not developed vegetative symptoms of depression, such as weight loss, anorexia, or fatigue. At the hospital, Lynn was diagnosed as having an adjustment disorder with depressed mood. He received brief supportive counseling and within days had returned to his usual level of functioning.

The potential therapeutic interventions for psychiatric sequelae of HIV infection are summarized in Table 21–5.

Clinical Management

Monitoring of mental status and evaluating cognitive impairment are important parts of the overall management of HIV-infected patients, in view of the common psychiatric and CNS sequelae. When HIV-related dementia is suspected, neuropsychological testing should be done. The results may show more or less impairment than was subjectively appreciated and will be helpful in treatment planning. Neuropsychological testing can also help to distinguish dementia from depression or anxiety. Depressive symptoms and suicide risk need to be assessed at each visit, especially because the rate of suicide in persons with AIDS is more than seven times higher than that in the general population; earlier studies had indicated even higher rates. Many patients benefit from supportive psychotherapy, where issues such as guilt associated with previous sexual practices or drug abuse, social isolation, and acknowledgment of the illness (along with the associated fear or anger) can be addressed. Stress management, such as relaxation training, and problem-solving techniques, may also benefit these patients. Cognitive techniques may help to correct the distorted thinking that patients with HIV disease often develop (e.g., "No one likes me because I am HIV positive").

Patients who develop psychiatric syndromes can benefit from medication. Benzodiazepines may be helpful to patients with generalized anxiety disorder or an adjustment disorder, and antidepressants—particularly those without anticholinergic effects (e.g., fluoxetine)—may be useful for patients with a major depression or panic disorder. Some investigators have used low-dose psychostimulants as a treatment for depression in AIDS patients (e.g., methylphenidate 10–40 mg daily in divided doses). Antipsychotics are helpful in treating the patient who develops hallucinations or delusions. Electroconvulsive therapy may be useful in depressed or manic AIDS patients who are unresponsive to medication.

Patient management should also include providing education about AIDS, information about etiology and modes of transmission, and practical precautions regarding safe sex and safe needle use by drug abusers. Support groups organized by local AIDS outreach organizations (e.g., Shanti) can be helpful in buttressing social support. Physicians need to work with public health agencies to help patients obtain financial and physical assistance.

Table 21–5. Therapeutic interventions for psychiatric sequelae of HIV infection

Problem	Potential intervention
Worried well	Assessment of HIV risk and infection status Diagnosis and treatment of possible underlying psychiatric disorder Reassurance and counseling
Acute adjustment reaction to positive test results (or diagnosis)	Assessment and intervention for possible shock and/or suicide potential Provision of accurate medical and prognostic information Coordination of psychosocial care and treatment or referral for depression and anxiety Introduction to community support organizations Early diagnosis and treatment of any CNS disease
Anxiety	Assessment for use of caffeine, alcohol, and prescribed or illicit drugs Counseling of patient and patient's family or friends Introduction to community support organizations Pharmacological treatment for generalized anxiety disorder or adjustment disorder with anxiety
Depression	Workup to rule out secondary depression and CNS involvement, appropriate treatment if indicated Supportive or cognitive psychotherapy Pharmacological treatment for moderate to severe depression with low dosage of antidepressant
Hypochondriasis	Evaluation and treatment for underlying depressive, anxiety, or somatoform disorder Provision of reassurance and accurate medical information Behavioral therapy including relaxation training, desensitization, and avoidance conditioning
Psychosis	Evaluation and treatment for potential drug-induced or HIV-related organic brain disorder Evaluation and treatment for potential bipolar illness Low-dosage neuroleptic treatment for psychotic state Behavioral management to reduce stimulation and to minimize agitation Support and counseling for patient's family or lover, or both

Source. Adapted from Miller D: Diagnosis and treatment of acute psychological problems related to AIDS, in Behavioral Aspects of AIDS. Edited by Ostrow DJ. New York, Plenum, 1990, pp. 187–206.

Caring for the AIDS Patient

The problems of caring for the AIDS patient extend beyond the medical and psychiatric complications of the disease. Caring for patients with HIV disease is medically complex, time consuming, and physically demanding; caring for young patients with terminal illnesses is emotionally demanding. These aspects, combined with the ambivalence that caregivers may feel about the lifestyle of the patient, may lead some caregivers to burnout; some experts have compared this burnout with posttraumatic stress disorder. Group discussions among caregivers to ventilate their feelings and frustrations may be valuable. Health care workers may need to confront their own prejudices toward high-risk groups; prejudice can negatively affect the ability of care providers to offer their highest standard of care. Many doctors still believe that AIDS patients deserve their illness and that they are less deserving of sympathy than, for example, cancer patients. These views should not be tolerated.

Recommendations for treatment of the AIDS patient

1. Acceptance and a nonjudgmental attitude are essential in the care of patients infected with HIV.
   - There is no excuse for blaming or belittling patients for their predicament.
   - Caregivers need to separate their personal negative beliefs about the patient's lifestyle (e.g., homosexuality, drug abuse) from their care of the patient.
2. Be alert to neuropsychiatric symptoms that can signal involvement of the CNS, including neurological signs (e.g., tingling, numbness, weakness) and psychiatric symptoms (e.g., depression, mania, confusion).
3. AIDS patients need much emotional support, especially because many will have lost their traditional supports after having revealed simultaneously their homosexuality (or drug addiction) and their development of a fatal and communicable illness.
   - Many patients need practical assistance in solving everyday problems. Many will need to be referred to social service agencies.
   - The therapist must help the patient deal with issues of death and dying in a realistic and humane way.
   - Support groups are available in most communities for HIV-positive patients and the worried well.
4. Many patients will benefit from specific treatment for depression, anxiety, or psychosis (e.g., antidepressants, anxiolytics, antipsychotics).
5. Educate yourself, other staff members, and the patient about AIDS and its transmission.
   - Despite great publicity and public educational efforts, some persons (including medical personnel) stubbornly cling to inaccurate beliefs (e.g., AIDS can be transmitted by casual contact).

Bibliography

Atkinson JH, Grant I, Kennedy CJ, et al: Prevalence of psychiatric disorders among men infected with human immunodeficiency virus. Arch Gen Psychiatry 45:859–864, 1988

Blendon RJ, Donelan K, Knox RA: Public opinion and AIDS—lessons for the second decade. JAMA 267:981–986, 1992

Burack JH, Barrett DC, Stall RD, et al: Depressive symptoms and CD4$^+$ lymphocyte decline among HIV-infected men. JAMA 270:2568–2573, 1993

Centers for Disease Control: 1993 revised classification system for HIV infection and expanded surveillance case definition for AIDS among adolescents and adults. MMWR CDC Surveill Summ 41(RR-17):1–19, 1992

Coté TR, Biggar RJ, Dannenberg AL: Risk of suicide among persons with AIDS: a national assessment. JAMA 268:2066–2068, 1992

Dilley JW, Ochitill HN, Pearl M, et al: Findings in psychiatric consultations with patients with acquired immune deficiency syndrome. Am J Psychiatry 142:82–86, 1985

Faulstich ME: Psychiatric aspects of AIDS. Am J Psychiatry 144:551–556, 1987

Geleziunas R, Schipper HM, Wainberg MA: Pathogenesis and therapy of HIV-1 infection of the central nervous system. AIDS 6:1411–1426, 1992

Heaton RK, Velin RA, McCutchan JA, et al: Neuropsychological impairment in human immunodeficiency virus-infection—implications for employment. Psychosom Med 56:8–17, 1994

Johnston MI, Hoth DF: Present status and future prospects for HIV therapies. Science 260:1286–1293, 1993

Levy JA: Human immunodeficiency virus and the pathogenesis of AIDS. JAMA 161:2997–3006, 1989

Lyketsos CG, Hoover DR, Guccione M, et al: Depressive symptoms as "predictors of medical outcomes in HIV infection." JAMA 270:2563–2567, 1993

Miller D: Diagnosis and treatment of acute psychological problems related to AIDS, in Behavioral Aspects of AIDS. Edited by Ostrow DJ. New York, Plenum, 1990, pp 187–206

Navia BA, Choo ES, Petito CK: The AIDS dementia complex, II: neuropathology. Ann Neurol 19:525–535, 1986

Navia BA, Jordan BD, Price RW: The AIDS dementia complex, I: clinical features. Ann Neurol 19:517–524, 1986

Ostrow DJ: Psychiatric consequences of AIDS: an overview. Int J Neurosci 32:669–676, 1987

Perry SW: Organic mental disorders caused by HIV: update on early diagnosis and treatment. Am J Psychiatry 147:696–710, 1990

Perry SW, Markowitz JC: Counseling for HIV testing. Hosp Community Psychiatry 39:731–739, 1988

Sande MA, Carpenter CCJ, Cobbs CG, et al: Antiretroviral therapy for adult HIV-infected patients. JAMA 270:2583–2589, 1993

Schmitt FA, Bigley JW, McKinnis R, et al: Neuropsychological outcome of zidovudine (AZT) treatment of patients with AIDS and AIDS-related complex. N Engl J Med 319:1573–1578, 1988

Sewell DD, Jeste DV, Atkinson JH, et al: HIV associated psychosis: a study of 20 cases. Am J Psychiatry 151:237–242, 1994

Silverman DC: Psychosocial impact of HIV-related caregiving on health providers—a review and recommendations for the role of psychiatry. Am J Psychiatry 150:705–712, 1993

Self-Assessment Questions

1. What is HIV? How is HIV transmitted?
2. What are the major risk groups for HIV, and how have they changed over the years?
3. What are the diagnostic criteria for AIDS? How is HIV disease staged?
4. What are the testing procedures for HIV?
5. What neuropsychiatric symptoms have been reported in cases of AIDS?
6. What symptoms affect the worried well?
7. What are the common psychiatric disorders that affect persons with HIV?
8. How does prejudice affect the caregiver?

Chapter 22

Disorders of Childhood and Adolescence

Children sweeten labors, but they make misfortunes more bitter. They increase the cares of life, but they mitigate the remembrance of death.

Francis Bacon

As any 17-year-old will testify, the distinction between childhood and adulthood is arbitrary, often ludicrous, and frequently fluctuating in response to the needs of the person invoking the distinction. Psychiatric nosology and classification are no exception to this rule. Many of the disorders described in other chapters (not classified among childhood disorders in the DSM-IV) occur rather frequently in children. Mood disorders and anxiety disorders are especially common. Schizophrenia often arises during adolescence and occasionally during childhood. In inner cities, crack cocaine is traded on the grade school playground. Children and adolescents display signs and symptoms of personality disorder. Indeed, there is probably no adult disorder from which children are exempt.

Nevertheless, the DSM-IV nosology does set aside a group of disorders that are considered to be relatively specific to children and adolescents, in that they typically *arise* during that period of life, rather than simply *occur* during childhood and adolescence. The overall summary of this group of disorders appears in Table 22–1, and a more detailed overview has already been provided in Chapter 2. These disorders are both diverse and numerous. Some are not very common

Table 22–1.   Disorders usually first diagnosed in infancy, childhood, or adolescence

Mental retardation	**Attention-deficit and disruptive behavior disorders**
Mild	
Moderate	Attention-deficit/hyperactivity disorder
Severe	Conduct disorder
Profound	Oppositional defiant disorder
Learning disorders	**Feeding and eating disorders of infancy and early childhood**
Reading	
Mathematics	**Tic disorders**
Written expression	Tourette's disorder
Motor skills	**Elimination disorders**
Communication disorders	**Other disorders**
Pervasive developmental disorders	Separation anxiety disorder

(e.g., communication disorders such as selective mutism), and some are seen more frequently in pediatrics clinics than in child psychiatry clinics (e.g., elimination disorders such as encopresis and enuresis). To permit more complete coverage of the most important disorders, we selectively review only some of them in this chapter, focusing on those that are most frequently seen in child psychiatry clinics or in a family practice setting. These include mental retardation, learning disorder, autistic disorder, attention-deficit/hyperactivity disorder (ADHD), conduct disorder, oppositional defiant disorder, Tourette's disorder, and separation anxiety disorder. In addition, a brief overview is provided of those adult disorders that are commonly seen in children (e.g., mood disorders, schizophrenia) and of physical, emotional, and sexual abuse.

Child psychiatry is one of the most challenging and interesting areas of specialization within psychiatry. Because it requires working with multiple individuals and groups (e.g., the child, the parents, the school system), it is in many respects a primary care specialty. Because the child psychiatrist must know a great deal about other childhood illnesses, maturational processes, and developmental disorders, it is also closely allied with pediatrics and requires a good knowledge of general medicine. Because cognitive development is an important aspect of child psychiatry as well, child psychiatry is tied to cognitive psychology. Further, the clinician working in child psychiatry has an opportunity to catch disorders at their earliest; because children are adaptable, fresh in outlook, and pleasantly unpredictable, working with them and helping them overcome their problems can be particularly rewarding. Finally, the childhood mental illnesses are quite common. Estimates of prevalence vary depending on breadth or narrowness of definition, but it is probably a reasonable estimate that between 5% and 15% of children will experience an illness that is sufficiently severe to require treatment or to impair their functioning during the course of a year.

Special Aspects of the Assessment of Children

Although there are many continuities between adult and child psychiatry, there are also important differences in emphasis and approach. These include techniques of assessment, the importance of flexible norms or criteria, involvement of family or significant others, an increased role of nonphysicians in the health care team, and the frequent occurrence of comorbidity. These aspects of assessment must be kept in mind as the clinician attempts to evaluate the presence or absence of the various disorders listed in Table 22–1.

Trajectories of Development

Although the lives of adults change with time and are affected by surrounding life situations, the pace of change and the impact of life events are much greater in children. Consequently, in working with children, it is important to emphasize a longitudinal and developmental approach, rather than the cross-sectional approaches that are typically used in assessing adults. This developmental approach must take into account the growth and maturational processes that all children undergo, assessing them in the light of each particular child's life situation and strengths and weaknesses. Any mental illness that arises in children must be treated within this context. Each child has a natural trajectory of development that will be completed through the process of passing from infancy to adulthood. The development of mental illness and the experience of environmental stressors will have very different effects depending on the place where a given child is in that trajectory of development. As each child is evaluated, the clinician must ask these questions:

- What level of emotional and intellectual maturity does this child have?
- What are his or her particular strengths?
- How do they provide a protective and healing element?
- What particular weaknesses are present?
- What stresses are impacting on the child?
- How do those stresses impact on him or her at this particular stage of life?
- How do gender-specific challenges affect the expression of illness and its treatment?

For example, parental divorce or even abandonment has become an all-too-common experience for children, at least in the United States. What difference does it make if the father walks out or the mother walks out? If the parent walks out or dies? What is the difference in impact if the child is a boy or a girl? What difference does it make if the child is 2, 10, or 16 years old? What difference does it make if the remaining parent is strong and capable versus weak and immature? What impact does the child's place in a sibship have on him or her? How much success and self-esteem has the child achieved up to this time?

Obviously, maternal death would have a very different impact on each child in a family of five children, the oldest of whom is a 16-year-old-girl (who is likely to assume the maternal role) and the youngest of whom is 2 years old. The impact would be different for the children whose surviving father is unemployed and alcoholic than it would be for the children whose surviving father is a high-functioning blue- or white-collar worker. The impact would also be different depending on whether the eldest child is herself highly functional or has some mental illness, such as autism or conduct disorder. The impact on each child would vary depending on the availability of other social supports, such as an extended family with grandparents, a good versus a weak school system, and a safe environment versus one characterized by crime, violence, and drug use. All things being constant, a 2-year-old has a very different understanding of parental loss or abandonment than does an older child, because the younger child has had little time to build either a self-image incorporating that parent or a conceptual structure that can be used to comprehend parental loss.

Who Is the Patient?

Children rarely pick up the phone and make an appointment to see a child psychiatrist. Usually they are brought in at someone else's request. Invariably, someone else is paying the bill. All these things make child psychiatry a different ball game than adult psychiatry. The child may be unwilling, uncompliant, distrusting, or resentful. In this instance, the assessment is likely to be particularly challenging, because the clinician must win the child's trust. Even if the child is the identified patient, the parents are usually interviewed and evaluated as well. Sometimes it becomes clear that the parents themselves have serious problems, which they have ignored or projected onto the child. In this instance, it may be necessary to reassess and to suggest treatment of the parents in addition to (or even instead of) the child. Further, in child psychiatry, as in few other medical specialties, the clinician is likely to feel ambivalent and confused from time to time about the appropriate role to play. Extraordinary maturity is required on the part of a good child psychiatrist, who typically has chosen this specialty because of a liking for children and who will feel frustrated at the lack of astuteness toward the patient shown by parents, teachers, or others. The child will usually be the identified patient, even though others may be in greater need of intervention and yet do not seek or accept it.

The Assessment of Children

Childhood disorders can be diagnosed in individuals ranging from infants through people in their late teens or early 20s. Obviously, standard approaches to interviewing and assessment, described in Chapter 3, do not apply well to infants, children, and young teenagers. Standard techniques for the psychiatric assessment of adults, which may be applicable to the patients in their late teens and are applicable to patients in their early 20s, emphasize the use of questioning, self-report, and introspection. These approaches require verbal skills not yet achieved in the maturational process of children, the capacity to separate and step back from oneself to describe feelings and behavior, and the ability to form abstractions about cognition, behavior, or emotions. For example, young children may not be able to respond to questions about concepts such as depression, loneliness, or anger. The interviewer often needs to talk to children at a much more concrete level. Questions of the following type are helpful in interviewing children:

- Do you feel like crying?
- What kinds of things make you feel like crying?
- Do you ever want to hit people?
- Who do you feel like hitting?
- Who are your best friends?
- How often do you see them?
- What kinds of things do you do together?
- Do they like you?

In addition to interviewing, playing games with the child often gives the clinician some insight into the child's ability to function interpersonally, to tolerate frustration, and to focus his or her attention. Imaginative play, using dolls that can represent important figures in the child's life, may also give some sense as to his or her feelings toward and relationships with others. Taking turns in telling stories may also elicit interesting information. For example, if the clinician suspects that the child may be feeling anxious about something, he or she may tell a story about "how Jimmy is afraid of going to school because the other children make fun of him." When the child then tells his or her own story, he or she may be able to describe his or her own fears in this indirect manner. Direct observation of activity level, motor skills, verbal expression, and vocabulary are also fundamental components of assessment.

Application of Norms and Criteria

In assessing children, the clinician must have a good sense of what is normal for a given child at a given age, as well as an awareness that norms may vary widely. Younger clinicians who are completing medical school or a residency usually have not had the experience of rearing their own children or of watching a large number of younger siblings develop. Thus, they must get their sense of norms from textbooks, from observing large numbers of children, and from recalling their own experiences in the process of growing up. The latter approach may be particularly helpful in the assessment of teenagers, although the average medical student or physician must recognize that he or she is likely to be much more uptight, obsessional, and compliant with authority than the average child. Nevertheless, remembering one's own growing pains often helps to increase empathy with the frustrations and struggles that many adolescents experience and seek help for.

Having a sense of what is normal and abnormal for a given child, in a given family, and in a given social and intellectual environment can be extremely difficult. For example, a typical normal 10-year-old has an IQ of 100, is able to read at a fourth-grade level, is able to perform addition and subtraction and some multiplication, and is able to throw, catch, and kick a ball with at least some accuracy. Some normal children have an IQ of only 85, however, whereas some have an IQ of 160. These children clearly differ from one another a great deal in their school performance. Boys and girls have quite different levels of maturation, both physically and mentally, and these differences are especially pronounced in younger children. Boys and girls have different maturational tasks as they go through puberty and enter adolescence, and consequently, they experience different stresses. Success and failure also mean different things to an inner-city child and a child from an affluent background.

Particularly in the area of child psychiatry, clinicians are likely to be asked over and over, "is this child normal?" or "is this behavior normal?" The clinician who experiences some doubt, ambiguity, and difficulty in answering those questions easily is definitely normal. Coming up with facile judgments about normality is probably an indication that the clinician has not been thinking hard enough or has too simple and authoritarian a notion of what constitutes normality. Extreme cases are simple, of course, but most are likely to be in the murky middle.

Involvement of Family and Significant Others

Clinicians who work with children usually need to work with their families and significant others as well. The degree of family involvement varies, of course, depending on the age of the child. In the case of very young children, the parents are likely to be the primary informants and probably will be important recipients of treatment as well, because they are likely to need both psychological support and assistance in learning behavioral techniques to manage their child's behavior. For grade school children, involvement of family members remains essential, but the child becomes an increasingly important protagonist in both assessment and treatment. Teenagers, who are going through important maturational changes as they move into adulthood, are usually brought to the forefront of the assessment and treatment process, although the family will also provide resources much of the time.

Deciding whether to maintain complete confidentiality or to share information becomes a crucial issue in the assessment of teenagers. In general, teenagers should be assured that the things they tell the clinician will end there, unless the teenager gives permission to share the information or can be encouraged to bring it out in a family or group setting. The assurance of confidentiality is important in establishing a bond of trust between teenager and clinician, because the patient otherwise is likely to see the therapist as a potentially antagonistic authority figure. Although this advice may seem easy in principle, it places a great burden of responsibility on the clinician, because he or she is likely to hear about things that parents would want to know and that the clinician instinctively feels he or she should discuss with them, such as suicidal thinking, sexual experimentation, lying, cheating, and drug use.

Only in situations dangerous to the child, such as a clear risk of suicide, should the rule of confidentiality be broken. This rule should be explained to the parents in a tactful manner so that they do not feel excluded. Depending on circumstances, the clinician may also choose to see the parents independently. Alternately, the clinician may refer the parents to another psychiatrist, psychologist, or social worker with whom he or she has a good working relationship. If the parents are referred elsewhere, maintaining some liaison in the continuing assessment and treatment process is quite important.

Involvement of Nonphysicians in the Health Care Team

Depending on the specific problem, the evaluation and treatment of children may require more knowledge and input than a single psychiatrist can provide. Child psychiatry is more difficult and complicated than adult psychiatry, because the problems of children tend to impinge on many different aspects of their lives, and treatment often involves a number of these different aspects. Children with some particular childhood disorder, such as ADHD, are likely to have difficulty with their parents, their siblings, their school performance, and their relationship with their peers. Most people who must interact with children who have ADHD are likely to find their high level of impulsivity, distractibility, and physical activity annoying and disruptive. These children themselves have a poor self-concept, produced in part by a sense of frustration and failure in all spheres of their lives.

In such instances, assessment involves determining how well the child is functioning in these various domains. That is, the clinician needs to talk to and observe the child. In addition, however, the clinician needs to talk to the parents and perhaps the entire family. With the permission of the child and family, the clinician may need to talk to the child's teacher and to obtain some assessment of his or her performance in the classroom. School records, as well as the child's scores on tests of educational achievement, are important aspects of assessment. Parents or teachers may also need to provide information about the child's interaction with his or her peers.

Because of the diversity of the domains involved, many clinicians working in the area of child psychiatry like to operate in the context of a health care team. This team may be relatively small, involving a psychologist or social worker in addition to the psychiatrist. In larger settings, however, it includes a psychiatrist (who works primarily with the child in psychotherapy and the prescription of medication), a social worker (who works primarily with the family), an educational specialist (who assesses the child's educational achievement and assists in designing a nonfrustrating remedial program as needed), and a psychologist (who develops programs for behavioral management, may do psychotherapy as needed, and may work with child, family, and school system as needed).

Comorbidity

Comorbidity, or the simultaneous occurrence of two or more diagnoses in the same patient, occurs in adults; for example, patients with depression often have problems with anxiety or substance abuse as well. Comorbidity tends to be the norm rather than the exception in children, however. For example, children with ADHD often have impairment in academic skills, such as specific disabilities in reading or arithmetic. They may also show symptoms of conduct disorder, oppositional defiant disorder, or anxiety disorder.

The clinician has to remain very alert to the likelihood of multiple problems and design his or her assessment and treatment plan accordingly. The commonness of comorbidity also makes child psychiatry somewhat more complex and difficult than adult psychiatry. On the positive side, however, is the hope that early intervention will prevent larger problems from developing and the addition of new diagnoses (e.g., substance abuse in addition to ADHD).

Testing in Child Psychiatry

Because of the complexity and ambiguity of child psychiatry, some selected objective assessment measures may be quite useful. Psychological tests, such as IQ tests, may be helpful in determining a child's specific areas of strength and weakness, as well as the level of academic performance that he or she can be expected to achieve. Some diagnoses in child psychiatry, such as mental retardation or the learning disorders, depend on knowledge of the child's IQ. Some disorders of childhood, such as Tourette's disorder or autism, have an organic quality to them that suggests a need to rule out an associated or underlying disorder, such as seizures. Other disorders, such as mental retardation, are often accompanied by a variety of medical problems (e.g., seizures, congenital anomalies, metabolic disorders). In these instances, laboratory tests are useful either in diagnosing the accompanying physical disorders or in monitoring their progress.

Psychological and Educational Testing in Child Psychiatry

Psychological and educational testing often plays a central role in the evaluation of children. Several tests that are commonly used in child psychiatry are listed in Table 22–2.

General intelligence. General intelligence may be assessed with the Stanford-Binet Intelligence Scale, the Wechsler Intelligence Scale for Children—Revised (WISC-R), or other well-validated instruments. The WISC-R was recently revised (1986) with new forms and items. The Stanford-Binet Intelligence Scale was one of the earliest IQ tests to be developed, and it is still appropriate for relatively young children, because its bottom threshold is lower and does not require extensive acquisition of knowledge. The Kaufman ABC and a new Wechsler Preschool and Primary Scale of Intelligence (WPPSI) have also become available recently and are very appropriate for assessing young children.

The WISC-R has now become established as the standard test for assessing the intelligence of school-age children. As in the Wechsler Adult Intelligence Scale—Revised (WAIS-R), the WISC-R consists of a group of verbal scales (information, vocabulary, similarities, arithmetic, and comprehension, plus digit span) and a set of performance tests (picture completion, picture arrangement,

Table 22–2. Cognitive, psychological, and educational tests used in child psychiatry

Factor	Test
Intelligence	Stanford-Binet Intelligence Scale, Wechsler Intelligence Scale for Children—Revised (WISC-R), Peabody Picture Vocabulary, Kaufman ABC, Wechsler Preschool and Primary Scale of Intelligence (WPPSI)
Educational achievement	Iowa Test of Basic Skills (ITBS), Iowa Test of Educational Development (ITED), Wide Range Achievement Test—Revised (WRAT-R), Woodcock-Johnson Psychoeducational Battery
Adaptive behavior	Vineland Adaptive Behavior Scales, Iowa Conner's Teacher Rating Scale
Perceptual-motor abilities	Draw-a-Person, Bender-Gestalt, Benton Visual Retention Test, Purdue Pegboard Test, Beery Developmental Test of Visual-Motor Integration
Personality	Thematic apperception test (TAT), Rorschach test

block design, object assembly, coding, and mazes). Thus, verbal and performance IQs can be derived separately, as well as a full-scale IQ.

Examining the scores on individual WISC-R subtests gives clinicians a sense of the child's overall intellectual skills and weaknesses. The test is scaled to have a mean of 100 and a standard deviation of 15. Sixty-seven percent of children have IQs that fall between 85 and 115, whereas 95% have IQs that fall between 70 and 130. Children from middle-class and culturally advantaged backgrounds tend to perform better on these tests. In such instances, the performance scales of the test may give a somewhat better indication of the child's "culture-free intelligence," although this clearly will not be helpful for those children who have performance deficits for some reason (e.g., visual-motor and/or perception difficulties). Interpretation of the WAIS-R must be made within the context of each child's social background and educational opportunities.

The Peabody Picture Vocabulary Test is a simpler and cruder test sometimes used to give a simple global measure of intelligence. Using pictures, it provides a measure of oral language comprehension, from which verbal intelligence can be inferred. In general, IQ based on the Peabody test tends to be an overestimate.

Educational achievement. Several standardized educational achievement tests are often used in the public school systems. Two of the most widely used are the Iowa Test of Basic Skills (ITBS) and the Iowa Test of Educational Development (ITED). The former is typically used for younger children, whereas versions of the latter are available for assessment until completion of high school. For the

ITBS and the ITED, national, state, and school specific norms are available, so that the child's achievement can be assessed within his or her specific environmental context. These achievement tests provide scores for specific areas such as reading, language arts, study skills, arithmetic, and social studies. Evaluating the pattern of achievement can provide some index as to whether the child has a learning disorder.

The ITBS and ITED are group tests. If a specific concern is present, the child may also be referred for individual testing by an educational specialist, which will often involve the Wide Range Achievement Test—Revised (WRAT-R). The Woodcock-Johnson Psychoeducational Battery is also a widely used individual test to assess skills such as reading or arithmetic. Children may perform poorly on group tests because of inattention or other problems; therefore, group tests may underestimate the child's true abilities.

Adaptive behavior.   Various standard questionnaires can be used to assess adaptive behavior. The Vineland Adaptive Behavior Scales were originally developed to evaluate children with mental retardation, but they are now widely used to provide a standardized measure of adaptive skills for children with a broader range of problems, including those with normal intelligence. The Iowa Connor's Teacher Rating Scale was developed to assess the child's behavior in the classroom. It is specifically targeted to assessing behavior that tends to be associated with ADHD, such as impulsivity, physical activity, or impaired attention. It also has subscales to assess social withdrawal and aggressive behavior.

Perceptual-motor skills.   Various standardized tests are used to assess perceptual-motor skills. For the assessment of young children, the Draw-a-Person Test is one of the most popular. The complexity and detail of the person drawn give a crude indication of the child's maturity, whereas the exhibited drawing skills allow assessment of the child's ability to translate his or her thoughts into a visual representation. The Bender-Gestalt and Benton Visual Retention Test assess the ability to copy a design or to recall it later, which are also fundamental aspects of perceptual-motor skills. The Purdue Pegboard Test is a somewhat pure test of manual dexterity, assessing the child's ability to place pegs in appropriate slots. The Beery Developmental Test of Visual-Motor Perception is popular with school systems.

Personality style and social adjustment.   Personality style and social adjustment are typically evaluated in children through projective tests. The thematic apperception test (TAT) uses a series of cards depicting obscure figures in ambiguous situations; the child is asked to describe what is happening and tell a story about it. The Rorschach test is the famous ink blot test. In this test, the child is shown cards containing ink blots that have ambiguous and suggestive shapes. The child is asked to identify and label what he or she sees and to indicate the basis for his or her perception. Although semistandardized scores can be applied, one of the most common applications of these tests is to provide a standardized structured stimulus to the child, using his or her response as an indication of interpersonal experiences, anxieties, fears, drives, and other important psychological components.

Other Tests

Other laboratory tests may also be useful in the assessment of children. The decision to order these tests will depend on the child's past history and the clinician's index of suspicion for finding an abnormality. For example, there is often comorbidity between seizure disorders and other childhood disorders, such as autism or mental retardation, and children with these diagnoses should probably be evaluated with an electroencephalogram (EEG). For other disorders in which seizures sometimes occur or in which EEG abnormalities have been noted, such as conduct disorders or ADHD, an EEG may be appropriate if the history indicates a possibility of seizures.

Evaluation of children with mental retardation typically includes an assessment for possible causes of the mental retardation. Karyotyping may be used to evaluate for the Fragile X syndrome, Down's syndrome, or XYY. Computed tomography (CT) or magnetic resonance imaging (MRI) may be appropriate in such patients, as well as in patients with autism or Tourette's disorder.

Physical Examination

A careful physical examination, incorporating some simple standardized neuropsychological tests, is also an important part of the evaluation. In addition to the standard physical examination, the clinician should carefully inspect the child for indications of congenital anomalies, such as a high-arched palate, low-set ears, single palmar creases, unusual carrying angle, webbing, abnormalities of the genitalia, and neuroectodermal anomalies. It is well recognized that congenital anomalies tend to occur together, and that midline or neuroectodermal anomalies are more likely to be associated with central nervous system anomalies. Observation of any such anomalies is an indication for CT or MRI.

The clinician should be attentive to assessment of neurological soft signs in children as well. A standardized repertoire should be developed for assessing graphesthesia, left-right discrimination, motor coordination, and simple perceptual-motor skills that can be evaluated at the bedside. For example, left-right discrimination can be examined systematically through a graded series of questions such as the following: "Hold up your right hand. Hold up your left foot. Put your right forefinger on your nose. Use your left forefinger to point to your right foot. Point to my right hand. Use your left forefinger to point to my left hand." Tongue twisters such as "Methodist-Episcopal" or "Luke Luck likes lakes" may be used to assess oral-motor coordination, whereas hopping, tandeming, and rapid alternating movements are used to evaluate other motor skills. Fine motor skills are evaluated through drawing and writing. After he or she has assessed a large number of children across a wide range of ages, the clinician will gradually develop a sense of what constitutes normal performance on these tests of neurological soft signs for a given child at a given age. Extensive neurological soft signs may serve as an indicator for ordering a more extensive laboratory workup, involving an EEG or a brain scan.

Mental Retardation

Mental retardation is a disorder characterized by subnormal intelligence, as measured by IQ, accompanied by deficits in adaptive functioning. IQ is defined as mental age (as assessed by a standard test such as the WISC-R) divided by chronological age and multiplied by 100. Thus, a child with an IQ of 50 might have a mental age of 5 and a chronological age of 10; in other words, he or she would be performing with the intellectual skills of a 5-year-old. The specific IQ cutoff point used to define mental retardation is 70; individuals who have an IQ below 70 are more than 2 standard deviations below the population mean. People with IQs between 70 and 85 (1 standard deviation below the mean) are sometimes considered to have borderline intellectual functioning but are not mentally retarded. The criteria also require that the individual have problems in coping with social and economic demands or exhibit abnormalities in interpersonal adjustment.

The criteria for mental retardation, which appear in Table 22–3, summarize this definition. They also require an onset before age 18 years. In general, mental retardation is typically observed and diagnosed long before age 18 and usually is considered to be present from very early in life. For example, a 13-year-old who sustains a head injury in a car accident and subsequently displays a marked decrement in IQ is considered to have a dementia induced by trauma rather than mental retardation.

Mental retardation is divided into four broad categories: mild, moderate, severe, and profound. Children with *mild mental retardation* have IQs between

Table 22–3.   DSM-IV criteria for mental retardation

A. Significantly subaverage intellectual functioning: an IQ of approximately 70 or below on an individually administered IQ test (for infants, a clinical judgment of significantly subaverage intellectual functioning)

B. Concurrent deficits or impairments in present adaptive functioning (i.e., the person's effectiveness in meeting the standards expected for his or her age by his or her cultural group) in at least two of the following areas: communication, self-care, home living, social/interpersonal skills, use of community resources, self-direction, functional academic skills, work, leisure, health, and safety

C. The onset is before age 18 years

Coding note: Code on degree of severity reflecting level of intellectual impairment:

     Mild mental retardation: IQ level 50–55 to approximately 70
     Moderate mental retardation: IQ level 35–40 to 50–55
     Severe mental retardation: IQ level 20–25 to 35–40
     Profound mental retardation: IQ level below 20 or 25
     Mental retardation, severity unspecified: when there is strong presumption of mental retardation but the person's intelligence is untestable by standard tests

approximately 50 and 70. They represent the majority of cases of mental retardation, constituting approximately 85% of individuals with IQs below 70. Children with IQs in this range are considered to be educable, and they are usually able to attend special classes and to work toward the long-term goal of being able to function in the community and to hold some type of job. They usually can learn to read, write, and perform simple arithmetical calculations. Children with *moderate mental retardation* have IQs ranging between 35 and 50 (between 3 and 4 standard deviations below the population mean), and constitute approximately 10% of the mentally retarded population. They are considered to be trainable, in that they can learn to talk, to recognize their name and other simple words, to perform activities of self-care such as bathing and doing their laundry, and to handle small change. They require management and treatment in special education classes. The ideal long-term goal for these individuals is care in a sheltered environment, such as a group home. Severely and profoundly mentally retarded children constitute the smallest groups. *Severe mental retardation* is defined as an IQ between 20 and 35, and *profound mental retardation* is defined as an IQ below 20. Individuals with IQs in this range almost invariably require care in institutionalized settings, usually beginning relatively early in life.

Epidemiology.   Mental retardation is very common, affecting between 1% and 2% of the population. Mental retardation is more common in males, with a male-to-female ratio of approximately 2:1. Mild mental retardation is more common in lower social classes, but moderate, severe, and profound mental retardation are equally common among all social classes.

Pathophysiology and etiology.   The pathophysiology and etiology of mental retardation are heterogeneous. Mental retardation is almost certainly a syndrome that represents a final common pathway produced by a variety of factors that injure the brain and affect its normal development. Those individuals with IQs below 55 often have an identifiable cause for their mental retardation, whereas those with IQs above 55 often do not and probably develop their mental retardation through some complex multifactorial and polygenetic combination. Down's syndrome is the most common cause of mental retardation. Fragile X syndrome is the most common heritable form of mental retardation and is second only to Down's syndrome in frequency. The fragile X gene has been discovered; it contains an unstable segment that expands as it is passed through generations and affects children differently depending on whether it is passed through fathers or mothers (imprinting). Inborn errors of metabolism account for a small percentage of cases; examples include Tay-Sachs disease and untreated phenylketonuria.

In addition to these clearly defined genetic causes, a substantial proportion of cases of mental retardation probably also reflect polygenic inheritance, possibly interacting with a variety of environmental factors such as nutrition and psychosocial nurturance. A variety of prenatal factors may also affect fetal development and lead to neurodevelopmental anomalies. The high rate of Down's syndrome (trisomy 21) in children born to older mothers is a prime example. Other prenatal factors that may affect fetal development include maternal substance abuse, exposure to other toxins such as radiation, and maternal illnesses such as diabetes, toxemia, or rubella. Perinatal and early postnatal factors may also contribute. Examples include traumatic deliveries that cause brain injury, malnutrition, exposure to toxins, infections such as encephalitis, and head injuries occurring during infancy or early childhood. Psychosocial factors obviously contribute to some of these biological factors, and some psychosocial factors may also contribute independently. Malnutrition, exposure to toxins such as lead, increased likelihood of maternal infection due to inadequate immunization, and poor prenatal and perinatal care are more likely to occur in children born in impoverished environments.

Course and outcome.   The long-term outcome of mental retardation is variable. Some severe and profound forms may be characterized by progressive physical deterioration and ultimately premature death, as early as the teens or early 20s (e.g., Tay-Sachs disease). Individuals with mild and moderate forms of mental retardation have a somewhat reduced life expectancy, but active intervention may enhance their quality of life. Like all children, children with mental retardation grow and develop, and they may show maturational spurts that could not be predicted at an earlier age. Typically, mentally retarded children progress through normal milestones, such as sitting, standing, talking, and learning numbers and letters, in a pattern similar to that of normal children but at a slower rate. Educable and trainable mentally retarded children are able to learn to read, write, and calculate at some level, as long as appropriately structured educational settings are provided.

Differential diagnosis.   As in other childhood disorders, the differential diagnosis of mental retardation (particularly mild mental retardation) can be complex, due to the frequent comorbidity of childhood disorders. The differential diagnosis includes ADHD, learning disorders, autism, and childhood psychoses or mood disorders, but all these conditions can occur with mental retardation. Seizure disorders are also very common in children with mental retardation. Children in whom mental retardation is suspected should be thoroughly evaluated with careful physical and neurological examinations, EEG, and CT (or MRI if available), as well as IQ testing.

Treatment.   The treatment of children with mental retardation is similar to the treatment of children with other serious chronic disorders, such as autism. After a thorough evaluation, a comprehensive program should be developed to determine the best situation in which to place and treat the child, taking the needs and abilities of both the child and the parents into account. Decisions may range from care in the home (supplemented by family support and special education), to placement in a foster or group home, to long-term institutionalization. Because the majority of mentally retarded children are mildly retarded, the majority will remain at home, at least initially. Because the parents of some of these children themselves have mental retardation, ongoing evaluation through social service agencies may be helpful and even necessary to ensure that the child's needs are being adequately met.

Whatever their own intellectual resources, the parents of mentally retarded children are confronted with a host of burdens and stresses and will benefit from both supportive counseling and training in behavioral techniques to assist in the management of their child's behavioral problems. Comorbid conditions such as seizures require medical management. Intellectual evaluation assists in determining the appropriate educational placement for the child, but this placement should be subjected to periodic review. At this stage, it is still not clear whether mildly mentally retarded children benefit more from placement in regular school programs (mainstreaming) or from placement in special settings where education is tailored to their specific needs. To a large extent, however, mainstreaming is currently the dominant trend.

Learning Disorders

The learning disorders are characterized by an inability to achieve in a specific area of learning (reading, writing, or arithmetic) at a level consistent with the person's overall IQ. Typically, individuals with these disorders have normal intelligence (although it may be borderline or high), but they have a specific inability to learn at least one of these academic skills, and sometimes several.

The DSM-IV criteria for *reading disorder* appear in Table 22–4. The definitions for *mathematics disorder* and *disorder of written expression* are similar. In each case, the diagnosis is made on the basis of educational testing that indicates that the individual is performing markedly below the level expected on the basis of his or her IQ. For example, a 14-year-old with reading disorder (developmental dyslexia) may be observed to have an IQ of 110 and to be reading at a third-grade level.

These disorders are relatively common. A specific disability in reading affects from 2% to 8% of school-age children; whereas the rates for writing and mathematics disabilities are not known, they are probably high as well. These disorders are from two to four times as common in boys as in girls.

Specific learning disabilities tend to be familial, but not uniformly or consistently so. They are assumed to represent a neurodevelopmental defect or cerebral injury affecting the particular brain region involved in developing the academic skill. For example, in the case of some developmental reading or writing disorders, the language regions in the brain (i.e., Broca's area, Wernicke's area, and the left hemisphere) are thought to be affected.

If not diagnosed and treated early and aggressively, learning disorders are extremely handicapping. Although children with these disorders typically have normal intelligence, they quickly come to view themselves as failures because of their inability to progress academically in a particular area. They may come to regard themselves as stupid and feel rejected by their peers.

Table 22–4.   DSM-IV criteria for reading disorder

A. Reading achievement, as measured by individually administered standardized tests of reading accuracy or comprehension, is substantially below that expected given the person's chronological age, measured intelligence, and age-appropriate education.

B. The disturbance in criterion A significantly interferes with academic achievement or activities of daily living that require reading skills.

C. If a sensory deficit is present, the reading difficulties are in excess of those usually associated with it.

Coding note: If a general medical (e.g., neurological) condition or sensory deficit is present, code the condition on Axis III.

The frustration associated with an impairment in academic skills can lead to a variety of complications, such as truancy, school refusal, conduct disorder, mood disorder, and substance abuse. Consequently, it is important to identify the condition early and treat it aggressively. Rather than being causal, learning disorders may also be comorbid with these conditions, as well as with ADHD. In this instance, it is important to recognize the multiple disorders and to treat both (or all) of them appropriately.

Educational intervention proceeds on two fronts. Children or teenagers usually need remedial instruction to shore up skill deficits, as well as instruction in developing "attack" skills that will assist them in learning strategies to compensate for the neural deficits that underlie their condition. With steady, sympathetic educational support, most children with these specific learning disabilities are able to develop acceptable skills in reading, writing, and arithmetic.

Autistic Disorder

Autistic disorder is the most important among the *pervasive developmental disorders*. The film *Rain Man*, through its sympathetic portrayal of a person with autism, has done much to help increase public understanding of this particular disorder. Although Raymond Babbit is not a perfectly typical autistic person because he is cognitively very gifted in specific isolated areas, he is not atypical. He displays all the characteristic features of autism: impaired social interactions, impaired ability to communicate, and a restricted repertoire of activities and interests.

Individuals with autism are usually noted to be developing abnormally relatively soon after birth. Within the first 3–6 months of these children's lives, their parents may note that they do not develop a normal pattern of smiling or responding to cuddling. The first clear sign of abnormality is usually in language. As they grow older, they do not progress through developmental milestones such as learning to say words and speak sentences. They seem aloof, withdrawn, and detached. Instead of developing patterns of relating warmly to their parents, they may instead engage in self-stimulating behavior, such as rocking or head banging. By age 2 or 3 years, it is usually clear that there is something severely wrong, and the features of the disorder continue to become more obvious over time as the child fails to develop normal verbal and interpersonal communication. Children with this disorder are referred to as autistic because they appear to be withdrawn and self-absorbed. Most of the defining features of autistic disorder reflect this autistic pattern of thinking, speaking, feeling, and behaving.

The DSM-IV criteria for autistic disorder appear in Table 22–5. The criteria

Table 22–5.   DSM-IV criteria for autistic disorder

A. A total of six (or more) items from 1, 2, and 3, with at least two from 1 and one each from 2 and 3:

   1. Qualitative impairment in social interaction, as manifested by at least two of the following:

      a. Marked impairment in the use of multiple nonverbal behaviors such as eye-to-eye gaze, facial expression, body postures, and gestures to regulate social interaction

      b. Failure to develop peer relationships appropriate to developmental level

      c. A lack of spontaneous seeking to share enjoyment, interests, or achievements with other people (e.g., by a lack of showing, bringing, or pointing out objects of interest)

      d. Lack of social or emotional reciprocity

   2. Qualitative impairments in communication as manifested by at least one of the following:

      a. Delay in, or total lack of, the development of spoken language (not accompanied by an attempt to compensate through alternative modes of communication such as gesture or mime)

      b. In individuals with adequate speech, marked impairment in the ability to initiate or sustain a conversation with others

      c. Stereotyped and repetitive use of language or idiosyncratic language

      d. Lack of varied, spontaneous make-believe play or social imitative play appropriate to developmental level

   3. Restricted repetitive and stereotyped patterns of behavior, interests, and activities, as manifested by at least one of the following:

      a. Encompassing preoccupation with one or more stereotyped and restrained patterns of interest that is abnormal either in intensity or focus

      b. Apparently inflexible adherence to specific, nonfunctional routines or rituals

      c. Stereotyped and repetitive motor mannerisms (e.g., hand or finger flapping or twisting, or complex whole-body movements)

      d. Persistent preoccupation with parts of objects

B. Delays or abnormal functioning in at least one of the following areas, with onset prior to age 3 years: 1) social interaction, 2) language as used in social communication, or 3) symbolic or imaginative play.

C. The disturbance is not better accounted for by Rett's disorder or childhood disintegrative disorder.

require that at least 6 from a list of 12 items be present; the items cover the three major domains involved in autism (i.e., social interaction, communication, and behavioral repertoire). The criteria provide an excellent comprehensive description of the symptoms of this disorder.

The *impairment in social interaction* is one of the first signs of the disorder. Autistic children appear to lack the ability to bond to their parents or others. In severe cases, these children seem totally withdrawn. In milder cases, they display some interaction but lack warmth, sensitivity, and awareness. Interactions, when they occur, tend to have a detached and mechanical quality to them. Displays of love and affection do not occur, nor do autistic children (or autistic adults) appear to respond to such displays from others.

The *failure to develop normal language* is usually the first thing that leads parents to realize the gravity of the problem and eventually to seek medical attention. The verbal impairments range from the complete absence of verbal speech to mildly deviant speech and language patterns. Even in patients who develop good facility in verbal expression, the speech has an empty, repetitive quality to it, and intonations may be singsong and monotonous. Autistic children and adults seem to lack the capacity to engage in conversation with others, sometimes talking spontaneously without an audience and at other times replying irrelevantly or inappropriately.

Finally, the *behavioral repertoire* is impaired. There is an intense and rigid commitment to maintaining specific routines, and autistic children tend to become quite distressed if routines are interrupted. They may have to sit in a particular chair, dress in a particular way, and eat particular foods.

Most autistic individuals (70%) show some evidence of mental retardation, but others have normal intelligence, and some have very specific talents or abilities, particularly in the areas of music and mathematics. IQ testing tends to show considerable scatter, and there is a tendency for patients with autism to perform better on performance scales than on verbal scales.

Children who present with symptoms suggestive of autism should receive comprehensive psychiatric and physical examinations, with emphasis on neurological evaluation as well. Children should be screened for metabolic disorders such as phenylketonuria, and karyotyping should also be done. Because these children present with profound social withdrawal, hearing and vision should be checked to rule out sensory defects as a cause. Because a substantial number of children with autism have a comorbid seizure disorder (25%) or develop one eventually, an EEG should also be obtained. IQ testing will assist in assessing the child's intellectual strengths and weaknesses.

Epidemiology.   Autism is relatively rare and has a prevalence of approximately 10–15 per 10,000. The disorder is more common in males than in females, with a ratio of 3 or 4:1. The onset of autism usually occurs in early childhood, and problems are typically noted during the first or second year of life.

Pathophysiology and etiology.   The pathophysiology and etiology of autism are uncertain, but the preponderance of evidence indicates that this disorder is due to some type of brain abnormality. The disorder is familial, but no clear mendelian pattern has been identified. The concordance rate in monozygotic twins has been estimated at 36%, compared to 0 in dizygotic twins, supporting a genetic component that is not totally penetrant. The fragile X chromosome has been noted in a small number of autistic patients, and there is a high rate of autism in individuals with tuberous sclerosis. Apart from these findings, data are not available to assist in defining the genetic anomaly more specifically.

Neuroanatomical and neuropathological studies have revealed a few positive findings. The most consistent abnormality noted with neuroimaging is ventricular enlargement. Neuropathological studies have reported small, densely packed (and presumably immature) cells in limbic structures and the cerebellum; there have also been a few reports of polymicrogyria. The neurochemistry and cerebral localization of autism have not been determined. Abnormalities in both the dopamine system and the serotonin system have been reported.

Course and outcome. Autism is associated with relatively severe morbidity. It is a chronic, lifelong disorder. Some children do show some improvement as they mature, although others may worsen. Very few individuals with autism (2%–3%) are able to progress normally through school or to live independently. Follow-up studies of a group of autistic individuals diagnosed in childhood and reevaluated in adulthood indicate that most autistic persons show some improvement in social interaction over time, but even the most functional of those persons never achieve normality. Nearly all of the defining features of the disorder tend to persist into adulthood, including social aloofness, language abnormalities, and rigid and ritualistic behavior. Good prognostic features include higher IQ and better language and social skills.

Differential diagnosis. The major differential diagnoses include childhood psychosis, mental retardation, and congenital deafness, blindness, or language disorders. The most important distinctions are between autism and mental retardation or language disorders such as selective mutism and expressive language disorder. These distinctions can be quite difficult, and the differential turns largely on the quality of the social interactions (in the context of the individual's particular intellectual abilities). Mentally retarded children also typically have pervasive intellectual impairments, whereas autistic children tend to have a much more uneven profile of functional intellectual abilities on the WISC-R and may be normal to superior in some areas. The major distinction between autism and childhood schizophrenia turns on the presence or absence of overt psychotic symptoms (delusions and hallucinations), which typically do not occur in autism, but are difficult to assess in the noncommunicative child.

Treatment. The treatment of autism requires assistance and support in the many different areas of functioning in which these children are impaired. Once the diagnosis is firmly made, the disorder should be described and explained to the parents, making it clear that their child has a neurodevelopmental disease and not a psychological disturbance that they caused through poor parenting. Guidelines for behavioral management should be provided, so that the parents can assist in reducing the rigid and stereotyped behaviors and improving language and social skills. Children with autism usually require special education or specialized day care programs that also emphasize improvement in social and language skills. Medications are often used as adjuncts to these supportive and behavioral approaches. Children who have seizures will require anticonvulsants. Among other medications, neuroleptics (e.g., haloperidol, in low doses ranging from 1 to 10 mg/day) have been empirically observed to decrease aggressive and self-stimulating behavior. Other medications found to be empirically helpful in some cases include clomipramine, naltrexone, fluoxetine, and carbamazepine.

Attention-Deficit and Disruptive Behavior Disorders

The attention-deficit and disruptive behavior disorders are the staples of child psychiatry. Children with these disorders are experienced as difficult to manage and therefore disruptive by those around them, including parents, teachers, and often peers. Sometimes this group of disorders is referred to as involving acting-out behavior, meaning that the child expresses his or her problems outwardly rather than holding them within. This group of behavior disorders is contrasted with the internalizing disorders, such as the anxiety disorders, in which the child is considered to turn his or her suffering inward. Although closer contact with many of the children who manifest disruptive behavior makes it clear that they too may suffer a great deal internally and may also experience considerable anxiety, this aspect of the disorder is not immediately obvious to those who must deal with these children on a day-to-day basis. On superficial contact, these children may seem hard to love and even hard to like. The three major classes of disruptive behavior disorders include ADHD, conduct disorder, and oppositional defiant disorder.

Attention-Deficit/Hyperactivity Disorder

ADHD has been recognized under various names for many years—probably for many centuries. Children with this disorder are a caricature of the active child. They are physically overactive, distractible, inattentive, impulsive, and hard to manage. Because they often show soft neurological signs and indices of slight delay in reaching developmental milestones, this disorder was originally referred to as *minimal brain dysfunction*. Later, as it became apparent that no objective evidence could be marshalled for the minimal brain dysfunction, the disorder was referred to as *hyperactivity* and the patient as a hyperactive child. These designations appear in the earlier DSM nomenclature. By the time the DSM-III was developed in 1980, child psychiatrists had reached a consensus that the basic deficit in this disorder is one of attention. Thus, it came to be known as *attention-deficit disorder*, and clinicians could also indicate whether hyperactivity was present or absent. By the time DSM-IV was produced, clinicians had decided that this distinction was arbitrary and began to refer to the disorder as ADHD, although it is possible to denote whether the presentation is mixed, predominantly inattentive, or predominantly hyperactive.

The DSM-IV criteria for ADHD are summarized in Table 22–6. The criteria require that at least 12 from a group of 18 symptoms be present for at least 6 months. These symptoms fall into two broad categories that characterize the overall syndrome: 1) difficulty focusing and maintaining attention and 2) hyperactivity and impulsivity. At least six symptoms must be present from the domain of attention and six from the domain of hyperactivity-impulsivity. The symptoms involving attention include being easily distracted, difficulty following instructions, difficulty sustaining attention in tasks, shifting attention from one uncompleted activity to another, not listening, losing things, and other similar problems. Those involving hyperactivity include fidgeting, difficulty sitting still, difficulty playing quietly, and talking excessively. Those involving impulsivity include difficulty waiting in turn, blurting out answers to questions, and interrupting or intruding on others.

The actual manifestation of these symptoms will vary depending on the age of the child. Younger children (in the 4- to 6-year age range) are "little terrors." They run from one part of the room to another, hop on furniture, knock objects off tables, explore the contents of visitors' handbags, talk incessantly, run outside without telling their parents where they are going, have difficulty learning to look both ways when crossing the street, lose and break toys, stay up late, wake up early, and generally exhaust their parents. When these children enter school and begin the task of learning, the difficulties in focusing attention become more obvious. They may miss things that the teacher says, be unable to finish assignments, forget their pencils or notebooks, and answer the teacher's questions without holding up a hand and often without even waiting to have the question completed. They may annoy their schoolmates by pushing ahead in line, grabbing equipment on the playground, and violating the rules of games without seeming to be aware of them. These children may begin to fall behind their peers in school and to develop a poor concept of themselves. Teachers may complain about their behavior to their parents and request that help be sought.

Table 22–6. DSM-IV criteria for attention-deficit/hyperactivity disorder

A. Either 1 or 2:

   1. Six (or more) of the following symptoms of **inattention** have persisted for at least 6 months to a degree that is maladaptive and inconsistent with developmental level:

   Inattention
   a. Often fails to give close attention to details or makes careless mistakes in schoolwork, work, or other activities
   b. Often has difficulty sustaining attention in tasks or play activities
   c. Often does not seem to listen when spoken to directly
   d. Often does not follow through on instructions and fails to finish schoolwork, chores, or duties in the workplace (not due to oppositional behavior or failure to understand instructions)
   e. Often has difficulty organizing tasks and activities
   f. Often avoids, dislikes, or is reluctant to engage in tasks that require sustained mental effort (such as schoolwork or homework)
   g. Often loses things necessary for tasks or activities (e.g., toys, school assignments, pencils, books, or tools)
   h. Is often easily distracted by extraneous stimuli
   i. Is often forgetful in daily activities

   2. Six (or more) of the following symptoms of **hyperactivity-impulsivity** have persisted for at least 6 months to a degree that is maladaptive and inconsistent with developmental level:

   Hyperactivity
   a. Often fidgets with hands or feet or squirms in seat
   b. Often leaves seat in classroom or in other situations in which remaining seated is expected
   c. Often runs about or climbs excessively in situations in which it is inappropriate (in adolescents or adults, may be limited to subjective feelings of restlessness)
   d. Often has difficulty playing or engaging in leisure activities quietly
   e. Is often "on the go" or often acts as if "driven by a motor"
   f. Often talks excessively

   Impulsivity
   g. Often blurts out answers before questions have been completed
   h. Often has difficulty awaiting turn
   i. Often interrupts or intrudes on others (e.g., butts into conversations or games)

B. Some hyperactive-impulsive or inattentive symptoms that caused impairment were present before age 7 years.

C. Some impairment from the symptoms is present in two or more settings (e.g., at school [or work] and at home).

D. There must be clear evidence of clinically significant impairment in social, academic, or occupational functioning.

E. The symptoms do not occur exclusively during the course of a pervasive developmental disorder, schizophrenia, or other psychotic disorder and are not better accounted for by another mental disorder (e.g., mood disorder, anxiety disorder, dissociative disorder, or a personality disorder).

Code based on type:

Attention-deficit/hyperactivity disorder, combined type: if both criteria A1 and A2 are met for the past 6 months

Table 22–6. DSM-IV criteria for attention-deficit/hyperactivity disorder *(continued)*

Attention-deficit/hyperactivity disorder, predominantly inattentive type: if criterion A1 is met but criterion A2 is not met for the past 6 months

Attention-deficit/hyperactivity disorder, predominantly hyperactive-impulsive type: if criterion A2 is met but criterion Al is not met for the past 6 months

Coding note: For individuals (especially adolescents and adults) who currently have symptoms that no longer meet full criteria, "in partial remission" should be specified.

The following is a relatively typical case history of a patient with ADHD.

Charlie was a 6-year-old boy brought in by his mother after a recent school conference in which it was pointed out that he seemed to be having difficulty in adjusting to first grade.

Charlie's mother described that he had always been a somewhat difficult child. He was the second of two, and his older sister Mary (age 9) had always been much quieter and more pliable. Charlie's mother had assumed that much of Charlie's disruptive behavior was due to the fact that "little boys tend to be more active." Whereas Mary had responded well to encouragement to put her toys away each evening and had kept their various components intact (e.g., puzzles in their boxes, Lincoln Logs in their containers), Charlie never seemed to be able to keep track of anything or put it away. He had been a whiny infant who had had colic. Even as an infant he was irritable and overactive. He learned to crawl at 7 months and was soon exploring the entire house, leaving a wake of emptied wastepaper baskets and disrupted cupboards behind him. He did not seem to be able to remember or follow through with parental instructions that he should keep his feet off the furniture, not walk on the tops of tables, and not run through the living room carrying melting chocolate popsicles. As he learned to talk, he seemed to talk incessantly and to be continuously in need of attention from his parents. Attempts to ignore his attention-seeking behavior seemed to have little effect on him. His parents complained that he was a "perpetual-motion machine."

He began to attend preschool at age 4. Teachers at that time complained that he was disruptive and impulsive, seeming to have little consideration for the other children in the school. The same noisy, attention-seeking behavior that occurred at home was noticed at the preschool. Similar complaints were registered by his teacher when he entered kindergarten the following year. After 3 months of first grade, the patience of the public school system was already exhausted. Charlie's teacher complained that it was difficult to even get through a routine class day because of Charlie's behavior. He would not sit in his seat like the other children and would often get up and run around the room. He could not work on an assignment for more than 5 minutes without being distracted. He would also distract his classmates by talking to them when they were supposed to be working quietly. None of the teacher's efforts seemed to be effective in quieting or calming Charlie.

On initial evaluation, Charlie was noted to indeed be quite active. He entered the doctor's office with a firm, aggressive step. He jumped on his chair rather than sitting down, finally squirming himself into a sitting position which he maintained for only 2 or 3 minutes. He then jumped up and began pulling books off the bookshelves, asking what they were for in a somewhat immature, whiny-sounding voice. When told that they belonged to the doctor and should be placed back on the shelf, he threw one or two on the floor and proceeded to the doctor's desk to examine the pens, pencils, and paperweights. Charlie's mother looked embarrassed and exasperated and tried to get him to sit back down.

An individual evaluation with Charlie alone, involving an attempt to put a puzzle together, indicated that Charlie did indeed have problems focusing his attention on a relatively simple task. He was given a five-piece puzzle that the average 6-year-old can complete quickly. Charlie put one piece in place and then lost interest, instead pounding another puzzle piece on the floor and then throwing the remainder across the room. He was unable to perform any tests of graphesthesia. After five tries, when asked to write the first six letters of the alphabet, he completed four with one letter reversal and then lost interest. He also reversed the letter "r" when writing his name. He could not distinguish between right and left at any level. Otherwise, his physical examination was totally normal.

A decision was made to try Charlie on methylphenidate. Within 1 week, his mother related that the effects were "amazing." Almost immediately, his behavior improved, and he showed a distinct increase in his ability to focus attention and a decrease in impulsive, overactive behavior. His teacher also noticed a distinct difference. He was able to complete the first grade with only minimal difficulty and was considered to have appropriate progress for his age in basic skills of learning to read and to do very simple arithmetic.

Epidemiology.   Because the definition of ADHD has changed over time, its prevalence is uncertain, but it is definitely common in young and school-age children. Estimates range from 3% to 10%. It is far more common in boys than in girls, with a sex ratio of approximately 3:1. The etiology and pathophysiology of ADHD are uncertain. Genetic, environmental, neurobiological, and social explanations have been proposed.

Pathophysiology and etiology.   ADHD runs in families. Not only does ADHD itself show familial aggregation, particularly in the males, but other psychiatric disorders tend to show familial aggregation with it as well. In particular, there appears to be an association with learning disorders, mood disorder, substance abuse, and antisocial personality disorder. Most of the existing evidence for familial aggregation is based on family studies. Twin studies have not yet been done. There may be a gender threshold effect, in that girls with ADHD tend to have a stronger family history of ADHD than do boys.

Environmental explanations tend to stress the possibility of perinatal problems, including maternal nutrition, maternal substance abuse, obstetrical complications during delivery, viral infections, and exposure to toxins. The possible role of such environmental factors is consistent with the higher prevalence of ADHD in boys, as well as the gender threshold effect described above, in that male children are more vulnerable to prenatal and perinatal injury. They are also consistent with the slight increase in neurological soft signs that has been observed in children with ADHD.

Other neurobiological markers have also been evaluated in children with ADHD. There is no specific diagnostic marker for the disorder, but a variety of findings have been observed. A decrease in norepinephrine metabolites (3-methoxy-4-hydroxyphenylglycol [MHPG]) has been argued to support a catecholamine hypothesis, whereas low levels of homovanillic acid have been thought to support the possibility of hypodopaminergic function. Approximately 20% of ADHD children show EEG abnormalities, and sleep EEG studies show decreased rapid eye movement latency and increased delta latency; the latter finding is consistent with the clinical observation that these children tend to have difficulty falling asleep.

Psychosocial explanations stress the role of parental anxiety and inexperience, as well as failure to extinguish undesirable behavior through ignoring it (often difficult to do with hyperactive children). Parents may become uncertain of their parenting skills when faced with a child who seems so difficult to control or shape, thereby conveying uncertainty or anxiety to him or her.

Course and outcome.   The long-term course and outcome of ADHD are variable. Approximately half of the children diagnosed with this disorder have a good outcome, completing school on schedule with acceptable grades consistent with their family background and family expectations. For a time, it was assumed that most children with ADHD would grow out of it. This assumption does not seem to be valid for many individuals, however, because approximately half of the patients diagnosed with ADHD during childhood continue to show some problems with attention and impulsivity as adults. In fact, a subset of these patients continue to need medication as adults, and a small number of individuals are occasionally diagnosed as having *adult attention-deficit disorder* (adult ADD). These individuals are sometimes treated with psychostimulants (e.g., dextroamphetamine, methylphenidate) by psychiatrists.

Some patients with ADHD have a relatively poor outcome. Twenty-five percent subsequently meet criteria for antisocial personality disorder as adults. Children given this diagnosis also have higher rates of substance abuse, more arrests, more suicide attempts, and more car accidents and complete fewer years of school. Problems with confidence and self-esteem may be prominent, because the disorder invites rejection by both parents and peers.

Differential diagnosis.   The differential diagnosis of ADHD includes a wide variety of disorders. In making a differential diagnosis, the clinician must also be aware that a child with this disorder may have comorbidity with other disorders common in childhood, such as seizure disorders, other disruptive behavior disorders (i.e., conduct and oppositional disorders), and learning disorders. When one of these disorders is present along with ADHD, it is often difficult to distinguish which disorder is primary and which is secondary. Other disorders that may cause similar symptoms include childhood bipolar disorder, childhood depression, conduct disorder, a normal response to a pathological or abusive home environment (e.g., physical abuse or neglect by the parents), and a neuroendocrine abnormality, such as thyroid disorder.

Treatment.   The treatment for ADHD often involves a combination of somatic therapy and behavioral management.

A majority of children respond favorably to psychostimulants. Methylphenidate in a dose of 10–60 mg/day is usually the first line of treatment, followed by D-amphetamine in a dose of 5–40 mg/day. If neither of these succeeds, pemoline (another psychostimulant) or tricyclic antidepressants (e.g., imipramine) may be used. Tricyclic doses range from 25 to 100 mg/day. In general, methylphenidate and D-amphetamine offer short-term effects, lasting 4–6 hours, whereas the effects of the antidepressants tend to last longer. Because psychostimulants may have long-term effects on weight gain and body size (i.e., to decrease or inhibit them), clinicians usually strive to use the lowest possible doses of these agents and, whenever possible, to restrict their use to periods of greatest need, such as during the school year. Sometimes it is possible to diminish or discontinue medication as the child enters puberty. Further information about the use of psychostimulants is found in Chapter 26.

Behavioral and environmental management is also important. Parents will benefit from learning basic techniques of behavioral management, such as the value of positive reenforcement and firm, nonpunitive limit setting. They can also be taught techniques for reducing stimulation, thereby diminishing distractibility and inattentiveness. For example, young hyperactive children do better playing with only one friend rather than in groups. Noisy and complex toys should be avoided, as should toys that encourage impulsivity and aggression. The parent may want to work closely with the child in completing homework tasks and to teach him or her the value of working on tasks in the single, small increments best suited to the child's relatively short attention span, mastering one completely before going on to another.

Conduct Disorder

Conduct disorder is characterized by a pattern of behavior that violates the rights of others, such as stealing, lying, or cheating. In terms of both behavior and diagnostic criteria, conduct disorder can be considered to be a forerunner of antisocial personality disorder in adults, because it involves similar antisocial behavior. Nevertheless, not all children who manifest conduct disorder develop antisocial personality disorder as adults. With appropriate treatment and rehabilitation, many of these juvenile delinquents go on to lead acceptable and normal adult lives.

The DSM-IV criteria for conduct disorder appear in Table 22–7. The criteria require the presence of 3 from a list of 15 antisocial behaviors and persistence of these behaviors for at least 1 year (with at least one criterion being present during the previous 6 months). The criteria define four major domains of relevant behavior: aggression to people and animals, destruction of property, deceitfulness or theft, and serious violations of rules. Individuals who manifest this delinquent behavior are further subdivided into two different types. The *childhood-onset type* begins before age 10 years and probably has a more guarded prognosis, whereas the *adolescent-onset type* begins after age 10 and is more likely to have a better outcome.

As is the case for antisocial personality disorder (the adult equivalent of conduct disorder), the DSM-IV criteria stress behavior in the definition of conduct disorder, as opposed to values, motives, or attitudes. Although the objective behavioral definition clearly improves reliability, some critics have expressed the concern that these behavioral definitions ignore the true core phenomena of delinquency and antisocial personality: shallowness of relationships and attachments, inability to feel for others, and an impaired capacity to feel guilt. A distinction between group delinquency and solitary aggressive behavior has been used to refine the definition by stressing that young delinquents who commit antisocial acts as part of a gang are able to form some ties to others. Recent episodes of "wilding" make it clear, however, that group delinquents can commit senseless acts of violence that also seem to indicate a fundamental and severe lack of moral sense.

Children and adolescents who present with signs and symptoms of conduct disorder are a very mixed group, and most clinicians regard this category as fundamentally quite heterogeneous, both with respect to etiology and with respect

Table 22–7. DSM-IV criteria for conduct disorder

A. A repetitive and persistent pattern of behavior in which the basic rights of others or major age-appropriate societal norms or rules are violated, as manifested by the presence of three (or more) of the following criteria in the past 12 months, with at least one criterion present in the past 6 months:

Aggression to people and animals
  1. Often bullies, threatens, or intimidates others
  2. Often initiates physical fights
  3. Has used a weapon that can cause serious physical harm to others (e.g., a bat, brick, broken bottle, knife, gun)
  4. Has been physically cruel to people
  5. Has been physically cruel to animals
  6. Has stolen while confronting a victim (e.g., mugging, purse snatching, extortion, armed robbery)
  7. Has forced someone into sexual activity

Destruction of property
  8. Has deliberately engaged in fire setting with the intention of causing serious damage
  9. Has deliberately destroyed others' property (other than by fire setting)

Deceitfulness or theft
  10. Has broken into someone else's house, building, or car
  11. Often lies to obtain goods or favors or to avoid obligations (i.e., "cons" others)
  12. Has stolen items of nontrivial value without confronting a victim (e.g., shoplifting, but without breaking and entering; forgery)

Serious violations of rules
  13. Often stays out at night despite parental prohibitions, beginning before age 13 years
  14. Has run away from home overnight at least twice while living in parental or parental surrogate home (or once without returning for a lengthy period)
  15. Is often truant from school, beginning before age 13 years

B. The disturbance in behavior causes clinically significant impairment in social, academic, or occupational functioning.

C. If the individual is age 18 years or older, criteria are not met for antisocial personality disorder.

Specify type based on age at onset:

  Childhood-onset type: Onset of at least one criterion characteristic of conduct disorder prior to age 10 years.

  Adolescent-onset type: Absence of any criteria characteristic of conduct disorder prior to age 10 years.

Specify severity:

  Mild: Few if any conduct problems in excess of those required to make the diagnosis **and** conduct problems cause only minor harm to others.

  Moderate: Number of conduct problems and effect on others intermediate between "mild" and "severe."

  Severe: Many conduct problems in excess of those required to make the diagnosis **or** conduct problems cause considerable harm to others.

to outcome. The child seen in a psychiatry clinic for conduct disorder is usually brought in at someone else's request after he or she has committed some kind of socially unacceptable behavior, such as lying, cheating, stealing, fighting, or assaulting. Some children who perform these acts come from families where this type of behavior is not unusual, but others come from families where these acts are unacceptable, thereby shocking and dismaying their parents. The degree to which parents support and assist the child in modifying his or her behavior varies substantially.

Children or adolescents with conduct disorder typically are angry, sullen, and resentful when placed in the context of the adult world, with its pressures to conform, stay in school, and persist in conspicuously dull activities. School performance is usually average to poor. These children or adolescents typically consider their schoolwork irrelevant or uninteresting, do not complete homework, and often cut class to joyride with buddies, smoke pot, or drink beer. When with their peers, their anger and sullenness often disappears, and they seem to be having a good time. Beneath the veneer of anger, toughness, and rebellion, however, they may often have profound feelings of self-doubt and worthlessness, although they may be reluctant to discuss these feelings with either adults or their peers. Some children with conduct disorder have experienced either physical or sexual abuse from their parents.

The following is a representative case history of a child with conduct disorder.

Heather, a 14-year-old girl, was brought to the child psychiatry clinic by her mother with the complaint that "Heather is getting out of hand. I just can't seem to discipline her anymore." Heather was the youngest of four children and the only girl in the family. She was the product of a normal pregnancy and delivery and had completed her developmental milestones on schedule. She had been an average student but had taken a particular interest in sports as a child. Her three older siblings were all boys, and she tended to tag along after them and play with them and their friends whenever they would permit. Her brother Tom, with whom she was closest, was 3 years older. Heather was noted to be somewhat stubborn and moody as a child and was occasionally defiant, but she had otherwise seemed completely normal.

Heather's father was a truck driver and was often away from the family, leaving the mother to rear the four children largely by herself. Heather's mother remained at home with the children until Heather was in second grade and then took a job as a clerk in a store. Both parents had completed high school and had similar expectations for their children. Although the two oldest boys had had some problems with drinking, using drugs, and truancy, both were able to complete high school. Both obtained jobs, married, and settled down. Tom, a high school senior, was currently showing behavior similar to that of his older brothers, but his school performance was adequate and he appeared to be due for graduation in the spring, with plans to join the military thereafter.

Heather's parents had separated and divorced 3 years earlier. This appeared to bother Heather much more than the boys, since she had always been "her father's little girl." Her father had developed a relationship with a woman in another city, had moved away, saw the children infrequently, and was not dependable in child support payments. Heather did not tell her sixth-grade friends about the separation and divorce for many months because she felt embarrassed and ashamed.

Heather's behavioral problems began when she entered junior high. She began to enter puberty in sixth grade, and by seventh grade her body was markedly feminized. Her mother reported that she seemed to react to this by "acting tougher instead of more like a girl." She started to hang out more with boys her own age or slightly older and began to smoke cigarettes secretly (although the evidence was smelled all over the house and on her clothes). Her grades, previously average, began to drop steadily. She also showed signs of increasingly devious behavior, lying to her mother about where she was going, returning at night well past predefined deadlines, and staying home "sick" without telling her mother (having called the school herself to report the "illness" in her mother's guise). Items that Heather could not afford began to appear in the house, such as expensive costume jewelry and cosmetics. Heather's mother suspected her of having stolen these things, but Heather insisted that they were gifts from friends. Several times marijuana was found in Heather's room. Whenever Heather's mother confronted her, Heather became angry and ran out of the house. Several times she stayed away overnight without telling her mother of her whereabouts.

When interviewed alone, Heather was initially evasive and defensive, looking at the floor and answering questions very briefly. She was an attractive, slightly overweight, dark-haired girl attired in conventional teenage garb with a slightly punk touch (multiple earrings in her ears, leather boots, sleeveless T-shirt showing a nude couple embracing and bearing the logo "too drunk to fuck"). Eventually she admitted to most of the conduct abnormalities that her mother described.

As a consequence of this assessment, it was concluded that Heather was indeed having difficulties, but that fortunately she had many strengths: a relatively intact childhood, normal intelligence, a history of adequate school performance, and a mother who appeared to genuinely care about her. Heather was seen in individual therapy on a weekly basis for 3–4 months, with a primary emphasis on supportive and relationship approaches. Heather responded well to this therapy and began to talk freely about her difficulties in adjusting to the loss of her father, her experience of puberty, and her confusion about whether it was better to relate to her male peers (from whom she desperately desired love and approval) as a "tough girl" or a "sexy girl." With Heather's permission, she was also seen jointly with her mother in family therapy, and on several occasions her older brother joined as well. Tom was able to assist his mother by assuming the role of a surrogate father and encouraging his "little sis" to be more honest, to attend school regularly, and to behave in ways that he and his older brothers could be proud of. Heather responded well to this increased attention and support, and it was possible to terminate the therapy successfully at the end of the school year.

Epidemiology.   Approximately 10% of males and 2% of females under the age of 18 years meet criteria for conduct disorder. The rate in females may be increasing.

Pathophysiology and etiology.   The etiology and pathophysiology of conduct disorder are almost certainly multifactorial. Family studies indicate that children with conduct disorder tend to come from families that have increased prevalence rates of antisocial personality disorder, mood disorder, substance abuse, and learning disorders. Adopted children may also have higher rates of conduct disorder, consistent with reports that the adopted offspring of female felons have a high rate of antisocial behavior, such as traffic violations or arrests for robbery, which suggests that there may be at least some genetic component to conduct disorder. Apart from a possible genetic component, no specific neurobiological factors have been identified in children with conduct disorders to any consistent degree, although a slight increase in neurological soft signs and psychomotor seizures has been observed.

Psychosocial factors probably play a major role in the development of conduct disorders. Psychosocial factors that have been shown to have some relationship to conduct disorders include parental separation or divorce; parental substance abuse; forms of poor parenting such as rejection, abandonment, abuse, inadequate supervision, and inconsistent or excessively harsh discipline; and association with a delinquent peer group.

Course and outcome.   The long-term course and outcome of conduct disorders are variable. To some extent, outcome depends on the degree of socialization and aggressiveness. Children with the "socialized" types of conduct disorder tend to have a much better outcome, as do children who are less aggressive. As children get older, the severity of the conduct disorder worsens in that teenagers or young adults get into increasingly serious problems that may eventually lead to incarceration. Nonetheless, between 25% and 40% of children with conduct disorders will develop adult antisocial personality disorder.

Differential diagnosis.   Conduct disorders have considerable comorbidity with other childhood disorders. Among those that often coexist with conduct disorder are learning disorders, ADHD, and mood disorders. These disorders will often be encountered as the clinician runs through a differential diagnosis for conduct disorder, because they are the ones that most commonly must be distinguished from conduct disorder. Sixty to seventy percent of the children who present with ADHD also meet criteria for conduct disorder. At least 10% of children with conduct disorder have specific learning disorders. In general, the greater the comorbidity, the more complicated the case, and the worse the outcome.

Treatment.   Treatment of conduct disorders varies greatly, depending on the age of the child, the symptoms with which he or she presents, the extent of comorbidity, the availability of family supports, and the child's intellectual and social assets. A relatively mild case of conduct disorder, such as was represented by Heather in the case history above, typically is treated with individual and family therapy. At the opposite extreme are those cases in which the child comes from a highly deviant family and engages in repeated antisocial acts that bring him or her to legal attention; such cases may require removal from the home and placement in a group home or perhaps even in a juvenile detention facility. Children and adolescents with conduct disorder who have comorbid disorders such as hyperactivity or seizures will benefit from medication to treat the comorbid condition; apart from such indications, however, medications are not typically used to treat patients with conduct disorder. Limit setting, consistency, and other techniques for behavioral management are essential components of the treatment of conduct disorder, both on the part of family members (when a supportive family is available) and on the part of the clinician. Testing limits and manipulating or defying the system are fundamental components of conduct disorder, and the clinician must be prepared to react to this behavior with firmness, but preferably without annoyance or rejection.

Oppositional Defiant Disorder

Oppositional defiant disorder is a relatively new diagnosis that attempts to provide a category for children and adolescents who demonstrate difficult behavior but who do not have full-blown conduct disorder. Since the establishment of this diagnosis, it has become apparent that many youngsters who would have been diagnosed as having good-prognosis or mild conduct disorder according to DSM-III are now being placed in this category. Table 22–8 summarizes the criteria for this disorder.

There is a fine line between normal naughtiness and oppositional defiant disorder. Most children lose their tempers, argue with their parents, refuse to clean their rooms, or fail to obey a curfew. Thus the proviso is added that these behaviors must be more frequent than those of most people at the same mental age. Clearly, however, there will be great variation in the definition of *more frequent*, depending on who is judging. Religiously conservative or authoritarian

Table 22–8. DSM-IV criteria for oppositional defiant disorder

A. A pattern of negativistic, hostile, and defiant behavior lasting at least 6 months, during which four (or more) of the following are present:

1. Often loses temper
2. Often argues with adults
3. Often actively defies or refuses to comply with adults' requests or rules
4. Often deliberately annoys people
5. Often blames others for his or her mistakes or misbehavior
6. Is often touchy or easily annoyed by others
7. Is often angry and resentful
8. Is often spiteful or vindictive

Note: Consider a criterion met only if the behavior occurs more frequently than is typically observed in individuals of comparable age and developmental level.

B. The disturbance in behavior causes clinically significant impairment in social, academic, or occupational functioning.

C. The behaviors do not occur exclusively during the course of a psychotic or mood disorder.

D. Criteria are not met for conduct disorder, and, if the individual is age 18 years or older, criteria are not met for antisocial personality disorder.

families are likely to be less tolerant of opposition and defiance than families with a background of behavioral abnormalities. Thus, to some extent, the appearance of children with this diagnosis in child psychiatry clinics may partially reflect a given family's threshold for accepting defiant behavior, which must be considered in treatment planning. Unlike conduct disorders, which specify that the child must have violated personal rights and social rules (making it more likely that the child's deviant behavior has come to the attention of people outside the immediate family), oppositional defiant disorder is defined almost totally on the basis of annoying, difficult, and disruptive behavior.

Because this is a new disorder, very little is known about its epidemiology, etiology, pathophysiology, comorbidity, and treatment. By definition, it cannot coexist with conduct disorder, but it may coexist with ADHD. Common sense dictates that management will emphasize individual and family counseling, with treatment of comorbid hyperactivity (or possibly mood disorder) with medications as needed.

Tourette's Disorder

Tourette's disorder is a condition that is characterized by the presence of multiple motor and vocal tics. By definition, there must be at least one form of vocal tic that has been present for at least 1 year. The vocal tics are most likely to cause psychological discomfort for the patient and to engage the attention of others. Vocal tics associated with Tourette's disorder most frequently consist of loud grunts or barks, but approximately 30% of the time they involve shouting words, and the words are sometimes obscenities such as "shit." The patient is aware that he or she is saying these phrases, is able to exert a mild degree of control over them, but ultimately has to submit to expressing them as an uncontrollable urge overwhelms him or her. Because of the patient's awareness, he or she finds the tics very embarrassing. Because the disorder is essentially unknown to the general public, the behavior is simply seen as inappropriate or bizarre. Motor tics include a variety of phenomena such as blinking, nodding, tongue protrusion, sniffing, or even squatting or hopping. The criteria for Tourette's disorder appear in Table 22–9.

Tourette's disorder usually begins during childhood or early adolescence, and motor tics usually antedate vocal tics. Thus, grade-school–aged children may display motor tics and some barks or grunts. During late grade school or early junior high, vocalization of obscenities (coprolalia) begins to appear. Twenty percent have a remission of motor and vocal tics during their third decade, and the majority of the remainder of the patients have a significant decrease in their symptoms as they grow older. Patients with Tourette's disorder may experience shame and embarrassment about their disorder, which may lead them to avoid public and social situations and even close interpersonal relationships.

Epidemiology.   Tourette's disorder is relatively rare, affecting 0.4% of the population. It is more common in males than in females, with a ratio of 3:1. As with

---

Table 22–9.   DSM-IV criteria for Tourette's disorder

A. Both multiple motor and one or more vocal tics have been present at some time during the illness, although not necessarily concurrently. (A *tic* is a sudden, rapid, recurrent, nonrhythmic, stereotyped motor movement or vocalization.)

B. The tics occur many times a day (usually in bouts) nearly every day or intermittently throughout a period of more than I year, and during this period there was never a tic-free period of more than 3 consecutive months.

C. The disturbance causes marked distress or significant impairment in social, occupational, or other important areas of functioning.

D. The onset is before age 18 years.

E. The disturbance is not due to the direct physiological effects of a substance (e.g., stimulants) or a general medical condition (e.g., Huntington's disease or postviral encephalitis).

ADHD, a gender threshold effect has been observed; that is, female patients with Tourette's disorder appear to have higher genetic loading than male patients with Tourette's disorder, suggesting that there is a lower penetrance for the disorder in females.

Pathophysiology and etiology. Tourette's disorder appears to be highly familial and appears to cotransmit with obsessive-compulsive disorder. The obsessive-compulsive phenomena tend to be more prominent in females in affected families, whereas the males manifest full-blown Tourette's disorder. These findings suggest that, in some instances, obsessive-compulsive behavior may be on a continuum with motor and vocal tic phenomena. The genetic pattern of transmission is not clear; in some, but not all, families it appears to follow an autosomal dominant pattern. The search for a Tourette's gene is under way.

For two decades it has been clear that symptoms of Tourette's disorder can be markedly improved through treatment with antipsychotic medication. Because these drugs exert a primary effect by blocking dopaminergic pathways in the brain, abnormalities in dopamine transmission are the most commonly hypothesized neurochemical abnormality. Because of the prominent motor component, investigators suspect that the primary abnormalities may lie within nigrostriatal projections, but given the complex feedback loops of the dopamine system (as described in Chapter 5), many other localizations are also possible.

Differential diagnosis. The evaluation of a patient presenting with Tourette's disorder should stress a comprehensive neurological evaluation to rule out other causes for the tics. The patient should be examined for stigmata of Wilson's disease, and a family history should be obtained to evaluate the possibility of Huntington's disease. An EEG is useful to rule out the possibility of seizure disorder. The patient should also be evaluated for other psychiatric conditions. Comorbidity with ADHD may occur, as may symptoms of mood disorder, anxiety disorders, or obsessive-compulsive disorder.

Treatment. The treatment of Tourette's disorder primarily stresses the use of neuroleptics. Haloperidol has been used for many years as the first-line treatment; doses are lower than those used to treat psychosis and tend to range from 1 to 5 mg/day. Pimozide, used for decades in Europe, is also effective; doses of 8–10 mg/day are used (maximum dose is 0.3 mg/kg/day, or a total of 20 mg/day). Although the treatment of Tourette's disorder stresses the use of medications, it is also important to educate the family about the disorder and to assist them in providing psychological support to the patient. Because of the social embarrassment that it produces, Tourette's disorder has the potential for serious long-term social complications, and supportive psychotherapy for the patient or family may assist in minimizing these problems.

Separation Anxiety Disorder

Separation anxiety disorder represents a more severe and disabling form of a maturational experience that all children normally have. Most infants and children experience fear at the possibility (or reality) of being separated from their parents. Once infants learn to recognize maternal and paternal faces and shapes, they also learn to cry when the parent leaves the room or hands them to a stranger. No doubt this pattern of behavior reflects some primal fear of loss or fear of the unknown. As the child grows older, he or she also experiences natural fears of being left with a baby-sitter, being sent to preschool, and entering kindergarten. Crying, tenseness, or physical complaints may appear and last for minutes, hours, or days in such situations.

As the DSM-IV criteria specify (see Table 22–10), separation anxiety disorder is defined largely by the persistence of such symptoms for a long enough duration to be considered pathological. Three from a list of eight characteristic symptoms must be present for at least 4 weeks. The characteristic symptoms include three types of distress or worry (distress at being separated from home, worry that some harm will come to the parents, and worry that the child will be lost or somehow separated from them), three types of behaviors (school refusal, sleep refusal, and clinging), and two physiological symptoms (nightmares and physical complaints such as headache or nausea).

Another clinically significant anxiety disorder observed in children is variously referred to as school phobia, school refusal, or school absenteeism. Although this particular anxiety disorder is classified among the adult disorders as a type of social phobia in DSM-IV, it is an important and common childhood anxiety disorder. In some cases, it may be related to separation anxiety disorder. Children with this problem develop a fear of going to school. It may begin with attendance at preschool or kindergarten, but more typically it develops during grade school or junior high. Typically, children who have previously been going to school (albeit with some anxiety) begin to develop methods for staying home. They may display repeated episodes of "illness" such as headache or nausea. Such children may be truant, leaving home with the appearance of going to school and then returning home without their parents' knowledge or going to some other environment that they experience as safe. They may simply refuse to go to school and give some vague explanation such as "I don't like it." These various reasons explain why the problem is variously referred to as a phobia, absenteeism, or

Table 22–10. DSM-IV criteria for separation anxiety disorder

A. Developmentally inappropriate and excessive anxiety concerning separation from home or from those to whom the individual is attached, as evidenced by three (or more) of the following:

1. Recurrent excessive distress when separation from home or major attachment figures occurs or is anticipated
2. Persistent and excessive worry about losing, or about possible harm befalling, major attachment figures
3. Persistent and excessive worry that an untoward event will lead to separation from a major attachment figure (e.g., getting lost or being kidnapped)
4. Persistent reluctance or refusal to go to school or elsewhere because of fear of separation
5. Persistently and excessively fearful or reluctant to be alone or without major attachment figures at home or without significant adults in other settings
6. Persistent reluctance or refusal to go to sleep without being near a major attachment figure or to sleep away from home
7. Repeated nightmares involving the theme of separation
8. Repeated complaints of physical symptoms (such as headaches, stomachaches, nausea, or vomiting) when separation from major attachment figures occurs or is anticipated

B. The duration of the disturbance is at least 4 weeks.

C. The onset is before age 18 years.

D. The disturbance causes clinically significant distress or impairment in social, academic (occupational), or other important areas of functioning.

E. The disturbance does not occur exclusively during the course of a pervasive developmental disorder, schizophrenia, or other psychotic disorder and, in adolescents and adults, is not better accounted for by panic disorder with agoraphobia.

Specify if:

Early onset: If onset occurs before age 6 years.

---

refusal. There is some controversy among child psychiatrists as to whether school refusal should be considered strictly a subset of separation anxiety disorder or should be defined more broadly to include all children who do not attend school, for whatever reason (e.g., truancy secondary to conduct disorder, avoidance of school as a complication of mood disorder, school avoidance secondary to a psychosis).

Once discovered, school avoidance should be thoroughly evaluated and treated as quickly as possible to prevent personal, social, and academic complications. The clinician should attempt to determine the reasons why the child does not want to go to school. These reasons may be expressed overtly (e.g., "the kids make fun of me because I'm stupid," "I'm afraid that Jimmy Taylor will beat me up"), but often considerable investigation will be needed. The child's intellectual and school performance should be evaluated to determine whether there is indeed some problem with academic skills, which may make the child feel inferior and avoidant. Teachers and parents need to be consulted about the child's relationships with his or her peers, and a specific effort should be made to determine whether there is a problem with teasing or bullying.

Other situations that children often find stressful may occur on the playground, in the gym, or in the school lunchroom. Young teenagers may be embarrassed about the appearance of their bodies, or they may be afraid that others will not sit with them in the lunchroom or on the bus. Clearly, the child's own self-esteem and self-concept need to be examined, and parental behavior needs to be explored to determine whether it is contributing to the child's problem or even causing it. Anxious, fearful, controlling parents may be communicating their own fears about separation to the child. They may be setting academic or social expectations so high that the child feels doomed to failure at school.

Treatment of school avoidance depends on the cause that has been identified. Often, the child will need encouragement and support from several directions: at home, at school, and from the clinician. If specific problems are identified with academic skills, remedial training should be initiated. Similar training may be appropriate for problems with athletic or social skills. Whatever the cause, however, it is important to impress on both the child and the family that the child must go to school regularly and that absenteeism and refusal will not be tolerated.

Other "Adult" Disorders
Frequently Seen in Children

Several other common adult disorders may have their first onset during childhood or adolescence. Because these are syndromally similar across all ages, they are classified among the adult disorders. Two common examples are schizophrenia and mood disorder. In general, children with these disorders meet the criteria that have been defined for adults. There may be subtle differences in presentation and management, however.

Schizophrenia often presents initially during adolescence, but there are rare instances when the onset is during childhood. Schizophrenia in adolescents often begins insidiously, with apathy, a change in personal hygiene, and withdrawal. Schizophrenia may be particularly difficult to distinguish from depression, and it is usually preferable to make an initial diagnosis of depression if there is any doubt; after an unsuccessful trial of several different antidepressants, the diagnosis of schizophrenia is more certain. The major challenge in assessing childhood schizophrenia involves determining the difference between normal childhood fantasies and frank delusions and hallucinations. In addition, the symptoms of disorganization of speech and behavior must be distinguished from abnormalities of speech and behavior that are simply due to developmental slowness or mental retardation. Children with a definite diagnosis of schizophrenia are usually treated with neuroleptic medications, but the dose is typically lower than that in adults.

Depression in adolescents is extremely common, and it is also more common in children than was thought several decades ago. A major difference between the two ages of onset is in suicide risk: the risk is high in adolescents, but much lower in children. In both age groups the patient may present initially with physical complaints rather than the psychological complaint of depression. In young children, the complaints may be abdominal pain, nightmares, or trouble sleeping. In teenagers, complaints of fatigue, insomnia or hypersomnia, headache, or tension are common. Depression may also present initially as a disruptive behavior disorder. The somatic treatment of depression in children and adolescents is similar to that in adults, but the need for psychotherapy or family therapy is much greater.

Physical, Emotional, and Sexual Abuse

Attitudes toward the abuse of children have evolved dramatically during the past several decades. The variability in attitudes toward the rights of children versus those of adults is a striking example of the extent to which the definitions of both mental illnesses and general medical disorders are culture bound. Until this century few adults anywhere in the world considered the possibility that children (or women, for that matter) might have any rights at all. Disciplining children through whipping and beating was considered to be good for them and to build character. Corporal punishment was routine not only at home, but also within the schools. The climate has changed—and is still changing—so rapidly that corporal punishment *even by parents* has been outlawed in Sweden, and teachers, physicians, and social workers in the United States are trained to be alert for signs of physical and emotional abuse in the children they see.

Within Western society, sexual activity in children was considered abnormal and was vigorously repressed until very recently. ("Masturbation will lead to blindness," as children and teenagers were sometimes taught as recently as 30 or 40 years ago.) At the other extreme, initiation into sexuality at the time of puberty, often by an older relative, has been and is still the norm in some non-Western societies. Thus, it is difficult to formulate absolute and immutable rules as to what constitutes physical, emotional, and sexual abuse and how this abuse should be assessed and treated. Nevertheless, these forms of abuse are of increasing concern to psychiatrists and primary care providers, who often must assume frontline responsibility for recognizing and managing them.

Given the problems of definition, the epidemiology of physical and emotional abuse is at best uncertain. Nevertheless, this abuse is common, and it may be increasing rather than decreasing. The National Center on Child Abuse recently estimated that 2%–3% of children have experienced abuse; approximately two thirds of the cases involved neglect, and approximately one quarter involved physical abuse.

Children who have experienced *physical or emotional abuse* are more likely to present with physical than psychological symptoms. At the farthest extreme is the child who has obvious signs of physical abuse—broken bones, cigarette burns, bruises, scars, and open wounds. The signs of physical neglect or emotional abuse may be more subtle—failure to thrive; somatic complaints such as abdominal pain, sleep disturbances, and nightmares; and marked anxiety and exaggerated startle responses. The physician who notices such signs and suspects abuse must proceed both carefully and appropriately; excessive vigilance in either overdiagnosing or underdiagnosing can lead to problems. The child should be carefully evaluated on several consecutive appointments, accompanied by tactful interviewing of both the child and the parents or caregivers concerning behavioral difficulties, disciplining practices, feeding and bathing routines, and other key aspects of parent-child interactions. If the evidence of physical or emotional abuse is consistent and clear, then social service agencies should be contacted to conduct further investigations.

The treatment of abuse varies depending on its nature. In extreme cases, the child is removed from the home and placed in foster care. Ideally, such children and their foster parents should be provided with supportive individual and family therapy to assist in recovery from the consequences of the abuse. Cases involving milder forms of abuse, with the child remaining in the home, should receive careful follow-up. Parents may need evaluation and treatment for problems that they are experiencing (e.g., depression, alcoholism, drug abuse), and family or marital therapy may assist in identifying interpersonal problems that trigger the abuse. Depending on the child's age and the nature of the problems, the child will also benefit from individual therapy that focuses on building confidence and coping with problems in feeling basic trust.

Sexual abuse is perhaps an even murkier area than physical and emotional abuse. Guidelines for norms in this area are also steadily evolving. On the one hand, in some subcultures, incest between siblings or between parents and children is common and is conveniently overlooked. On the other hand, some grandfathers are beginning to worry about being accused of child sexual abuse if they kiss and cuddle with their grandchildren. The definition of what constitutes sexual abuse is unclear on many fronts. Rape of a stepdaughter by a stepfather is obvious. So is seduction of a child by a teacher that involves sexual intercourse. So is a sex or prostitution ring organized by a "friendly neighbor" who frequently invites the neighborhood girls or boys to his house and rewards them with small gifts such as cosmetics, compact disc players, or drugs. But how many of the following also constitute child sexual abuse: frequent exposing of genitalia by a parent or stepparent of the opposite sex, children and parents getting into bed together on Sunday morning and reading together, taking children into opposite-sex locker rooms at a swimming pool after the age of 3 or 4 years, and intercourse between a 21-year-old male and a 16-year-old (or 12-year-old) female?

The epidemiology of sexual abuse is also unclear. Variable definitions obviously affect prevalence rates. Depending on the definition and the methods for assessment, lifetime prevalence rates range from 15% to as high as 70%. It is clear, however, that girls are more frequently victims than boys, probably with a ratio of approximately 5:1.

Assessment of sexual abuse in children involves careful history taking, accompanied by a physical examination. The methods for history taking vary depending on the age of the child and the way that he or she has come to attention. If a mother brings in a child complaining about abuse by a stepfather, the situation may be relatively straightforward (although one must be cautious about being caught in marital or other interpersonal cross fire even in such "obvious" situations). Younger children may lack the concepts or vocabulary to discuss their experiences, but can explain them through storytelling or the use of anatomically explicit dolls. Older children can usually describe their experiences more directly. A physical examination should be conducted (with the child's permission), and the child may be able to explain what has happened more easily in the context of this examination. Unfortunately, the exam will not necessarily confirm the diagnosis unless obvious evidence (e.g., semen) is found.

Although it was once safe to assume that a child would not make up allegations of abuse, media attention to this issue and the ugly quarrels that may occur in divorce cases have made it clear that the clinician must approach the stories of both adults and children with some caution and skepticism.

The long-term emotional impact of childhood sexual abuse is not clear. Reports of posttraumatic stress disorders and various personality disorders (e.g., borderline personality) secondary to childhood sexual abuse are steadily increasing. One must remember the early experience of Freud in relation to reports of childhood sexuality; originally, he believed the accounts of parental seduction that his patients reported, but he later realized that he was often hearing wish-fulfilling fantasies rather than actual experiences. Nevertheless, children who are clearly the victims of obvious and/or repeated abuse are likely to be significantly traumatized. Treatment varies depending on the situation. Most of the guidelines outlined above for physical and emotional abuse also apply to sexual abuse.

Management of Child and Adolescent Disorders

General suggestions for the management of disorders occurring in children and adolescents appear in the box.

Recommendations for management of children and adolescents

1. In assessing children and adolescents, be imaginative and meet each patient on his or her own terms.
   - Play games to evaluate problem-solving and motor skills.
   - Use dolls and toys with young children to create pretend situations that will provide insight about personal and social interactions.

2. Remember that normal maturational levels are highly variable in children and adolescents.

3. Remember that children and adolescents often do not have a level of cognitive development suitable for the insight-oriented and introspective approaches used with adults.

4. Establishing rapport with adolescents is difficult, but may be crucial to creating a therapeutic alliance.
   - Find out what the patient is interested in and relate to him or her through these interests.

5. Don't preach or judge.

6. Remember that the basic maturational task of adolescents is to disengage themselves from their parents, become independent, and define their own identities; reliance on peers is an important crutch for adolescents in this transitional period.

7. Remain neutral; try not to criticize either parents or peers.

8. Most work with adolescents will carry an inevitable transference component; the adolescents' first reaction will be to see you as a parent. You need to try to use this transference to a therapeutic advantage, or at least to prevent it from being a therapeutic handicap.

9. It is best to strike a balance between being perceived as a good parent or a good peer, but this balance cannot and should not (usually) be achieved by attacking the real parent or real peer.

10. Because the parents and peers of adolescents may vary in quality, the therapist needs to be flexible, insightful, and creative in dealing with transference components.

11. Be aware of the pervasiveness of comorbidity in childhood adolescent disorders.

Recommendations for management of children and adolescents
(continued)

- The more diagnoses there are, the more complicated the management.
- Drugs used for one condition may be detrimental to another condition (e.g., psychostimulants prescribed for attention-deficit/hyperactivity disorder [ADHD] may worsen Tourette's disorder; anticonvulsants prescribed for seizure may be sedating and affect school performance or worsen ADHD).
- Because comorbid disorders often interact with one another, identifying one that is serious and highly treatable may have a major impact on outcome (e.g., aggressive assistance with learning disorders may prevent the worsening of mild conduct disorders or school phobias).

12. Be prepared to use a team approach and to combine a variety of assessment and therapeutic techniques when working with most children and adolescents.
- Disorders often impinge on many aspects of the child's life (e.g., relationship with parents, relationships with peers, educational achievement).
- Special skills not possessed by physicians may be needed for management (e.g., consultation with an educational specialist).
- Use of cotherapists is often helpful in working with the patient and his or her family, because both need to feel that their special needs are being recognized and that they are receiving support and assistance.

Bibliography

Anderson JC, Williams S, McGee R, et al: DSM-III disorders in preadolescent children—prevalence in a large sample from the general population. Arch Gen Psychiatry 44:69–76, 1987

August GJ, Stewart MA: Is there a syndrome of pure hyperactivity? Br J Psychiatry 140:305–311, 1982

August GJ, Stewart MA, Holmes CS: A four-year follow-up of hyperactive boys with and without conduct disorder. Br J Psychiatry 143:192–198, 1983

Bailey AJ, Bolton P, Butler L, et al: Prevalence of the fragile X anomaly amongst autistic twins and singletons. J Child Psychol Psychiatry 34:673–688, 1993

Baroff GS: Mental Retardation—Nature, Cause and Management. New York, Hemisphere, 1986

Behar D, Stewart MA: Aggressive conduct disorder: the influence of social class, sex and age on the clinical picture. J Child Psychol Psychiatry 25:119–124, 1984

Berg I: School phobia in children of agoraphobic women. Br J Psychiatry 128:86–89, 1976

Biederman J, Munir K, Knee D, et al: High rate of affective disorders in probands with attention deficit disorder and in their relatives—a controlled family study. Am J Psychiatry 144:330–333, 1987

Campbell M, Green WH, Deutsch SI: Child and Adolescent Psychopharmacology. Beverly Hills, CA, Sage, 1985

Cantwell DP, Baker L: Developmental Speech and Language Disorders. New York, Guilford, 1987

Cohen D, Bruun R, Leckman J: Tourette's Syndrome. New York, Wiley, 1988

Cohen D, Donnellan A, Rhea P (eds): Handbook of Autism and Pervasive Developmental Disorders. New York, Wiley, 1987

Deutsch CK, Swanson JM, Bruell JH, et al: Overrepresentation of adoptees in children with the attention deficit disorder. Behav Genet 12:231–238, 1982

Famularo R, Fenton T: The effect of methylphenidate on school grades in children with attention deficit disorder without hyperactivity—a preliminary report. J Clin Psychiatry 48:112–114, 1987

Gittleman R: Anxiety Disorders of Childhood. New York, Guilford, 1986

Green WH, Campbell M, Hardesty AS, et al: A comparison of schizophrenic and autistic children. Journal of the American Academy of Child Psychiatry 4:399–409, 1984

Kanner L: Autistic disturbances of affective contact. Nervous Child 2:217–250, 1943

Kelso J, Stewart MA: Factors which predict the persistence of aggressive conduct disorder. J Child Psychol Psychiatry 27:77–86, 1986

Last CG, Francis G, Hersen M, et al: Separation anxiety and school phobia—a comparison using DSM-III criteria. Am J Psychiatry 144:653–657, 1987

Offord DR, Bennett KJ: Conduct disorder: long-term outcomes and intervention effectiveness. J Am Acad Child Adolesc Psychiatry 33:1069–1078, 1994

Pauls DL, Leckman JF: The inheritance of Gilles de la Tourette's syndrome and associated behaviors. N Engl J Med 315:993–997, 1986

Piven J, Nehme E, Siman J, et al: Magnetic resonance imaging in autism: measurement of the cerebellum, pons, and fourth ventricle. Biol Psychiatry 31:491–504, 1992

Popper CW: Disorders usually first evident in infancy, childhood, or adolescence, in The American Psychiatric Press Textbook of Psychiatry. Edited by Talbott JA, Hales RE, Yudofsky SC. Washington, DC, American Psychiatric Press, 1988, pp 649–735

Porrino LJ, Rapoport JL, Behar D, et al: A naturalistic assessment of the motor activity of hyperactive boys, I: comparison with normal controls. Arch Gen Psychiatry 40:681–687, 1983

Puig-Antich J: Major depression and conduct disorder in prepuberty. Journal of the American Academy of Child Psychiatry 21:118–128, 1982

Rapoport JL, Buchsbaum MS, Weingartner H, et al: Dextroamphetamine—its cognitive and behavioral effects in normal and hyperactive boys and normal men. Arch Gen Psychiatry 37:933–943, 1980

Rapoport JL, Conners CK, Reatig N: Rating scales and assessment instruments for use in pediatric psychopharmacology research. Psychopharmacol Bull 21:713–1125, 1985

Rumsey JM, Andreasen NC, Rapoport JL: Thought, language, communication, and affective flattening in autistic adults. Arch Gen Psychiatry 43:771–777, 1986

Rutter M: Pathways from childhood to adult life. J Child Psychol Psychiatry 8:1–11, 1989

Rutter M, Taylor E, Hersov L: Child and Adolescent Psychiatry, 3rd Edition. Oxford, England, Blackwell Scientific Publications, 1994

Shapiro E, Shapiro AK, Fulop G, et al: Controlled study of haloperidol, pimozide, and placebo for the treatment of Gilles de la Tourette's syndrome. Arch Gen Psychiatry 46:722–730, 1989

Stewart MA, deBlois S: Diagnostic criteria for aggressive conduct disorder. Psychopathology 18:11–17, 1985

Stewart M, Kelso J: A two-year follow-up of boys with aggressive conduct disorder. Psychopathology 20:296–304, 1987

Tsai L, Stewart MA, August G: Implication of sex differences in the familial transmission of infantile autism. J Autism Dev Disord 11:165–173, 1981

Yu S, Pritchard M, Kremer E, et al: Fragile X genotype characterized by an unstable region of DNA. Science 252:1179–1181, 1991

Self-Assessment Questions

1. Describe some techniques that are useful in assessing younger children and establishing rapport with them.
2. Describe some techniques that are useful in assessing adolescents and establishing rapport with them.
3. List the various types of nonphysician clinicians who may be helpful in assessing and managing children and adolescents; describe the types.
4. Give four examples of conditions that often are comorbid in children and adolescents.
5. What IQ range defines children within 1 standard deviation of the population mean of 100? What percentage of children fall in this range? What IQ range encompasses children between 1 and 2 standard deviations from the mean? What percentage of the population falls in this range? List the IQ levels that are used to define borderline intelligence and mild, moderate, severe, and profound mental retardation. Discuss the distinction between autism, mental retardation, and learning disorders. List three well-recognized causes of mental retardation.
6. Why is it important to obtain IQ testing and educational testing in some chil-

dren and adolescents? Describe three situations where the use of such testing may be crucial either to establishing a diagnosis or to planning treatment.

7. List three disorders of childhood or adolescence that may be comorbid with a seizure disorder and for which an EEG may be a useful laboratory assessment procedure.

8. List three disorders of childhood or adolescence for which karyotyping may be useful.

9. Describe four simple tests to assess soft neurological signs in children.

10. Define learning disorder and list the three skills that are commonly affected. How common is developmental dyslexia, and what is its sex ratio?

11. Describe the three major domains that are abnormal in autism, and give examples of signs and symptoms within these domains. How common is autism? What are its long-term course and outcome? What methods are used to treat it?

12. List the two broad categories of symptoms used to define ADHD, and give several examples of each. Describe the long-term course and outcome of ADHD. Identify two medications commonly used to treat ADHD and specify the appropriate dosage range.

13. Describe the four basic symptom categories of conduct disorder. What are the prevalence and sex ratio for conduct disorder? What are the long-term course and outcome of conduct disorder? Give two different case vignettes of conduct disorder, and describe appropriate treatment for each.

14. Describe the clinical features of Tourette's disorder. What are the hypothesized pathophysiology and etiology of this disorder? How common is it? Describe two pharmacological strategies for treating Tourette's disorder.

15. Describe oppositional defiant disorder and discuss its relationship to conduct disorder.

16. Describe separation anxiety disorder and discuss its relationship to school refusal (phobia, avoidance). List three factors that may predispose to the development of school avoidance. Describe three approaches to treating school avoidance.

17. Why do you think most disorders of childhood and adolescence are more common in boys than in girls? (The answer to this question is not really included in the chapter, and if you can come up with a definitive answer, you may be on your way to winning a Nobel prize.)

Chapter 23

Sleep Disorders

The woods are lovely, dark and deep.
But I have promises to keep,
and miles to go before I sleep.

Robert Frost

Sleep disorders are among the most common complaints that people report to physicians. More than 50 million Americans have sleep-related complaints, and about 20% of patients consulting a general practitioner report sleep disturbances. Insomnia is the most common sleep disorder; each year between 20% and 50% of adults report difficulty sleeping, and about 17% consider the problem serious. Because sleep disorders are so common, it is important for clinicians to be familiar with them.

The classification and management of sleep disorders have evolved over the past decade as physicians and researchers have learned more about them. DSM-IV divides the sleep disorders into two major subgroups: the *dyssomnias* and the *parasomnias*. The predominant disturbance in dyssomnias is in initiating and maintaining sleep. The predominant disturbance in parasomnias is an abnormal event occurring during sleep. A category exists for *sleep disorders related to another mental disorder*, such as major depression or borderline personality disorder. A residual category also exists for other sleep disorders that may result from a general medical condition or the direct physiological effects of a substance. The sleep disorders are listed in Table 23–1.

Although the diagnostic criteria do not include data from laboratory proce-

Table 23–1.   DSM-IV sleep disorders

Dyssomnias
- Primary insomnia
- Primary hypersomnia
- Narcolepsy
- Breathing-related sleep disorder
- Circadian rhythm sleep disorder
- Dyssomnia not otherwise specified

Parasomnias
- Nightmare disorder (dream anxiety disorder)
- Sleep terror disorder
- Sleepwalking disorder
- Parasomnia not otherwise specified

Sleep disorders related to another mental disorder
- Insomnias related to an Axis I or Axis II disorder
- Hypersomnia related to an Axis I or Axis II disorder

Other sleep disorders
- Sleep disorder due to a general medical condition
- Substance-induced sleep disorder

---

dures such as polysomnography (a procedure in which electroencephalographic [EEG], electrooculographic, and electromyographic tracings are recorded during sleep), these data may be necessary in some patients to thoroughly investigate their disorder. An extensive discussion of the physiology of the various sleep stages is beyond the scope of this text. However, a basic understanding of the sleep stages is helpful in learning about the different sleep disorders.

Normal Sleep and Sleep Architecture

The average healthy adult requires about 7½ hours of sleep per night, although some persons require more and some less to feel sufficiently rested. Normal sleep can be influenced by a variety of factors; for example, young persons require more sleep than elderly persons, who show a decrease in total sleep time due to frequent awakenings. Further, the longer a person has been awake, the more quickly he or she falls asleep (i.e., sleep latency).

Sleep stages are divided into rapid eye movement (REM) sleep and non-rapid eye movement (NREM) sleep. These two stages of sleep alternate with one another in a cycle that lasts between 70 and 100 minutes. There are generally four to six NREM/REM cycles nightly. Although the first REM period lasts from

5–10 minutes, REM periods tend to become longer and closer together and show progressively greater density of rapid eye movements.

The sleep stages are as follows:

Stage 0 is a period of wakefulness with eyes closed, which occurs just before sleep onset. The EEG mainly demonstrates sinusoidal alpha waves, which have a frequency of 8–12 cycles per second (CPS) and a fairly low amplitude (or voltage). Beta waves (13–35 CPS) are intermixed. Muscle tone tends to be increased. Alpha activity decreases with increasing drowsiness.

Stage 1 is called the sleep-onset stage, because it provides a brief transition from wakefulness to sleep. Alpha activity diminishes to less than 50% of the EEG recording. There is a low-amplitude, mixed-frequency signal, comprised mostly of beta and the slower theta (4–8 CPS) activity. Stage 1 accounts for about 5% of the total sleep period.

Stage 2 generally represents the onset of true sleep and is dominated by theta activity. High-voltage delta waves (1–4 CPS) may comprise up to 20% of EEG activity. This stage is also characterized by the appearance of two types of intermittent events. *Sleep spindles* are a brief burst of rhythmic (12–14 CPS) waves with a duration of $\frac{1}{2}$ to $1\frac{1}{2}$ seconds. They may persist into stages 3 and 4, but are not seen in REM sleep. *K complexes* may also occur; these are sharp, negative, high-voltage EEG waves, followed by slower, positive activity. They are thought to represent central nervous system evoked responses to internal stimuli; they can also be elicited during sleep with external stimuli, such as loud noises. Muscle tone is increased, but eye movements are absent. Stage 2 usually accounts for between 45% and 55% of the total sleep time.

Stage 3 is characterized by 20%–50% high-voltage delta wave activity. Increased muscle tone is present, but eye movements are absent. This stage accounts for about 15%–20% of the sleep period. Stage 3 is often combined with stage 4, due to the lack of documented physiological differences between the stages. Collectively, stages 3 and 4 are often referred to slow-wave sleep, delta sleep, or deep sleep.

Stage 4 is defined by high-voltage delta waves comprising more than 50% of the EEG recording. Increased muscle tone may be present, but there are no eye movements. This stage accounts for about 15%–20% of the total sleep period.

REM sleep is characterized by an EEG recording similar to that in stage 1, along with a burst of rapid conjugate eye movements and a reduced level of muscle activity. REM sleep comprises between 20% and 25% of the total sleep period and is also known as desynchronized sleep.

Figure 23-1 depicts a polysomnographic recording during the various stages of sleep.

A normal young adult goes from waking into a period of NREM sleep lasting

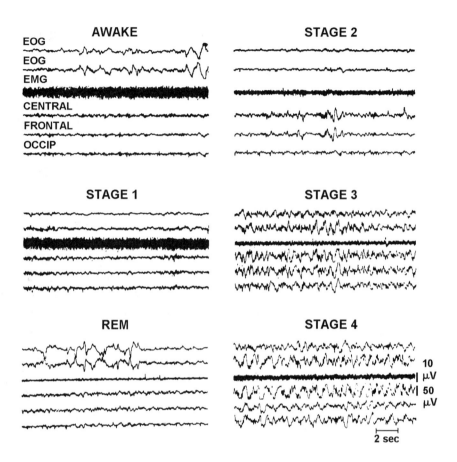

Figure 23-1.   Polysomnographic recording during the various stages of sleep. Notice the high electromyogram (EMG) and eye movements during wakefulness, the slow eye movements but absence of rapid eye movements (REMs) during descending stage 1, and REMs with low EMG during stage REM. Stages 2, 3, and 4 are characterized by the slowing of frequency and an increase in amplitude of the electroencephalogram (EEG). Reprinted with permission from Bixler EO, Vela-Bueno A: Normal sleep: physiological, behavioral, and clinical correlates. Psychiatric Annals 17:437–445, 1987.

approximately 90 minutes before the first REM period; this portion of NREM sleep is referred to as REM latency. In an ideal situation, the sequence of sleep stages is as follows: NREM stages 1, 2, 3, 4, 3, and 2; at this point the first REM period occurs, followed by a repetition of NREM stages 2, 3, 4, 3, and 2 and then another REM episode.

The sleep cycle (REM time to REM time) is shorter in infants than in adults. REM periods emerge every 50–60 minutes during the sleep of infants and gradually increase to the adult sleep cycle length of 70–100 minutes during adolescence. At birth, REM and NREM periods are equally dispersed throughout the sleep period; as the person ages, REM periods become more confined to the final third of the night. Figure 23-2 depicts typical sleep architecture and demonstrates the effects of age on the various stages of sleep.

Although the biochemistry and neuroanatomy of sleep are not well understood, serotonin-containing nuclei and pathways play an important role in regulating NREM sleep, and noradrenergic systems are principally involved in the control of REM sleep. The serotonin-containing neurons are mainly located in the group of nuclei in the lower midbrain and upper pons, referred to as the *raphe nuclei*. Activation of these neurons regulates NREM sleep. This knowledge is based on animal models in which destruction of the raphe nuclei induces total insomnia and on models in which animals were injected with parachlorophenylalanine, which inhibits serotonin synthesis.

Noradrenergic neurons are found throughout the brain stem, but achieve their highest concentration in the *locus coeruleus* in the pons. The locus coeruleus is thought to regulate REM sleep; this inference is primarily based on animal research in which lesions of neurons in the locus coeruleus abolish REM sleep and lead to hyperactive behavior. REM suppression is brought about by injecting animals with α-methylparatyrosine, a substance that inhibits the synthesis of norepinephrine.

Acetylcholine also plays a major role in sleep, and the reciprocal interaction between serotonergic and noradrenergic systems on the one hand and cholinergic systems on the other hand may underlie the basic oscillation of the NREM-REM cycle.

Dyssomnias

The essential feature of these disorders is a disturbance in the amount, quality, and timing of sleep. The dyssomnias include the *insomnias,* which are disorders of initiating or maintaining sleep or of not feeling rested after sleep; *hypersomnias,* or disorders of excessive daytime sleepiness or sleep attacks; *breathing-related sleep abnormalities*; and *circadian rhythm sleep disorder,* in which there is a mismatch between the person's sleep-wake pattern and the pattern that is normal for his or her environment. The category *dyssomnias not otherwise specified* is used when a dyssomnia is present but cannot be better classified.

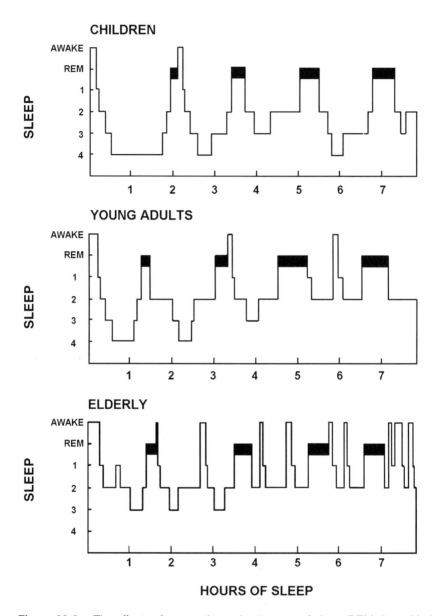

Figure 23-2. The effects of age on the various stages of sleep. REM sleep *(darkened area)* occurs cyclically throughout the night at intervals of approximately 90 minutes in all age groups. REM sleep shows little variation in the different age groups, whereas stage 4 sleep decreases with age. In addition, the elderly have frequent awakenings and a marked increase in total wake time. Reprinted with permission from Bixler EO, Vela-Bueno A: Normal sleep: physiological, behavioral, and clinical correlates. Psychiatric Annals 17:437–445, 1987.

Primary Insomnia

Primary insomnia is characterized by difficulty initiating or maintaining sleep, or having nonrestorative or nonrestful sleep, for at least 1 month, which is not due to another mental disorder, a general medical condition, or the direct physiological effects of a substance (see Table 23–2). The subjective report of poor or nonrefreshing sleep may or may not be associated with any objective sleep disturbance, and may not accurately reflect the magnitude of the objective disturbances of sleep when they are present. The objective evidence of disturbed sleep is often relatively minor, because subjective estimates of sleep latency and total sleep time tend to exaggerate the degree of any disturbance present. Many persons with primary insomnia are reported to be anxious worriers, who exhibit increased alertness and hyperarousal.

As indicated earlier, insomnia is relatively common in the general population and is even more common among psychiatric patients; yet only a small proportion of those persons with insomnia consult a physician. Sleep difficulty occurs more frequently as people age, in women, among individuals of lower educational and socioeconomic status, and in persons with chronic or multiple medical problems.

The duration of insomnia is the most helpful factor in evaluating the patient's problem. Transient insomnia (no more than a few nights) typically occurs in persons who usually sleep normally. This form of insomnia occurs at times of acute psychological stress, such as during bereavement. Other situations typically associated with transient insomnia include a hospital admission, a public-speaking engagement, and a scheduled examination. In these cases, insomnia is rarely brought to medical attention, because it is not regarded as pathological and tends to correct itself.

Primary insomnia lasts more than 4 weeks and is more likely to come to a

Table 23–2. DSM-IV criteria for primary insomnia

A. The predominant complaint is difficulty initiating or maintaining sleep, or nonrestorative sleep, for at least 1 month.

B. The sleep disturbance (or associated daytime fatigue) causes clinically significant distress or impairment in social, occupational, or other important areas of functioning.

C. The sleep disturbance does not occur exclusively during the course of narcolepsy, breathing-related sleep disorder, circadian rhythm sleep disorder, or a parasomnia.

D. The disturbance does not occur exclusively during the course of another mental disorder (e.g., major depressive disorder, generalized anxiety disorder, a delirium).

E. The disturbance is not due to the direct effects of a substance (e.g., a drug of abuse, a medication) or a general medical condition.

physician's attention. An estimated one-third to one-half of patients with chronic insomnia have an underlying psychiatric disorder that is responsible for the disturbance; therefore, they do not have primary insomnia. Sleep disorders associated with specific mental disorders are discussed later in the chapter.

The patient with primary insomnia requires a thorough medical and psychiatric evaluation (see Table 23–3). The medical history should include a detailed review of drug and medication use. It may be helpful to have the patient maintain a sleep log. Patients should record their bedtime, sleep latency (estimated time required to fall asleep), awake time, number of awakenings, daytime naps, and use of drugs or medications. It may be useful to interview the bed partner to learn about the presence of snoring, breathing difficulties, and leg jerks.

"Sleep hygiene" measures have been developed for patients with chronic insomnia. These measures include the following:

- Waking up and going to bed at the same time every day, even on weekends
- Avoiding long periods of wakefulness in bed
- Not using the bed as a place to read, watch television, or work
- Leaving the bed and not returning until drowsy if sleep does not begin within a set period (such as 20–30 minutes)
- Avoiding napping
- Exercising at least three or four times a week (but not in the evening if this interferes with sleep)
- Discontinuing or reducing the consumption of alcoholic beverages, beverages containing caffeine, cigarettes, and sedative-hypnotic drugs

Table 23–3. Sleep history outline

Elicit sleep data during assessment: obtain data from patient, chart, and nursing staff
Review medication history, including illicit drugs, alcohol, and use of hypnotic medication
Obtain information on the following sleep characteristics:

- Usual sleep pattern
- Characteristics of disturbed sleep (for insomnia, difficulty falling asleep, difficulty staying asleep, and early-morning awakenings)
- The clinical course: onset, duration, frequency, severity, and precipitating and relieving factors
- 24-hour sleep-wake cycle (corroborate with staff and chart)
- History of sleep disturbances, including childhood sleep pattern and pattern of sleep when under stress
- Family history of sleep disorders
- Personal history of other sleep disorders
- Sleep pattern at home as described by bed partner

Some aspects of the program may be difficult for the patient, such as quitting smoking; other aspects, such as caffeine withdrawal, may lead to temporary headaches and sluggishness. However, patients who are motivated to improve their daytime functioning are generally willing to make an effort to follow these simple measures.

Although sedative-hypnotic medications (i.e., sleeping pills) do not cure insomnia, they can provide dramatic temporary relief. They should be thought of as an adjunctive measure only for transient and short-term insomnia, in the context of a doctor-patient relationship and in combination with the sleep hygiene steps outlined above. Although they may be of benefit initially, intermediate to long-term benefits are unpredictable and hard to document. Furthermore, some patients may become dependent on them. In general, the benzodiazepines are the main choice for reasons of safety and efficacy; they have relatively few side effects, and most have a low potential for addiction. Tolerance to their sleep-promoting effects appears to develop less often than it does with barbiturates, barbiturate-like compounds, and antihistamines. A new alternative to the benzodiazepines is zolpidem, which appears to produce little tolerance; it does not impair daytime alertness or cause rebound insomnia, problems often associated with benzodiazepines. Further details about the rational use of benzodiazepines and zolpidem are found in Chapter 26.

Other compounds are frequently used as sleeping aids. Chloral hydrate is a nonbarbiturate sedative-hypnotic, known more for the fact that it is markedly potentiated by alcohol and forms the basis for knockout drops (i.e., a Mickey Finn). Certain antihistamines, such as diphenhydramine, hydroxyzine, and doxylamine, are used as hypnotic agents, but they are not as potent as the benzodiazepines. Sedative antidepressants, such as amitriptyline or doxepin, are often used in low doses at bedtime as hypnotic agents for patients with primary insomnia. Because of their potential danger in overdose, it is best to avoid them as hypnotics. Most over-the-counter sleeping aids contain relatively low doses of an anticholinergic agent or antihistamine and are not very effective.

Primary Hypersomnia

Although excessive daytime somnolence is less common than insomnia, it still affects about 5% of the adult population, including similar numbers of men and women. According to DSM-IV, the excessive sleepiness lasts at least 1 month, as evidenced by either prolonged sleep episodes or daytime sleep episodes occurring almost daily; the excessive sleepiness causes significant impairment or distress; and it is not accounted for by another sleep disorder, a general medical condition, or the direct physiological effects of a substance (see Table 23–4).

Table 23–4.   DSM-IV criteria for primary hypersomnia

A. The predominant complaint is excessive sleepiness for at least 1 month (or less if recurrent) as evidenced by either prolonged sleep or daytime sleep episodes occurring almost daily.

B. The excessive sleepiness causes clinically significant distress or impairment in social, occupational, or other important areas of functioning.

C. The excessive sleepiness is not better accounted for by insomnia and does not occur exclusively during the course of another sleep disorder (e.g., narcolepsy, breathing-related sleep disorder, circadian rhythm sleep disorder, or a parasomnia) and cannot be accounted for by an inadequate amount of sleep.

D. The disturbance does not occur exclusively during the course of another mental disorder.

E. The disturbance is not due to the direct physiological effects of a substance (e.g., a drug of abuse, medication) or a general medical condition.

Specify if:

Recurrent: If there are periods of excessive sleepiness lasting at least 3 days occurring several times a year for at least 2 years

---

Primary hypersomnia usually involves prolonged, but polysomnographically normal, nocturnal sleep and continual daytime drowsiness. Nearly one-half of the patients report sleep drunkenness (i.e., excessive grogginess) on wakening, which may last for hours. Patients may report taking one or two naps daily (which can last more than an hour), unlike the short naps of narcoleptic patients.

Treatment of primary hypersomnia involves a combination of sleep hygiene measures, stimulant drugs, and maintenance of a daily log of sleep hours. Naps may need to be included, according to the patient's needs and ongoing responsibilities. Stimulants may be helpful in maintaining wakefulness, particularly dextroamphetamine and methylphenidate, both of which have relatively short half-lives and must be taken in multiple divided doses. Pemoline, a longer-acting stimulant, is also used. Nonsedating tricyclic antidepressants (e.g., protriptyline) have also been reported to be helpful. Unfortunately, because stimulants carry substantial abuse potential, their use needs to be carefully monitored.

One of our patients had this condition; his case is described below.

Chris, a 24-year-old college student, was being treated for obsessive-compulsive disorder, consisting mainly of intrusive and unwanted thoughts of harming others. On paroxetine, a serotonin reuptake inhibitor, his symptoms were minimal.

Although obsessive-compulsive disorder was his main complaint, his mother, who usually accompanied him to the clinic, reported that his excessive sleeping and napping were even more of a problem. She described how Chris would typically sleep 12–14 hours nightly and often took afternoon naps. Chris admitted he was frequently late for class, often fell asleep in class, and was too sleepy to study in the evening.

Chris was referred to a sleep disorders clinic. His polysomnography was normal, and as there was no evidence of sleep attacks, cataplexy, sleep paralysis, or hypnogogic hallucinations, he received a diagnosis of primary hypersomnia. He was treated with methylphenidate. On this regimen, he was able to remain awhile and alert most of the day, without napping. He was more alert in class, and his academic performance improved.

Narcolepsy

Narcolepsy is an unusual condition characterized by excessive sleepiness associated with irresistible sleep attacks that occur either as the only symptoms or perhaps in combination with one or more auxiliary symptoms including cataplexy, sleep paralysis, and hypnagogic hallucinations. This condition affects about 1 in 1,000 persons; men and women are equally affected.

The symptoms of narcolepsy are quite striking in that the sleep attacks may last from a few seconds to half an hour or more and may be precipitated by sedentary and monotonous activity, such as watching television. However, narcoleptic patients may experience sleep attacks at work, during conversations, or under other circumstances normally considered stimulating, such as having sexual intercourse. Up to 80% of narcoleptic patients experience episodes of *cataplexy*, in which sudden loss of muscle control occurs. This may cause the person to collapse (as if fainting) without loss of consciousness. This loss of muscle tone may occur in reaction to strong emotional experiences, such as laughter or surprise.

Sleep paralysis and hypnogogic hallucinations are less frequent than cataplexy. Both symptoms have a relatively brief duration and occur during the transitional period between wakefulness and sleep. *Sleep paralysis* causes a temporary loss of muscle tone with a resulting inability to move. *Hypnogogic hallucinations* are vivid hallucinatory perceptions, usually visual or auditory, that occur while one is falling asleep. Although these symptoms occur infrequently in psychiatrically normal persons, patients with narcolepsy may experience them as often as several times a week. These auxiliary symptoms generally appear several years after the onset of sleep attacks. The exact mechanism for these symptoms is unknown, but sleep attacks and other narcoleptic symptoms appear to be closely related to the neurophysiological mechanisms underlying REM sleep. Narcolepsy may have a hereditary basis, because up to half of patients with narcolepsy have a first-degree relative with the disorder.

A careful sleep history is helpful in making the diagnosis of narcolepsy, as are descriptions provided by parents, spouses, and bed partners. The diagnosis is relatively easy to make when the auxiliary symptoms (e.g., cataplexy) are present. Polysomnographic recordings are indicated when the diagnosis is unclear or when a breathing-related sleep disorder is suspected. Persons with narcolepsy tend to have REM at sleep onset rather than after 90–120 minutes, which is more normal. Patients may have additional psychiatric or psychological problems due to the severe consequences that narcolepsy may have on the patient's family life, job situation, and social interactions; these problems will also need exploration.

The management of narcolepsy involves separate treatments for sleep attacks and for the auxiliary symptom of cataplexy. Stimulants, particularly methylphenidate, are the preferred drugs for treating sleep attacks because of their prompt action and relative lack of side effects. Methylphenidate is given in multiple divided doses starting with 5 mg; the dose may be gradually increased to 60 mg. Tricyclic antidepressants are often used. These drugs tend to alleviate sleep paralysis, but have little effect on sleep attacks. The dose for controlling the sleep disorder is much lower than that used for treating depression (e.g., imipramine 10–75 mg nightly).

The physician needs to explain the nature of the disorder to the patient and his or her family. Social acquaintances and employers may also need education to understand that the symptoms of narcolepsy are beyond the patient's volitional control. The cooperation of an employer can be enormously helpful, as one or two brief naps daily may reduce job difficulties and decrease the dose requirement for stimulant medication. Patients need to be warned that an occurrence of symptoms while driving or engaging in other activities requiring constant alertness could be dangerous, just as epileptic patients need to be warned. Physicians should learn their state and local laws regarding the legal responsibility for reporting narcoleptic patients.

Breathing-Related Sleep Disorder

Several conditions lead to sleep disruption caused by distorted breathing mechanisms. These conditions are important because of their potentially serious medical, social, and psychological consequences. This form of sleep disorder is generally called *sleep apnea*. Sleep apnea is characterized as central, obstructive, or of mixed origin. Central apnea presents a failure of the respiratory center to initiate sufficient peripheral respiratory effort. In obstructive apnea, respiratory efforts persist, but are rendered ineffective by upper-airway blockage. Obstructive apnea is more common than central apnea.

Breathing-related sleep disorder is characterized by episodes of breathing cessation for 10 seconds or more during sleep; these episodes can occur 30 or more times during the night. Other nocturnal signs include snoring, gasping and snorting sounds, excessive body movements, night sweats, and morning headaches. Daytime symptoms include excessive sleepiness or sleep attacks. The disorder can have severe psychological consequences, including a general slowing of thought processes, memory impairment, and inattention. Patients frequently develop anxiety, depressed mood, or multiple physical complaints. The typical patient with sleep apnea is an overweight, middle-aged man who snores heavily, is prone to hypertension, and has excessive daytime sleepiness.

A thorough medical evaluation is a necessary part of the assessment and may include a sleep laboratory evaluation with recording of respiration and monitoring of nocturnal oxygen desaturation. Because surgery may be the therapy of choice when obstructive apnea is present, sleep laboratory data must be accurate and complete. In mild cases, obese patients are urged to reduce their weight, which may be sufficient to relieve the apnea. Tricyclic antidepressant medication (e.g., protriptyline at doses between 10 and 60 mg nightly) has been used; there are reports that buspirone may also be beneficial. Benzodiazepines should not be used due to their tendency to inhibit alerting responses and depress respiration at higher doses.

In severe cases, continuous positive airway pressure applied through the nostrils can be helpful; surgical options include removal of excess tissue in the pharynx and tracheotomy.

Circadian Rhythm Sleep Disorder (Sleep-Wake Schedule Disorder)

Disrupted sleep may be caused when the sleep-wake cycle is not correctly synchronized with a person's daily schedule. For example, persons with night shift work or frequently changing shift work (e.g., nurses, factory workers) may develop circadian rhythm sleep disorder. Persons who travel frequently and cross time zones also develop disrupted sleep, commonly known as *jet lag*. Persons with these disorders may never feel rested. When they want to sleep, they cannot, and when they are expected to be awake and alert, they may be excessively sleepy and drowsy.

The best way to avoid these problems is to avoid shift work. Industrial plants have gradually become more aware of these problems, and many have redesigned their schedules, finding that productivity has increased and personnel turnover has decreased. Because some persons will always be intolerant to shifting work schedules and will have chronic fatigue as a result, they should probably be urged to seek other types of employment.

Persons who travel frequently probably cannot avoid jet lag. Because of the human circadian time-keeping system (which has an innate period of about 25 hours), it is usually easier for persons to adjust when the cycle is lengthened, rather than shortened, traveling west rather then east. Because the internal system is normally longer than the solar day, by traveling east, persons must impose a shorter day on themselves, creating even greater demand than usual on the circadian time-keeping system.

The treatment for jet lag, other than tincture of time, involves the recommendation that usual sleep hours be maintained in the new time zone. Conventional wisdom is that it takes about 1 day to adjust to each eastward time zone crossed, and slightly less after westward travel. Travelers may minimize the loss of sleep by judicious use of low doses of hypnotic agents and by avoiding alcohol and other substances that interfere with sleep.

Parasomnias

Parasomnias consist of sleepwalking (or somnambulism), night terrors, and nightmares. All three disorders are relatively common in children, but they rarely lead to medical attention unless they are frequent and intense. These disorders resolve by late adolescence in most cases; when a parasomnia persists into adulthood, it should be brought to the attention of a psychiatrist.

Nightmare Disorder (Dream Anxiety)

This condition consists of repeated awakenings with detailed recall of extended and extremely frightening dreams, typically involving threats to survival, security, and self-esteem (see Table 23–5). The awakenings usually occur in the second half of the sleep period. On awakening, the person rapidly becomes alert and oriented. This condition is estimated to affect as many as 5% of the general population, and it can become chronic.

Table 23–5. DSM-IV criteria for nightmare disorder (dream anxiety disorder)

A. Repeated awakenings from the major sleep period or naps with detailed recall of extended and extremely frightening dreams, usually involving threats to survival, security, or self-esteem. The awakenings generally occur during the second half of the sleep period.

B. On awakening from the frightening dreams, the person rapidly becomes oriented and alert (in contrast to the confusion and disorientation seen in sleep terror disorder and some forms of epilepsy).

C. The dream experience, or the sleep disturbance resulting from the awakening, causes clinically significant distress or impairment in social, occupational, or other important areas of functioning.

D. The nightmares do not occur exclusively during the course of another mental disorder (e.g., a delirium, posttraumatic stress disorder) and are not due to the direct physiological effects of a substance (e.g., a drug of abuse, a medication) or a general medical condition.

Nightmares tend to occur during REM sleep and may take place at any time during the night. They are more frequent in the second half of the night, when REM cycles are increased in frequency and duration. In childhood, nightmares are often related to specific developmental phases and are particularly common during the preschool and early school years. In that age group, children may be unable to distinguish reality from dream content.

Nightmares have also been associated with febrile illness and delirium, particularly in elderly and chronically ill persons. Withdrawal from certain drugs, such as the benzodiazepines, may also result in nightmares. The increase in REM sleep after withdrawal of barbiturates or alcohol may be associated with a temporary increase in the intensity of dreaming and nightmares. More recently, the serotonin reuptake inhibitors (e.g., sertraline, paroxetine) have been associated with vivid dreams.

The main differential diagnoses for nightmare disorder are the presence of a psychiatric illness that could lead to nightmares (e.g., major depression), the effects of a medication, or withdrawal from medication. When the psychiatric illness is diagnosed and treated, the nightmares may disappear. Nightmares caused by psychologically traumatic events may respond to short-term counseling.

Sleep Terror Disorder

Night terrors, or *pavor nocturnus*, are a sudden, partial arousal from delta sleep associated with screaming and frantic motor activity. According to DSM-IV, these episodes occur during the first third of the major sleep episode and begin with a terrifying scream followed by intense anxiety and signs of autonomic hyperarousal, such as tachycardia and rapid breathing (see Table 23–6). Persons with night terrors may not fully awaken after an episode and usually have no

Table 23–6.   DSM-IV criteria for sleep terror disorder

A. Recurrent episodes of abrupt awakening from sleep, usually occurring during the first third of the major sleep episode and beginning with a panicky scream.

B. Intense anxiety and signs of autonomic arousal, such as tachycardia, rapid breathing, and sweating, during each episode.

C. Relative unresponsiveness to efforts of others to comfort the person during the episode.

D. No detailed dream is recalled, and there is amnesia for the episode.

E. The episodes cause clinically significant distress or impairment in social, occupational, or other important areas of functioning.

F. This disturbance is not due to the direct physiological effects of a substance (e.g., a drug of abuse, a medication) or a general medical condition.

detailed recall of the event the following morning. Any attempt to restrain the person may result in injury either to the person suffering the terrors or to the person attempting the restraint.

The cause of night terrors is unknown, but they often co-occur with sleepwalking, which is discussed later. Both conditions tend to be familial and are present in a high percentage of first-degree relatives. The disorders may begin in childhood and terminate by late adolescence; when the episodes occur frequently or present in late adolescence or adulthood, it is likely that significant psychopathology will be found, such as an anxiety or mood disorder.

Sleepwalking (Somnambulism)

Sleepwalking is also considered a disorder of impaired arousal. It is more likely to occur in children than in adults. Nearly 15% of children have had at least one episode of sleepwalking, whereas fewer than 3% experience night terrors. Fewer than 5% of healthy adults have a problem with sleepwalking.

Sleepwalking is defined as repeated episodes of arising from sleep and walking about. It usually occurs during the first third of the sleep episode (see Table 23–7). During sleepwalking, the person generally has a blank stare, is relatively unresponsive to the efforts of others to communicate, and can only be awakened with great difficulty. On awakening, the person has amnesia for the episode and within minutes is generally alert and oriented. The episodes of sleepwalking and night terrors generally occur within 3 hours of falling asleep. EEG recordings show extremely high amplitude slow waves preceding the muscular activation that triggers the attack; sleepwalking occurs in association with stages 3 and 4 NREM sleep.

Table 23–7.   DSM-IV criteria for sleepwalking disorder

A. Repeated episodes of rising from bed during sleep and walking about, usually occurring during the first third of the major sleep episode.

B. While sleepwalking, the person has a blank, staring face, is relatively unresponsive to the efforts of others to communicate with him or her, and can be awakened only with great difficulty.

C. On awakening (either from the sleepwalking episode or the next morning), the person has amnesia for the episode.

D. Within several minutes after awakening from the sleepwalking episode, there is no impairment of mental activity or behavior (although there may initially be a short period of confusion or disorientation).

E. The sleepwalking causes clinically significant distress or impairment in social, occupational, or other important areas of functioning.

F. The disturbance is not due to the direct physiological effects of a substance (e.g., a drug of abuse, a medication) or a general medical condition.

Sleepwalking episodes typically last less than 10 minutes. Persons may move about clumsily without purpose, and they are indifferent to their environment. Sleepwalkers usually have the ability to maneuver around objects and perform simple tasks such as opening doors or windows, a fact that makes sleepwalking so potentially dangerous.

The most important consideration in managing patients with sleepwalking or night terror episodes is protection from injury. Attempts to actively interrupt episodes should be avoided, because intervention may confuse or frighten the patient. Special precautions may include placing latches on outside doors and bedroom windows and moving sleep accommodations to the first level. Parents need to be told that their child's problem will probably be outgrown by late adolescence. In adults, sleepwalking is often associated with the presence of a major psychiatric disorder, such as depression.

Certain drugs that suppress stages 3 and 4 sleep, primarily the benzodiazepines, may be prescribed for adults with sleepwalking or night terrors. Relapse is likely when the drugs are discontinued, particularly at times of stress. Tricyclic antidepressants may also be effective in reducing the frequency of sleepwalking and night terror episodes. Improved sleep hygiene may lead to the resolution of minor disorders.

Sleep Disorders Related to Another Mental Disorder

This category was created to acknowledge the fact that sleep disorders are regularly associated with specific mental disorders, including psychotic, mood, and anxiety disorders. Sleep disorders may also be related to a general medical condition or the direct physiological effects of a substance. When a relationship can be demonstrated, the patient should receive a diagnosis of *sleep disorder related to another mental disorder* or *other sleep disorder* if related to a general medical condition or substance use. A summary of typical sleep disorders related to other conditions follows.

Psychoses

The primary sleep disturbances in psychotic patients are insomnia and excessive sleepiness. Schizophrenic patients, for instance, may experience severe disruption of their sleep during psychotic episodes. Changes include reduced total sleep time, variability in REM time, and increased REM density. A reduction in stage 4 NREM sleep is the most frequently replicated finding.

Mood Disorders

The insomnia of depression is typically described as early morning awakening (i.e., waking earlier than usual and being unable to fall back asleep). Hypersomnia is sometimes observed, particularly in patients with bipolar depression or dysthymia. Manic and hypomanic patients may go without sleep or have shorter sleep durations due to their reduced need for sleep.

Polysomnographic changes in sleep in depressed patients may include prolonged sleep latency, increased nocturnal awakenings, and early-morning awakenings; diminished slow-wave sleep (stages 3 and 4); and changes in REM sleep, including the occurrence of REM sleep earlier in the night (i.e., shortened REM latency) and increased frequency of eye movements during REM sleep.

Table 23–8. Common EEG sleep characteristics in mental disorders

Diagnosis	General sleep findings
Psychoses	
Schizophrenia	Marked variability in sleep continuity Reduced REM sleep after REM sleep deprivation Reduced slow-wave sleep
Mood disorders	Sleep continuity disturbances Decreased slow-wave sleep Shifting of REM sleep to earlier in the night
Anxiety disorders	Difficulty falling asleep Difficulty staying asleep Reduced total sleep time
Panic disorder	Difficulty falling asleep Difficulty staying asleep Reduced total sleep time Sleep "panic attacks" may occur during stage 2 or 3 sleep
Alcoholism	
Acute use	Reduced wakefulness and REM sleep, with increased delta sleep in first half of the night, rebound of REM sleep, and increased wakefulness in second half of the night
Chronic use	Fragmented sleep with frequent arousals
Abstinence	Continued fragmentation and reduced slow-wave sleep
Personality disorders	
Borderline	REM sleep changes may be related to concurrent mood disorder
Dementia	Sleep continuity disruptions Polyphasic sleep-wake schedule

Note. REM = rapid eye movement.
Source. Adapted from Nofzinger EA, Buysse DJ, Reynolds CF, et al: Sleep disorders related to another mental disorder: a DSM-IV literature review. J Clin Psychiatry 54:244–255, 1993.

Anxiety Disorder

Anxiety disorders are frequently associated with delayed sleep onset or trouble remaining asleep. Polysomnographic features include nonspecific changes in sleep latency, decreased sleep efficiency, increased amounts of stages 1 and 2 sleep, and decreased slow-wave sleep.

Posttraumatic stress disorder may lead to insomnia and disturbing dreams, but polysomnographic changes are not specific. Panic disorder may be associated with sudden awakenings from sleep, which may be the main complaint. Polysomnographic features include marginally increased sleep latency and decreased sleep efficiency.

Alcohol Abuse or Dependence

Alcohol dependence may lead to insomnia or excessive sleepiness. The effects of alcohol differ depending on use. Acute use induces sleepiness and reduces wakefulness for the first 3–4 hours of sleep, with subsequent increases in wakefulness and anxiety dreams in the latter half of the night. With chronic use, sleep becomes fragmented, with short periods of deep sleep interrupted by brief arousal periods. With abstinence, sleep is initially disrupted; insomnia and nightmares

Table 23–9. Medical and neurological conditions and substances associated with sleep disorders

Medical and neurological disorders	Drugs
Alzheimer's disease	Antidepressants
Angina	Antipsychotics
Asthma	Lithium
Coronary artery disease	Sedative-hypnotics
Diabetes mellitus	Anticonvulsants
Dysthymias	Opioids
Eczema	Psychostimulants
Gastrointestinal reflux	Hallucinogens
Hypertension	Alcohol
Hyperthyroidism	
Myotonic dystrophy	
Muscular dystrophy	
Paroxysmal nocturnal hemoglobinuria	
Peptic ulcer disease	
Pregnancy	
Obstructive lung disease	
Progressive supranuclear palsy	
Pain syndromes	
Shy-Drager syndrome	
Uremia	

may occur. Sleep improves over time, but light sleep and increased vulnerability to other sleep-disrupting factors may persist even after 2 weeks of abstinence.

Other Psychiatric Disturbances

Delirium may lead to agitation, combativeness, and wandering during early-evening or nighttime hours. Clinically, sleep may be fragmented with frequent awakenings, initial insomnia, or early-morning awakenings The polysomnographic findings include sleep fragmentation, lower sleep efficiency, decreased stages 3 and 4 sleep, and a decreased percentage of REM sleep.

Table 23–8 summarizes EEG sleep characteristics in mental disorders.

Treatment recommendations for sleep disorders

1. For accurate diagnosis, a thorough sleep history is essential including:
   - Drug use pattern
   - Use of caffeine
   - An interview with the patient's bed partner
2. For patients with insomnia, the sleep hygiene measures outlined in this chapter in the section "Primary Insomnia" are the simplest and most overlooked strategy.
3. Complaints of disturbed sleep should alert the clinician to the possibility of a major psychiatric illness. Depression and alcoholism are probably the most common causes of sleep disturbance.
4. Prescribing benzodiazepine hypnotics for patients with sleep complaints is inappropriate without having first made a diagnosis. For primary insomnia, patients should be told that the sleeping pills are for temporary use only.
5. Temazepam and estazolam probably have the best therapeutic properties for a hypnotic: rapid absorption, lack of metabolites, and an intermediate half-life that will allow a full night's sleep. Zolpidem is a good alternative to the benzodiazepine hypnotics.
6. In patients with narcolepsy or primary hypersomnia, methylphenidate is the first medication to use. Titrate up to 60–80 mg/day. Keep track of pill use, because some patients may be tempted to abuse them.
7. If patients have unusual sleep complaints or disorders, a referral should be made to a sleep disorders clinic for a more complete evaluation, which may include polysomnography.

Sleep Disorders Due to a General Medical Condition or Substances Other Than Alcohol

A variety of medical and neurological conditions may lead to disturbed or disrupted sleep. Examples are hypertension or cardiovascular insufficiency, hyperthyroidism, rheumatological conditions, Parkinson's disease, esophageal reflux, asthma, and head injury. Patients with coronary artery disease may report that anginal pain and breathing problems disrupt their sleep; patients with arthritis may report that a painful joint prevents them from sleeping well. Pregnant women may experience difficulty sleeping due to urinary frequency, fetal movements, and trouble finding a comfortable position.

A variety of substances, both legal and illegal, have the ability to disturb sleep. For example, persons who abuse stimulants (e.g., cocaine) may have difficulty falling or remaining asleep. Prescription medication may also lead to sleep disturbance; for example, a patient with a seizure disorder taking carbamazepine may report excessive sleep. A variety of medical conditions and substances can cause sleep disturbances; a list of the more common ones appears in Table 23–9.

Bibliography

Coleman R, Roffwarg H, Kennedy S, et al: Sleep-wake disorders based on polysomnographic diagnosis—a national cooperative study. JAMA 247:997–1003, 1982

Culebras A: Update on disorders of sleep and the sleep-wake cycle. Psychiatr Clin North Am 15:467–486, 1992

Dahl RE: The pharmacologic treatment of sleep disorder. Psychiatr Clin North Am 15:161–178, 1992

Driver HS, Shapiro CM: ABC of sleep disorders and parasomnias. Br Med J 306:921–923, 1993

Ford DE, Kamerow DB: Epidemiologic study of sleep disturbances and psychiatric disorders: an opportunity for prevention? JAMA 262:1479–1484, 1989

Gillin JC, Byerley WF: The diagnosis and management of insomnia. N Engl J Med 322:239–248, 1990

Jacobs EA, Reynolds CF, Kupfer DJ, et al: The role of polysomnography in the differential diagnosis of chronic insomnia. Am J Psychiatry 145:346–349, 1988

Kales A, Madow L: Office management of sleep disorder patients. Psychiatric Annals 17:479–483, 1987

Kales A, Soldatos CR, Kales JD: Sleep disorders: insomnia, sleepwalking, night terrors, nightmares, and enuresis. Ann Intern Med 106:582–592, 1987

Kales A, Vela-Bueno A, Kales JD: Sleep disorders: sleep apnea and narcolepsy. Ann Intern Med 106:434–443, 1987

Kyger H, Roth T, Dement WO (eds): Principles and Practice of Sleep Medicine. Philadelphia, PA, WB Saunders, 1989

Lugares E, Zucconi M, Bixler EO: Epidemiology of sleep disorders. Psychiatric Annals 17:446–453, 1987

Morin CM, Culbert JP, Schwartz SM: Non-pharmacological interventions for insomnia: a meta-analysis for treatment efficacy. Am J Psychiatry 151:1172–1180, 1994

Nofzinger EA, Buysse DJ, Reynolds CF, et al: Sleep disorders related to another mental disorder: a DSM-IV literature review. J Clin Psychiatry 54:244–255, 1993

Regestein QR, Dambrosia J, Hallett HM, et al: Daytime alertness in patients with primary insomnia. Am J Psychiatry 150:1529–1534, 1993

Regestein QR, Monk TH: Is the poor sleep of shift workers a disorder? Am J Psychiatry 148:1487–1493, 1991

Reynolds CF, Kupfer D (eds): Sleep disorders, in American Psychiatric Press Review of Psychiatry, Vol 13. Edited by Oldham J, Riba M. Washington, DC, American Psychiatric Press, 1994, pp 619–777

Reynolds CF, Kupfer DJ, Buysse DJ, et al: Subtyping DSM-III primary insomnia: a literature review by the DSM-IV work group on sleep disorders. Am J Psychiatry 148:432–438, 1991

Salin-Pascuel RJ, Roehrs TA, Merlott LA, et al: Long-term study of the sleep of insomnia patients with sleep state misperceptions and other insomnia patients. Am J Psychiatry 149:904–908, 1992

Shapiro CM, Flanigan MJ: ABC of sleep disorders-function of sleep. Br Med J 306:383–385, 1993

Waterhouse J: ABC of sleep disorders: circadian rhythms. Br Med J 306:448–451, 1993

Williams RL, Karacan I, Moore CA (eds): Sleep Disorders: Diagnosis and Treatment, 2nd Edition, New York, Wiley, 1988

Young T, Palta M, Dempsey J, et al: The occurrence of sleep disordered breathing among middle-aged adults. N Engl J Med 328:1230–1235, 1993

Self-Assessment Questions

1. What are the major categories of sleep disorders?
2. Describe the different dyssomnias.
3. What are sleep hygiene measures?
4. What are the REM and NREM stages? What is their significance?
5. Describe the appropriate use of hypnotic agents. Which are preferred?
6. Distinguish between nightmare disorder and sleep terrors.
7. Does sleepwalking have the same significance in a child that it does in an adult? Describe simple measures that can be taken to reduce the chance of injury in the sleepwalker.
8. How is hypersomnia managed?
9. Do other psychiatric disorders, such as depression, disrupt sleep? What about general medical conditions or substances?

Chapter 24

Legal Issues in Psychiatry

Lawsuit, n. a machine which you go into as a pig and come out as a sausage.

Ambrose Bierce, Devil's Dictionary

Psychiatrists have a unique role among medical specialists regarding the law, because they have regular contact with lawyers, courts, and legal issues. Whether they like it or not, psychiatrists must regularly confront sensitive issues. Should this patient be committed to the hospital for treatment against his or her will? Should this patient be forcibly medicated? Can I release information to my patient's parents without his or her permission? These are examples of situations that nonpsychiatric physicians rarely encounter.

Because our society values individual freedom and civil liberties, questions about involuntary hospitalization, the right to treatment (or the right to refuse treatment), confidentiality, and other legal issues have no easy answers. What may seem right may not be legally permissible. What may be legal may not make any practical sense. The right of a man with schizophrenia to live on the streets, for instance, loses its meaning when he clearly has lost his capacity to make important decisions. Thus, the psychiatrist often gets caught in the middle between what may be legally right (i.e., leaving the schizophrenic patient to fend for himself on the streets) and what may be ethically right (i.e., bringing the schizophrenic patient to the hospital for proper care). Because of this interface with the law, physicians treating psychiatric patients need to have an understanding of fundamental legal issues and the typical problems they will face as practitioners.

615

Legal issues pertaining to mental illness are best conceptualized by dividing them into three broad categories: civil, criminal, and personal issues. *Civil issues* have primarily to do with involuntary hospitalization, the right that patients have to treatment (as well as the right to refuse treatment), and a patient's competency to assist in treatment decisions. *Criminal issues* tend to focus on a patient's competency to stand trial or to bear criminal responsibility (i.e., whether the person accused of a crime is legally competent or insane). *Personal issues* involve a wide range of problems that have to do with the doctor-patient relationship and include confidentiality, informed consent, and malpractice (Table 24–1).

In this chapter, we focus primarily on civil and personal issues, because these are the problems that physicians are most likely to encounter in their day-to-day work. Although we will touch on criminal issues, persons seeking comprehensive information are referred to *Clinical Psychiatry and the Law.* Forensic psychiatry, a subspecialty within psychiatry, focuses on the interface between psychiatry and the law. Psychiatrists working in this subspecialty spend much of their time dealing with criminal issues, including testifying in court and examining persons to determine criminal responsibility; most practicing psychiatrists rarely encounter these issues.

Although general legal principles and concepts may be universal across the United States, specific laws differ from state to state and even from region to region within a state, depending on how the law is interpreted. Furthermore, laws are always being changed by legislatures or being reinterpreted by courts. Therefore, it is essential to become familiar with relevant laws that apply in one's region.

Civil Law

A fundamental responsibility of psychiatrists is to provide for the safety of both their patients and others who may be affected by their patients. Therefore, if a

Table 24–1.   Categories of legal issues affecting psychiatrists

Civil	Personal
• Involuntary hospitalization	• Physician-patient relationship
• Right to treatment	• Confidentiality
• Right to refuse treatment	• Informed consent
Criminal	• Malpractice
• Competency to stand trial	
• Competency to bear criminal responsibility	

patient is believed to be a threat to self or others and refuses hospitalization, the psychiatrist will have to seek a court order for involuntary hospitalization, or *civil commitment*. In the past, it was relatively easy for a psychiatrist to have a patient committed to a hospital, usually with a signature or a phone call. Legislatures and courts have gradually backed away from the once freewheeling nature of mental health commitment. In response to the civil rights movement, which included the rights of mentally ill persons, most states now carefully regulate civil commitment for the purpose of inpatient psychiatric care. The appropriateness of this shift toward an emphasis on civil rights versus the right to humane care has been hotly debated. It is sometimes said that the homeless are being allowed to "die with their rights on."

Most commitment laws employ the concepts of mental illness, dangerousness, and disability. First, the law requires the presence of mental illness, although the precise definition of mental illness may differ from place to place. A diagnosis of personality disorder, for example, may be insufficient for commitment in some areas; a diagnosis of alcoholism or substance abuse may not be accepted in other areas. The law may specify that the mental illness be treatable, which may complicate matters, because many disorders are only partially treatable, and some untreatable disorders are still very dangerous. The concept of dangerousness usually requires that persons be an imminent danger to themselves or others. An example would be a patient who is thought likely to commit suicide or homicide within the next 24 hours if not hospitalized. Evidence of past dangerousness is usually insufficient for commitment. Because physicians are unable to accurately predict dangerousness except in the most obvious of situations, this requirement can be difficult to apply. Disability is a measure of patients' inability to properly care for themselves by virtue of their mental illness. Some states use the term *gravely disabled* to imply that persons are unable to take care of personal grooming and dress, to take adequate hydration, and to feed themselves. This criterion has only recently been added as an alternative to dangerousness for the purpose of commitment. Clearly, persons who are gravely disabled may not be in imminent danger of harming themselves, but they still need hospitalization and treatment.

Most states allow for patients to be hospitalized on an emergency basis to provide short-term intervention; this period may range from 1 to 20 days. Civil commitments either after the emergency hospitalization or on direct petition from the community provide for a longer period of involuntary hospitalization. These commitments are done with judicial approval and due process protection. In most states, a variety of due process protections for mentally ill persons are standard. These include an adequate notice of legal action, the right to a timely hearing, the right to appear at all legal proceedings, the right to be represented by an attorney, formal rules of evidence, and privilege against self-incrimination. The burden of proof is placed on the state to establish the reason for commitment, and the patient is guaranteed the right to appeal. These requirements contribute to the tension between the individual's need for legal protection and the desire of society to provide necessary treatment.

These due process protections differ substantially among the states. Thus, in many areas, hearsay testimony is admissible, and hearings may be closed to the public and conducted in treatment facilities; a hearing officer may be used rather than a judge or jury. In Iowa, for example, civil commitment hearings are conducted informally in the hospital, and formal rules of evidence do not apply. The case is presented to a hospitalization magistrate, who makes a decision based on "clear and convincing evidence," not on the more strict standard of "beyond a reasonable doubt." The hearing is not thought of as an adversarial proceeding, and the decision is supposed to favor the best interest of the patient. Once committed, the patient is deemed incapable of participating in treatment decisions, which the physicians are then empowered to make.

Outpatient commitment, which is now permitted in many states, is generally recommended for chronically noncompliant patients, most of whom are severely mentally ill. Because noncompliance will result in rehospitalization, patients have an incentive to follow through on treatment plans. We personally have found that outpatient commitments can be enormously helpful in the care of many chronically ill patients and have seen how these commitments can reduce the frequency of their hospitalizations.

In the past, many patients were involuntarily hospitalized, and there was no explicit right to receive treatment. Although most patients can be helped, a substantial number of involuntarily hospitalized patients are unlikely to improve with any treatment. The person with antisocial personality disorder, for instance, may be mentally ill and dangerous, but no proven treatments exist for the condition. Paralleling the decisions about right to treatment have been legal decisions about the right to refuse treatment. Thus, a person may be involuntarily hospitalized and still be deemed competent to refuse treatment. Psychiatrists find this situation particularly frustrating and ironic; an ill and dangerous person may be involuntarily hospitalized and under their care, yet they are powerless to provide treatment.

A great deal of litigation has concerned the right of civilly committed persons to refuse psychotropic medication in nonemergency situations. (Voluntarily hospitalized patients have almost always been allowed to refuse medication except in emergency situations.) Much of this concern has centered on antipsychotic medication, due to the potential risk of serious side effects such as tardive dyskinesia. Unfortunately, some courts have emphasized the potential risk of treatment rather than its potential benefit; some have even elevated treatment with antipsychotic medication to the status of an "extraordinary" form of medical therapy requiring special judicial scrutiny. In some states, a patient retains the right to refuse medication until the medical treatment team has petitioned the local court to declare the patient incompetent to consent to or refuse medication. In other states, such as Iowa, physicians are permitted to medicate patients on the basis of the commitment hearing alone.

As a practical matter, when should the clinician make a decision to involuntarily hospitalize a patient? The most typical scenario is that the police bring a person alleged to be mentally ill to the emergency room. The psychiatrist is then contacted to assess the patient and to make an appropriate decision about disposition. If the person is deemed mentally ill, dangerous, and/or disabled and refuses hospitalization, the decision is relatively easy to make: the hospitalization magistrate is contacted, and an order for involuntary hospitalization is sought. From the physician's perspective, it is probably better to err on the side of safety rather than to allow someone who is potentially dangerous to leave the emergency room.

Another common scenario occurs when a patient admitted voluntarily requests discharge but is thought to be a continuing danger to self or others (e.g., a person who has admitted to having suicidal plans). In these situations, a court order should be sought for continued hospitalization.

Personal Issues

Confidentiality

Maintaining confidentiality is one of the most important obligations the psychiatrist has to patients. What passes between doctor and patient should remain private and should not be divulged without the patient's permission, because disclosure could be socially embarrassing or harmful. As a practical matter, this means that before information is given to a third party, the patient must provide written permission.

Some exceptions have created a *duty to protect* for the psychiatrist. In the course of treating a patient, a psychiatrist may learn of potential harm to a third party. In that case, the psychiatrist has a legal responsibility to break confidentiality and warn the third party. This is called the *Tarasoff* rule, named after a 1976 decision by a California court. A therapist was held responsible for harm done to a third party by his patient, because it had been revealed that the therapist was aware of this potential threat.

How this ruling should be implemented by psychiatrists and other mental health professionals has been debated. In practice, once the psychiatrist believes that a patient will become violent, hospitalization is the best course. If violence is believed to be a distinct possibility, but is not imminent, the best course is to warn the intended victim.

Once a decision has been made to warn the intended victim, a phone call is appropriate, because it allows him or her to ask questions. Sometimes psychiatrists will phone in the patient's presence, which may help to head off suspicious ideas about the psychiatrist acting duplicitously. A trusted third party may sometimes act as a go-between for the psychiatrist and the intended victim. The psychiatrist should always discuss the warning with the patient before giving it.

Although a psychiatrist may need to repair the damage done to the therapeutic relationship by the breach of confidentiality, some patients may actually feel relieved by the issuance of the warning. Moreover, a patient who is ambivalent about harming another person may decide not to carry out the threat after learning that the intended victim has been warned.

Confidentiality can be waived for other reasons as well. In some states, mental health codes give mental health care providers the right to disclose information to close family members when it is deemed to be in the best interest of the patient. Further, utilization review groups and third-party payers often demand access to hospital charts. When signing into the hospital, a patient will waive his or her right to confidentiality, so as to allow these bodies to review the records.

Informed Consent

Informed consent should be obtained from all patients before any treatment, although formal written consent is probably necessary only before electroconvulsive therapy (ECT). In addition, many hospitals now require written informed consent before medications, especially antipsychotics, are initiated, because they carry the long-term risk of tardive dyskinesia. Patients should be apprised of the indications and contraindications for the treatment, adverse reactions, and alternative therapies. The physician should take care to carefully document the fact that the patient has given consent. A problem with informed consent arises when the patient is not competent to provide consent. In these cases, it is advisable for the patient to have a court-appointed guardian who can make health care decisions.

Malpractice

Malpractice is negligence in the conduct of one's professional duties. The number of malpractice suits filed in the United States seems to climb each year; it is now estimated that every physician will experience at least one malpractice law-suit during his or her professional lifetime. Fortunately, psychiatrists have rela-tively few malpractice suits filed against them. Consequently, their malpractice premiums are less costly than those of other physicians.

There are many reasons why psychiatrists are sued less frequently than other physicians. However, one of the main reasons is that the psychiatrist, by virtue of the disorders treated and the types of treatments provided, is less likely to do physical harm to a patient; a surgeon, for example, has the ability to kill or maim. Psychiatric patients are also reluctant to publicize their mental disorders and treatments, and there are typically no witnesses to the alleged mistreatment.

Although no study has ever shown that psychiatrists are able to predict sui-cides, the courts and the public tend to blame the psychiatrist for failing to pre-dict or prevent a patient's self-injury or death. Suicides that occur during hospitalization are probably the ones most likely to result in litigation because they are seen as entirely preventable; suicidal behavior may, in fact, be the reason the patient was in the hospital. Potential errors include failure to take an ade-quate history of suicidal behavior, failure to provide adequate protection in the hospital (e.g., one-on-one supervision), or failure to communicate changes in the patient's condition to other doctors and nurses.

Unfortunately, sexual activity between doctors and patients is all too fre-quent. The problem occurs in many specialties (e.g., gynecology), but litigation against psychiatrists for sexual activity with current or former patients has be-come relatively common. In addition to legal sanctions, a psychiatrist may be expelled from professional associations and have his or her license suspended or revoked. The American Psychiatric Association has made it clear that sexual conduct with patients at any time is inappropriate and unethical. No matter how seductive the patient is, or how much time has elapsed since the physician treated the patient, there is never an excuse for a sexual relationship with a patient.

Another reason psychiatrists are sued is failure to obtain informed consent. Patients may claim that the information provided to them was inadequate, that alternatives were omitted, or that the consent was never obtained. Again, it be-hooves the clinician to maintain careful records about what happens during an appointment, particularly as it pertains to obtaining consent and providing in-formation.

Psychiatrists are occasionally sued by patients who sustain injuries from psychotropic medications. Situations that have led to claims include failure to disclose relevant information to the patient about adverse effects, failure to obtain an adequate history, and prescription of a drug or drug combination when it is not indicated or when potentially harmful drug interactions might occur.

The development of tardive dyskinesia is one of the major complications that results in litigation. It is generally recommended that prescribing physicians regularly monitor patients for the presence and severity of tardive dyskinesia and repeatedly present information to the patient and family members (or guardian) about the risks of treatment, as well as the continuing need for antipsychotic medication.

Psychiatrists are sometimes sued for abandonment, defined as improperly terminating a doctor-patient relationship despite the continuing need for treatment. Abandonment can give rise to actions for both negligence and breach of contract. These claims are likely to come about because the patient fails to cooperate with treatment, fails to pay bills, threatens or assaults the psychiatrist, or presents a difficult management problem.

Claims involving ECT are relatively rare, but they do occur and involve allegations of failure to obtain informed consent, inappropriate or improper treatment, and injury resulting from treatment, such as memory loss. Liability can be minimized by using ECT in accordance with accepted standards and monitoring and supervising patients very carefully between treatments.

Criminal Issues

For most practicing psychiatrists, situations involving criminal law are rarely encountered. The two main issues in this area are competency to stand trial and criminal responsibility. To receive a fair trial, persons must be able to understand the nature of the charges against them, the possible penalty, and the legal issues and procedures; they must also be able to work with the attorney to participate in preparing the defense. In most areas, competency is decided by a judge, who may base his or her decision on expert testimony. If the court determines that the defendant is incompetent to stand trial, he or she may be transferred to a psychiatric hospital for treatment to achieve competence to stand trial, which occurs after clinical improvement.

Defendants determined by the courts to be incompetent to be sentenced (or executed) are managed in the same way as those who are alleged or determined to be incompetent to stand trial; they may be transferred for psychiatric treatment to restore their competency. This, of course, presents the ironic scenario of a person sent for psychiatric treatment that on his or her improvement will lead to execution!

The presence of a psychiatric disorder, even a severe psychosis, does not generally render defendants incapable of standing trial; most patients referred for competency evaluation are able to understand the nature and quality of their acts and to participate in their own defense, the usual measures for determining legal competence to stand trial.

Criminal responsibility has to do with the subject's state of mind at the time of a crime. Under our current system, criminal responsibility occurs only in the presence of a blameworthy state of mind.

There are three general categories of traditional criminal defense in which evidence of a psychiatric condition is used. First, evidence of a psychiatric disorder at the time of the alleged offense can be used to negate the requirement for criminal intent. Second, the defense may claim that the defendant's mental condition at the time of the act relieves him or her of criminal responsibility through the special verdict of not guilty by reason of insanity. According to the M'*Naghten* rule used in many states, defendants can establish an insanity defense when, at the time of the alleged offense, they were laboring under such defective reasoning caused by a disease of the mind that they did not know the nature and quality of the criminal act. The rule is named after Daniel M'Naghten, who in 1843 shot and killed Edward Drummond, private secretary to the prime minister Sir Robert Peel, the intended victim. M'Naghten had harbored delusions for many years and believed he was persecuted by the Tory Party and their leader Peel.

The American Law Institute standard is used in many states and incorporates a volitional test: a person is not responsible for criminal conduct if, at the

---

Recommendations for handling legal situations

1. When seeking commitment, there must be evidence of a treatable mental illness, recent (or potential for) harm to self or others, or evidence of grave disability.
   - Know your state laws.
   - Know your local magistrate who handles civil commitments.
   - Outpatient commitments are useful in patients who are chronically noncompliant and a nuisance to the community.
2. Understand your state laws on confidentiality and informed consent.
3. Breaking confidentiality under *Tarasoff* may involve contacting the threatened party.
   - Although breaking confidentiality may harm the therapeutic alliance, many patients will feel a sense of relief.
4. Malpractice lawsuits are frequent in our litigious society; have adequate insurance.
   - The best defense against claims of malpractice is to maintain proper records and documentation.
5. Most psychiatrists do not routinely conduct competency evaluations to determine whether a patient can stand trial. You should get to know the forensic psychiatrists in your region.

time of such conduct and as a result of mental disease, he "lacks substantial capacity either to appreciate the criminality of his conduct, or to conform his conduct to the requirements of the law."

Finally, the third traditional criminal defense is that a defendant's psychiatric disorder can be used to find the defendant guilty of the charges against him or her but mentally ill. Although this standard is used less frequently, it provides that the defendant has been found to have a mental illness at the time of the alleged offense, but that the mental illness is not sufficient to acquit him or her of culpability for that offense. Defendants found guilty but mentally ill are customarily transferred to correctional facilities, where psychiatric treatment may or may not be provided.

The verdict of guilty but mentally ill has become more popular since John Hinckley's verdict of not guilty for his shooting of President Ronald Reagan. Critics have charged that excusing Hinckley and others from responsibility lessens society's ability to deal with potentially dangerous persons and knowingly encourages further use of the insanity defense, which they feel makes a mockery of our system of justice.

The verdict of guilty but mental ill recognizes the obvious in certain cases: although a crime was committed and a person was found guilty of that crime, the person was also mentally ill at the time of the act.

Bibliography

American Law Institute: Model Penal Code, sec. 401 [responsibility for criminal conduct in the case of mental disease]. Philadelphia, PA, American Law Institute, 1974

American Medical Association Board of Trustees: Insanity defense in criminal trials and limitations of psychiatric testimony. JAMA 251:2967–2981, 1984

American Medical Association Committee on Medico-Legal Problems: Insanity defense in criminal trials and limitations of psychiatric testimony. JAMA 251:1967–2981, 1984

Appelbaum PS: Tarasoff and the clinician: problems in fulfilling the duty to protect. Am J Psychiatry 142:425–429, 1985

Appelbaum PS: Resurrecting the right to treatment. Hosp Community Psychiatry 38:703–704, 1987

Appelbaum PS, Roth LH: Clinical issues in the assessment of competency. Am J Psychiatry 138:1462–1467, 1981

Drane JF: Competency to give informed consent—a model for making clinical assessments. JAMA 252:925–927, 1984

Faust D, Ziskin J: The expert witness in psychology and psychiatry. Science 241:31–35, 1988

Felthous AR: Duty to warn or protect: current status for psychiatrists. Psychiatric Annals 21:591–597, 1991

Gutheil TG, Appelbaum PS: Clinical Handbook of Psychiatry and the Law. New York, McGraw-Hill, 1982

Lamb HR: Incompetency to stand trial. Arch Gen Psychiatry 44:754–758, 1987

Leong GB, Eth S, Silva JA: The psychotherapist as witness for the prosecution: the criminalization of Tarasoff. Am J Psychiatry 149:1011–1015, 1992

Miller RD: Need for treatment criteria for involuntary civil commitment: impact on practice. Am J Psychiatry 149:1380–1384, 1992

Simon RI: Clinical Psychiatry and the Law. Washington, DC, American Psychiatric Press, 1992

Simon RI, Sadoff RL: Psychiatric Malpractice: Cases and Comments for Clinicians. Washington, DC, American Psychiatric Press, 1992

Self-Assessment Questions

1. What is forensic psychiatry?
2. What are the three main categories of legal issues psychiatrists face?
3. What are the major concepts that most civil commitment laws contain?
4. Explain the right to treatment and the right to refuse treatment. Why is the latter so frustrating to psychiatrists?
5. Explain the *Tarasoff* ruling and the "duty to protect."
6. Why is confidentiality important? List several situations in which it can be waived.
7. What are the usual reasons behind malpractice lawsuits filed against psychiatrists?
8. How may a psychotic patient be competent to stand trial?
9. Explain the M'Naghten standard.
10. What is the guilty but mentally ill verdict about?

Section IV

Treatments

Chapter 25

Psychosocial Treatments

The mind is its own place, and in itself
Can make a heav'n of hell, a hell of heav'n.

John Milton, Paradise Lost

Although the use of medication has become increasingly important in psychiatry, clinicians who care for patients with the broad range of mental illnesses must also develop a high level of skill in talking with their patients, listening to their problems, instilling confidence and a sense of support, helping them have insight into abnormal patterns of behavior, and assisting them in learning new ways to correct or alter maladaptive or painful behavior, emotions, and attitudes. Because psychiatrists deal with diseases that are especially human, involving thoughts, feelings, and relationships, it is essential that they maintain a humanistic, empathetic, and caring attitude toward their patients and that they become skilled in treating patients with therapies directed at the mind in addition to the brain. Although the empathic relationship used in many types of psychotherapy is in principle the same as that used by a caring and involved family practitioner or medical specialist, it is more prominent and pervasive in psychiatric practice due to the nature of the illnesses.

Because writing a prescription is both easier and more obviously medical than performing psychotherapy, beginning students often wonder whether there is any need to do psychotherapy at all. There is, however, a substantial empirical base that confirms the effectiveness of psychosocial treatments. For some disorders (e.g., eating disorders), they are first-line treatments, and they have been repeatedly demonstrated to produce good outcomes. For many other disorders (e.g., schizophrenia, mood and anxiety disorders), they have been shown to be an important adjunct to medications because they deal with issues such as compliance, education of patients about symptoms and expected outcome, and provision of insight and support to deal with the psychological consequences of a severe illness.

This chapter provides a brief overview of the major classes of psychotherapy used by specialists who care for mentally ill patients. Some of these psychosocial treatments require extensive experience and training, on a scale that is outside the range of description of a single chapter. Students who want to explore specific types of psychosocial treatments in more detail may want to read material cited in the bibliography at the end of this chapter. The various psychosocial treatments that are often used for major mental illnesses include behavior therapy, cognitive therapy, the individual psychotherapies that draw on psychodynamic principles, group therapy, family therapy, and social skills training. The major classes of psychosocial treatments are summarized in Table 25–1.

Behavior Therapy

The theoretical underpinnings of behavior therapy derive from British empiricism, Pavlov's studies of conditioning, and subsequent research on stimulus-response relationships conducted by other leading behaviorists such as Skinner, Wolpe, and Eysenck. Behaviorists stress the importance of working with objective, observable phenomena, usually referred to as behavior, including physical activities such as eating, drinking, talking, and completing the serial-sequential activities that lead to habit formations and social interactions. In contrast to psychodynamic psychotherapies, discussed below, behavioral techniques do not necessarily help the patient to understand his or her emotions or motivations. Instead of working on the patient's thoughts and feelings, the behavior therapist works on *what the patient does*. Indeed, some clinicians using behavioral ap-

Table 25–1.　Types of psychosocial therapy

• Behavior therapy	• Insight-oriented psychotherapy
• Cognitive therapy	Relationship psychotherapy
• Individual therapy	Interpersonal psychotherapy
• Classical psychoanalysis	Supportive psychotherapy
• Psychodynamic psychotherapy	• Group therapy
	• Family therapy
	• Social skills training

proaches argue that changing a patient's behavior may lead to substantial changes in how the patient thinks and feels and that correcting pathological behavior may be more effective than correcting pathological emotions. The motto for this approach is "Change the behavior, and the feelings will follow."

Behavior therapies are particularly effective for disorders that are associated with clearly abnormal behavioral patterns in need of correction. These disorders include alcohol and drug abuse, eating disorders, anxiety disorders, and particularly phobias and obsessive-compulsive behavior. A general knowledge of the principles of behaviorism may be useful in dealing with a broad range of patients, however, including patients with dementias, psychoses, adjustment disorders, childhood disorders, and personality disorders.

The concept of conditioning is fundamental to the various behavior therapies. Two types of conditioning have been described: classical (Pavlovian) and operant. Early in the twentieth century, the Russian physiologist Pavlov described the first controlled experiments with conditioning. He demonstrated that through pairing stimuli, such as striking a bell at the same time that dogs were given food, he could eventually produce a conditioned reflex in the animals in the absence of the original triggering stimulus. For example, if the two stimuli (food and the ringing of a bell) were paired frequently enough, the dog would eventually learn to salivate when it heard the bell alone. In this model, the food is regarded as the unconditioned stimulus, the bell as the conditioned stimulus, and salivation in response to the bell the conditioned reflex.

The concept of stimulus pairing can obviously be used both to explain the development of psychopathology and to create behavioral therapies through conditioning patients to alter their response patterns.

The study and use of *operant conditioning* involve examining responses that are produced within the subject, rather than produced by some outside stimulus. A therapist using operant conditioning seeks to understand the forces that trigger and modify specific behaviors, rather than beginning with a predetermined conditioned stimulus. Operant responses, in contrast to conditioned reflexes, are voluntary. For example, a young child sitting in a high chair quickly learns that banging a spoon on his tray gets his mother's attention and is likely to produce gratification of some desire, such as more milk in his cup or another piece of toast. By varying the amount of banging, he may also learn that if he bangs too much his mother may become annoyed, take away his spoon, and remove him from his high chair before a dessert is provided. Thus, the child learns to change both his behavior and his environment in relation to the responses that his behavior elicits in a manner that is under his voluntary control.

The study of operant conditioning has created an enormous experimental literature that explores the various ways that learning occurs and that behaviors are reinforced or extinguished. The concepts of positive and negative reinforcement are fundamental. A *positive reinforcer* (e.g., giving a reward) is one that strengthens the response, and a *negative reinforcer* (e.g., giving a punishment) diminishes the response. An extensive behavioral literature now suggests that positive reinforcement is more effective in sustaining behavior than negative reinforcement, that failure to provide reinforcements will usually extinguish a behavior, and that variable and unpredictable schedules of reinforcement may be more effective in maintaining behavior than fixed, regular reinforcements. For example, pathological gamblers receive the positive reinforcement of winning only occasionally, but they continue to gamble and are rarely deterred by threats of punishment or even by punishment itself, such as loss of their financial assets or incarceration. If they won every time they gambled, they would very likely lose interest eventually; likewise, they would lose interest if they never won at all.

Some of the established forms of behavior therapy that use these principles are listed in Table 25–2. They include relaxation training, systematic desensitization, flooding, and behavior modification. These principles can also be used to shape the behavior of patients (and of one's children, colleagues, and friends) in spontaneous and creative ways.

Relaxation Training

Relaxation training is used to teach patients control over their bodies and mental states. Relaxation training is a simple and straightforward procedure; the patient is instructed to move through the muscle groups of the body and make them tense and then completely relaxed. Through this procedure, patients learn how to achieve voluntary control over feelings of tension and relaxation. Relaxation training can be done simply through providing patients with an instructional audiotape that they can listen to in order to practice the techniques on their own. Relaxation training can be used in isolation to help patients who have anxiety or various problems involving pain (e.g., headache, low back pain), or it can be used in conjunction with systematic desensitization.

Systematic Desensitization

Systematic desensitization is a behavioral technique that involves teaching the patient how to reduce or control the fear elicited by specific stimuli. This tech-

Table 25–2. Established forms of behavior therapy

Relaxation training	Flooding
Systematic desensitization	Behavior modification techniques

nique is particularly useful for patients with specific fears, such as agoraphobia and the various social phobias. The therapist may use any one of a variety of techniques to train the patient to reduce her tense and anxious response to the feared stimulus. For example, the therapist may ask the agoraphobic patient to imagine what it is like to leave her house and visit the shopping mall where she typically develops panic attacks, thereby leading the patient to experience the panic attack. The patient is then encouraged to use relaxation techniques to diminish the sensation of panic and place it under voluntary control. The patient will gradually become able to enter the feared situation—that is, actually go to the shopping mall—and use relaxation techniques while in the feared setting. In complex and difficult situations, the therapist may need to lead the patient gradually to a sense of control by developing a hierarchy of stimuli that increasingly approximate the feared stimulus (e.g., moving from imagination to photographs to photographs plus recorded noises, and finally to the actual situation itself).

Flooding

Flooding involves teaching patients to extinguish anxiety produced by a feared stimulus through placing them in continuous contact with the stimulus and helping them learn that the stimulus does not in fact lead to any feared consequences. For example, a patient with a disabling fear of riding on airplanes may be asked to take repeated flights until the fear is extinguished. The patient with a fear of snakes may be requested to go to the zoo and stand in front of the snake cage until her anxiety is completely gone. A patient with obsessions about harming children may be asked to think of nothing else; the anxiety produced by the stimulus is gradually extinguished.

A variant of flooding, also used to treat obsessions and compulsions, is referred to as *paradoxical intention*. The therapist asks the patient to perform the rituals regularly and to keep a daily record of the rituals. When encouraged to perform them, the patient gradually becomes aware of their inherent ludicrousness and their ineffectiveness as a method for reducing anxiety and therefore is able to voluntarily abandon them.

Behavior Modification Techniques

Behavior modification techniques tend to use the concept of reinforcement as a way of shaping behavior—in particular, to reduce or eliminate undesirable behavior and to replace it with healthier behaviors or habits. Behavior modification techniques are especially appropriate for disorders of impulse control, such as alcoholism, substance abuse, eating disorders, and conduct disorders.

Individual programs must be designed to suit the particular patient, using stimuli that are specific positive and negative reinforcers for that individual. For example, the long-term goal for a patient with anorexia nervosa is weight gain. Intermediate goals are to become less preoccupied with food and body image. Patients with anorexia nervosa typically enjoy exercise. A particular anorectic patient may also enjoy reading mystery novels and chewing gum. A specific program would be developed for such a patient in which she would be provided with three regular, well-balanced meals per day and told that access to her specific preferred pleasures would be contingent on going to the dining room for meals, eating them, and demonstrating a regular pattern of weight gain. A schedule of reinforcers would be developed to encourage her compliance with eating regularly. For example, she might be initially restricted to her room between meals and given no access to exercise, mystery novels, and chewing gum. After she gains 5 pounds, she will be allowed to leave her room. After she gains an additional 5 pounds, she will be given access to mystery novels. After the gain of an additional 5 pounds, she will be allowed access to chewing gum. After she reaches her desired target weight (involving a total weight gain of 20 pounds), she will be allowed to exercise regularly. To be permitted to continue exercising, however, she must maintain her target weight for 2 weeks while exercising as much as she desires. If her weight drops, positive reinforcers will gradually be removed until the weight gain is reestablished. In such a program, negative reinforcers, such as tube feeding, may also be built in. As mentioned above, however, it is well recognized that these negative reinforcers are much less effective than the positive reinforcers.

Different mixtures of behavior modification techniques are required for different disorders. For example, a program similar to the one above, but involving a different schedule of reinforcers and different targets, might be appropriate for the obese patient. Behavior modification programs for patients with substance abuse are more likely to stress teaching the patient the various stimuli that tend to trigger his craving, such as diminishing the pent-up irritation of a long day at work by dropping by the bar and socializing with the boys. The patient would be taught to substitute other positive reinforcers in their place, such as dropping by an exercise spa and releasing his hostility by hitting a punching bag, followed by drinking copious amounts of his favorite nonalcoholic beverage with a new set of friends developed through contacts with Alcoholics Anonymous (AA).

Combining Therapies

Originally, proponents of behavior therapy were purists, and they tended to denigrate mixing behavior therapy with various types of psychotherapy or with the use of medications. Increasingly, however, various types of therapy are being combined. Thus, the treatment of panic disorder and agoraphobia may involve the use of antidepressants or alprazolam along with systematic desensitization. Behavior therapy may also be combined with psychodynamic psychotherapy; for example, a patient with anorexia nervosa may benefit from a behavior modification program and from efforts to help her understand the underlying fears that make her seek a bodily appearance that most people find quite unattractive. A patient with comorbid anxiety and depression may benefit from a program of relaxation training, cognitive therapy, and antidepressant medication.

Cognitive Therapy

The theoretical support for cognitive therapy derives from a variety of sources, including cognitive psychology, Freudian psychodynamic theory, and some aspects of behaviorism. The theory and techniques of cognitive therapy were developed principally by Aaron Beck. The techniques of cognitive therapy are based on the assumption that *cognitive structures* or *schemata* shape the way people react and adapt to a variety of situations that they encounter in their lives. An individual's particular cognitive structures derive from a variety of constitutional and experiential factors (e.g., physical appearance, loss of a parent early in life, previous achievements or failures at school or with friends). Each person has her own specific set of cognitive structures that determines how she will react to any given stressor in any particular situation. A person develops a psychiatric syndrome, such as anxiety or depression, when these schemata become overactive and predispose her to developing a pathological or negative response.

The most widespread use of cognitive therapy is for the treatment of depression. In this instance, the individual is typically found to have schema that lead to negative interpretations. Beck designated the three major cognitive patterns observed in depression as the *cognitive triad*. These consist of a negative view of oneself, a negative interpretation of experience, and a negative view of the future. Patients with these cognitive patterns are predisposed to react to situations by interpreting them in the light of these three negative sets. For example, a woman who applied for a highly competitive job and did not receive it, and whose perceptions are shaped by such negative sets, may conclude, "I didn't get it because I'm not really bright, in spite of my good school record, and the employer was able to figure that out" (negative view of self). "Trying to find a decent job is so hopeless that I might as well just give up trying" (negative view of experience). "I'm always going to be a failure. I'll never succeed at anything" (negative view of future).

The techniques of cognitive therapy focus on teaching patients new ways to change these pathological schemata. Cognitive therapy tends to be relatively short term and highly structured. Its goal is to help patients restructure their negative cognitions so that they can perceive reality in a less distorted way and learn to react accordingly.

The actual practice of cognitive therapy combines a group of behavioral techniques with a group of cognitive restructuring techniques. The behavioral techniques include a variety of homework assignments and a graded program of activities designed to teach patients that their negative schemata are incorrect and that they are in fact able to achieve small successes and interpret them as such.

For example, the woman described above who failed to obtain the job might be asked to keep a record of her daily activities during the course of a week. Together, therapist and patient would then review this diary and (in the context of other information about her) develop a set of assignments to be completed during the ensuing week. The diary of activities might indicate a very limited range of social contacts, based on the patient's fear and expectation of rejection. The patient might be assigned to make at least five social contacts during the course of the week by talking to neighbors, phoning friends, and going out on at least one social engagement. These activities, along with the patient's notes about her responses to the various contacts, would also be recorded in a diary and reviewed the following week with the therapist. She would be helped to see that she tended to initiate each contact with a negative hypothesis or expectation, which typically was disconfirmed by her actual experience. In fact, the contacts were largely affirmative. As therapy progresses and confidence builds, the assignments would gradually be made more difficult, until the patient achieved an essentially normal level of behavior and expectation. The diary would serve as a comforting reminder to the patient that, based on past experience, negative hypotheses are typically disconfirmed. The patient would, of course, have some negative experiences, and the therapist would assist her in understanding that such negative experiences are not a consequence of her own deficiencies and that even negative experiences can be surmounted.

These behavioral techniques are complemented with a variety of cognitive techniques that assist the patient in identifying and correcting the dysfunctional schemas that shape the patient's perception of reality. These techniques involve identifying a variety of cognitive distortions that the patient is prone to make and *automatic thoughts* that intrude into the patient's consciousness and produce negative attitudes. Six typical cognitive distortions, identified by Beck, are listed in Table 25–3.

Arbitrary inference involves drawing an erroneous conclusion from an expe-

Table 25–3. Typical cognitive distortions treated through cognitive therapy

Distortion	Definition
Arbitrary inference	Drawing an erroneous conclusion from an experience
Selective abstraction	Taking a detail out of context and using it to denigrate the entire experience
Overgeneralization	Making general conclusions about overall experiences and relationships based on a single instance
Magnification and minimization	Altering the significance of specific events in a way that is structured by negative interpretations
Personalization	Interpreting events as reflecting on the patient when they have no relationship to him or her
Dichotomous thinking	Seeing things in an all-or-none way

rience. For example, if the patient's hairdresser suggests that she may want to try a new hairstyle, the patient assumes that the hairdresser believes she is becoming older appearing and unattractive. *Selective abstraction* involves taking a detail out of context and using it to denigrate the entire experience. For example, while playing tennis, the patient may hit the ball out of the court, losing it in a grassy area, and reach the conclusion "That just proves I'm a lousy tennis player." *Overgeneralization* involves making general conclusions about overall experiences and relationships based on a single interaction. For example, after a disagreement with another employee at his current (less desirable) job, the patient concludes, "I'm a failure. I can't get along with anybody." *Magnification and minimization* involve altering the significance of specific small events in a way that is structured by negative interpretations. For example, the significance of a success may be minimized (a good grade on an exam is considered to be trivial because the exam was easy), and the significance of a failure may be maximized (losing a tennis game is seen as indicating that the patient will never succeed at anything). *Personalization* involves interpreting events as reflecting on the patient when they in fact have no specific relationship to him or her. For example, a frown from a grouchy traffic policemen is seen as a recognition of the patient's overall lack of skill as a driver and general worthlessness. *Dichotomous thinking* represents a tendency to see things in an all-or-none way. For example, an A– student with high expectations receives a B in a course and concludes, "That just proves it. I'm really a terrible student after all."

In addition to these erroneous interpretations, patients are also often troubled with a variety of automatic thoughts that spontaneously intrude into their flow of consciousness. The specific automatic thoughts vary from one individual to another, but they involve negative themes of self-denigration and failure (e.g., "You're so stupid," "You never do anything right," "People wouldn't want to talk to you"). These thoughts intrude spontaneously and produce an accompanying dysphoria. Patients are encouraged to identify these automatic thoughts and to learn ways to counteract them. Such techniques include replacing the automatic thoughts with positive counterthoughts, testing the hypotheses embedded in the thoughts through behavioral techniques as described above, and identifying and testing the assumptions behind the thoughts.

The goal of the cognitive component of cognitive-behavior therapy is to identify and restructure the various negative schemata that shape the patient's perceptions. The cognitive goal is achieved like the behavioral goals: the patient is encouraged to do homework, to complete assignments that identify the occurrence of dysfunctional cognitions, and to steadily test and correct these cognitions. The therapist also reviews these aspects of the patient's diary and helps formulate an organized program for restructuring the dysfunctional cognitive sets, providing ample empathy and positive reinforcement.

Cognitive therapy is particularly effective for patients with depression. Its techniques can also be adapted to treat various anxiety disorders through identifying cognitive schema characterized by fear. It may be used either alone for the treatment of relatively mild psychopathology or in conjunction with medications for patients with more severe disorders.

Individual Psychotherapy

The term *individual psychotherapy* covers a broad range of psychotherapeutic techniques. Both behavior therapy and cognitive therapy are usually done individually (i.e., a single therapist working with a single patient). The historical roots of individual psychodynamic psychotherapy derive from Freudian psychodynamic approaches. In addition, however, simpler, briefer approaches to individual psychotherapy have been developed, which may draw either directly or indirectly on psychodynamic approaches. There are countless schools of psychotherapy that offer a variety of approaches. The description below provides a simplified and selective overview.

The various psychotherapies do share some common elements. These include the following, which are characteristic of all psychotherapies:

1. Based on an interpersonal relationship
2. Use of verbal communication between two (or more) people as a healing element
3. Specific expertise on the part of the therapist in using communication and relationships in a healing way

4. Based on a rationale or conceptual structure that is used to understand the patient's problems
5. Use of a specific procedure in the relationship that is linked to the rationale
6. Structured relationship (i.e., contact time, frequency, and duration are pre-specified)
7. Expectation of improvement

Classical Psychoanalysis and Psychodynamic Psychotherapy

Psychoanalysis was originally developed by Sigmund Freud during the early twentieth century. This technique arose from Freud's experience in attempting to treat patients with hysterical conversion symptoms, such as pains and paralyses. Following the lead of Charcot, his initial efforts involved the use of hypnosis. He observed, however, that this treatment was not always effective and that there was a high recurrence and relapse rate. He began to suspect that these conversion symptoms reflected some sort of painful early psychological experience that had been repressed. Instead of hypnosis, he began to experiment with the technique of having the patient lie down and relax while he placed his hand on her forehead and encouraged her to talk about whatever came into her mind and to release the repressed thoughts.

This treatment developed at a time when Victorian puritanism and hypocrisy still reigned supreme, and even Freud must have been astonished at the thoughts that flowed from his patients' minds, covering a variety of sexual fantasies and experiences. Based on his many years of experience in applying this approach, initially to conversion symptoms but subsequently to a range of symptoms including anxiety disorders and even psychoses, Freud developed a systematic theory to describe the structure and operations of the human psyche. Basic concepts include stages of psychosexual development (oral, anal, phallic, and genital), the structure of conscious and unconscious thoughts (primary versus secondary process thinking), the structure of drives and motivations (id, ego, and superego), the symbolism inherent in dreams, theories of infant sexuality, and a host of other concepts that the lay person associates with Freudianism.

Subsequent psychoanalysts elaborated and modified Freud's original work in a variety of ways, such as developing theories of ego psychology and expanding understanding of the mental mechanisms involved in defense, coping, and adaptation. These various ideas and theories are major resources for clinicians trained in either psychoanalysis or psychodynamic psychotherapy. Use of these approaches requires extensive experience and training under the supervision of a qualified psychoanalyst.

Classical psychoanalysis is currently used only in relatively special situations and settings. The form of treatment is best adapted to individuals who are fundamentally healthy (both psychologically and financially) and who have sufficient adaptive resources to go through the intensive process of self-scrutiny required by psychoanalysis. Typical reasons for seeking psychoanalysis include difficulties in relationships and persistent and recurrent anxiety, although neither should be so severe as to be incapacitating.

The core component of classical psychoanalysis is the development of a *transference neurosis*. That is, the patient transfers to the therapist all the thoughts and feelings that he experienced during early life; through this transference, he is able to make conscious the various unconscious drives and emotions that are troubling him and ultimately to modify and heal them, as the analyst makes appropriate interpretations during the course of the psychoanalysis.

The patient is typically asked to lie on a couch and to free-associate, saying whatever comes into his mind without any type of censorship. The analyst sits behind the patient, remaining a relatively shadowy and neutral figure to encourage the development of transference. (If the analyst becomes too human or "real," then transference cannot develop.) To maintain an appropriate level of intensity, the patient must be seen four or five times per week for 50-minute sessions. The process typically requires 2–3 years. Because the analyst becomes a repository of large quantities of intimate and highly personal information, it is essential that she be both psychologically and ethically trustworthy. Analysts must go through an extensive period of psychoanalysis themselves to understand their own psychological vulnerabilities—particularly the nature of the counter-transference that they are likely to develop in relation to their patients.

Psychodynamic psychotherapy uses many of the concepts embodied in psychoanalytic theory, but these concepts are used in ways that make them more suitable for the treatment of larger numbers of patients. Treatment is not necessarily less intensive, in the sense of attempting to focus on and correct problems, but it does not involve the relatively rigidly defined techniques (e.g., use of the couch) that characterize classical psychoanalysis.

Psychodynamic psychotherapy is used to treat patients with a variety of problems, including personality disorders, sexual dysfunctions, somatoform disorders, anxiety disorders, and mild depression. Psychodynamic psychotherapy is typically conducted face to face. Depending on the frequency and duration of therapy, a transference neurosis may or may not occur. The therapist attempts to help the patient in a neutral but empathic way. The patient is encouraged to review early relationships with parents and significant others, but may also focus on the here and now. As in classical psychoanalysis, the patient is expected to do the bulk of the talking, while the psychodynamic psychotherapist occasionally interjects clarifications to assist the patient in understanding the underlying dynamics that shape her behavior. Psychodynamic psychotherapy typically involves sessions one or two times a week and may involve 2–5 years of treatment.

Insight-Oriented and Relationship Psychotherapy

Insight-oriented psychotherapy and relationship psychotherapy are two other variants of individual psychotherapy that may be somewhat less intensive or long term.

Insight-oriented psychotherapy draws on many basic psychodynamic concepts, but focuses even more on interpersonal relationships and here-and-now situations than does purely psychodynamic psychotherapy. Patients are typically seen once a week for 50 minutes. During the sessions they are encouraged to review and discuss relationships, attitudes toward themselves, and early life experiences. The therapist maintains an involved and supportive attitude and occasionally assists patients with interpretations that will help them achieve insights. This form of psychotherapy does not encourage transference, regression, and abreaction. Instead of reexperiencing and reliving, patients are encouraged to achieve an intellectual understanding of the mainsprings of their behavior that will assist them in changing it as needed.

In *relationship psychotherapy* the therapist assumes a more active role. The stress is on achieving a corrective emotional experience, with the therapist serving as a loving and trustworthy surrogate parent who assists the patient in confronting unrecognized needs and unresolved drives.

The patient is typically seen once per week, and the therapy may last from 6 months to several years, depending on the patient's problems and level of maturity. As in insight-oriented psychotherapy, the content of the sessions focuses primarily on current situations and relationships, with some looking backward to early life experiences. Although the patient may achieve insight, the most important component of this type of psychotherapy is the empathic and caring attitude of the therapist.

Interpersonal Therapy

Interpersonal therapy (IPT) is a specific type of psychotherapy that was developed for the treatment of depression, although it is potentially useful for the treatment of other conditions as well, such as personality disorders. Drawing on the ideas of thinkers such as Harry Stack Sullivan, who stressed that mental illnesses may reflect and be expressed in problems with relationships (as opposed to the intrapsychic conflict stressed by psychodynamic approaches), IPT emphasizes working on improving interpersonal relationships during the process of psychotherapy.

During IPT, the emphasis is on the here and now rather than on the past. Using a process of exploration, the therapist helps the patient identify specific problem areas that may be interfering with self-esteem and interpersonal interactions. These usually involve four general domains: grief, interpersonal disputes, role transitions, and interpersonal deficits. After the exploration and identification process, the therapist works systematically with the patient to facilitate the learning of new adaptive behaviors and communication styles.

IPT is usually conducted in weekly sessions, and the overall course of therapy lasts from 3 to 4 months. It is one of the few forms of psychotherapy that has been subjected to rigorous empirical testing of its efficacy. In well-controlled acute and maintenance studies of depression, it has been shown to be superior to no active treatment and to medication alone when used in combination with amitriptyline.

Supportive Psychotherapy

Supportive psychotherapy is used to help patients get through difficult situations. Components of supportive psychotherapy may be incorporated into any of the other types of psychotherapy described in this section, with the exception of classical psychoanalysis.

In conducting supportive psychotherapy, the therapist maintains an attitude toward the patient of sympathy, interest, and concern. Patients describe and discuss the various problems they are confronting, which could range from marital discord all the way to psychotic experiences such as persecutory delusions. Supportive psychotherapy is appropriate for the full spectrum of psychiatric disorders, ranging from adjustment disorders through the psychoses and even dementia.

As in relationship psychotherapy, the therapist may function like a healthy and loving parent who provides the patient with encouragement and direction as needed. The goal of supportive therapy is to help the patient cope with difficult situations, experiences, or periods of adjustment. Patients typically describe their problems, and the therapist counters with encouragement and even specific advice. The therapist may suggest specific techniques that patients can use in coping with their problems, such as developing new interests or hobbies, trying new activities that may expand their range of social contacts, achieving emancipation from their parents by moving into independent living circumstances, and developing more organized study habits to improve their school performance. Psychotic patients may be taught to refrain from discussing their delusional ideas, except with the therapist. Alcoholic patients may receive praise and encouragement for refraining from drinking, as well as suggestions about ways to increase their self-esteem by achieving mastery and control, such as through improving their skills in a particular sport or developing a new creative hobby. As the above examples indicate, the clinician involved in conducting supportive therapy needs to tailor the therapy sessions to the individual needs of each particular patient.

Supportive psychotherapy, which is typically done weekly, is often done in conjunction with other treatments, particularly the somatic therapies. It may be relatively brief, as when it is used for crisis intervention in patients with adjustment disorders. On the other hand, it may be very long term (although it may be less frequent than weekly) when it is used as a treatment modality for patients with more chronic or protracted mental illnesses, such as schizophrenia, recurrent mania or depression, and various anxiety disorders.

Defense and Coping Mechanisms

Defense and coping mechanisms are techniques that both patients and psychiatrically normal people use to help themselves deal with difficult situations and emotional experiences. These techniques are divided into *defense mechanisms* (which are considered less mature and more primitive and therefore less healthy) and *coping mechanisms* (which represent a higher adaptive level and are considered to be mature ways to cope with life's stresses and problems) (Table 25–4). The clinician can observe these mechanisms in operation in a variety of medical settings, ranging from the emergency room to the recovery room. Understanding these mechanisms assists the clinician both in providing most types of psychosocial treatments for psychiatric patients and in providing general medical care.

Table 25–4.   Some common defense and coping mechanisms

Defense mechanisms (immature)	Coping mechanisms (mature)
Denial	Sublimation
Projection	Religiousness
Regression	Humor
Repression	Altruism
Splitting	Mastery and control
Reaction formation	
Undoing	
Isolation	
Displacement	

Defense Mechanisms

Defense mechanisms are used to ward off or avoid painful feelings and thoughts that are difficult to confront. They are usually considered to be neurotic and immature.

Denial is characterized by ignoring an undesirable situation or piece of information and behaving as if it did not exist. For example, a man with established coronary artery disease may insist that he feels fine and refuse to comply with instructions to diet, lose weight, stop smoking, and exercise. A patient with recurrent mania may refuse to admit the presence of periods of pathological euphoria.

Projection involves attributing to others unwanted ideas or feelings that are experienced within oneself. Archetypally, this mechanism involves attributing to others the negative emotions that one has toward them; for example, a paranoid patient who feels angry with her doctor (an unacceptable emotion) believes instead that the doctor is angry with her and is tormenting her by insisting that she take medication. On a more everyday level, projection is often seen as a mechanism by which patients refuse to accept responsibility for their own mistakes and instead place the blame on others. For example, a person who is having difficulty at work because of procrastination and failure to meet deadlines says to himself, "It isn't my fault. They're all being too demanding. If only my co-workers would be more helpful, I'd be able to get my work done."

Regression is withdrawal to a more primitive level of adaptation in response to some overwhelming stressor. For example, a woman with a mild dementia may be able to cope at a minimal but acceptable level, but she regresses to an infantile state characterized by inability to feed herself or maintain her toilet habits when confronted with the death of the husband who has supported her for the past 50 years. A 40-year-old woman in intensive psychotherapy may relate to her therapist in a childlike, dependent way, treating the therapist as if he is a father (a regression that may be appropriate in the context of intensive psychodynamic therapy).

Repression involves suppressing from awareness emotions and memories experienced as painful. For example, a patient dying from cancer may go through a period when he feels quite cheerful, even though he is consciously aware that his illness is terminal, simply because he feels an uncontrollable need to ward off the recognition of his inevitable and impending death.

Splitting involves keeping emotions and past experiences in stereotyped univalent logic-tight compartments, preventing recognition and integration of the nuances and complexities of relationships and experiences (i.e., everything is either good or bad). For example, a woman who feels angry with her mother for divorcing her father and remarrying may be unable to develop a much-needed reconciliation because she has split away the good affects (based on the periods of genuine happiness that she shared with her mother) and can recognize only the bad affects of anger and estrangement.

Reaction formation involves substituting an opposite attitude for one that is experienced as psychologically painful. For example, a patient with hemophilia may take up motorcycle racing and skydiving as a way of counteracting the painful fact of his disease. A patient with obsessive-compulsive personality disorder, who feels angry that her meticulousness and diligence are not recognized by her boss, may maintain an air of affection and cheerfulness toward the boss.

Undoing involves the substitution of one behavior for another, in an effort to change or modify the initial behavior. Undoing is particularly common in obsessive-compulsive disorder and is thought to reflect the patient's basic ambivalence and indecisiveness. For example, a person may become angry with a supervisor or teacher and express this anger by making a critical comment. Later, he may try to undo this behavior by performing an opposite one, such as giving the supervisor or teacher a small gift or praising him in some way.

Isolation (intellectualization) is a defense technique for coping with painful affects; the affect is separated from its content, often by treating it objectively rather than experientially. Thus, a patient who is prone to experience intense anxiety about some topic, such as sexuality or emotional intimacy, will avoid placing herself in situations where she will be forced to confront this anxiety. Instead, she may pursue research on the mating habits of frogs or bees. In a clinical therapy setting, this defense is most commonly noted when the patient talks about her problems in an intellectual, overly abstract manner and has difficulty describing, recalling, and experiencing her actual feelings.

Displacement involves the resolution of a conflict about some particular relationship or event by shifting the emotion attached to it onto some other relationship or event. For example, a woman who feels intense anger toward her father or her husband because of neglect or mistreatment may direct her anger toward her young male child (or even her female child), because she perceives her husband or father as more powerful than she is and thus feels unable to express her anger directly.

Coping Mechanisms

Coping mechanisms are considered to be on a somewhat higher adaptational level than defense mechanisms. Although coping mechanisms may also ward off unpleasant or unconscious emotions and experiences, they are usually productive and helpful to both the patient and those around him.

Sublimation involves using past traumatic or unpleasant experiences and emotions as well as basic "id drives" in a way that both reduces anxiety and is not injurious to society. For example, a person with high levels of sexual energy may choose to work long hours.

Religiousness involves making painful past experiences more acceptable by experiencing them as part of God's will. For example, a dying patient may come to terms with her impending death by seeing it as simply part of a universal pattern ordained by God.

Humor involves counteracting painful affects by seeing the comic side of the human situation. Sometimes the comedy may be black, but other times it may be positive. Jokes made in the anatomy laboratory, the operating room, and the military trenches are all examples.

Altruism involves taking a negative experience and turning it into a socially useful or positive one. For example, a reformed alcoholic person may obtain great satisfaction by helping others in the context of Alcoholics Anonymous.

Mastery and control involve gaining a sense of control over a painful situation by confronting it directly and developing techniques that prevent feelings of being overwhelmed. For example, a medical student confronted with an enormous mass of information and responsibility (which makes him feel psychologically threatened and powerless) throws himself intensively into his work, eventually reducing his anxiety and increasing his sense of self-worth and internal strength by learning as much as he can. Some individuals choose to go into medicine as a way of gaining mastery and control. Having experienced illness or death within their immediate family, they may seek to gain control over it by choosing a profession that involves working toward reducing illness and death.

Group Therapy

Group therapy provides a highly effective way for clinicians to follow and monitor relatively large numbers of patients. It also provides patients with a social environment or even surrogate peer group that will help them to learn new and constructive ways to interact with others in a controlled and supportive environment.

Yalom, one of the major leaders of the group therapy movement in the United States, enumerated a variety of factors that summarize the therapeutic mechanisms that occur during the process of group therapy. These include instilling hope, developing socializing skills, imitative behavior, catharsis, interpersonal learning, imparting of information, behaving altruistically through attempting to help other members of the group, experiencing a corrective recapitulation of the primary family group, developing a sense of group cohesiveness, "universality" (diminishing feelings of isolation), and learning through feedback how one's behavior affects others ("interpersonal learning").

There are many different kinds of group therapy. The types vary depending on the individuals who compose the group, the problems or disorders that they are confronting, the setting in which the group meets, the type of role that the group leader takes, and the therapeutic goals that have been established.

In many hospital settings, a group therapy program is established for inpatients. Such groups are typically led by a physician, nurse, social worker, or some combination thereof. In very large inpatient hospital settings, several groups may run concurrently and be composed of patients with similar types of problems. For example, one group might consist of relatively high-functioning individuals with personality problems or depression. Another group might consist of patients with severe mood and psychotic disorders, and yet another group might consist of individuals with eating disorders. Such groups provide patients with a forum to share their problems, diminish their sense of isolation and loneliness, enable them learn new techniques to cope with their problems either through other patients or through the group leader, and provide support, inspiration, and hope. Such groups may also assist patients in improving interpersonal and social skills; for example, patients with schizophrenia and other psychoses may improve their social skills in relating to others, and patients with personality disorders may receive useful feedback from other group members concerning counterproductive behavior.

In many clinical settings, such inpatient groups are supplemented by outpatient or aftercare groups, where patients receive continued follow-up, pursuing goals similar to those described above, but in the more stressful environment of the real world. These outpatient groups represent an attempt to consolidate and support the learning and skills already developed in the inpatient setting.

Some groups are oriented largely toward providing support. Such groups may or may not have a professional leader. Examples of such support groups include Alcoholics Anonymous meetings, family support groups such as those organized by chapters of the Alliance for the Mentally Ill (an organization composed of the family members of patients with serious mental illnesses), support groups for individuals who conceive of themselves as minorities in a particular setting (e.g., women professionals, women medical students, black students), groups composed of Vietnam veterans, and groups composed of individuals who have experienced some serious medical illness or difficult surgery (e.g., patients with diabetes, women who have experienced mastectomies, individuals receiving dialysis). Such groups provide a forum for sharing information, giving encouragement and support, and instilling hope through diminishing feelings of isolation.

Groups are also constituted to conduct group psychotherapy. Such groups are typically under the leadership of a therapist with extensive experience in group psychotherapy and are often conducted with a cotherapist. These groups aim to achieve goals similar to those of insight-oriented and interpersonal psychotherapy, but within the context of a group setting. Psychotherapy groups are typically more highly structured than the other groups described above. The group leaders take an active role in organizing each session, often prescribe exercises within the session, establish ground rules for membership within the group (e.g., no tardiness, regular attendance), resolve conflicts between members of the group, and assume responsibility for providing summaries of each session and access to videotapes of the sessions. Patients are typically carefully screened before being admitted to a psychotherapy group to ensure that they will be able to participate effectively. Such groups are particularly helpful for individuals with the same sorts of problems that lead them into individual psychotherapy, such as interpersonal and relationship problems, anxiety, mild depression, and personality disorders.

Marital Therapy and Family Therapy

Some problems for which patients seek treatment clearly involve other people. A man may present with feelings of depression and inadequacy because his wife has returned to work and is requesting that he assume his fair share of household duties and child care, a situation that he finds demeaning and inappropriate. A young teenager may present with mild symptoms of acting-out behavior, such as truancy from school and experimenting with alcohol, and indicate that she is seeking support from peers because she is having difficulty coping with her parents' inappropriately high expectations and overprotective smothering. In such situations, although the patient may come in initially as an individual case, the clinician usually will rapidly determine that he or she needs to be seen within the context of the larger family unit, which would be husband and wife in the first example (marital counseling) and parents and child in the second example (family therapy).

These two types of therapy may be done by psychiatrists but are also often done by psychologists, social workers, and nurses. Depending on the specific problems of the presenting individual, family therapy or marital counseling may be done in addition to individual therapy and medication management. Both these types of therapy are usually relatively short term, lasting from weeks to months, and both are oriented toward identifying and resolving specific, clearly defined problems as quickly as possible. All physicians should have at least a superficial familiarity with these types of therapy, because they must recognize that nearly all their patients live within the context of a family. In specific instances, the internist, pediatrician, or family physician must be able to recognize the need for family therapy or marital counseling and to refer the patient appropriately (usually through additional screening and assessment by a psychiatrist, who will evaluate the need for a referral and may conduct the treatment).

Marital Therapy

Marital therapy involves working with two people who see themselves as partners in a marital relationship to help them stabilize and improve their relationship. This therapy once involved seeing a husband and wife only. In contemporary society, however, the partners seeking treatment may be unmarried or homosexual. Depending on the commitment of the two partners, there are many variations to marital therapy. Ideally, both partners are willing and cooperative participants who are anxious to initiate change. Sometimes, however, marital therapy is sought because of a crisis: one of the partners may have lost interest in the relationship (and may or may not want to get out), whereas the other is hanging on tight and trying to save the relationship. In the latter instance, one possible outcome might be the eventual decision to end the relationship, and therapy might turn into divorce mediation and counseling; if children are involved, then what began as marital therapy might turn into family therapy as the couple attempts to work out an equitable arrangement in the context of the larger number of people who will be affected. In some instances, a dysfunctional sexual relationship between the couple will become apparent, and the couple may want referral to a sex therapy clinic for treatment of impotence or anorgasmia. The treatment of sexual disorders is described in Chapter 17.

An individual conducting marital therapy must take care to maintain an atmosphere of fairness, neutrality, and impartiality. Each partner will be particularly sensitive to the possibility that the therapist may take sides and treat him or her unfairly. The gender of the therapist may seem quite significant to either of the partners, even though the therapist may feel quite comfortable with his or her ability to be impartial. The women's movement has left both achievements and scars in its wake, sometimes causing individuals to conceptualize members of the opposite sex as potential enemies. Women may believe that only a woman therapist is able to understand their point of view and may feel quite defensive if asked to work with a male therapist. Male partners may have similar attitudes or problems.

Marital counseling typically begins with identifying the specific problem. Each partner is asked to identify specific areas in which he or she would like to see change in the other. The therapist attempts to assist the couple in implementing changes in a gradual, graded way, attacking one problem at a time. Typically, in the early sessions, a single, salient problem is the focus of attention. For example, a wife may express feelings of being ignored, whereas a husband may complain of his wife's whining expressions of dependency. Each will identify specific target behaviors in the other that need modification. They then contract with one another to modify these behaviors. Subsequent marital sessions focus on the steps they have taken to achieve improvement and on continuing work in new areas of concern.

This type of graded behavioral change is the minimum component of marital therapy. Often, couples also benefit from discussing their hopes for and expectations of one another in the context of personal values, prior family experiences, (i.e., role expectations about men and women, based on the behavior of their own parents), changing social norms about the roles of men and women, and the needs for both intimacy and independence that occur within the context of male-female relationships.

Family Therapy

Family therapy tends to focus on the larger family unit—at a minimum, one parent and the child (in single-parent families), but more typically both parents and the child (or a parent and stepparent, two separated parents, or other parental pairings depending on the family environment in which the child lives), or one or more parents and the child plus siblings. Typically, the child is brought in initially for treatment of a specific problem, such as school difficulties, hyperactivity, delinquency, or aggressive behavior. Often, it rapidly becomes clear that these problems exist in the overall context of the family setting. The family should not necessarily be regarded as dysfunctional, however. Because of changing circumstances or demands (e.g., a recent move), the parents may have difficulty in determining methods for coping with the child's behavior or understanding why it is occurring.

It is important for the therapist to be fair and impartial in family therapy, just as it is in marital therapy. In this instance, however, the therapist is not dealing with two potential equals, but rather with a hierarchy in which parents are expected to assume some authority and responsibility for the behavior of their child. The degree of hierarchy in the family will vary depending on the age of the child. For adolescents and teenagers, one important problem for the family may be the challenge that the "child's" growing independence is adding to this hierarchical structure.

As is the case with marital therapy, behavioral approaches are a mainstay of family therapy. The therapist usually begins by focusing on here-and-now problems. Parents and child discuss openly the nature of the problem that has brought about the need for therapy. For example, a 12-year-old boy may be intermittently truant from school, tell lies about his activities, and seek out parties on the weekends where he has been known to drink beer occasionally. The child may complain of parental pressure and repeated criticism while the parents express their fears about the child's unreliability and his poor school performance. As in marital therapy, graded areas of priority are identified, and contracts are made about changes that both parents and child will implement. Parents are given tactful but explicit suggestions about the value of positive reinforcement instead of criticism as a way of modifying behavior, and the child is led to realize that some hierarchy and structure will remain in his life, although to a gradually lessening degree as he demonstrates mature and dependable behavior.

Family therapy may also be used as a means of helping families in which at least one member has a relatively serious mental illness, such as schizophrenia, mania, or recurrent depression. In this type of family therapy, it is important to work firmly within the medical model and to emphasize that the patient has an illness for which neither the patient nor the family can be considered responsible. This approach minimizes guilt, scapegoating, and castigation, and it permits both the patient and the family members to seek methods for coping with the symptoms of the illness that may be more consoling and constructive. A young schizophrenic patient living at home may need some assistance from her family in developing social skills (see "Social Skills Training" below), and family members may need assistance in learning ways to cope with outbursts of anger and periods of emotional disengagement and withdrawal. Families with high levels of involvement (referred to as high "expressed emotion") may need counseling on ways to be less intensely involved, because it has been shown that in some instances high expressed emotion may be experienced as stressful by the schizophrenic patient and lead to relapse. Thus, families may need assistance in finding the right balance between providing needed support and encouragement and setting up excessively high expectations. Education about the symptoms of the illness is also an important component of family therapy for both the patient and the family members.

Social Skills Training

Social skills training is a specific type of psychotherapy that focuses primarily on developing abilities in relating to others and in coping with the demands of daily life. It is used primarily for patients with severe mental illnesses such as schizophrenia, which are often accompanied by marked impairments in social skills.

Social skills training may be done initially on an inpatient basis, but the bulk of the effort is typically done with outpatients, because the long-term goal of social skills training is to assist patients in learning to live in the real world. Social skills training is typically done by nurses, social workers, and psychologists. It may be done individually, but it more typically is accompanied by some group work as well, and it may occur in the context of day hospitals or sheltered workshops.

The techniques of social skills training are also primarily behavioral. Specific problems are identified and addressed in a sequentially integrated manner. Severely handicapped patients may need assistance initially in grooming and hygiene. They may need encouragement in learning to shave or bathe daily, to keep their clothes laundered, and to eat regular meals. They may also need help in learning how to approach other people and to talk with them appropriately. At higher levels of functioning, they may need assistance in learning how to apply for a job, complete job interviews, and relate to employers and co-workers. Because long-term institutional care is no longer available to most patients with psychotic illnesses, these individuals are literally being forced to learn to live in the community. Many cannot do so without receiving training and assistance in activities of daily living, such as grooming, managing money, and achieving at least a minimal level of social interaction with others. Although the development of such skills may seem elementary or minimal, for some patients it can lead to a substantial improvement in their quality of life.

Bibliography

Beck AT, Emery G, Greenberg BL: Anxiety Disorders and Phobias: A Cognitive Perspective. New York, Basic Books, 1985

Beck AT, Rush AJ, Shaw BF, et al: Cognitive Therapy of Depression. New York, Guilford, 1979

Bowen M: Family Therapy in Clinical Practice. New York, Jason Aronson, 1978

Corsini RJ (ed): Current Psychotherapies, 3rd Edition. Itasca, IL, FE Peacock, 1984

Davanloo H (ed): Short-Term Dynamic Psychotherapy. New York, Jason Aronson, 1980

Fenichel O: The Psychoanalytic Theory of Neurosis. New York, WW Norton, 1945

Freud A: The Ego and the Mechanisms of Defense. New York, International Universities Press, 1965

Freud S: The dynamics of transference (1912), in The Standard Edition of the Complete Psychological Works of Sigmund Freud, Vol 12. Translated and edited by Strachey J. London, Hogarth Press, 1958, pp 97–108

Freud S: On beginning the treatment (1913), in The Standard Edition of the Complete Psychological Works of Sigmund Freud, Vol 12. Translated and edited by Strachey J. London, Hogarth Press, 1958, pp 121–144

Gabbard GO: Psychodynamic Psychiatry in Clinical Practice. Washington, DC, American Psychiatric Press, 1990

Klerman GL, Weissman MM, Rounsaville BJ, et al: Interpersonal Psychotherapy of Depression. New York, Basic Books, 1984

Leff J, Vaughan C: Expressed Emotion in Families. New York, Brunner/Mazel, 1979

Nichols M: Family Therapy: Concepts and Methods. New York, Gardner, 1984

Satir V: Conjoint Family Therapy. Palo Alto, CA, Science and Behaviour Books, 1967

Vaillant GE: Theoretical hierarchy of adaptive ego mechanisms. Arch Gen Psychiatry 24:107–118, 1971

Vaillant GE: Adaptation to Life. New York, Little, Brown, 1977

Vaillant GE: An empirically derived hierarchy of adaptive mechanisms and its usefulness as a potential diagnostic axis, in Diagnosis and Classification in Psychiatry: A Critical Appraisal of DSM-III. Edited by Tischler G. New York, Cambridge University Press, 1987, pp 464–476

Vaillant GE, Bond M, Vaillant CO: An empirically validated hierarchy of defense mechanisms. Arch Gen Psychiatry 43:786–794, 1986

Weiner M: Practical Psychotherapy. New York, Brunner/Mazel, 1986

Weissman MM, Markowitz JC: Interpersonal psychotherapy: current status. Arch Gen Psychiatry 51:599–606, 1994

Yalom ID: Inpatient Group Psychotherapy. New York, Basic Books, 1980

Yalom ID: The Theory and Practice of Group Psychotherapy, 3rd Edition. New York, Basic Books, 1985

Self-Assessment Questions

1. What is the difference between classical conditioning and operant conditioning?
2. What is the definition of a positive reinforcer? A negative reinforcer?
3. Describe four common techniques for conducting behavior therapy.
4. Describe cognitive therapy. What is the cognitive triad? What are automatic thoughts?
5. Describe classical psychoanalysis. How does it differ from psychodynamic psychotherapy? What is transference?

6. Describe the concept of a corrective emotional experience in psychotherapy.
7. Describe two different types of group therapy and enumerate some situations in which they would be appropriate.
8. Describe the role of the therapist in marital and family therapy.

Chapter 26

Somatic Treatments

The desire to take medicine is perhaps the greatest feature
which distinguishes man from animals.

Sir William Osler

The modern treatment era in psychiatry began with the introduction of effective psychotropic medication in the early 1950s. Until that time, the mainstay of treatment was psychotherapy, although prefrontal leukotomy and electroconvulsive therapy (ECT) had been recently introduced—each accompanied by the excitement that any new treatment generates. Their limitations soon became apparent, and after the introduction of antipsychotics and antidepressants, leukotomy fell into disuse, and the use of ECT became limited to a relatively small group of patients with severe illnesses, such as major depression.

Before the availability of these new somatic treatments, psychiatrists were greatly limited in their ability to help patients, and overcrowded mental hospitals were common. The introduction of medication revolutionized psychiatry and led to the era of deinstitutionalization, a period in which mental patients were released from state hospitals in large numbers to be cared for in the community. The wisdom of this movement is now being critically assessed.

Antipsychotics

Chlorpromazine was first introduced in 1952 by two French psychiatrists, Jean Delay and Pierre Deniker, after it had become clear that the drug had powerful calming effects on agitated psychotic patients. Delay and Deniker soon discovered that the drug was especially effective in patients with schizophrenia. Not only were agitated schizophrenic patients calmed, but the new drug seemed to eradicate or markedly diminish their terrifying hallucinations and troubling delusional thoughts.

Since chlorpromazine was introduced, many antipsychotic drugs have been developed and marketed. Antipsychotics, with minor exceptions, are similar in action and efficacy and differ primarily in their side effects and potency. Antipsychotics ameliorate the symptoms of psychotic illnesses, including hallucinations, delusions, bizarre behavior, disordered thinking, and agitation. Although they are collectively referred to as *major tranquilizers*, this term is a misnomer, because the drugs do not produce a state of tranquillity in either psychiatrically normal or psychotic persons, and in fact, in psychiatrically normal persons, they produce a rather unpleasant state. The term *antipsychotic* is more appropriate in that the drugs are helpful in ameliorating symptoms of psychoses.

Although their use is primarily confined to schizophrenia and related illnesses (e.g., schizophreniform disorder, schizoaffective disorder), they are also prescribed to psychotic patients with mood disorders. Additionally, antipsychotics have been used to reduce agitated, aggressive, and inappropriate behavior in mentally retarded patients, patients with borderline personality disorder, and patients with delirium or dementia. They are also prescribed to patients with Tourette's disorder to diminish the frequency and severity of vocal tics. Because they may induce severe and possibly irreversible side effects (e.g., tardive dyskinesia), other indications requiring nonspecific sedation are probably not appropriate (e.g., generalized anxiety disorder).

There are 10 classes of antipsychotic drugs, each differing in molecular structure. The most important class, the phenothiazines, has a three-ring nucleus, but the three subtypes within the class differ by nature of the side chains joined to the nitrogen atom in the middle ring. The phenothiazine subtypes are the aliphatics (e.g., chlorpromazine), the piperazines (e.g., trifluoperazine), and the piperidines (e.g., thioridazine). Other classes of antipsychotics include the thioxanthenes (e.g., thiothixene), the dibenzoxazepines (e.g., loxapine), the dihydroindolones (e.g., molindone), the butyrophenones (e.g., haloperidol), the benzamides (e.g., sulpiride, not available in the United States), the dibenzodiazepines (e.g., clozapine), the benzisoxazoles (e.g., risperidone), the rauwolfia alkaloids (e.g., reserpine, no longer used to treat psychoses), and the diphenylbutylpiperidines (e.g., pimozide, used to treat Tourette's disorder).

Clozapine and risperidone are examples of atypical antipsychotics, which may be more effective than other antipsychotics in some patients. They represent a new generation of antipsychotic medication that appears to benefit up to

30% of treatment-refractory schizophrenic patients, while producing relatively few of the extrapyramidal side effects (EPS) typical of nearly all other antipsychotic agents.

Mechanism of Action of Antipsychotics

The potency of antipsychotic compounds correlates closely with their affinity for the dopamine 2 (D_2) receptor, blocking the effect of endogenous dopamine at this site. The pharmacological profile of clozapine and risperidone differs from that of more typical antipsychotics in that they are weaker D_2 receptor antagonists, but are potent serotonin type 2 (5-HT_2) receptor antagonists and have significant anticholinergic and antihistaminic activity as well. A central 5-HT_2 receptor antagonism is believed to broaden the therapeutic effect of the drug, while reducing the incidence of EPS associated with D_2 antagonists. Antipsychotic agents appear to exert their influence at mesocortical and mesolimbic dopaminergic pathways. Although positron-emission tomographic (PET) studies have demonstrated that antipsychotics block these receptors almost immediately, onset of antipsychotic action takes weeks to develop. Furthermore, although all antipsychotics block these same receptors, a patient may respond to one antipsychotic but not to another. These observations suggest that antipsychotics have other effects on the brain that may actually be responsible for the antipsychotic action, such as an action on second-messenger systems.

Although many side effects of these drugs can be directly attributed to their dopamine-blocking properties (e.g., EPS, galactorrhea in women), these drugs also block noradrenergic (α, α_2, β), cholinergic, and histaminic receptors to different degrees, accounting for the unique side-effect profile of each agent. See Table 26–1 for a comparison of commonly used antipsychotics.

Pharmacokinetics of Antipsychotics

Absorption of orally administered medication is variable, but clinical effects generally appear within 30–60 minutes. Rate of absorption differs among agents and may be complicated by the presence of food, antacids, smoking, and even anticholinergic agents. Intramuscular administration usually produces effects within 10 minutes (e.g., sedation), because injectable antipsychotics have much greater bioavailability than oral medication. For example, intramuscular chlorpromazine is 4–10 times more bioavailable than an equivalent oral dose. Metabolism occurs almost entirely in the liver, largely by oxidation, so that these highly lipid-soluble agents are converted to water-soluble metabolites and excreted through the kidneys. Excretion of antipsychotics tends to be slow as a result of drug accumulation in fatty tissue. Most antipsychotic agents have a

Table 26–1. Common antipsychotic agents

Category	Drug (trade name)	Sedative potency	Orthostatic hypotensive potency	Anticholinergic potency	Extrapyramidal potency	Equivalent dosage (mg)	Dosage range (mg/day)
Phenothiazines							
Aliphatics	Chlorpromazine (Thorazine)	High	High	High	Low	100	50–1,200
Piperidines	Mesoridazine (Serentil)	High	High	High	Low	50	50–400
	Thioridazine (Mellaril)	High	High	Very high	Low	95	50–800
Piperazines	Fluphenazine (Prolixin)	Low	Low	Low	Moderate	2	2–20
	Fluphenazine decanoate	Low	Low	Low	Moderate	—[a]	12.5–50 mg q 2 wk
	Perphenazine (Trilafon)	Low	Low	Low	Moderate	10	12–64
	Trifluoperazine (Stelazine)	Low	Low	Low	Moderate	5	5–40+
Thioxanthenes	Thiothixene (Navane)	Moderate	Low	Low	High	5	5–60
Dibenzoxazepines	Loxapine (Loxitane)	Moderate	Moderate	Moderate	High	15	20–250
Butyrophenones	Haloperidol (Haldol)	Low	Low	Low	High	2	2–60
	Haloperidol decanoate	Low	Low	Low	High	—[a]	50–250 mg q 4 wk
Dihydroindolones	Molindone (Moban)	Low	Low	Low	Low	10	50–400
Dibenzodiazepines	Clozapine (Clozaril)	High	Very high	High	Very low	50	200–900
Benzisoxazoles	Risperidone (Risperidol)	Low	Low	Moderate	Very low	Unknown	2–6

[a]Long-acting ester; dosage is not directly comparable with that of standard compounds.

half-life of 24 hours or longer and have many active metabolites with longer half-lives; depot formulations have even longer elimination half-lives. This has made it difficult to correlate blood levels with therapeutic response. As a result, no dose-response curve has ever been demonstrated for the antipsychotics. A treatment range for chlorpromazine, for instance, has been estimated to vary nearly 40-fold. Antipsychotics also differ greatly in potency. For example, 100 mg of chlorpromazine is approximately equal therapeutically to 2 mg of haloperidol. The relative potencies of the various antipsychotics are compared in Table 26–1.

Plasma concentrations can be measured reliably for many antipsychotic agents (e.g., chlorpromazine, thioridazine, fluphenazine, thiothixene, clozapine, haloperidol), but studies attempting to correlate plasma levels with response are inconsistent. This inconsistency may be due to the fact that active metabolites are available for many, but not all (e.g., haloperidol), of these drugs. Haloperidol and clozapine levels in blood have been correlated with clinical response; haloperidol may have a therapeutic window between 5 and 15 ng/ml, and clozapine levels greater than 500 ng/ml are associated with a two- to fivefold greater response rate than lower levels.

Except for clozapine and risperidone, all antipsychotics are more or less similar in pharmacological action and efficacy. Therefore, there is little reason to prescribe more than one agent at a time. Further, there is no evidence that a specific agent should be prescribed for a specific subtype of schizophrenia. Selection of an agent should rest on predicted side effects, prior treatment response, and history of compliance.

Once a drug has been selected, a trial should last 4–6 weeks; a patient who fails to respond should receive a trial of a second or third agent. Because blood level measurements optimize dosing, a reasonable strategy is to prescribe haloperidol with the aim of achieving a blood level of 5–15 ng/ml for 4–6 weeks. If the patient fails to respond, a trial of risperidone (6 mg/day) for 4–6 weeks should follow, because risperidone is highly effective and has minimal side effects. The next option in this treatment algorithm is a trial of clozapine at a dose producing blood levels greater than 500 ng/ml. Because of its expense and propensity to cause agranulocytosis, clozapine cannot be considered a first-line drug.

Use of Antipsychotics in Acute Psychosis

For the treatment of acute psychosis, a daily dose of 10–20 mg of haloperidol (or 500–600 mg of chlorpromazine) orally usually produces improvement; a daily dose of 5 mg of haloperidol (or 200 mg of chlorpromazine) is considered a minimal therapeutic dose. Higher doses do not add to therapeutic response and only increase the likelihood of adverse effects. In general, the acutely agitated psychotic patient can be started on 5 mg of haloperidol (or its equivalent) daily. The medication is increased as needed at the rate of 2–5 mg of haloperidol per day. Doses may be divided when initiating therapy, a practice that may help to reduce the incidence and severity of side effects and may help to sedate the patient. One week after a stable dose is achieved, the medication can be given once daily, usually at bedtime.

The uncontrollable patient should be given frequent, equally spaced doses of an antipsychotic every 1/2–2 hours until agitation is under control. Haloperidol or other high-potency antipsychotics are recommended, because low-potency compounds (e.g., chlorpromazine) may cause serious hypotension. Seldom is more than 20–30 mg of haloperidol required in a 24-hour period for this indication. Combinations of an antipsychotic agent and a benzodiazepine may work even better in subduing patients (e.g., combining 5 mg of haloperidol and 2–4 mg of lorazepam).

Maintenance Treatment With Antipsychotics

Once the patient has been stabilized on a dose of an antipsychotic and the target symptoms (e.g., hallucinations, agitation) are under control, the dose may be gradually reduced to one-half to one-third the maximal dose, but generally not falling below 5 mg of haloperidol (or its equivalent) per day. Schizophrenic patients should receive maintenance therapy for at least 1–2 years after an initial psychotic episode, which will reduce the risk of relapse by a factor of nearly fourfold. After two such episodes, a patient should probably have at least 5 years of treatment. Beyond this point, data are incomplete, but lifelong treatment should be considered for patients who pose a danger to themselves or others.

When it is time to reassess the need for medication, an attempt should be made to withdraw the medication slowly (e.g., over weeks or months). Should symptoms reoccur, the drug should immediately be reinstituted and the dose increased. Some patients will remain well for months or years without medication, although controlled studies show that with maintenance treatment, relapse is much less likely. Because many of the medications have long-acting metabolites, relapse often may not occur for months after a drug is withdrawn. Research suggests that risk of relapse while on medication is greater with oral than with intramuscular antipsychotics, probably because of noncompliance.

The patient with tardive dyskinesia, a side effect discussed later, presents special problems, because the treatment of choice is to stop the offending drug. However, many patients will decompensate without the medication; they (and their relatives) may choose to continue treatment with the antipsychotic regardless of the tardive dyskinesia because life may be intolerable without medication. In this situation, there are no simple answers, and patients and their relatives need to be consulted. Further information about the use of antipsychotics in the treatment of schizophrenia is found in Chapter 7.

For patients who are unable to take medication on a regular basis or who are noncompliant, long-acting preparations are available, such as fluphenazine decanoate or haloperidol decanoate. There is no universally accepted method for converting a patient from oral to long-acting dose forms, and dosing with sustained-release preparations must be individualized. Usually patients are started on a dose of 6.25 mg of fluphenazine decanoate (Prolixin) intramuscularly every 2 weeks, and the dose is titrated upward or downward based on the patient's therapeutic response and the side effects. For haloperidol, a 400-mg loading dose in the first month, followed by a maintenance dose of 250 mg per month, produces a blood level of about 10 ng/ml (the middle of the therapeutic range), and a dose of 150 mg per month produces a blood level between 5 and 6 ng/ml.

There are generally no good reasons to use antipsychotics as maintenance treatment in patients with psychotic mood disorders. Instead, an antidepressant or mood stabilizer such as lithium carbonate should be used. An occasional patient with a psychotic mood disorder will benefit from continuing antipsychotic treatment, but as this indication has been poorly studied, the decision to use antipsychotics for maintenance will be based on trial and error. These caveats also apply to patients with schizoaffective disorder.

Adverse Effects of Antipsychotics

Despite their effectiveness in managing psychotic syndromes, antipsychotics have a variety of potentially troublesome adverse effects, especially EPS mediated by dopamine blockade. The severity of these effects differs from drug to drug and corresponds with the drug's ability to affect a particular neurotransmitter system (e.g., dopaminergic, noradrenergic, cholinergic, histaminic). Risperidone doses under 10 mg/day and clozapine appear less likely to cause EPS than conventional antipsychotics. The treatment of EPS is discussed later in this chapter.

Tardive dyskinesia is the most dreaded complication of treatment with antipsychotic medication; it is usually untreatable and often irreversible. All antipsychotics have the potential to cause tardive dyskinesia; cases have even been reported with clozapine or risperidone therapy. Elderly patients, women, and patients with mood disorders appear to be more susceptible to developing tardive dyskinesia, and it has been reported to occur in up to 15% of all patients using antipsychotics for more than a year. It is generally advisable to use the lowest effective doses of antipsychotic medication possible. Tardive dyskinesia consists of abnormal involuntary movements, usually of the mouth and tongue, although other parts of the body, including the trunk and extremities, may become involved. In most patients, the movements are mild and tolerable, but some patients develop a more malignant form of the disorder that may be totally disabling. There is some evidence that vitamin E (i.e., 1200–1600 IU daily) may help to alleviate the abnormal movements to some extent, particularly in patients with tardive dyskinesia of more than 5 years' duration. Therefore, prophylactic vitamin E therapy might be reasonable, especially in predisposed patients.

Patients receiving long-term antipsychotic medication should be regularly monitored for the development of tardive dyskinesia. The Abnormal Involuntary Movement Scale (AIMS) has been developed to help clinicians and researchers rate the severity of tardive dyskinesia. A copy of this instrument is included in the Appendix.

Antipsychotic medications are also frequently associated with the development of *pseudoparkinsonism*. Although this side effect may take 3 or more weeks to develop, patients develop symptoms of Parkinson's disease, including tremor, rigidity, and hypokinesia. *Akathisia* is another side effect that may not appear immediately, but typically has an onset in the first few weeks of treatment with antipsychotics. This condition consists of subjective feelings of anxiety and objective fidgetiness and agitation. Patients report that they feel compelled to pace, to move around in their chairs, or to tap their feet. Treatment for both pseudoparkinsonism and akathisia generally consists of reducing the dose of antipsychotic if possible and/or adding an antiparkinsonian drug (e.g., benztropine) to the medication regimen. Akathisia has been treated with β-blockers (e.g., propranolol 40–160 mg daily in divided doses) or amantadine, a drug that potentiates the release of dopamine in the basal ganglia. Clonidine has also been used to treat akathisia (e.g., 0.2–0.8 mg daily) with some success, but it may cause sedation and orthostatic hypotension.

Another potential neurological side effect is the *acute dystonic reaction*, which usually occurs during the first 4 days of treatment with antipsychotics. A dystonia is a sustained contraction of the muscles of the neck, mouth, tongue, eyes, or occasionally other muscle groups that is subjectively distressing and often painful. Acute dystonias usually respond dramatically to intravenous benztropine (e.g., 1–2 mg) or diphenhydramine (e.g., 25–50 mg). After the dystonia resolves, a 2-week course of benztropine 2 mg twice a day or another antiparkinsonism agent usually prevents recurrences. Patients with a history of dystonic reactions can benefit from a week of prophylactic benztropine when they are restarted on antipsychotics.

The most common cardiovascular effect of the antipsychotics is *postural hy-*

potension, mediated by α-adrenergic blockade. This side effect is caused more frequently by low-potency compounds (e.g., chlorpromazine, thioridazine). Antipsychotics generally do not cause arrhythmogenic effects when used in standard doses. Chlorpromazine, thioridazine, and pimozide have been reported to produce broad, flattened T waves and can prolong the Q-T interval; these changes are of uncertain clinical significance.

Low-potency antipsychotics may also induce *seizures*, especially at higher doses (e.g., more than 1 g of chlorpromazine daily), but high-potency drugs (e.g., haloperidol) are usually safe. Clozapine has also been reported to cause seizures, particularly at high doses. The drugs are not contraindicated in epileptic patients, as long as these patients are adequately treated with anticonvulsants.

Agranulocytosis, a side effect associated with the use of low-potency antipsychotics, is rare, and its incidence peaks during the first 2 months of treatment. The best prevention is clinical alertness for the appearance of malaise, fever, and sore throat early in the course of therapy; routine blood counts are usually not necessary. Clozapine causes agranulocytosis at a higher rate than other antipsychotics, usually between weeks 6 and 24 of treatment. Because of this potentially fatal side effect, patients receiving clozapine must have weekly blood counts as long as they take the medication.

Other miscellaneous side effects include sedation, nonspecific skin rashes, retinitis pigmentosa (especially with doses of thioridazine greater than 800 mg/day), fever (with clozapine), pigmentary changes in the skin (i.e., a blue, gray, or tan color), weight gain, cholestatic jaundice (1% of patients treated with chlorpromazine), and sexual dysfunction including reduced libido, retarded or retrograde ejaculation (especially with thioridazine), impotence, and anorgasmia in women. Antipsychotics appear to be safe during pregnancy, but as a general rule they should be avoided. Because antipsychotics can be excreted in breast milk, breast-feeding is not recommended either.

Antipsychotics, particularly low-potency compounds such as chlorpromazine, commonly cause anticholinergic side effects. Anticholinergic effects include dry mouth, tachycardia, urinary retention, blurry vision, and constipation. Anticholinergics may also exacerbate narrow-angle glaucoma. These side effects are best treated by reducing the dose of medication or switching to a more potent agent (e.g., haloperidol). Antiparkinsonian drugs (e.g., benztropine) used to treat extrapyramidal symptoms can exacerbate these side effects. If urinary retention continues to be a problem, small doses of bethanechol (Urecholine) (e.g., 15 mg three times daily) may help the patient empty his or her bladder more efficiently, and bulk laxatives will help with constipation.

All antipsychotics have the potential to cause the *neuroleptic malignant syndrome*, a rare idiosyncratic reaction that does not appear to be dose related. Usually considered a medical emergency, the syndrome is characterized by rigidity, high fever, delirium, and marked autonomic instability. There are no pathognomonic laboratory abnormalities, although elevations of creatinine phosphokinase and liver enzymes are common. The muscle relaxant dantrolene and the dopamine agonist bromocriptine have been used to treat neuroleptic malignant syndrome, although some experts believe that merely stopping the offending agent and providing supportive care is just as effective. Although earlier reports suggested an alarming 20% mortality rate, the current estimated mortality rate is about 4%. Once the patient has recovered, antipsychotics may be cautiously reintroduced after a 2-week wait, although an agent from a different antipsychotic class is advisable (e.g., chlorpromazine rather than haloperidol, if haloperidol caused the neuroleptic malignant syndrome).

Rational use of antipsychotics

1. Adequate dosages should produce improvement in 4–6 weeks.
   - Improvement should be monitored by following target symptoms (e.g., hallucinations, delusions, hostility).
   - If the patient does not improve, the dosage should be increased.
2. Each drug trial should last at least 4–6 weeks.
   - If response is unsatisfactory, even after the dosage increase, then the drug should be discontinued.
3. There is no reason to use combinations of antipsychotics, particularly because combinations will increase side effects without adding to efficacy.
4. Drug holidays, once advocated for reducing risk of tardive dyskinesia, are ineffective and only increase risk of relapse.
5. Because all antipsychotics (except clozapine and risperidone) are equally effective, the choice of drug depends mainly on side effects.
   - An agitated patient may do best with a sedating antipsychotic (e.g., chlorpromazine); an elderly patient may not tolerate anticholinergic side effects of low-potency agents (e.g., chlorpromazine).
6. Clozapine and risperidone may be more effective than other antipsychotics and have fewer extrapyramidal side effects; clozapine should be reserved for patients considered to be treatment refractory or who have severe extrapyramidal side effects from other agents, but risperidone may be a first-line treatment, because of its high efficacy and minimal side effects.
   - Clozapine has the potential to induce agranulocytosis, and blood counts must be obtained weekly.

Antidepressants

Not long after chlorpromazine appeared, the antidepressant imipramine was synthesized in an attempt by researchers to find additional compounds for the treatment of schizophrenia. It was soon learned, however, that although imipramine had little effect on hallucinations and delusions, it clearly alleviated depression in patients who were both psychotic and depressed. Thus, another class of drugs was created: the tricyclic antidepressants (TCAs). Other modifications of the three-ring structure followed as other TCAs were produced, including amitriptyline and desipramine.

About the same time TCAs were being discovered, the antidepressant properties of the monoamine oxidase inhibitors (MAOIs) were being discovered as well. In this case, iproniazid, an antibiotic used to treat tuberculosis, was noted to bring relief to depressed tuberculosis patients. Later work showed that the drug was also effective in relieving depression in a broad range of psychiatric patients. Although iproniazid is no longer used as an antidepressant, it has been succeeded by other more effective MAOIs, such as phenelzine and tranylcypromine.

A second and third generation of antidepressants have since been developed, some of which differ structurally from both the tricyclics and the MAOIs. All antidepressants, with minor exceptions, are equally efficacious and differ primarily in their potency and side effects. Three groups of antidepressants are commonly recognized: the TCAs, the MAOIs, and the newer agents. Several of the newer agents (e.g., fluoxetine, fluvoxamine, paroxetine, sertraline) are collectively known as the *serotonin reuptake inhibitors* (SRIs). Although tricyclics, MAOIs, and the newer agents are all classified as antidepressant medications and are effective in relieving depressive symptoms, they are used to treat a wide variety of disorders. Hence, the term *antidepressant* is a misnomer.

Indications for Antidepressants

Antidepressants are useful in treating many different psychiatric disorders. The primary indication for antidepressants, however, is the treatment of depressive syndromes. The efficacy of antidepressants is unequivocal, and approximately 70% of the patients treated with TCAs and 65% of the patients treated with MAOIs respond to treatment within 6 weeks. (The placebo response rate in depression is approximately 25%–40%.) Depressed patients with melancholic symptoms (e.g., diurnal variation, psychomotor agitation or retardation, terminal insomnia, pervasive anhedonia) appear to respond better than depressed patients without these features. Secondary depressions (i.e., depressions that follow or complicate other psychiatric disorders), or depressions accompanied by neurotic features (e.g., anxiety, somatization, hypochondriasis) or personality disorders do not respond as well to antidepressants as depressions without these features.

Other disorders treated with antidepressants include the depressed phase of bipolar disorder, dysthymic disorder, panic disorder and agoraphobia, obsessive-compulsive disorder, chronic pain (in selected patients), social phobia, generalized anxiety disorder, certain sleep disorders (e.g., sleep apnea), premenstrual syndrome, and a few childhood conditions (e.g., attention-deficit/hyperactivity disorder, enuresis, school phobia). Antidepressants are also used for maintenance therapy in unipolar depression. New indications for antidepressants include the treatment of bulimia nervosa and facilitation of withdrawal from cocaine.

MAOIs have been recommended as the treatment of choice in cases of *atypical depression*. Patients with this condition usually have a mixture of anxiety and depression and often have reversal of diurnal variation (i.e., worse in evening), hypersomnia, mood lability, hyperphagia, and personal problems such as oversensitivity to rejection. Clomipramine, a TCA, and the SRIs are antiobsessional and are of special value in the treatment of obsessive-compulsive disorder.

Mechanism of Action of Antidepressants

It is widely believed that antidepressants work as a result of their ability to alter levels of the central nervous system (CNS) neurotransmitters. TCAs affect both norepinephrine and serotonin levels by blocking their reuptake at the presynaptic nerve ending. These activities form the cornerstone of the so-called *biogenic amine hypothesis* of the mood disorders. The tertiary amines (e.g., amitriptyline, imipramine, doxepin) tend to block serotonin reuptake to a greater extent, and the secondary amines (e.g., desipramine, nortriptyline, protriptyline) tend to block norepinephrine reuptake.

MAOIs inhibit monoamine oxidase (MAO), an enzyme responsible for the oxidation of tyramine, serotonin, dopamine, and norepinephrine. Blocking this enzymatic process leads to an increase in CNS levels of norepinephrine and serotonin. Two types of MAO have been identified: MAO A, found in the brain, liver, gut, and sympathetic nerves, and MAO B, found in the brain, liver, and platelets. MAO A acts primarily on serotonin and norepinephrine, and MAO B acts primarily on phenylethylamine; both act on dopamine and tyramine. It is thought that inhibitors of MAO A may be more effective as antidepressants.

The newer antidepressants also affect CNS neurotransmitter levels. Maprotiline and amoxapine primarily block reuptake of norepinephrine, and trazodone blocks serotonin reuptake. The mechanism of action of bupropion is unknown, although it does provide weak dopamine receptor blockade. The SRIs selectively block serotonin reuptake by presynaptic receptors and generally have little effect on other neurotransmitter systems. Venlafaxine blocks serotonin reuptake, but it also blocks norepinephrine and dopamine reuptake. Nefazodone blocks serotonin reuptake and is a $5\text{-}HT_2$ agonist.

Pharmacokinetics of Antidepressants

All antidepressants are metabolized by the liver. The TCAs and many newer antidepressants have active metabolites, but MAOIs do not. There is as much as a 10-fold variation in steady-state plasma levels of TCAs among individuals, due primarily to individual variation in the way the liver metabolizes the drugs. In general, the medications are well absorbed orally, undergo an enterohepatic cycle, and develop peak plasma levels 2–4 hours after ingestion. TCAs are highly bound to plasma and tissue proteins and are fat soluble. Free TCA comprises about 1% of the total body load of antidepressants.

All antidepressants are excreted by the kidneys, and their half-lives range from several hours to more than 5 days for fluoxetine. Steady-state plasma levels are achieved after five half-lives, which in turn depend on metabolism by hepatic microsomal enzymes. Blood levels tend to be increased by drugs that inhibit the cytochrome P450 system, including chlorpromazine and other antipsychotics, disulfiram, cimetidine, estrogens, and methylphenidate. The SRIs (primarily fluoxetine and paroxetine, but not sertraline) have been shown to elevate TCA plasma levels through this mechanism. Because fluoxetine and its metabolite norfluoxetine have particularly lengthy half-lives, women of childbearing age should be warned that they should stop the drug about 6 weeks before attempting to conceive. Likewise, before a trial of MAOIs is initiated, the patient on fluoxetine should have a 5- to 6-week washout, because the combination of these compounds is potentially dangerous.

Blood Levels of Antidepressants

Meaningful plasma blood levels are available for imipramine, nortriptyline, and desipramine. Plasma blood levels may be measured for other antidepressants (e.g., fluoxetine), but they are not clinically meaningful. Plasma levels should be obtained 12 hours after the last dose. The established therapeutic range for imipramine (the total for imipramine plus its metabolite desipramine) is between 175 and 350 ng/ml; for desipramine, plasma levels greater than 115 ng/ml; and for nortriptyline, plasma levels between 50 and 150 ng/ml. Research suggests that meaningful plasma levels will also be found for clomipramine.

Plasma levels should not be obtained routinely, particularly if the patient is doing well. Reasons for obtaining blood levels include failure to respond adequately, significant symptoms of toxicity, cases of suspected patient noncompliance, establishment of a therapeutic window (e.g., with nortriptyline), and perhaps the presence of significant cardiac or other medical disease, when it is desirable to keep the blood level at the lower range of the therapeutic value. Blood levels are also valuable in cases of drug overdose.

Adverse Effects of Antidepressants

The most common side effects of TCAs are sedation, orthostatic hypotension, and the anticholinergic side effects (e.g., constipation, urinary hesitancy, dry mouth, visual blurring). Each TCA differs somewhat in its propensity to cause these effects. (See Table 26–2 for a comparison of the antidepressants and their adverse effects.) Tertiary amines (e.g., amitriptyline, imipramine, doxepin) tend to cause more prominent side effects. Tolerance usually develops to anticholinergic side effects and sedation, but TCAs should be used with caution in patients with prostatic enlargement and narrow-angle glaucoma. Elderly patients should have their blood pressure carefully monitored, because drug-induced hypotension can lead to falls and resultant fractures.

Antihistaminic effects of TCAs include sedation and weight gain; α-adrenergic blockade causes orthostatic hypotension and reflex tachycardia. Miscellaneous side effects of TCAs include tremors, pedal edema, myoclonus, restlessness or hyperstimulation, insomnia, nausea and vomiting, electroencephalographic changes, rashes or allergic reactions, confusion, and seizures. Sexual dysfunction, including erectile and ejaculation disturbances in men and anorgasmia in women, is relatively frequent with TCAs.

Cardiovascular side effects tend to be the most worrisome. All TCAs prolong cardiac conduction, much like quinidine or procainamide. In fact, clinical trials have favorably compared imipramine with these type I antiarrhythmics. Thus, TCAs carry the risk of exacerbating existing conduction abnormalities. Patients with low-grade abnormalities such as a first-degree atrioventricular (AV) block or right bundle branch block should use these medications cautiously; increase in dose should be accompanied by serial electrocardiograms. Patients with a higher block (e.g., a second-degree AV block) should not be given TCAs. Doxepin has been recommended as having less cardiovascular toxicity, but this recommendation was based on data in early studies that used inadequate doses. In patients with cardiac conduction defects, newer antidepressants that do not prolong cardiac conduction (e.g., trazodone, fluoxetine) should be used.

A discontinuation syndrome occurs in some patients who have been taking high doses of TCAs for weeks or months. If the medication is stopped abruptly, symptoms may begin within days; these include anxiety, insomnia, headache, myalgia, chills, malaise, and nausea. This syndrome can usually be prevented by a gradual medication taper (e.g., 25–50 mg per week). If this gradual tapering is not possible, use of small doses of anticholinergic medication such as diphenhydramine (e.g., 25 mg two to three times a day) may help alleviate symptoms. A discontinuation syndrome has recently been observed with the shorter-half-life (e.g., fluvoxamine, paroxetine) SRIs, although it is probably uncommon with

Table 26–2. Commonly used antidepressants

Category	Drug (trade name)	Sedative potency	Anticholinergic potency	Orthostatic hypotension potency	Cardiac arrhythmogenic potency	Active metabolites	Half-life (h)	Target dosage (mg)	Dosage range (mg/day)
Tricyclics									
Tertiary amines	Doxepin (Sinequan, Adapin)	Very high	Moderate	Moderate	Yes	Yes	8–25	200	50–300
	Amitriptyline (Elavil)	Very high	Very high	High	Yes	Yes	9–46	150	50–300
	Imipramine (Tofranil)	Moderate	Moderate	High	Yes	Yes	6–28	200	50–300
	Trimipramine (Surmontil)	High	Moderate	Moderate	Yes	Yes	16–40	150	50–300
	Clomipramine (Anafranil)	High	High	High	Yes	Yes	23–122	150	50–300
Secondary amines	Protriptyline (Vivactil)	Low	High	Low	Yes	No	54–198	30	10–60
	Nortriptyline (Pamelor)	Moderate	Low	Low	Yes	No	18–56	100	20–150
	Desipramine (Norpramin)	Low	Low	High	Yes	No	12–28	150	50–300
Monoamine oxidase inhibitors									
	Phenelzine (Nardil)	Low	Low	High	Low	No	—[a]	60	15–90
	Tranylcypromine (Parnate)	Low	Low	High	Low	No	—[a]	30–40	20–90
	Isocarboxazid (Marplan)	Low	Low	High	Low	No	—[a]	30	10–50

(continued)

Table 26–2. Commonly used antidepressants (*continued*)

Category	Drug (trade name)	Sedative potency	Anticholinergic potency	Orthostatic hypotension potency	Cardiac arrhythmogenic potency	Active metabolites	Half-life (h)	Target dosage (mg)	Dosage range (mg/day)
Newer agents									
	Amoxapine (Asendin)	Low	Low	Moderate	Yes	Yes	8	200	100–600
	Maprotiline (Ludiomil)	Moderate	Low	Moderate	Yes	Unknown	51	150	75–300
	Trazodone (Desyrel)	High	Very low	High	Low	Yes	6–11	400	300–800
	Bupropion (Wellbutrin)	Very low	Very low	Low	Low	Yes	12	300	150–450
	Nefazodone (Serzone)	Moderate	Very low	Low	Low	Yes	?	300	100–600
	Venlafaxine (Effexor)	Low	Very low	Low	Low	Yes	3–5	225	75–375
Serotonin reuptake inhibitors	Fluoxetine (Prozac)	Very low	Very low	Low	Low	Yes	7–9 days	20	20–80
	Sertraline (Zoloft)	Low	Very low	Low	Low	No	2–4 days	100	50–200
	Paroxetine (Paxil)	Low	Low	Low	Low	No	24	20	20–50
	Fluvoxamine (Luvox)	Low	Low	Low	Low	No	14–22	200	100–300

aMaximal inhibition by monoamine oxidase inhibitors is achieved in 5–10 days.

fluoxetine because of its long half-life. The syndrome, which consists of irritability, dizziness, headache, and nausea, can probably be prevented by tapering the medication over 1–2 weeks.

The MAOIs have minimal anticholinergic and antihistaminic effects. They are, however, potent α-adrenergic blockers, resulting in a high frequency of orthostatic hypotension. Other common side effects include sedation or hyperstimulation (e.g., agitation), insomnia, dry mouth, weight gain, and impotence in men and anorgasmia in women. The most serious side effect results from the concomitant ingestion of a MAOI and substances containing tyramine. Because tyramine, a pressor agent, is usually broken down by MAO, a buildup will lead to severe hypertension and (rarely) death or stroke.

In addition to interacting with foods, MAOIs can interact with sympathomimetics (e.g., amphetamines) to produce a hypertensive crisis. For these reasons, patients must follow a special low-tyramine diet and must also be aware of potential interactions with prescribed and over-the-counter sympathomimetic medications. A list of foods and substances to be avoided is found in Table 26–3.

Table 26–3. Dietary instructions for patients taking monoamine oxidase inhibitors (MAOIs)

Foods to avoid
- Cheese: all cheeses except for cottage cheese, farmer cheese, and cream cheese
- Meat and fish: caviar; liver; smoked, dried, pickled, cured, or preserved meats and fish
- Vegetables: overripe avocados, fava beans
- Fruits: overripe fruits, canned figs
- Other foods: yeast extracts
- Beverages: chianti wine, beers that contain yeast

Foods to use in moderation
- Chocolate
- Coffee

Medications to avoid
- Over-the-counter pain medications except for plain aspirin, acetaminophen, and ibuprofen
- Cold or allergy medications
- Nasal decongestants and inhalers
- Cough medications; plain guaifenesin elixir may be taken, however
- Stimulants and diet pills
- Sympathomimetic drugs
- Meperidine
- Serotonin reuptake inhibitors (e.g., fluoxetine, fluvoxamine, paroxetine, sertraline)

Adapted from Hyman SE, Arana GW: Handbook of Psychiatric Drug Therapy. Boston, MA, Little, Brown, 1987.

MAOIs also have a potentially lethal interaction with meperidine, the mechanism of which is not fully understood but may have to do with serotonin agonism. If symptoms of hypertensive crisis do occur (e.g., headache, nausea, vomiting), patients should be instructed to immediately seek medical attention. Patients can be treated with intravenous phentolamine (e.g., 5 mg). Patients who do not have easy access to medical care should be advised to carry a 10-mg tablet of nifedipine with them. Nifedipine's α-blocking properties, which act to lower blood pressure when the drug is taken sublingually, make it a useful stopgap measure. The combination of a MAOI and an SRI should be avoided as well because of the possibility of inducing a *serotonin syndrome*, consisting of fever, diaphoresis, confusion, myoclonus, hypertension, tremor, and diarrhea. The syndrome can easily be mistaken for neuroleptic malignant syndrome in the emergency room.

All physicians and dentists must be informed when their patients are taking MAOIs, especially if surgery or dental work is indicated, so that drugs that interact adversely with these agents can be avoided. It is generally advisable to wait 2 weeks after discontinuing a MAOI before resuming a normal diet or using a TCA or other medications that may have an adverse interaction with the MAOI.

The TCAs and MAOIs have no association with fetal abnormalities, and the use of these agents is probably safe during pregnancy. However, common sense suggests they be avoided, especially in the first trimester, unless the medication is absolutely necessary. The newer agents are probably safe in pregnancy as well, although very few studies address this issue. TCAs and paroxetine may be excreted in breast milk, exposing newborns to potentially hazardous antidepressant levels. Little is known about the excretion of other antidepressants in breast milk. As a general rule, women taking these medications should not breast-feed their infants.

Newer antidepressants (e.g., trazodone, fluoxetine, venlafaxine) have little or no anticholinergic potential, and none seem to cause cardiac toxicity or to be fatal in overdose. Amoxapine and maprotiline, however, have mild anticholinergic side effects and can cause postural hypotension and cardiac arrhythmias. The main side effects of trazodone are postural hypotension, nausea, and sedation; a rare but troublesome side effect of trazodone is priapism. Men given this drug should be warned to report any abnormal erections to their physician immediately, because priapism can lead to permanent erectile dysfunction. The main side effects of the SRIs are transient nausea, vomiting, insomnia, and hyperstimulation (e.g., agitation, nervousness). Sexual dysfunction, which appears to be relatively common with SRIs, includes erectile and ejaculatory disturbance in men and anorgasmia in women. These may subside when the dose is lowered. Case reports suggest that the addition of low-dose bethanechol (e.g.,

20 mg taken 30–60 minutes before intercourse) may help, whereas cyprohep-tadine (e.g., 4–8 mg taken 30–60 minutes before intercourse) is useful for an-orgasmia. Yohimbine is also reported to be of some benefit. Venlafaxine and nefazodone are well tolerated; the most common side effects with venlafaxine are nausea, somnolence, and insomnia; and nefazodone is associated with nausea and sedation.

Antidopaminergic effects such as dystonia, parkinsonism, and akathisia are rare side effects of antidepressants. Amoxapine has a greater potential to cause these EPS because its major metabolite has antipsychotic properties. For these reasons, amoxapine is not recommended as a first-line treatment.

Use of Antidepressants

In the past, clinicians generally selected a TCA as the first-line treatment for depressed patients, unless the patient had a history of good response to a MAOI. Because the newer antidepressants, especially the SRIs, are effective, well toler-ated, and relatively safe in overdose, they should now be considered first-line treatments as well, if cost is not a consideration. Patients with a history of a cardiac conduction defect should receive a MAOI or one of the newer antide-pressants. Impulsive patients or those with suicidal urges should receive one of the newer agents (e.g., fluoxetine, sertraline) because they are unlikely to be fatal in overdose. Elderly patients may also do best with a newer agent, because they may not tolerate TCAs or MAOIs very well. Of course, when treating pa-tients, clinicians must be aware of the cost differential among agents; some of the newer medications may not be affordable for some patients.

Once a medication has been selected, the drug should be prescribed for a trial lasting 6–8 weeks. If the clinician chooses to prescribe a TCA, nortriptyline, imipramine, or desipramine should be used because meaningful plasma levels can be assessed. Most patients can be started on 50 mg of imipramine at bedtime, increasing the dose by 50 mg every 3–4 days as tolerated up to 150 mg/day. If no therapeutic response is seen within 1 week of this dose, the dose should be in-creased to 200 mg. If no response occurs within 1 week, the dose should be grad-ually increased to 300 mg. Alternatively, the patient may be given a morning dose of 20 mg of fluoxetine, an SRI. This dose will be sufficient for most patients, negating the need for dose titration. If no response occurs after 3–4 weeks, the dose should be increased to 40 mg daily.

Recommended target doses for the different antidepressants are found in Table 26–2. These should be considered the minimum effective doses for most patients; dose ranges are also shown in the table. These ranges are rough guide-lines to help with dosing decisions. Some patients may respond to doses at the lower end of the range, but others will need doses at the high end. Doses must be individualized to the patient, and much skill and experience are needed to learn how to adjust medication properly. Dosing is key to the therapeutic efficacy of antidepressants, particularly the TCAs and MAOIs.

If a depressed patient fails to respond to an antidepressant after 6–8 weeks of treatment at the target dose shown in Table 26–2, an alternative treatment—another TCA, a MAOI, a newer antidepressant, or ECT—should be considered. (These treatments are effective in 60%–70% of refractory patients.) If a MAOI is selected to follow a TCA, allow a 2-week washout. Lithium augmentation may be tried if these strategies fail. The addition of lithium to an antidepressant increases the likelihood of response in about 50% of patients. Response to lithium augmentation is often evident in a week. Doses similar to those for bipolar patients (e.g., 300 mg 3 times daily) may give the best results. Lithium has been used successfully to augment the effects of TCAs, MAOIs, and SRIs.

Rational use of antidepressants

1. If there is no contraindication, a tricyclic antidepressant (TCA) or serotonin reuptake inhibitor (SRI) should be used initially; monoamine oxidase inhibitors (MAOIs) and the other agents should be reserved for nonresponders. Patients with conduct disturbances should be treated with trazodone, bupropion, or an SRI. Impulsive patients or those with a history of suicide attempt should receive an SRI or one of the other new antidepressants that are relatively safe in overdose.

2. Doses should be carefully adjusted, and each drug trial should last 6–8 weeks.

3. TCAs can be administered as a single dose, usually at bedtime. MAOIs are usually prescribed twice daily, but not at bedtime, as they can cause insomnia. Bupropion is administered in two to three divided doses to minimize its propensity to cause seizures. SRIs are generally given once daily.

4. Although adverse effects appear within days of starting a drug, therapeutic effects may require 2–4 weeks to become apparent.
   • Improvement should be monitored by following target symptoms (e.g., mood, energy, appetite).

5. Antidepressants should not be used in patients with grief reactions (uncomplicated bereavement) or adjustment disorder with depressed mood, because these disorders are self-limiting.

6. TCAs should be tapered slowly (e.g., weeks to months) due to their tendency to cause withdrawal reactions. There is no clinically significant withdrawal reaction from MAOIs, but a taper over 5–7 days is sensible. If possible, SRIs should also be tapered (except for fluoxetine, due to its long half-life), as there is some evidence that they induce withdrawal syndromes in some patients.

7. Use of two different antidepressants simultaneously will not boost efficacy and will only worsen side effects. In rare cases, the combined use of a TCA and a MAOI is justified, or a TCA and an SRI, but these combinations should never be routinely used.

Other agents have been used to augment the effect of TCAs, including tri-iodothyronine (e.g., 25–50 µg daily), L-tryptophan (e.g., 0.5–2 g daily), and methylphenidate (e.g., 10–40 mg daily), but the effect of these agents in augmenting response has not been adequately studied. L-Tryptophan is currently unavailable, after having been withdrawn from the market in 1989 by the Food and Drug Administration. A contaminated batch of tryptophan led to an outbreak of the potentially fatal eosinophilia-myalgia syndrome.

Some patients may benefit from a combination of a TCA and an SRI; the dose of the tricyclic should be kept low because the SRI inhibits the tricyclic's metabolism. Other patients may benefit from a combination of a TCA and a MAOI. Precautions must be taken to avoid potentially dangerous complications, such as a hypertensive crisis. Generally, the two drugs should be started together, preferably after a medication-free period (e.g., 2 weeks if the patient had been taking a TCA). The doses are gradually increased.

Antimanic Agents

By 1970, another major type of drug was added to the psychiatrist's therapeutic arsenal—lithium carbonate, a naturally occurring salt. Its first use in medicine (in the form of lithium chloride) was as a salt substitute for people with hypertension who needed a low-sodium diet; its use was soon abandoned after it was discovered to make some people sick. In the late 1940s, the Australian John Cade found that lithium seemed to sedate agitated psychotic patients. Later, it was learned that lithium was particularly effective in people with mania and was free of many of the unwanted side effects of chlorpromazine. A Danish researcher, Mogens Schou, observed that not only was lithium effective in relieving the target symptoms of mania, but it also seemed to have a prophylactic effect. Lithium is now the treatment of choice for acute mania and for the maintenance treatment of bipolar affective disorder.

Carbamazepine and sodium valproate, both anticonvulsants, are now being used to treat bipolar illness. Other compounds have also been used to treat bipolar illness (e.g., calcium channel blockers, clonidine), but they are still considered experimental.

Lithium Carbonate

Despite much research, the precise mechanism of action of lithium is not known. Lithium has many effects on intracellular processes, such as inhibiting the enzyme inositol-1-phosphatase within neurons. The inhibition leads to decreased cellular responses to neurotransmitters that are linked to the phosphatidylinositol second-messenger system.

The onset of action of lithium often takes 5–7 days to become fully apparent. Antipsychotics, which work more quickly, may be preferred when rapid behavioral control is needed, although benzodiazepine-induced sedation may be as effective. The usual plasma level for the treatment of acute mania is 0.9–1.4 mEq/L, although individual patients may do well outside this range. Lithium is also the medication of choice for prophylaxis in patients with bipolar disorders.

Maintenance doses may be smaller, aiming for a blood level in the range of 0.6–0.8 mEq/L. Lithium has no proven role in the acute treatment of unipolar depression, although the bipolar depressed patient or patient with a family history of bipolar illness may respond to lithium alone. Lithium is also used to augment the effect of antidepressants used in the treatment of unipolar depression.

The most dramatic effect of lithium is in the prophylaxis of manic and depressive episodes in bipolar patients, although lithium appears to work best at reducing the frequency and severity of manic episodes. Prevention of episodes with lithium is not absolute, and patients may still have breakthrough episodes. Lithium has also been shown to be as effective as antidepressants in preventing recurrences of depression in unipolar patients.

The use of lithium in the treatment of schizoaffective disorders and schizophrenia has not been adequately studied, although it is reported that about half of schizophrenic patients will show improvement if lithium is added to their antipsychotic medication. The response rate among schizophrenic patients may be higher when there is a strong affective component to their illness. Mood symptoms are the most likely symptoms to respond, but there may be some improvement in core schizophrenic symptoms (e.g., thought disorder, psychosis). It may be worthwhile to add lithium to an antipsychotic on a trial basis in treatment-refractory schizophrenic patients.

Other uses of lithium include treatment of alcoholic persons to enhance abstinence (discussed in Chapter 14) and treatment of aggression in patients with dementia or a personality change due to a substance or general medical condition, mental retardation, or a personality disorder (e.g., borderline, antisocial). These indications are based on case reports and small case series, so further study is needed before any recommendations can be made for the use of lithium in these situations.

Pharmacokinetics.   Lithium carbonate is administered orally as a salt, most commonly in the form of a 300-mg capsule. It is also available in liquid form as lithium citrate. Lithium carbonate is rapidly absorbed, and peak blood levels are obtained about 2 hours after ingestion. The elimination half-life is about

8–12 hours in patients with acute mania and in the 18- to 36-hour range in euthymic patients. Lithium is not protein bound, nor does it have metabolites. It is almost entirely excreted through the kidney and is present in all body fluids (e.g., saliva, semen). Lithium levels may be monitored in any body fluid, but plasma levels 12 hours after the last dose are the most easily obtained.

Slow-release preparations are available and are indicated when there is gastrointestinal toxicity or when twice-daily dosing would enhance compliance. Lithium is usually administered two to three times daily in patients with acute mania, whereas once-daily dosing with extended-release preparations is recommended in patients receiving the drug prophylactically. Some investigators believe that once-daily dosing offers some protection to the kidneys, but a single large dose daily often causes gastric irritation. Lithium is usually begun at 300 mg three times daily in the average individual and is then titrated by blood levels until a target level is achieved. Adjustments in dose may be made every 3–5 days. Lithium may be discontinued abruptly without a characteristic withdrawal.

Adverse effects.   Minor side effects occur frequently after initiating treatment with lithium. Approximately 50% of patients report thirst or polyuria, 40% tremor, 20% diarrhea, 20% weight gain, and 10% edema. Side effects tend to diminish over time. Many patients gain weight on lithium and should be warned of this possibility. About 5%–15% of patients undergoing long-term treatment may develop clinical signs of hypothyroidism, a side effect more common in women that tends to occur during the first 6 months of treatment. Patients can be managed effectively with thyroid replacement if hypothyroidism develops. Baseline thyroid assays should be obtained before starting lithium; thyroid-stimulating hormone should be measured on a semiannual basis, or whenever there is a clinical suspicion of abnormality. Thyroid dysfunction reverses after lithium is discontinued.

Lithium is excreted through the kidneys and is reabsorbed in the proximal tubule with sodium and water. When the body is sodium depleted, the kidneys compensate by reabsorbing more sodium than normal in the proximal tubules. Lithium is absorbed along with sodium, leading to risk of lithium toxicity. Thus, patients should be instructed to avoid becoming dehydrated from exercise, fever, or other causes of increased sweating. Sodium-depleting diuretics (e.g., thiazides) should be avoided because they may elevate lithium levels.

Long-term lithium patients may develop increased calcium, ionized calcium, and parathyroid hormone levels, although these elevations are usually clinically insignificant. High levels of calcium, however, can cause lethargy, ataxia, and dysphoria, symptoms that may be attributed to depression rather than hypercalcemia.

Although most patients treated with lithium do not experience cardiovascular side effects, about one quarter develop reversible, nonspecific T-wave changes similar to those seen with hypokalemia. Arrhythmias are rare, but sinus node dysfunction has been reported. Many patients develop acne, and those with acne may have an exacerbation. Psoriasis may also be worsened. Lithium has been reported to cause hair loss in some patients. Lithium induces a reversible leukocytosis with white blood cell counts of 13,000–15,000 mm^3. The increase is usually in neutrophils and represents a step-up of the total body count rather than demargination.

Lithium has the potential to cause nephrogenic diabetes insipidus, because it reduces the ability of the kidneys to concentrate urine. As a result, lithium-treated patients produce large volumes of dilute urine; this may be clinically significant for some patients, particularly if output exceeds 4 liters per day. Significant polyuria may be difficult for some patients to tolerate. If it is necessary to reduce urine output, diuretics such as amiloride (e.g., 5 mg twice daily) or hydrochlorothiazide (e.g., 50 mg twice daily) may paradoxically reduce urine output.

Lithium-treated patients rarely develop a nephrotic syndrome due to glomerulonephritis. This complication typically reverses when lithium is discontinued. Taken long-term, lithium can cause a small decrease in the glomerular filtration rate; significant decreases are uncommon. The decreased glomerular filtration rate is thought to be due to a tubulointerstitial nephropathy, perhaps caused by a patient's cumulative exposure to lithium; therefore, it is wise to use the lowest effective dose possible. Serum creatinine measurement and urinalysis should be done at baseline and semiannually afterward. If there is any evidence of proteinuria or a rise in creatinine, additional tests should be performed.

Parkinsonian-like symptoms, such as cogwheeling, hypokinesis, and rigidity, can develop in patients receiving lithium, although these symptoms are unusual. Cognitive effects, such as distractibility, poor memory, and confusion, can occur at therapeutic levels of lithium. In this case, the dose should be lowered.

Contraindications. Patients with severe renal disease (e.g., glomerulonephritis, pyelonephritis, polycystic kidneys) should not receive lithium because it is primarily excreted through the kidney; dangerous blood levels may result in these patients. In patients who have had myocardial infarction, lithium should be discontinued for at least 10–14 days. If treatment with lithium is necessary during the postinfarct period, low doses and cardiac monitoring may be necessary.

Lithium is also contraindicated in the presence of myasthenia gravis, because in therapeutic doses it blocks the release of acetylcholine. Because lithium may aggravate or cause pseudoparkinsonism, patient with Parkinson's disease should be closely monitored when lithium is administered. Lithium should be given cautiously in the presence of diabetes mellitus, ulcerative colitis, psoriasis, and senile cataracts. Due to the increased incidence of cardiovascular malformation in infants of mothers taking lithium (Ebstein's deformity), lithium should be discontinued during the first trimester of pregnancy. Because lithium is secreted in breast milk, mothers taking the drug should not breast-feed.

Carbamazepine

Carbamazepine (Tegretol), an anticonvulsant used to treat complex-partial and tonic-clonic seizures, has a structure similar to that of the TCAs. It is used as an alternative to lithium in the treatment of bipolar illness. Carbamazepine has a therapeutic profile similar to that of lithium. It appears to be effective in treating acute mania and may be effective as a prophylaxis for bipolar illness. Some data indicate that it has a role in the treatment of bipolar depression, but it does not have any known role in the treatment of unipolar depression.

Although the precise mechanism of action for carbamazepine is unknown, it has multiple effects on the CNS. Of theoretical interest is its dampening effect on kindling, a process in which repetitive stimuli may lead to either a behavior or convulsive activity. In mood disorders, repeated biochemical or psychological stressors are thought to result in abnormal excitability of limbic neurons, which carbamazepine dampens through its antikindling action.

When carbamazepine is used to treat mania, its efficacy is reported to be comparable to that of both chlorpromazine and lithium. There is generally a delay of 5–7 days before its full effect is apparent. Carbamazepine may be combined with antipsychotics, especially when behavioral control is necessary. It may be more effective in patients who cycle rapidly (i.e., more than four episodes per year) and who tend not to respond well to lithium. Although a dose-response curve has not been established, the usual custom is to aim for typical blood anticonvulsant levels of 8 –12 µg/ml.

Side effects of carbamazepine include a skin rash in 10%–15% of patients, which is a cause for discontinuation. Other side effects may include impaired coordination, drowsiness, dizziness, slurred speech, and ataxia. Many of these symptoms can be avoided by increasing the dose slowly. A transient leukopenia causing as much as a 25% decrease in the white blood cell count occurs in 10% of patients. A smaller reduction in the white blood cell count may persist in some patients as long as they are on the drug, but this is not a reason for discontinuation. In rare patients, aplastic anemia can develop, but the estimated prevalence of this complication is less than 1 per 50,000 patients exposed.

The drug should be started with 200 mg twice daily and increased to three times daily after 3–5 days. A blood level should be determined 5 days later,

12 hours after the last dose. Most patients require between 600 and 1,600 mg daily.

Before starting carbamazepine, the patient should have a complete blood count (CBC) and an electrocardiogram. While the dose is being adjusted, a CBC should be obtained weekly for 4 weeks; once the dose is stabilized, a CBC should be obtained every 3 months. The patient should be warned about the hematological side effects, and any indication of infection, anemia, or thrombocytopenia (e.g., petechiae) should be investigated. Carbamazepine levels should be checked weekly during the first 4 weeks and every 3 months thereafter. Hyponatremia may be associated with carbamazepine; therefore, convulsions or undue drowsiness should be cause for obtaining measurements of serum electrolytes. Because carbamazepine has been linked with fetal malformations similar to those seen with phenytoin, the drug should be avoided in pregnant women, especially during the first trimester. Breast-feeding by women taking this drug is not recommended.

Patients who do not respond to lithium alone or carbamazepine alone may respond to both taken together. Other pharmacological alternatives that have been studied include clonazepam, clonidine, sodium valproate, and calcium channel blockers (e.g., verapamil, diltiazem). Of the alternatives, sodium valproate is the best studied and is now widely used to treat mania.

Sodium Valproate

Sodium valproate, a simple branched-chain carboxylic acid, is commonly used as an anticonvulsant. Research has shown that it is also effective for treating the manic phase of bipolar illness and for long-term maintenance. It is considered a second- or third-line treatment for patients who do not respond to lithium or carbamazepine, or for those who do not tolerate these agents.

The mechanism of its action is unknown, although it enhances CNS levels of γ-aminobutyric acid (GABA) by inhibiting its degradation and stimulating its synthesis and release. Sodium valproate is rapidly absorbed after oral ingestion, and its bioavailability is nearly complete. Peak concentrations occur in 1–4 hours; it is rapidly distributed and highly (90%) protein bound.

The half-life of sodium valproate ranges from 8 to 17 hours. The drug is metabolized in the liver, primarily through glucuronide conjugation. Less than 3% is excreted unchanged. In contrast to carbamazepine, sodium valproate does not induce its own metabolism. The plasma concentration required for anticonvulsant activity is about 50–125 µg/ml, but this level does not correlate with antimanic activity. The response to sodium valproate may be associated with rapid-cycling illness (more than four episodes per year), the presence of non-paroxysmal electroencephalogram abnormalities, and to a lesser extent, a history of closed head trauma occurring before the onset of the mood disorder.

The enteric coated form of sodium valproate (Depakote) is generally well tolerated and has a low incidence of adverse effects. Commonly reported side effects include gastrointestinal complaints (e.g., nausea, poor appetite, vomiting, diarrhea), asymptomatic serum hepatic transaminase elevation, tremor, and sedation. Less frequent side effects include rashes and hematological abnormalities. Hepatic transaminase elevation can occur in more than 40% of patients and is dose related; it generally subsides spontaneously.

Neural tube defects have been reported with the use of sodium valproate during use in the first trimester of pregnancy; therefore, its use in pregnant women is not recommended. Finally, coma and death have occurred from sodium valproate overdoses with serum levels over 2,000 µg/ml.

Before sodium valproate treatment is begun, a CBC and a liver enzyme measurement should be done, the latter repeated frequently (e.g., every 1–4 weeks) for the first 6 weeks and every 3–6 months thereafter. The drug is begun at 500–1,000 mg daily in two to four divided doses. Serum levels can be obtained after 3–4 days. Depending on the level, the dose can be adjusted further. Most patients need between 1,000 and 2,000 mg daily.

Rational use of antimanic agents

1. Lithium should be used initially (along with an antipsychotic and/or benzodiazepine in highly agitated patients). Carbamazepine or sodium valproate should be used in lithium nonresponders.

2. A clinical trial of lithium in mania lasts 3 weeks at therapeutic blood levels (i.e., 0.9–1.4 mEq/L). A trial of carbamazepine or sodium valproate lasts 3 weeks, but blood levels have not been well correlated with response.

3. Lithium may be given as a single daily dose at bedtime if the amount is less than 1,200 mg. Lithium should be given with food to minimize gastric irritation.

4. Because there is no withdrawal syndrome, lithium can be abruptly withdrawn.

5. Both carbamazepine and sodium valproate may be combined with lithium safely and may be of value in lithium nonresponders. Both agents are thought to be particularly effective in rapid cyclers (i.e., more than three episodes/year).

Anxiolytics

Anxiolytics are the most widely prescribed group of drugs. This class of drugs includes the barbiturates, the nonbarbiturate sedative-hypnotics (e.g., meprobamate), the benzodiazepines, and buspirone. Currently, only the benzodiazepines and buspirone can be recommended because of their superior safety record. The use of anxiolytics probably peaked in the 1970s and has since dropped by about one-third, perhaps as a result of the increased awareness of their abuse potential. There is still a great sense among the general population that these medications are overused by psychiatrists and other physicians. Despite their reputation, benzodiazepines are generally prescribed for short periods, are prescribed for rational indications, and are not overused by the vast majority of patients.

Benzodiazepines

Benzodiazepines—an important class of drugs with clear superiority over the barbiturates and nonbarbiturate sedative-hypnotics—have been marketed in the United States since 1964. They have a high therapeutic index, little toxicity, and few drug interactions. All benzodiazepines can serve as antianxiety agents, sedatives, muscle relaxants, and anticonvulsants. Their approved indications reflect subtle differences among them (e.g., side effects, potency) and marketing strategy. Common benzodiazepines are compared in Table 26–4.

Benzodiazepines are believed to exert their effects by binding to specific benzodiazepine receptors in the brain. The receptors are intimately linked to receptors for GABA, a major inhibitory neurotransmitter. By binding to benzodiazepine receptors, the drugs potentiate the actions of GABA, leading to a direct anxiolytic effect on the limbic system.

Indications.　　The benzodiazepines are indicated for treatment of anxiety syndromes, sleep disturbances, musculoskeletal disorders, seizure disorders, and alcohol withdrawal and for inducing anesthesia.

Benzodiazepines are useful in the treatment of generalized anxiety disorder, especially in persons with severe anxiety. Although some patients may need long-term maintenance treatment with benzodiazepines, their chronic use has been poorly studied, and it is probably best to treat the patient for a short period (e.g., weeks or months), withdraw the medication, and reevaluate. Many patients need benzodiazepines for a relatively short time, during periods when their anxiety is most acute and most problematic. Patients with mild anxiety may not need medication and can probably be successfully managed with behavioral interventions (e.g., progressive muscle relaxation). Further information about the treatment of generalized anxiety disorder is found in Chapter 10.

Alprazolam has been shown to have an antipanic effect, a property that may be shared by other benzodiazepines. Alprazolam also appears to work as an antidepressant in cases of mild to moderate depression; however, it is best to use a traditional antidepressant in the initial treatment in patients with major depression.

Table 26–4. Commonly used benzodiazepines

Drug (trade name)	Rate of onset	Half-life (h)	Long-acting metabolite	Equivalent dosage (mg)	Dosage range (mg/day)
Alprazolam (Xanax)	Intermediate	6–20	No	0.5	1–4
Chlordiazepoxide (Librium)	Intermediate	20–100	Yes	25.0	15–60
Clorazepate (Tranxene)	Rapid	30–100	Yes	7.5	15–45
Diazepam (Valium)	Rapid	30–100	Yes	5.0	5–40
Estazolam (ProSom)	Rapid	10–24	No	1.0	1–2 hs
Flurazepam (Dalmane)	Rapid	50–100	Yes	30.0	15–30 hs
Lorazepam (Ativan)	Intermediate	10–20	No	1.0	2–6
Oxazepam (Serax)	Slow	5–20	No	15.0	30–120
Prazepam (Centrax)	Slow	60–70	Yes	7.5	20–60
Quazepam (Doral)	Rapid	15–35	Yes	7.5	7.5–15 hs
Temazepam (Restoril)	Intermediate	8–18	No	15.0	15–30 hs
Triazolam (Halcion)	Rapid	2–3	No	0.25	0.125–0.5 hs

Note. hs = at bedtime.

Anxiety may also complicate depression. Although the depression should be treated with an antidepressant, accompanying anxiety is more quickly relieved by the use of a benzodiazepine. In some patients, it is wise to combine an antidepressant with a benzodiazepine to provide quick symptomatic relief. When the antidepressant begins to take effect, the benzodiazepine can be safely withdrawn.

Benzodiazepines are effective in alleviating situational anxiety. These conditions, termed *adjustment disorders with anxiety* in DSM-IV, are characterized by anxiety symptoms (e.g., tremors, palpitations) that appear to occur in reaction to a stressful event. Adjustment disorders are generally brief; therefore, treatment with benzodiazepines will be time limited.

Benzodiazepines have established efficacy in the short-term treatment of insomnia unrelated to identifiable medical or psychiatric illness. Most patients with insomnia do not require long-term treatment, and there are few hazards with well-monitored therapy of limited duration. Five benzodiazepines are indicated specifically for the treatment of insomnia (i.e., estazolam, flurazepam, quazepam, temazepam, triazolam), although other anxiolytics are probably as effective. Most patients with insomnia report difficulty falling asleep, so the rate of absorption is a critical determinant of efficacy in this form of insomnia. All of these agents are rapidly absorbed except temazepam. Accumulation of compounds with long half-lives increases the likelihood of continued efficacy during repeated dose and minimizes the probability that rebound insomnia will occur on discontinuation of the drug. The likelihood of daytime drowsiness and impairment of performance is increased, but is partly offset by clinical adaptation or tolerance. Nonaccumulating hypnotics with short half-lives, such as triazolam, have a reduced likelihood of causing daytime grogginess.

Zolpidem (Ambien), a nonbenzodiazepine hypnotic that has recently become available, is indicated for the short-term treatment of insomnia. It is rapidly absorbed, has a half-life of 2–3 hours, and has no active metabolites. The usual dose is 10 mg. This compound does not impair daytime alertness or cause rebound insomnia or tolerance, problems associated with benzodiazepine hypnotics. However, it may cause more adverse effects than benzodiazepines (e.g., gastrointestinal complaints, CNS stimulation, amnesia). Further information on insomnia and its treatment is found in Chapter 23.

Diazepam is approved for the treatment of muscle spasms and musculoskeletal disorders and is also used to treat spasticity associated with spinal cord injury. Its efficacy in these disorders probably results from its nonspecific sedative and anxiolytic effects, because patients with muscle spasm and low back pain commonly experience anxiety or agitation that may exacerbate pain and spasm.

Parenteral diazepam remains the drug of choice for the treatment of status epilepticus. Lorazepam probably has similar efficacy, although onset of action may be slightly slower than that of diazepam. However, lorazepam's activity may last longer because its peripheral distribution is more limited. (Diazepam is extensively distributed in peripheral tissues.) Clonazepam is used to treat certain seizure disorders in childhood. Its use is limited, however, by a relatively high incidence of side effects (e.g., sedation) and development of tolerance.

The alcohol withdrawal syndromes described in Chapter 14 are commonly treated with benzodiazepines, particularly chlordiazepoxide. Benzodiazepines are also used before the initiation of inhalant anesthesia. Benzodiazepines are a logical choice as induction agents before general anesthesia because they carry a low risk of cardiovascular and respiratory depression compared with barbiturates.

Pharmacokinetics.   Benzodiazepines are rapidly absorbed from the gastrointestinal tract and, with the exception of lorazepam, are poorly absorbed intramuscularly. Several of these compounds are available for parenteral use (e.g., diazepam). Midazolam, a short-acting agent used to induce anesthesia, is not available orally. Benzodiazepines are metabolized chiefly by hepatic oxidation. Lorazepam, oxazepam, and temazepam, however, are metabolized by glucuronide conjugation, have no active metabolites, are relatively shorter acting, and are therefore the preferred benzodiazepines in elderly patients.

There is a difference in the half-lives between single-dose and steady-state kinetics. Rapid-onset drugs tend to be very lipophilic, a property that facilitates rapid transit across the blood-brain barrier. Drugs differ markedly in their half-lives; drugs with longer half-lives accumulate more slowly and take a longer time to reach steady state. Washout of the drug is similarly prolonged. Drugs with shorter half-lives reach steady state much more rapidly, but also have less total accumulation. Drugs with long half-lives tend to have active metabolites. Because of the differences in metabolism and half-lives, the best therapeutic results are obtained when the needs of the patient and the situation are taken into account. When prescribing, these three parameters (i.e., half-life, presence of metabolites, and route of elimination) largely determine which drug should be selected. For example, in elderly patients, the clinician would want to select a benzodiazepine with a short half-life, few metabolites, and renal excretion—all in an effort to reduce the possibility that the drug would accumulate, leading to undesirable side effects such as excessive sedation.

Adverse effects.   CNS depression is the most common side effect with benzodiazepines. Specific manifestations depend on the sensitivity of the individual. Commonly reported side effects include drowsiness, excessive somnolence, impairment of intellectual function, reduced motor coordination, and impairment of memory and recall. When these symptoms complicate long-term therapy, they usually occur early in the course of therapy and gradually diminish as a result of adaptation or tolerance, or after reduction of dosage.

All benzodiazepines have a potential for abuse and addiction, although their tendency to produce these effects is exaggerated in the media. Most patients who take these drugs benefit from them, even when they are taken for long periods, and evidence of drug abuse or excessive escalation of dosage is rare. True psychological addiction can occur, most commonly when high doses are prescribed, but it can occur with usual therapeutic doses. Because physiological dependence is more likely to occur with longer drug exposure, minimizing the duration of continuous treatment should reduce this possibility.

Discontinuation of benzodiazepine treatment after long-term use usually leads to recurrence of symptoms, but these symptoms do not suggest addiction. Withdrawal symptoms seem to appear rapidly, reach a peak, and then diminish over time. Symptoms of withdrawal may include tremulousness, sweating, sensitivity to light and sound, insomnia, abdominal distress, and systolic hypertension. Serious withdrawal syndromes and seizures are relatively uncommon. Symptom recurrence appears to have a more rapid onset after discontinuation of short-acting benzodiazepines, and the impact of drug discontinuation can be minimized by tapering rather than abruptly discontinuing treatment. A slow taper is particularly important for benzodiazepines with short half-lives. In fact, when discontinuing a short-acting benzodiazepine, it is often helpful to switch the patient to a long-acting medication before initiating a taper (e.g., from alprazolam to diazepam).

The patient should be advised to avoid alcohol when taking benzodiazepines because of their tendency to interact and cause greater depression of the CNS together than either given alone.

The benzodiazepines appear to be safe during pregnancy, but as a rule they should be avoided. Benzodiazepines are secreted in breast milk, so mothers taking these drugs should be instructed not to breast-feed.

The least controversial aspect of benzodiazepines is their tremendous index of safety. When taken alone, massive quantities of benzodiazepines can be ingested with little or no hazard of prolonged or serious CNS depression. Fatal overdose with benzodiazepines taken alone is almost unheard of. Therapy of benzodiazepine overdose beyond the usual supportive measures is usually not necessary.

Buspirone

Buspirone is used primarily in treating generalized anxiety disorder. It has not been found useful in treating panic disorder, agoraphobia, obsessive-compulsive disorder, or other specific anxiety disorders. Structurally unlike other anxiolytics, buspirone does not interact with the benzodiazepine receptor, cannot be used to treat alcohol withdrawal, and appears to have little abuse potential. Its mechanism of action is unknown, although it alters dopamine receptors. It is relatively nonsedating, does not alter seizure threshold, does not interact with alcohol, and is not a muscle relaxant. Buspirone is well absorbed orally and is metabolized by hepatic oxidation. Its half-life ranges from 2 to 11 hours. Drowsiness, headache, and dizziness are the most commonly reported complaints.

Research has shown that buspirone's effect on chronic anxiety (i.e., generalized anxiety disorder) is equal to that of diazepam, although its effects are not apparent for 1–2 weeks. The drug is no more effective than placebo in the treatment of panic disorder, however. Optimal results are obtained with 20–30 mg daily in divided doses.

Rational use of anxiolytics

1. In general, the benzodiazepines should be used for limited periods (e.g., weeks to months) to avoid the problem of dependency, because most conditions they are used to treat are probably self-limiting.
   - Occasionally, certain patients will benefit from long-term benzodiazepine administration. Long-term administration can be safely carried out, but the patient should be periodically assessed for its continuing need.
2. The benzodiazepines have similar clinical efficacy, so the choice of a specific agent depends on its half-life, the presence of metabolites, and the route of administration.
3. In most clinical situations, multiple daily dosing of benzodiazepines is not necessary for adequate effect, and once- or twice-daily dosing may be sufficient.
   - A dose given at bedtime will eliminate any need for a separate hypnotic.
   - Short-acting agents (e.g., alprazolam) are an exception, because their dosing interval is determined by their half-lives.
4. Buspirone is not effective on an as-needed (PRN) basis and is useful only for the treatment of chronic anxiety (e.g., generalized anxiety disorder).

Agents Used to Treat Extrapyramidal Syndromes

Anticholinergic agents closely resemble atropine in their ability to block muscarinic receptors, and all are similar in action and efficacy for alleviating antipsychotic-induced EPS, especially pseudoparkinsonism. Anticholinergics are believed to diminish or eliminate EPS by reestablishing dopamine-acetylcholine equilibrium, which they do by blocking acetylcholine in the corpus striatum. An equilibrium of dopaminergic (inhibitory) and cholinergic (excitatory) neuronal activity in the corpus striatum is thought to be necessary for normal motor functioning. Antipsychotics cause dopamine reuptake blockage and an absolute decrease in dopamine and hence a relative increase in interneuronal acetylcholine, which results in EPS.

The anticholinergic agent benztropine should be started at a dose of 1–2 mg/day. Smaller doses should be used with geriatric patients. The maximum allowable dose is 6 mg/day of benztropine or its equivalent, because a delirium can occur at higher doses. Benztropine can be administered once daily, preferably at bedtime because it can cause sedation. Clinicians should remember that the anticholinergic side effects (e.g., dry mouth, blurry vision, constipation, urinary hesitancy) of these medications are additive with those of the antipsychotic. Most of the anticholinergics are similar in action and efficacy. Table 26–5 shows common agents used to treat EPS and their dose ranges.

Parenteral benztropine (1–2 mg) or diphenhydramine (25–50 mg) works within minutes to alleviate acute dystonic reactions. Diazepam (5–10 mg iv) also seems to work. Benztropine is the preferred agent because it usually does not cause sedation.

Other agents commonly used to treat EPS are amantadine and propranolol. Amantadine acts to increase CNS concentrations of dopamine by blocking its reuptake and increasing its release from presynaptic fibers. This action is thought to restore the dopamine-acetylcholine balance in the striatum. Amantadine is primarily useful in treating the symptoms of pseudoparkinsonism, such as tremors, rigidity, and hypokinesia. One advantage of amantadine is its lack of anticholinergic properties, so that it can be safely combined with antipsychotics without concern about the development of an anticholinergic delirium. Treatment is initiated at 100 mg daily and increased to 200–300 mg daily. Onset of action occurs within 1 week. Adverse effects include orthostatic hypotension, livedo reticularis, ankle edema, gastrointestinal upset, and (rarely) visual hallucinations.

Propranolol and other β-blockers have been used successfully to treat akathisia, which is usually not alleviated with an anticholinergic. Divided doses of propranolol (e.g., 10–20 mg three to four times daily), or another equivalent centrally acting β-blocker, seem to work well, with benefit occurring within 36 hours to 5 days. Propranolol is well tolerated, and up to 65% of patients benefit. Discontinuation will result in a return of symptoms within 3–5 days.

Clonidine, an α_2-receptor agonist, has also been used to treat akathisia. The drug is usually given in divided doses ranging from 0.2 to 0.8 mg daily. The main side effects are orthostatic hypotension and sedation. Clonidine should be used as a second-line drug for patients unresponsive to propranolol.

In treating EPS, the clinician should begin by reducing the dose of the anti-

Table 26–5.   Common agents used to treat extrapyramidal syndromes

Category	Drug (trade name)	Dosage range (mg/day)	Comments
Anticholinergics	Benztropine (Cogentin)	0.5–6	Use 1–2 mg iv of benztropine or 25–50 mg iv of diphenhydramine for acute dystonia. Anticholinergics tend to work better at relieving the tremor of pseudoparkinsonism than hypokinesia.
	Biperiden (Akineton)	2–6	
	Diphenhydramine (Benadryl)	12.5–150	
	Procyclidine (Kemadrin)	2.5–22.5	
	Trihexyphenidyl (Artane)	1–15	
Dopamine facilitators	Amantadine (Symmetrel)	100–300	Useful in situations in which anticholinergic side effects need to be avoided.
β blockers	Propranolol (Inderal)	10–80	Works well for treating akathisia.
α agonists	Clonidine (Catapres)	0.2–0.8	May cause orthostatic hypotension; therefore, dose should be increased slowly. Works well for treating akathisia.

psychotic if at all possible, or switching to an antipsychotic with less tendency to cause EPS. If these steps fail, anticholinergics, amantadine, or propranolol can be useful adjuncts. Because EPS are unpleasant and reduce the likelihood that the patient will remain compliant with treatment, agents used to treat them can make a significant difference in the patient's subjective comfort.

Psychostimulants

Amphetamines were introduced for clinical use in the 1930s and were soon used for dozens of conditions. As their abuse potential became apparent, governmental regulations became highly restrictive, so that medical use of these agents today has been confined to a few specific indications (e.g., narcolepsy, childhood attention-deficit/hyperactivity disorder [ADHD], refractory obesity). However, interest remains strong in using psychostimulants for the treatment of a variety of other psychiatric disorders.

Amphetamine is an indirect-acting sympathomimetic agent that exerts a host of pharmacological effects, including CNS stimulation, anorexia, vasoconstriction, and hypothermia. Development of tolerance has been documented for certain effects, such as anorexia, although not for CNS-stimulant properties. The

D-isomer is more active than the L form, is highly lipophilic, and is rapidly absorbed from the intestine. Onset of clinical effects is rapid, and peak plasma levels after oral dosing are achieved in 1–3 hours. Renal excretion occurs after hepatic biotransformation. Plasma half-life is about 12 hours. Amphetamine exerts its action through direct neuronal release of dopamine and norepinephrine, as well as the blockade of catecholamine reuptake.

Methylphenidate is structurally related to amphetamine and has similar pharmacological actions, although it is a somewhat milder stimulant. An oral dose is rapidly absorbed, peaks in the plasma in about 2 hours, and has a half-life of about 2 hours. Pemoline is structurally different from amphetamine and is a very mild CNS stimulant with minimal sympathomimetic activity. Its half-life is about 13 hours, and an oral dose peaks in the plasma in about 3 hours. The mode of excretion is primarily renal. The drug has little or no abuse potential.

The main use for these compounds in psychiatry is to treat ADHD in children and selected sleep disorders. As noted earlier in the chapter, psychostimulants have also been used to augment the effects of TCAs in patients with refractory depression. They have been used with some success in treating depression in elderly and medically ill patients (e.g., patients with acquired immunodeficiency syndrome), but they have not been adequately studied for these indications. Their use in treating sleep disorders is discussed in Chapter 23.

Parents, teachers, and clinicians rate 75% of hyperactive children with ADHD to be improved on stimulants compared to 40% of placebo-treated children. Stimulants tend to decrease physical activity, particularly at times when children are expected to be less active (e.g., during school), to improve handwriting, and to decrease vocalization, noise, and disruptive activity. Stimulants improve compliance with adult commands, improve attention span and short-term memory, and reduce distractibility and impulsivity. Common psychostimulants used to treat ADHD are listed in Table 26–6.

Stimulant medication should be initiated at a low dose and titrated weekly according to response and side effects within the recommended range. Stimulants should be given after meals to reduce the likelihood of suppressing appetite. Beginning therapy with a morning dose may be useful in assessing the drug effect, because morning and afternoon school performances may then be compared. The need for medication on weekends and after school must be determined on an individual basis. Pulse and blood pressure should be taken initially and at times of dose change. Weight should be followed during the initial titration, and weight and height should be measured several times annually.

Common side effects that usually disappear within 2–3 weeks of initiating therapy, or in response to a dose reduction, include anorexia, weight loss, irritability, abdominal pain, and insomnia. Occasional patients may develop mild dys-

Table 26–6. Common psychostimulants used to treat attention-deficit/
hyperactivity disorder

Drug (trade name)	Half-life (h)	Dosage range mg/kg/day (mg/day)	Comments
Dextroamphetamine (Dexedrine)	6–7	0.3–1.25 (5–40)	Associated with growth retardation
Methylphenidate (Ritalin)	2–4	0.6–1.7 (10–60)	Most commonly used and best studied; high doses (1 mg/kg) may impair cognitive performance.
Pemoline (Cylert)	Acute: 2–12 Chronic: 14–34	0.5–3.0 (37.5–112.5)	May take weeks for effects to become apparent; less abuse potential.

phoria and social withdrawal at higher doses. Children may (rarely) develop a mild to moderate depression requiring discontinuation of stimulants. A major concern has been the potential for these agents to retard growth, which may be due to the effect that stimulant agents have on cartilage metabolism. This side effect has been associated with dextroamphetamine to a greater extent than with methylphenidate or pemoline. The effect on growth reaches clinical significance in a small proportion of patients and can be minimized by using drug holidays. A potentially serious side effect is the development of motor or vocal tics, which may persist after the withdrawal of medication. Stimulants should be used with great caution in patients with a personal or family history of tics or Tourette's disorder and should be discontinued if tics develop.

Other miscellaneous side effects include dizziness, nausea, nightmares, dry mouth, constipation, lethargy, anxiety, hyperacusis, and fearfulness. Rebound effects consisting of excitability and overtalkativeness approximately 5 hours after a dose are commonly found as the last dose of the day wears off or for up to several days after the sudden withdrawal of high doses of stimulants.

Further information about the use of stimulants in children with ADHD is found in Chapter 22.

Electroconvulsive Therapy

ECT is a procedure in which an electric current is applied across scalp electrodes to induce a grand mal seizure. Interestingly, the treatment developed after the erroneous observation was made that schizophrenic patients improved after spontaneous seizures. ECT was introduced in 1938 in Italy by Cerletti and Bini to replace less reliable convulsive therapies that used liquid chemicals or gases. ECT is one of the oldest medical treatments available, a fact that attests to its safety and efficacy. Its mechanism of action remains a mystery, although it is known to produce multiple effects on the CNS, including the downregulation of β-receptors, a property that ECT has in common with most antidepressants. No other therapy has been demonstrated to be more effective than ECT in the treatment of depression.

Indications for ECT

When introduced, ECT was used indiscriminately to treat patients with all types of problems and diagnoses. It became clear, however, that certain types of patients responded much better than others; patients with mood disorders and specific forms of schizophrenia seemed to respond best. ECT is now used almost exclusively for the treatment of depression. It is generally reserved for depressed patients who fail one or more trials of antidepressant medication, patients at high risk for suicide, patients who are debilitated by their failure to take in adequate food and fluids, and patients who may be at risk for cardiovascular collapse.

ECT is an excellent alternative for antidepressant nonresponders; it is reported that about 70%–80% of drug nonresponders receiving ECT will improve. Research has shown that certain depressive symptoms are associated with a good response to ECT. These symptoms include psychomotor agitation or retardation; nihilistic, somatic, or paranoid delusions; and acute onset of illness. ECT has never been very useful in patients with chronic illnesses and depressed patients with neurotic tendencies (e.g., anxiety, somatization, hypochondriasis) or personality disorders.

Mania refractory to medication also responds well to ECT. In the past, it had been suggested that mania required between 12 and 20 treatment sessions, but research shows that mania responds to the same number of treatment sessions as depression (i.e., 6–12). The presence of mixed manic and depressive symptoms and severe manic behavior predict a good response to ECT.

Schizophrenic patients are occasionally treated with ECT, particularly when a superimposed depression or a catatonic syndrome is present. Anecdotally, catatonia often responds to fewer than five treatments, and we have seen catatonic patients respond to a single treatment. Cases of schizophrenia that have a relatively recent onset (i.e., less than 18 months in duration) and have not adequately responded to antipsychotic medication may respond to ECT; once the illness has become chronic, ECT is of little value. Indications for ECT are summarized in Table 26–7.

Table 26–7. Indications for electroconvulsive therapy (ECT)

• Medication-refractory depression	• Catatonic syndromes
• Suicidal depression	• Acute forms of schizophrenia
• Depression accompanied by refusal to eat or take fluids	• Mania unresponsive to medication
• Depression during pregnancy	• Psychotic or melancholic depression unresponsive to medication
• History of positive response to ECT	

Pre-ECT Workup

Although ECT is classified as a surgical procedure, it is relatively uncomplicated. Routine laboratory tests including a CBC, serum electrolytes, urinalysis,
an electrocardiogram, a chest X ray, and a physical examination are performed
to rule out physical disorders that may contraindicate ECT. Although obtaining
spine films is no longer a routine practice, the films may nevertheless be of value
in documenting the condition of the vertebrae before ECT, especially in elderly
patients and patients with arthritis. The only absolute contraindication for ECT
is increased intracranial pressure, because a physiological rise in cerebrospinal
fluid pressure during treatment could lead to brain herniation. Relative contraindications include recent myocardial infarction, coronary artery disease, cardiac failure, hypertensive cardiovascular disease, bronchopulmonary disease,
and venous thrombosis.

ECT Procedure

Patients are not allowed food or fluids after midnight to minimize the risk of
aspiration. At the ECT site the following morning, patients are anesthetized
with a short-acting anesthetic (e.g., methohexital), receive oxygen to prevent
hypoxia, receive atropine to reduce secretions and bradyarrhythmias, and receive succinylcholine as a muscle relaxant to attenuate convulsions. After the
patient is anesthetized, electrodes are placed on the scalp. Although bitemporal
electrode placement is most widely used, unilateral placement on the non-
dominant hemisphere is also popular because it has been found to reduce memory impairment after treatment. The only drawback to unilateral placement is
that it may be less effective.

A brief stimulus is applied after placement of the electrodes. The amount of
electricity applied is approximately equivalent to that required to light a 20-watt
bulb for 2 seconds. A brief pulse of electrical stimulus is usually used, rather than
a continuous sinusoidal waveform, because brief pulse stimulation is less likely to
cause cognitive impairment. Stimulation usually produces a 30- to 60-second

tonic-clonic seizure. This seizure is accompanied by a period of bradycardia, with a fall in blood pressure lasting about 60 seconds, followed by tachycardia and a rise in blood pressure. A rise in cerebrospinal fluid pressure parallels the rise in blood pressure. These responses are alleviated when ECT is performed under anesthesia. Minor arrhythmias are frequent but are rarely a problem.

Most depressed patients receive a series of 6–12 treatments, although the exact number is individualized. In the past, extra treatments were often administered to reduce the risk of relapse, but research has shown that this practice is ineffective.

Adverse Effects of ECT

As with any medical or surgical procedure, ECT is associated with adverse effects. During treatment, these effects can include brief episodes of hypotension or hypertension, bradyarrhythmias, and tachyarrhythmias; these effects are rarely serious. Fractures were widely reported to occur during ECT-induced seizures in the past, but are uncommon now because of the use of muscle relaxants. Other possible adverse effects include prolonged seizures (which are easily terminated with intravenous diazepam), laryngospasm, and prolonged apnea due to pseudocholinesterase deficiency, a rare genetic disorder. Patients often experience transient confusion immediately after the treatment; headache, nausea, and muscle pain may also be experienced.

The most troublesome long-term effect of ECT is memory impairment, which has led to the concern that ECT may cause brain damage. Several groups of investigators have looked at memory loss and cognitive impairment, and their findings are consistent in showing that the complaints of memory loss are often associated with continuing or untreated depression. Also, ECT can cause a retrograde amnesia involving a short period before and during the hospitalization and can sensitize patients to the normal process of forgetting. Thus, patients who have undergone ECT may be more aware of minor memory disturbance than patients who did not have such treatment. There is little evidence that ECT affects anterograde memory and subsequent learning. Therefore, although ECT may cause a limited retrograde amnesia, there is no lasting effect on anterograde memory. Finally, not all patients experience amnesia, and modifications in ECT, including unilateral electrode placement and brief pulse stimulation, help to minimize any memory loss that occurs.

Acceptance of ECT

Surveys of patients receiving ECT have generally found high acceptance levels. In one study, nearly 80% of patients felt they were helped by ECT, and 80% said they would not be reluctant to have it again. A substantial minority reported approaching treatment with anxiety, but in retrospect, over 80% found it no more anxiety producing than a dental appointment.

Amobarbital Sodium (Amytal) Interview

Amobarbital sodium, thiopental, and pentobarbital have been used for many years to produce a sedated state during which an interview (Amytal interview) may be conducted that is of value both diagnostically and therapeutically. Despite its long history, indications for the Amytal interview are relatively few.

The technique consists of administering 200–500 mg of amobarbital sodium intravenously at a rate of 25–50 mg/minute. The interviewer talks with the patient as the drug is being administered and halts the drug temporarily when the desired level of sedation is obtained (i.e., when lateral nystagmus develops during light sedation or slurred speech develops during deeper sedation). The interview should continue for 30–60 minutes, or until sufficient material has been produced for diagnostic purposes or therapeutic goals have been reached.

One indication for the Amytal interview is the evaluation of mute patients. Patients whose muteness is due to a catatonic syndrome often recover spontaneously and begin to speak. The speech may reveal a formal thought disorder, hallucinations, or delusions that are useful in diagnosing the underlying disorder. When the sedation wears off, the muteness will return. Occasional patients are immobilized by acute anxiety or panic and may talk about their concern when sedated. Dissociative amnesia, dissociative fugue, and conversion disorders are often temporarily relieved by amobarbital sodium; useful information may then be obtained (e.g., amnesic patients may reveal their name and address). The interview has also been felt to be helpful in separating cognitive impairment associated with a dementing illness or delirium from that caused by a mood or psychotic disorder. Patients who are confused or disoriented from a delirium or dementia tend to worsen when given amobarbital sodium, but patients whose impairment is due to major depression or a psychotic disorder will often temporarily improve.

There are several medical and psychiatric contraindications for use of the Amytal interview. Medical contraindications include a history of barbiturate allergy or addiction; severe liver, renal, or cardiac disorders; and upper-respiratory infections. A thorough psychiatric history, physical examination, and screening laboratory examination should identify these conditions. It is unwise to use the interview in paranoid patients, who may misinterpret its use, nor should it be used in unwilling patients, because cooperation is key to the procedure. Overeager patients are poor candidates, because they may use the test for their own (possibly manipulative) purposes or may have unrealistic expectations for the procedure.

Bibliography

Addonizio G, Susman VL, Roth SB: Neuroleptic malignant syndrome: review and analysis of 115 cases. Biol Psychiatry 22:1004–1020, 1987

Adler LA, Angrest B, Peselow E, et al: Clonidine in neuroleptic induced akathisia. Am J Psychiatry 144:235–236, 1987

Adler LA, Peselow E, Rotrosen J, et al: Vitamin E treatment of tardive dyskinesia. Am J Psychiatry 150:1405–1407, 1993

Aman MG: Efficacy of psychotropic drugs for reducing self-injurious behavior in the development disabilities. Annals of Clinical Psychiatry 5:171–188, 1993

American Psychiatric Association, Task Force on the Use of Laboratory Tests in Psychiatry: Tricyclic antidepressants—blood level measurements and clinical outcome: an APA Task Force report. Am J Psychiatry 142:155–162, 1985

Belongia EA, Hedberg CW, Gleich GJ, et al: An investigation of the cause of the eosinophilia-myalgia syndrome associated with tryptophan use. N Engl J Med 323:357–365, 1990

Black DW, Wesner R, Gabel J: The abrupt discontinuation of fluvoxamine in patients with panic disorder. J Clin Psychiatry 54:146–149, 1993

Borison RL, Pathiraja AP, Diamond BI, et al: Risperidone: clinical safety and efficacy in schizophrenia. Psychopharmacol Bull 28:213–218, 1992

Bowden CL, Brugger AM, Swann AC, et al: Efficacy of Divalproex vs lithium and placebo in the treatment of mania. JAMA 271:918–924, 1994

Chiarello RJ, Cole JO: The use of psychostimulants in general psychiatry: a reconsideration. Arch Gen Psychiatry 44:249–250, 1987

Chouinard G, Jones B, Remington G, et al: A Canadian multicenter placebo-controlled study of fixed doses of risperidone and haloperidol in the treatment of chronic schizophrenic patients. J Clin Psychopharmacol 13:25–40, 1992

Cohen LS, Friedman JM, Jefferson JW, et al: A reevaluation of risk of in utero exposure to lithium. JAMA 272:146–150, 1994

Consensus Conference: Electroconvulsive therapy. JAMA 254:2103–2108, 1985

Crowe RR: Electroconvulsive therapy—a current perspective. N Engl J Med 311:163–167, 1984

Devanand DP, Dwork AJ, Hutchinson ER, et al: Does ECT alter brain structure? Am J Psychiatry 151:971–978, 1994

Dilsaver SC: Antidepressant withdrawal syndromes, phenomenology and pathophysiology. Acta Psychiatr Scand 79:113–117, 1989

Fawcett J, Kravitz HM: The long-term management of bipolar disorders with lithium, carbamazepine, and antidepressants. J Clin Psychiatry 46:58–60, 1985

Feighner JP, Boyer WF, Tyler DL, et al: Adverse consequences of fluoxetine. MAOI combination therapy. J Clin Psychiatry 51:222–225, 1990

Fontaine R, Ontiveros A, Elie R, et al: A double-blind comparison of nefazodone, imipramine, and placebo in major depression. J Clin Psychiatry 55:234–241, 1994

Gerner RH, Stanton A: Algorithm for patient management of acute manic states: lithium, carbamazepine, or valproate? J Clin Psychopharmacol 12:57S–63S, 1992

Hyman SE, Arana GW: Handbook of Psychiatric Drug Therapy. Boston, MA, Little, Brown, 1987

Jabbari B, Brian GE, Marsh EE, et al: Incidence of seizures with tricyclic antidepressants. Arch Neurol 42:480–481, 1985

Jacobsen FM: Fluoxetine-induced sexual dysfunction and an open trial of yohimbine. J Clin Psychiatry 53:119–122, 1992

Jefferson JW, Greist JH, Ackerman DL, et al: Lithium Encyclopedia for Clinical Practice. Washington, DC, American Psychiatric Press, 1987

Joffe RT, Singer W, Levitt AJ, et al: A placebo controlled comparison of lithium and triiodothyronine augmentation of tricyclic antidepressants in unipolar refractory depression. Arch Gen Psychiatry 50:387–393, 1993

Jones KL, Lacro RV, Johnson KA, et al: Pattern of malformations in the children of women treated with carbamazepine during pregnancy. N Engl J Med 320:1661–1666, 1989

Kane J, Honigfeld G, Singer J, et al: Clozapine for the treatment-resistant schizophrenic—a double-blind comparison with chlorpromazine. Arch Gen Psychiatry 45:789–796, 1988

Kane JM, Woerner MG, Pollack S, et al: Does clozapine cause tardive dyskinesia? J Clin Psychiatry 54:327–330, 1993

Kaplan HI, Sadock BJ: Pocket Handbook of Psychiatric Drug Treatment. Baltimore, MD, Williams & Wilkins, 1993

Kocsis JH, Frances AJ, Voss C, et al: Imipramine treatment for chronic depression. Arch Gen Psychiatry 45:253–257, 1988

Kupfer DT, Carpenter LL, Frank E: Possible role of antidepressants in precipitating mania and hypomania in recurrent depression. Am J Psychiatry 145:804–808, 1988

Lerer B, Moore M, Meyendorf FE, et al: Carbamazepine versus lithium in mania. J Clin Psychiatry 48:89–93, 1987

Levenson DF, Simpson GM: Neuroleptic induced extrapyramidal symptoms with fever—heterogeneity of the "neuroleptic malignant syndrome." Arch Gen Psychiatry 43:839–848, 1986

Lipinsky JF, Zubenko G, Cohen BM, et al: Propranolol in the treatment of neuroleptic-induced akathisia. Am J Psychiatry 141:412–415, 1984

Little KY: D-Amphetamine versus methylphenidate effects in depressed inpatients. J Clin Psychiatry 54:349–355, 1993

Lusznat RM, Murphy DP, Nunn CMH: Carbamazepine vs lithium in the treatment and prophylaxis of mania. Br J Psychiatry 153:198–204, 1988

McCormick S, Olin J, Bortman AW: Reversal of fluoxetine-induced anorgasmia by cyproheptadine in 2 patients. J Clin Psychiatry 51:383–384, 1991

Merlotti L, Roehrs T, Koshorek G, et al: The dose effects of zolpidem on the sleep of healthy normals. J Clin Psychopharmacol 1:9–14, 1989

Miller LJ: Psychiatric medication during pregnancy: understanding and minimizing risk. Psychiatric Annals 24:69–75, 1994

Nair NPV, Suranyi-Cadotte B, Schwartz G, et al: A clinical trial comparing intramuscular haloperidol decanoate and oral haloperidol in chronic schizophrenic patients: efficacy, safety and dosage equivalents. J Clin Psychopharmacol 6:30S–37S, 1986

Noyes R, Anderson DJ, Clancy J, et al: Diazepam and propranolol in panic disorder and agoraphobia. Arch Gen Psychiatry 41:287–292, 1984

Noyes R, Garvey MJ, Cook BL, et al: Benzodiazepine withdrawal: a review of the evidence. J Clin Psychiatry 49:382–389, 1988

Olajide D, Lader M: A comparison of buspirone, diazepam, and placebo in patients with chronic anxiety states. J Clin Psychiatry 75:148–152, 1987

Pastuszak A, Schick-Boschetto B, Zuber C, et al: Pregnancy outcome following first trimester exposure to fluoxetine (Prozac). JAMA 269:2246–2248, 1993

Perry JC, Jacobs D: Overview: clinical applications of the amytal interview in psychiatric emergency settings. Am J Psychiatry 139:552–559, 1982

Perry PJ, Alexander B. Liskow BI: Psychotropic Drug Handbook, 6th Edition. Cincinnati, OH, Harvey Whitney Books, 1991

Pope HG, McElroy SL, Keck PE, et al: Valproate in the treatment of acute mania. Arch Gen Psychiatry 48:62–68, 1992

Preskorn S: Pharmacokinetics of antidepressants: why and how are they relevant to treatment. J Clin Psychiatry 54 (suppl 9):14–34, 1993

Quitkin FM, Stewart JW, McGrath PJ, et al: Phenelzine versus imipramine in the treatment of probable atypical depression: defining syndrome boundaries of selective MAOI responders. Am J Psychiatry 145:306–311, 1988

Rickels K, Feighner JP, Smith WT: Alprazolam, amitriptyline, doxepin, and placebo in the treatment of depression. Arch Gen Psychiatry 42:134–141, 1985

Rickels K, Fox IL, Greenblatt DJ, et al: Clorazepate and lorazepam: clinical improvement and rebound anxiety. Am J Psychiatry 145:312–317, 1988

Rickels K, Schweizer E: Clinical overviews of serotonin reuptake inhibitors. J Clin Psychiatry 51 (12, suppl B):9–12, 1990

Rickels K, Schweizer E, Case G, et al: Long-term therapeutic use of benzodiazepines, I: effects of abrupt discontinuation. Arch Gen Psychiatry 47:899–907, 1990

Roose SP, Glassman AH, Giardina EGV, et al: Tricyclic antidepressants in depressed patients with cardiac conduction disease. Arch Gen Psychiatry
44:273–275, 1987

Rosebush P, Stewart T: A prospective analysis of 24 episodes of neuroleptic malignant syndrome. Am J Psychiatry 146:717–725, 1989

Rothschild AJ, Sampson JA, Bessette MP, et al: Efficacy of the combination of
fluoxetine and perphenazine in the treatment of psychotic depression. J Clin
Psychiatry 54:338–342, 1993

Schweizer E, Feighner J, Mandos LA, et al: Comparison of venlafaxine and imipramine in the acute treatment of major depression in out-patients. J Clinical
Psychiatry 55:104–108, 1994

Small JG, Klapper MH, Kellams JJ, et al: Electroconvulsive treatment compared
with lithium in the management of manic states. Arch Gen Psychiatry 45:727–
732, 1988

Stein G, Bernadt M: Lithium augmentation therapy in tricyclic-resistant depression. Br J Psychiatry 162:634–640, 1993

Stokes PE: Fluoxetine: a five-year review. Clin Ther 15:216–243, 1993

Tyrer P, Murphy S: The place of benzodiazepines in psychiatric practice. Br J Psychiatry 151:719–723, 1987

Self-Assessment Questions

1. What is the mechanism of action of the antipsychotics?

2. What are the common indications for antipsychotics?

3. How are the antipsychotics used in the treatment of acute psychosis? How are
   they used in maintenance treatment?

4. What are the common extrapyramidal side effects that occur with antipsychotics? Describe the syndromes and discuss their clinical management.

5. What disorders can be treated with antidepressants? How is the term antidepressant a misnomer?

6. What is the putative mechanism of action of the TCAs? Of the MAOIs? Of
   the newer agents?

7. Are blood levels of TCAs meaningful? When should they be obtained?

8. What are the common side effects of the TCAs? Of the MAOIs? Of the newer
   agents?

9. What agent is associated with the occurrence of priapism? Why is this worrisome?

10. What are the typical plasma level ranges for lithium carbonate for acute treat-
    ment of mania? For prophylaxis?

11. What are the common side effects of lithium carbonate?

12. What is carbamazepine used to treat? What are its side effects?

13. Benzodiazepines may be used to treat several clinical conditions. What are these?
14. What are the advantages of benzodiazepines over the barbiturates? What are their pharmacokinetics?
15. What conditions are treated with psychostimulants?
16. What are the relative advantages and disadvantages of dextroamphetamine, methylphenidate, and pemoline?
17. Describe how electroconvulsive therapy (ECT) is administered? What is the purpose of atropine? Succinylcholine? Methohexital?
18. What conditions respond well to ECT?
19. What are the side effects of ECT?
20. Describe the Amytal interview. When is this technique useful?

Appendix

Brief Psychiatric Rating Scale

DIRECTIONS: Place an X in the appropriate box to represent level of severity of each symptom.

	Not Present	Very Mild	Mild	Moderate	Mod. Severe	Severe	Extremely Severe
SOMATIC CONCERN—preoccupation with physical health, fear of physical illness, hypochondriasis.	☐	☐	☐	☐	☐	☐	☐
ANXIETY—worry, fear, overconcern for present or future, uneasiness.	☐	☐	☐	☐	☐	☐	☐
EMOTIONAL WITHDRAWAL—lack of spontaneous interaction, isolation deficiency in relating to others.	☐	☐	☐	☐	☐	☐	☐
CONCEPTUAL DISORGANIZATION—thought processes confused, disconnected, disorganized, disrupted.	☐	☐	☐	☐	☐	☐	☐
GUILT FEELINGS—self-blame, shame, remorse for past behavior.	☐	☐	☐	☐	☐	☐	☐
TENSION—physical and motor manifestations of nervousness, overactivation.	☐	☐	☐	☐	☐	☐	☐
MANNERISMS AND POSTURING—peculiar, bizarre unnatural motor behavior (not including tic).	☐	☐	☐	☐	☐	☐	☐
GRANDIOSITY—exaggerated self-opinion, arrogance, conviction of unusual power or abilities.	☐	☐	☐	☐	☐	☐	☐
DEPRESSIVE MOOD—sorrow, sadness, despondency, pessimism.	☐	☐	☐	☐	☐	☐	☐
HOSTILITY—animosity, contempt, belligerence, disdain for others.	☐	☐	☐	☐	☐	☐	☐
SUSPICIOUSNESS—mistrust, belief others harbor malicious or discriminatory intent.	☐	☐	☐	☐	☐	☐	☐
HALLUCINATORY BEHAVIOR—perceptions without normal external stimulus correspondence.	☐	☐	☐	☐	☐	☐	☐
MOTOR RETARDATION—slowed, weakened movements or speech, reduced body tone.	☐	☐	☐	☐	☐	☐	☐
UNCOOPERATIVENESS—resistance, guardedness, rejection of authority.	☐	☐	☐	☐	☐	☐	☐
UNUSUAL THOUGHT CONTENT—unusual, odd, strange, bizarre thought content.	☐	☐	☐	☐	☐	☐	☐

	Not Present	Very Mild	Mild	Moderate	Mod. Severe	Severe	Extremely Severe
BLUNTED AFFECT—reduced emotional tone, reduction in formal intensity of feelings, flatness.	☐	☐	☐	☐	☐	☐	☐
EXCITEMENT—heightened emotional tone, agitation, increased reactivity.	☐	☐	☐	☐	☐	☐	☐
DISORIENTATION—confusion or lack of proper association for person, place, or time.	☐	☐	☐	☐	☐	☐	☐

Global Assessment Scale (Range 1–100)_____

Source.　Reprinted with permission from Overall JE: The Brief Psychiatric Rating Scale (BPRS): recent developments in ascertainment and scaling. Psychopharmacol Bull 24:97–99, 1988.

Scale for the Assessment of Negative Symptoms (SANS)

0 = None   1 = Questionable   2 = Mild   3 = Moderate   4 = Marked   5 = Severe

AFFECTIVE FLATTENING OR BLUNTING

1 *Unchanging Facial Expression*
The patient's face appears wooden, changes less than expected as emotional content of discourse changes.

0 1 2 3 4 5

2 *Decreased Spontaneous Movements*
The patient shows few or no spontaneous movements, does not shift position, move extremities, etc.

0 1 2 3 4 5

3 *Paucity of Expressive Gestures*
The patient does not use hand gestures, body position, etc., as an aid to expressing his ideas.

0 1 2 3 4 5

4 *Poor Eye Contact*
The patient avoids eye contact or "stares through" interviewer even when speaking.

0 1 2 3 4 5

5 *Affective Nonresponsivity*
The patient fails to smile or laugh when prompted.

0 1 2 3 4 5

6 *Lack of Vocal Inflections*
The patient fails to show normal vocal emphasis patterns, is often monotonic.

0 1 2 3 4 5

7 *Global Rating of Affective Flattening*
This rating should focus on overall severity of symptoms, especially unresponsiveness, eye contact, facial expression, and vocal inflections.

0 1 2 3 4 5

ALOGIA

8 *Poverty of Speech*
The patient's replies to questions are restricted in *amount*, tend to be brief, concrete, and unelaborated.

0 1 2 3 4 5

0 = None   1 = Questionable   2 = Mild   3 = Moderate   4 = Marked   5 = Severe

9 *Poverty of Content of Speech*   0 1 2 3 4 5
    The patient's replies are adequate in amount but
    tend to be vague, overconcrete, or overgeneralized,
    and convey little information.

10 *Blocking*   0 1 2 3 4 5
     The patient indicates, either spontaneously or
     with prompting, that his train of thought was
     interrupted.

11 *Increased Latency of Response*   0 1 2 3 4 5
     The patient takes a long time to reply to questions;
     prompting indicates the patient is aware of the
     question.

12 *Global Rating of Alogia*   0 1 2 3 4 5
     The core features of alogia are poverty of speech
     and poverty of content.

AVOLITION-APATHY

13 *Grooming and Hygiene*   0 1 2 3 4 5
     The patient's clothes may be sloppy or soiled, and
     he may have greasy hair, body odor, etc.

14 *Impersistence at Work or School*   0 1 2 3 4 5
     The patient has difficulty seeking or maintaining
     employment, completing school work, keeping house,
     etc. If an inpatient, cannot persist at ward activities,
     such as occupational therapy, playing cards, etc.

15 *Physical Anergia*   0 1 2 3 4 5
     The patient tends to be physically inert. He may sit
     for hours and does not initiate spontaneous activity.

16 *Global Rating of Avolition-Apathy*   0 1 2 3 4 5
     Strong weight may be given to one or two
     prominent symptoms if particularly striking.

ANHEDONIA-ASOCIALITY

17 *Recreational Interests and Activities*   0 1 2 3 4 5
     The patient may have few or no interests. Both
     the quality and quantity of interests should be
     taken into account.

0 = None   1 = Questionable   2 = Mild   3 = Moderate   4 = Marked   5 = Severe

18 *Sexual Activity*   0 1 2 3 4 5
   The patient may show a decrease in sexual interest
   and activity, or enjoyment when active.

19 *Ability to Feel Intimacy and Closeness*   0 1 2 3 4 5
   The patient may display an inability to form close
   or intimate relationships, especially with the opposite
   sex and family.

20 *Relationships With Friends and Peers*   0 1 2 3 4 5
   The patient may have few or no friends and
   may prefer to spend all of his time isolated.

21 *Global Rating of Anhedonia-Asociality*   0 1 2 3 4 5
   This rating should reflect overall severity, taking
   into account the patient's age, family status, etc.

ATTENTION

22 *Social Inattentiveness*   0 1 2 3 4 5
   The patient appears uninvolved or unengaged.
   He may seem spacey.

23 *Inattentiveness During Mental Status Testing*   0 1 2 3 4 5
   Tests of "serial 7s" (at least five subtractions) and
   spelling *world* backwards: Score: 2 = 1 error;
   3 = 2 errors; 4 = 3 errors.

24 *Global Rating of Attention*   0 1 2 3 4 5
   This rating should assess the patient's overall
   concentration, clinically and on tests.

Source. Available from Nancy C. Andreasen, M.D., Ph.D., Department of Psychiatry, College of Medicine, The University of Iowa, Iowa City, IA 52242. Copyright 1984 Nancy C. Andreasen. Reprinted with permission.

Scale for the Assessment of Positive Symptoms (SAPS)

0 = None   1 = Questionable   2 = Mild   3 = Moderate   4 = Marked   5 = Severe

HALLUCINATIONS

1 *Auditory Hallucinations*
The patient reports voices, noises, or other
sounds that no one else hears.

0 1 2 3 4 5

2 *Voices Commenting*
The patient reports a voice which makes a
running commentary on his behavior or
thoughts.

0 1 2 3 4 5

3 *Voices Conversing*
The patient reports hearing two or more
voices conversing.

0 1 2 3 4 5

4 *Somatic or Tactile Hallucinations*
The patient reports experiencing peculiar
physical sensations in the body.

0 1 2 3 4 5

5 *Olfactory Hallucinations*
The patient reports experiencing unusual
smells which no one else notices.

0 1 2 3 4 5

6 *Visual Hallucinations*
The patient sees shapes or people that
are not actually present.

0 1 2 3 4 5

7 *Global Rating of Hallucinations*
This rating should be based on the duration
and severity of the hallucinations and their
effects on the patient's life.

0 1 2 3 4 5

DELUSIONS

8 *Persecutory Delusions*
The patient believes he is being conspired
against or persecuted in some way.

0 1 2 3 4 5

0 = None   1 = Questionable   2 = Mild   3 = Moderate   4 = Marked   5 = Severe

9 *Delusions of Jealousy*
   The patient believes his spouse is having
   an affair with someone.

0 1 2 3 4 5

10 *Delusions of Guilt or Sin*
   The patient believes that he has committed some
   terrible sin or done something unforgivable.

0 1 2 3 4 5

11 *Grandiose Delusions*
   The patient believes he has special powers or abilities.

0 1 2 3 4 5

12 *Religious Delusions*
   The patient is preoccupied with false
   beliefs of a religious nature.

0 1 2 3 4 5

13 *Somatic Delusions*
   The patient believes that somehow his
   body is diseased, abnormal, or changed.

0 1 2 3 4 5

14 *Delusions of Reference*
   The patient believes that insignificant remarks or
   events refer to him or have some special meaning.

0 1 2 3 4 5

15 *Delusions of Being Controlled*
   The patient feels that his feelings or actions
   are controlled by some outside force.

0 1 2 3 4 5

16 *Delusions of Mind Reading*
   The patient feels that people can read
   his mind or know his thoughts.

0 1 2 3 4 5

17 *Thought Broadcasting*
   The patient believes that his thoughts are broadcast
   so that he himself or others can hear them.

0 1 2 3 4 5

18 *Thought Insertion*
   The patient believes that thoughts that are not
   his own have been inserted into his mind.

0 1 2 3 4 5

19 *Thought Withdrawal*
   The patient believes that thoughts have
   been taken away from his mind.

0 1 2 3 4 5

20 *Global Rating of Delusions*
   This rating should be based on the duration
   and persistence of the delusions and their
   effect on the patient's life.

0 1 2 3 4 5

0 = None   1 = Questionable   2 = Mild   3 = Moderate   4 = Marked   5 = Severe

BIZARRE BEHAVIOR

21 *Clothing and Appearance*
   The patient dresses in an unusual manner or does
   other strange things to alter his appearance.

   0 1 2 3 4 5

22 *Social and Sexual Behavior*
   The patient may do things considered
   inappropriate according to usual social
   norms (e.g., masturbating in public).

   0 1 2 3 4 5

23 *Aggressive and Agitated Behavior*
   The patient may behave in an aggressive,
   agitated manner, often unpredictably.

   0 1 2 3 4 5

24 *Repetitive or Stereotyped Behavior*
   The patient develops a set of repetitive
   actions or rituals that he must perform
   over and over.

   0 1 2 3 4 5

25 *Global Rating of Bizarre Behavior*
   This rating should reflect the type of
   behavior and the extent to which it
   deviates from social norms.

   0 1 2 3 4 5

POSITIVE FORMAL THOUGHT DISORDER

26 *Derailment*
   A pattern of speech in which ideas slip off track
   onto ideas obliquely related or unrelated.

   0 1 2 3 4 5

27 *Tangentiality*
   Replying to a question in an oblique or irrelevant
   manner.

   0 1 2 3 4 5

28 *Incoherence*
   A pattern of speech which is essentially
   incomprehensible at times.

   0 1 2 3 4 5

29 *Illogicality*
   A pattern of speech in which conclusions are
   reached which do not follow logically.

   0 1 2 3 4 5

30 *Circumstantiality*
   A pattern of speech which is very indirect
   and delayed in reaching its goal idea.

   0 1 2 3 4 5

0 = None   1 = Questionable   2 = Mild   3 = Moderate   4 = Marked   5 = Severe

31 *Pressure of Speech*   0 1 2 3 4 5
    The patient's speech is rapid and difficult
    to interrupt; the amount of speech produced
    is greater than that considered normal.

32 *Distractible Speech*   0 1 2 3 4 5
    The patient is distracted by nearby stimuli
    which interrupt his flow of speech.

33 *Clanging*   0 1 2 3 4 5
    A pattern of speech in which sounds rather than
    meaningful relationships govern word choice.

34 *Global Rating of Positive Formal Thought Disorder*   0 1 2 3 4 5
    This rating should reflect the frequency of
    abnormality and degree to which it affects
    the patient's ability to communicate.

INAPPROPRIATE AFFECT

35 *Inappropriate Affect*   0 1 2 3 4 5
    The patient's affect is inappropriate or
    incongruous, not simply flat or blunted.

Hamilton Rating Scale for Depression

For each item select the "cue" which best characterizes the patient.

1: DEPRESSED MOOD (Sadness, hopeless, helpless, worthless)
   0   Absent
   1   These feeling states indicated only on questioning
   2   These feeling states spontaneously reported verbally
   3   Communicates feeling states nonverbally—i.e., through facial expression, posture, voice, and tendency to weep
   4   Patient reports VIRTUALLY ONLY these feeling states in his spontaneous verbal and nonverbal communication

2: FEELINGS OF GUILT
   0   Absent
   1   Self-reproach, feels he has let people down
   2   Ideas of guilt or rumination over past errors or sinful deeds
   3   Present illness is a punishment. Delusions of guilt
   4   Hears accusatory or denunciatory voices and/or experiences threatening visual hallucinations

3: SUICIDE
   0   Absent
   1   Feels life is not worth living
   2   Wishes he were dead or any thoughts of possible death to self
   3   Suicide ideas or gesture
   4   Attempts at suicide (any serious attempt rates 4)

4: INSOMNIA EARLY
   0   No difficulty falling asleep
   1   Complains of occasional difficulty falling asleep—i.e., more than ¼ hour
   2   Complains of nightly difficulty falling asleep

5: INSOMNIA MIDDLE
   0   No difficulty
   1   Patient complains of being restless and disturbed during the night
   2   Waking during the night—any getting out of bed rates 2 (except for purpose of voiding)

6: INSOMNIA LATE
    0 No difficulty
    1 Waking in early hours of the morning but goes back to sleep
    2 Unable to fall asleep again if gets out of bed

7: WORK AND ACTIVITIES
    0 No difficulty
    1 Thoughts and feelings of incapacity, fatigue or weakness related to activities, work, or hobbies
    2 Loss of interest in activity, hobbies, or work—either directly reported by patient, or indirect in listlessness, indecision and vacillation (feels he has to push self to work or activities)
    3 Decrease in actual time spent in activities or decrease in productivity. In hospital, rate 3 if patient does not spend at least three hours a day in activities (hospital job or hobbies) exclusive of ward chores
    4 Stopped working because of present illness. In hospital, rate 4 if patient engages in no activities except ward chores, or if patient fails to perform ward chores unassisted

8: RETARDATION (Slowness of thought and speech; impaired ability to concentrate; decreased motor activity)
    0 Normal speech and thought
    1 Slight retardation at interview
    2 Obvious retardation at interview
    3 Interview difficult
    4 Complete stupor

9: AGITATION
    0 None
    1 "Playing with" hands, hair, etc.
    2 Hand-wringing, nail biting, hair pulling, biting of lips

10: ANXIETY PSYCHIC
    0 No difficulty
    1 Subjective tension and irritability
    2 Worrying about minor matters
    3 Apprehensive attitude apparent in face or speech
    4 Fears expressed without questioning

11: ANXIETY SOMATIC
    0 Absent
    1 Mild
    2 Moderate

Physiological concomitants of anxiety, such as:

Gastrointestinal—dry mouth, wind,

3	Severe	indigestion, diarrhea, cramps, belching
4	Incapacitating	Cardiovascular—palpitations, headaches
		Respiratory—hyperventilation, sighing
		Urinary frequency
		Sweating

12: SOMATIC SYMPTOMS GASTROINTESTINAL

0 None
1 Loss of appetite but eating without staff encouragement. Heavy feelings in abdomen
2 Difficulty eating without staff urging. Requests or requires laxatives or medication for bowels or medication for G.I. symptoms

13: SOMATIC SYMPTOMS GENERAL

0 None
1 Heaviness in limbs, back or head. Backaches, headache, muscle aches. Loss of energy and fatigability
2 Any clear cut symptom rates 2

14: GENITAL SYMPTOMS

0	Absent	Symptoms such as:
1	Mild	Loss of libido
2	Severe	Menstrual disturbances

15: HYPOCHONDRIASIS

0 Not present
1 Self-absorption (bodily)
2 Preoccupation with health
3 Frequent complaints, requests for help, etc.
4 Hypochondriacal delusions

16: LOSS OF WEIGHT

A: WHEN RATING BY HISTORY
0 No weight loss
1 Probable weight loss associated with present illness
2 Definite (according to patient) weight loss

B: ON WEEKLY RATINGS BY WARD PSYCHIATRIST, WHEN ACTUAL WEIGHT CHANGES ARE MEASURED
0 Less than 1 lb. weight loss in week
1 Greater than 1 lb. weight loss in week
2 Greater than 2 lb. weight loss in week

17: INSIGHT
  0 Acknowledges being depressed and ill
  1 Acknowledges illness but attributes cause to bad food, climate, overwork, virus, need for rest, etc.
  2 Denies being ill at all

18: DIURNAL VARIATION
  A.M.   P.M.
  0   0   Absent   If symptoms are worse in the morning
  1   1   Mild   or evening, note which it is and rate
  2   2   Severe   severity of variation

19: DEPERSONALIZATION AND DEREALIZATION
  0 Absent
  1 Mild   Such as:
  2 Moderate   Feelings of unreality
  3 Severe   Nihilistic ideas
  4 Incapacitating

20: PARANOID SYMPTOMS
  0 None
  1
  2 Suspiciousness
  3 Ideas of reference
  4 Delusions of reference and persecution

21: OBSESSIONAL AND COMPULSIVE SYMPTOMS
  0 Absent
  1 Mild
  2 Severe

22: HELPLESSNESS
  0 Not present
  1 Subjective feelings which are elicited only by inquiry
  2 Patient volunteers his helpless feelings
  3 Requires urging, guidance, and reassurance to accomplish ward chores or personal hygiene
  4 Requires physical assistance for dress, grooming, eating, bedside tasks, or personal hygiene

23: HOPELESSNESS
  0 Not present
  1 Intermittently doubts that "things will improve" but can be reassured
  2 Consistently feels "hopeless" but accepts reassurances

3 Expresses feelings of discouragement, despair, pessimism about future, which cannot be dispelled

4 Spontaneously and inappropriately perseverates "I'll never get well" or its equivalent

24: WORTHLESSNESS (Ranges from mild loss of esteem, feelings of inferiority, self-depreciation to delusional notions of worthlessness)

0 Not present

1 Indicates feelings of worthlessness (loss of self-esteem) only on questioning

2 Spontaneously indicates feelings of worthlessness (loss of self-esteem)

3 Different from 2 by degree. Patient volunteers that he is "no good," "inferior," etc.

4 Delusional notions of worthlessness—i.e., "I am a heap of garbage" or its equivalent

---

Source. Reprinted with permission from Hamilton M: A rating scale for depression. J Neurol Neurosurg Psychiatry 23:56–62, 1960.

Hamilton Anxiety Rating Scale

Patient's Name

Date of First Report

Diagnosis

Date of This Report

Current Therapy

Instructions   This checklist is to assist the physician in evaluating each
patient with respect to degree of anxiety and pathological
condition. Please fill in the appropriate rating.

0   None
1   Mild
2   Moderate
3   Severe
4   Severe, grossly disabling

Item	Rating	Descriptions
Anxious Mood		Worries, anticipation of the worst, fearful anticipation, irritability.
Tension		Feelings of tension, fatigability, startle response, moved to tears easily, trembling, feelings of restlessness, inability to relax.
Fear		Of dark, of strangers, of being left alone, of animals, of traffic, of crowds.
Insomnia		Difficulty in falling asleep, broken sleep, unsatisfying sleep and fatigue on waking, dreams, nightmares, night terrors.
Intellectual (Cognitive)		Difficulty in concentration, poor memory.
Depressed Mood		Loss of interest, lack of pleasure in hobbies, depression, early waking, diurnal swing.
Behavior at Interview		Fidgeting, restlessness or pacing, tremor of hands, furrowed brow, strained face, sighing or rapid respiration, facial pallor, swallowing, belching, brisk tendon jerks, dilated pupils, exophthalmos.

Item	Rating	Descriptions
Somatic (Sensory)		Tinnitus, blurring of vision, hot and cold flushes, feelings of weakness, picking sensation.
Cardiovascular Symptoms		Tachycardia, palpitations, pain in chest, throbbing of vessels, fainting feelings, missing beat.
Respiratory Symptoms		Pressure or constriction in chest, choking feelings, sighing, dyspnea.
Gastrointestinal Symptoms		Difficulty in swallowing, wind, abdominal pain, burning sensations, abdominal fullness, nausea, vomiting, borborygmi, looseness of bowels, loss of weight, constipation.
Genitourinary Symptoms		Frequency of micturition, urgency of micturition, amenorrhea, menorrhagia, development of frigidity, premature ejaculation, loss of libido, impotence.
Autonomic Symptoms		Dry mouth, flushing, pallor, tendency to sweat, giddiness, tension headache, raising of hair.
Somatic (Muscular)		Pains and aches, twitchings, stiffness, myoclonic jerks, grinding of teeth, unsteady voice, increased muscular tone.
Total Score		

Source. Reprinted with permission from Hamilton M: The assessment of anxiety states by rating. Br J Med Psychol 32:50–55, 1959.

Abnormal Involuntary Movement Scale (AIMS)

		None	Minimal	Mild	Moderate	Severe
FACIAL AND ORAL MOVEMENTS	1: Muscles of Facial Expression e.g., movements of forehead, eyebrows, periorbital area, cheeks; include frowning, blinking, smiling, grimacing	0	1	2	3	4
	2: Lips and Perioral Area e.g., puckering, pouting, smacking	0	1	2	3	4
	3: Jaw e.g., biting, clenching, chewing, mouth opening, lateral movement	0	1	2	3	4
	4: Tongue Rate only increase in movement both in and out of mouth, NOT inability to sustain movement	0	1	2	3	4
EXTREMITY MOVEMENTS	5: Upper (arms, wrists, hands, fingers) Include choreic movements (i.e., rapid, objectively purposeless, irregular, spontaneous), athetoid movements (i.e., slow, irregular, complex, serpentine). Do NOT include tremor (i.e., repetitive, regular, rhythmic)	0	1	2	3	4
	6: Lower (legs, knees, ankles, toes) e.g., lateral knee movement, foot tapping, heel dropping, foot squirming, inversion and eversion of foot	0	1	2	3	4
TRUNK MOVEMENTS	7: Neck, shoulders, hips e.g., rocking, twisting, squirming, pelvic gyrations	0	1	2	3	4
	8: Severity of abnormal movements	0	1	2	3	4
GLOBAL JUDGMENT	9: Incapacitation due to abnormal movements	0	1	2	3	4

10: Patient's awareness of abnormal movements
Rate only patient's report

- No awareness — 0
- Aware, no distress — 1
- Aware, mild distress — 2
- Aware, moderate distress — 3
- Aware, severe distress — 4

11: Current problems with teeth and/or dentures
- No — 0
- Yes — 1

12: Does patient usually wear dentures?
- No — 0
- Yes — 1

Examination Procedures for AIMS

Either before or after completing the Examination Procedure observe the patient unobtrusively, at rest (e.g., in waiting room). The chair to be used in this examination should be a hard, firm one without arms.

1: Ask patient whether there is anything in his/her mouth (i.e., gum, candy, etc.) and if there is, to remove it.

2: Ask patient about the *current* condition of his/her teeth. Ask patient if he/she wears dentures. Do teeth or dentures bother patient *now*

3: Ask patient whether he/she notices any movements in mouth, face, hands, or feet. If yes, ask to describe and to what extent they *currently* bother patient or interfere with his/her activities.

4: Have patient sit in chair with hands on knees, legs slightly apart, and feet flat on floor. (Look at entire body for movements while in this position.)

5: Ask patient to sit with hands hanging unsupported. If male, between legs, if female and wearing a dress, hanging over knees. (Observe hands and other body areas.)

6: Ask patient to open mouth. (Observe tongue at rest within mouth.) Do this twice.

7: Ask patient to protrude tongue. (Observe tongue at rest within mouth.) Do this twice.

*8: Ask patient to tap thumb, with each finger, as rapidly as possible for 10–15 seconds; separately with right hand, then with left hand. (Observe facial and leg movements.)

9: Flex and extend patient's left and right arms (one at a time). (Note any rigidity and rate on NOTES.)

10: Ask patient to stand up. (Observe in profile. Observe all body areas again, hips included.)

*11: Ask patient to extend both arms outstretched in front with palms down. (Observe trunk, legs, and mouth.)

*12: Have patient walk a few paces, turn, and walk back to chair. (Observe hands and gait.) Do this twice.

---

* Activated movements.

Source. Reprinted from Guy W: ECDEU: assessment manual for psychopharmacology (DHEW Publ No 76–338). Washington, DC, Department of Health, Education, and Welfare, Psychopharmacology Research Branch, 1976.

Simpson-Angus Rating Scale

1. **GAIT:** The patient is examined as he walks into the examining room; his gait, the swing of his arms, his general posture, all form the basis for an overall score for this item. This is rated as follows:
   0 Normal.
   1 Diminution in swing while the patient is walking.
   2 Marked diminution in swing with obvious rigidity in the arm.
   3 Stiff gait with arms held rigidly before the abdomen.
   4 Stooped shuffling gait with propulsion and retropulsion.

2. **ARM DROPPING:** The patient and the examiner both raise their arms to shoulder height and let them fall to their sides. In a normal subject a stout slap is heard as the arms hit the sides. In the patient with extreme Parkinson's syndrome the arms fall very slowly.
   0 Normal, free fall with loud slap and rebound.
   1 Fall slowed slightly with less audible contact and little rebound.
   2 Fall slowed, no rebound.
   3 Marked slowing, no slap at all.
   4 Arms fall as though against resistance; as though through glue.

3. **SHOULDER SHAKING:** The subject's arms are bent at a right angle at the elbow and are taken one at a time by the examiner who grasps one hand and also clasps the other around the patient's elbow. The subject's upper arm is pushed to and fro and the humerus is externally rotated. The degree of resistance from normal to extreme rigidity is scored as follows:
   0 Normal.
   1 Slight stiffness and resistance.
   2 Moderate stiffness and resistance.
   3 Marked rigidity with difficulty in passive movement.
   4 Extreme stiffness and rigidity with almost a frozen shoulder.

4. **ELBOW RIGIDITY:** The elbow joints are separately bent at right angles and passively extended and flexed, with the subject's biceps observed and simultaneously palpated. The resistance to this procedure is rated. (The presence of cogwheel rigidity is noted separately.) Scoring is from 0 to 4, as in the Shoulder Shaking test.
   0 Normal.
   1 Slight stiffness and resistance.

2 Moderate stiffness and resistance.

3 Marked rigidity with difficulty in passive movement.

4 Extreme stiffness and rigidity with almost a frozen shoulder.

5. **FIXATION OF POSITION OR WRIST RIGIDITY:** The wrist is held in one hand and the fingers held by the examiner's other hand, with the wrist moved to extension flexion and both ulnar and radial deviation. The resistance to this procedure is rated as in Items 3 and 4.

0 Normal.

1 Slight stiffness and resistance.

2 Moderate stiffness and resistance.

3 Marked rigidity with difficulty in passive movement.

4 Extreme stiffness and rigidity with almost a frozen shoulder.

6. **LEG PENDULOUSNESS:** The patient sits on a table with his legs hanging down and swinging free. The ankle is grasped by the examiner and raised until the knee is partially extended. It is then allowed to fall. The resistance to falling and the lack of swinging form the basis for the score on this item:

0 The legs swing freely.

1 Slight diminution in the swing of the legs.

2 Moderate resistance to swing.

3 Marked resistance and damping of swing.

4 Complete absence of swing.

7. **HEAD DROPPING:** The patient lies on a well-padded examining table and his head is raised by the examiner's hand. The hand is then withdrawn and the head allowed to drop. In the normal subject the head will fall upon the table. The movement is delayed in extrapyramidal system disorder, and in extreme Parkinsonism it is absent. The neck muscles are rigid and the head does not reach the examining table. Scoring is as follows:

0 The head falls completely, with a good thump as it hits the table.

1 Slight slowing in fall, mainly noted by lack of slap as head meets the table.

2 Moderate slowing in the fall, quite noticeable to the eye.

3 Head falls stiffly and slowly.

4 Head does not reach examining table.

8. **GLABELLA TAP:** Subject is told to open his eyes wide and not to blink. The glabella region is tapped at a steady, rapid speed. The number of times patient blinks in succession is noted:

0 0 to 5 blinks

1 6 to 10 blinks

2 11 to 15 blinks

3 16 to 20 blinks

4 21 or more blinks

9. **TREMOR:** Patient is observed walking into examining room and then is reexamined for this item:

0 Normal.

1 Mild finger tremor, obvious to sight and touch.

2 Tremor of hand or arm occurring spasmodically.

3 Persistent tremor of one or more limbs.

4 Whole body tremor.

10. **SALIVATION:** Patient is observed while talking and then asked to open his mouth and elevate his tongue. The following ratings are given:

0 Normal.

1 Excess salivation to the extent that pooling takes place if the mouth is open and the tongue raised.

2 When excess salivation is present and might occasionally result in difficulty in speaking.

3 Speaking with difficulty because of excess salivation.

4 Frank drooling.

Source. Reprinted with permission from Simpson GM, Angus JWS: A rating scale for extrapyramidal side effects. Acta Psychiatr Scand Suppl 212:11–19, 1970.

"Mini-Mental State"

ORIENTATION

5   ( )   What is the (year) (season) (date) (day) (month)?

5   ( )   Where are we: (state) (country) (town) (hospital) (floor)?

REGISTRATION

3   ( )   Name 3 objects: 1 second to say each. Then ask the patient all 3 after you have said them. Give 1 point for each correct answer. Then repeat them until he learns all 3. Count trials and record.
Trials _____

ATTENTION AND CALCULATION

5   ( )   Serial 7s. 1 point for each correct. Stop after 5 answers. Alternatively spell "world" backwards.

RECALL

3   ( )   Ask for the 3 objects repeated above. Give 1 point for each correct.

LANGUAGE

9   ( )   Name a pencil, and watch (2 points)

Repeat the following, "No ifs, ands, or buts." (1 point)

Follow a 3-stage command:
"Take a paper in your right hand, fold it in half, and put it on the floor"
(3 points)

Read and obey the following:
CLOSE YOUR EYES (1 point)
Write a sentence (1 point)
Copy design (1 point)

Total score _____

ASSESS level of consciousness along a continuum _____

Alert   Drowsy   Stupor   Coma

INSTRUCTIONS FOR ADMINISTRATION OF MINI-MENTAL STATE EXAMINATION

ORIENTATION

(1) Ask for the date. Then ask specifically for parts omitted, e.g., "Can you also tell me what season it is?" One point for each correct.

(2) Ask in turn "Can you tell me the name of this hospital?" (town, county, etc.). One point for each correct.

REGISTRATION

Ask the patient if you may test his memory. Then say the names of 3 unrelated objects, clearly and slowly, about one second for each. After you have said all 3, ask him to repeat them. This first repetition determines his score (0–3) but keep saying them until he can repeat all 3, up to 6 trials. If he does not eventually learn all 3, recall cannot be meaningfully tested.

ATTENTION AND CALCULATION

Ask the patient to begin with 100 and count backwards by 7. Stop after 5 subtractions (93, 86, 79, 72, 65). Score the total number of correct answers.

If the patient cannot or will not perform this task, ask him to spell the word "world" backwards. The score is the number of letters in correct order, e.g., dlrow = 5, dlorw = 3.

RECALL

Ask the patient if he can recall the 3 words you previously asked him to remember. Score 0–3.

LANGUAGE

Naming: Show the patient a wrist watch and ask him what it is. Repeat for pencil. Score 0–2.

Repetition: Ask the patient to repeat the sentence after you. Allow only one trial. Score 0 or 1.

3-Stage command: Give the patient a piece of plain blank paper and repeat the command. Score 1 point for each part correctly executed.

Reading: On a blank piece of paper print the sentence "Close your eyes," in letters large enough for the patient to see clearly. Ask him to read it and do what it says. Score 1 point only if he actually closes his eyes.

Writing: Give the patient a blank piece of paper and ask him to write a sentence for you. Do not dictate a sentence, it is to be written spontaneously. It must contain a subject and verb and be sensible. Correct grammar and punctuation are not necessary.

Copying: On a clean piece of paper, draw intersecting pentagons, each side about 1 in., and ask him to copy it exactly as it is. All 10 angles must be present and 2 must intersect to score 1 point. Tremor and rotation are ignored.

Estimate the patient's level of sensorium along a continuum, from alert on the left to coma on the right.

Source.   Reprinted with permission from Folstein MF, Folstein SE, McHugh PR: "Mini-Mental State": a practical method for grading the cognitive state of patients for the clinician. J Psychiatr Res 12:189–198, 1975. Copyright 1975 Pergamon Press PLC.

Global Assessment Scale (GAS)

Rate the subject's lowest level of functioning in the last week by selecting the lowest range which describes his functioning on a hypothetical continuum of mental health-illness. For example, a subject whose "behavior is considerably influenced by delusions" (range 21–30) should be given a rating in that range even though he has "major impairment in several areas" (range 31–40). Use intermediary levels when appropriate (e.g., 35, 58, 63). Rate actual functioning independent of whether or not subject is receiving and may be helped by medication or some other form of treatment.

100 No symptoms, superior functioning in a wide range of activities, life's problems never seem to
| get out of hand, is sought out by others because of his warmth and integrity.
91

90 Transient symptoms may occur, but good functioning in all areas, interested and involved in a
| wide range of activities, socially effective, generally satisfied with life, "everyday" worries that
81 only occasionally get out of hand.

80 Minimal symptoms may be present but no more than slight impairment in functioning, varying
| degrees of "everyday" worries and problems that sometimes get out of hand.
71

70 Some mild symptoms (e.g., depressive mood and mild insomnia) OR some difficulty in several
| areas of functioning, but generally functioning pretty well, has some meaningful interpersonal
61 relationships and most untrained people would not consider him "sick."

60 Moderate symptoms OR generally functioning with some difficulty (e.g., few friends and flat
| affect, depressed mood, and pathological self-doubt, euphoric mood and pressure of speech,
51 moderately severe antisocial behavior).

50 Any serious symptomatology or impairment in functioning that most clinicians would think
| obviously requires treatment or attention (e.g., suicidal preoccupation or gesture, severe
41 obsessional rituals, frequent anxiety attacks, serious antisocial behavior, compulsive drinking).

40 Major impairment in several areas, such as work, family relations, judgment, thinking, or mood
| (e.g., depressed woman avoids friends, neglects family, unable to do housework), OR some
| impairment in reality testing or communication (e.g., speech is at times obscure, illogical, or
31 irrelevant), OR single serious suicide attempt.

30 Unable to function in almost all areas (e.g., stays in bed all day), OR behavior is considerably
| influenced by either delusions or hallucinations, OR serious impairment in communication
21 (e.g., sometimes incoherent or unresponsive) or judgment (e.g, acts grossly inappropriately).

20 Needs some supervision to prevent hurting self or others, or to maintain minimal personal
| hygiene (e.g., repeated suicide attempts, frequently violent, manic excitement, smears feces),
11 OR gross impairment in communication (e.g., largely incoherent or mute).

10 Needs constant supervision for several days to prevent hurting self or others, or makes no
| attempt to maintain minimal personal hygiene.
1

Source. Reprinted with permission from Endicott J, Spitzer RL, Fleiss JL, et al: The Global Assessment Scale: a procedure for measuring overall severity of psychiatric disturbance. Arch Gen Psychiatry 33:766–771, 1976. Copyright 1976/78, American Medical Association.

Yale-Brown Obsessive-Compulsive Scale

For each item circle the number identifying the response which best characterizes the patient.

1. **Time Occupied by Obsessive Thoughts**
   How much of your time is occupied by obsessive thoughts? How frequently do the obsessive thoughts occur?
   0 = None
   1 = Mild (less than 1 hr day) or occasional (intrusion occurring no more than 8 times a day)
   2 = Moderate (1 to 3 hrs day) or frequent (intrusion occurring more than 8 times a day, but most of the hours of the day are free of obsessions)
   3 = Severe (greater than 3 and up to 8 hrs day) or very frequent (intrusion occurring more than 8 times a day and occurring during most of the hours of the day)
   4 = Extreme (greater than 8 hrs day) or near consistent intrusion (too numerous to count and an hour rarely passes without several obsessions occurring)

2. **Interference Due to Obsessive Thoughts**
   How much do your obsessive thoughts interfere with your social or work (or role) functioning? Is there anything that you don't do because of them?
   0 = None
   1 = Mild, slight interference with social or occupational activities, but overall performance not impaired
   2 = Moderate, definite interference with social or occupational performance but still manageable
   3 = Severe, causes substantial impairment in social or occupational performance
   4 = Extreme, incapacitating

3. **Distress Associated with Obsessive Thoughts**
   How much distress do your obsessive thoughts cause you?
   0 = None
   1 = Mild, infrequent and not too disturbing

2 = Moderate, frequent and disturbing but still manageable
3 = Severe, very frequent and very disturbing
4 = Extreme, near constant and disabling distress

4. **Resistance Against Obsessions**
How much of an effort do you make to resist the obsessive thoughts? How often do you try to disregard or turn your attention away from these thoughts as they enter your mind?
0 = Makes an effort to always resist, or symptoms so minimal doesn't need to actively resist
1 = Tries to resist most of the time
2 = Makes some effort to resist
3 = Yields to all obsessions without attempting to control them, but does so with some reluctance
4 = Completely and willingly yields to all obsessions

5. **Degree of Control Over Obsessive Thoughts**
How much control do you have over your obsessive thoughts? How successful are you in stopping or diverting your obsessive thinking?
0 = Complete control
1 = Much control, usually able to stop or divert obsessions with some effort and concentration
2 = Moderate control, sometimes able to stop or divert obsessions
3 = Little control, rarely successful in stopping obsessions
4 = No control, experienced as completely involuntary, rarely able to even momentarily divert thinking

6. **Time Spent Performing Compulsive Behaviors**
How much time do you spend performing compulsive behaviors? How frequently do you perform compulsions?
0 = None
1 = Mild (less than 1 hr day performing compulsions) or occasional (performance of compulsions occurring no more than 8 times a day)
2 = Moderate (1 to 3 hrs day performing compulsions) or frequent (performance of compulsions occurring more than 8 times a day, but most of the hours of the day are free of compulsive behaviors)
3 = Severe (greater than 3 and up to 8 hrs day performing compulsions) or very frequent (performance of compulsions occurring more than 8 times a day and occurring during most of the hours of the day)
4 = Extreme (greater than 8 hrs day performing compulsions) or near consistent performance of compulsions (too numerous to count and an hour rarely passes without several compulsions being performed)

7. **Interference Due to Compulsive Behaviors**
   How much do your compulsive behaviors interfere with your social or work (or role) functioning? Is there anything that you don't do because of the compulsions?
   0 = None
   1 = Mild, slight interference with social or occupational activities, but overall performance not impaired
   2 = Moderate, definite interference with social or occupational performance but still manageable
   3 = Severe, causes substantial impairment in social or occupational performance
   4 = Extreme, incapacitating

8. **Distress Associated With Compulsive Behavior**
   How would you feel if prevented from performing your compulsions? How anxious would you become? How anxious do you get while performing compulsions until you are satisfied they are completed?
   0 = None
   1 = Mild, only slightly anxious if compulsions prevented or only slightly anxious during performance of compulsions
   2 = Moderate, reports that anxiety would mount but remain manageable if compulsions prevented or that anxiety increases but remains manageable during performance of compulsions
   3 = Severe, prominent and very disturbing increase in anxiety if compulsions interrupted or prominent and very disturbing increases in anxiety during performance of compulsions
   4 = Extreme, incapacitating anxiety from any intervention aimed at modifying activity or incapacitating anxiety develops during performance of compulsions

9. **Resistance Against Compulsions**
   How much of an effort do you make to resist the compulsions?
   0 = Makes an effort to always resist, or symptoms so minimal doesn't need to actively resist
   1 = Tries to resist most of the time
   2 = Makes some effort to resist
   3 = Yields to all compulsions without attempting to control them, but does so with some reluctance
   4 = Completely and willingly yields to all compulsions

10. **Degree of Control Over Compulsive Behavior**
    0 = Complete control
    1 = Much control, experiences pressure to perform the behavior but usually

able to exercise voluntary control over it
2 = Moderate control, strong pressure to perform behavior, can control it only with difficulty
3 = Little control, very strong drive to perform behavior, must be carried to completion, can only delay with difficulty
4 = No control, drive to perform behavior experienced as completely involuntary

---

Source.   Goodman WK, Price LH, Rasmussen SA, et al. The Yale-Brown Obsessive-Compulsive Scale, I: development, use, and reliability. Arch Gen Psychiatry 46:1006–1011, 1989.

Index

*Page numbers printed in **bold** type refer to tables or figures.*